FRONTIERS IN CARDIOVASCULAR HEALTH

PROGRESS IN EXPERIMENTAL CARDIOLOGY

Edited by Naranjan S. Dhalla, Ph.D., M.D. (Hon.), D.Sc. (Hon.)

1. S. Mochizuki, N. Takeda, M. Nagano, N.S. Dhalla (eds.): *The Ischemic Heart.* 1998.
   ISBN 0-7923-8105-X
2. N.S. Dhalla, P. Zahradka, I. Dixon, R. Beamish (eds.): *Angiotensin II Receptor Blockade: Physiological and Clinical Implications.* 1998.
   ISBN 0-7923-8147-5
3. N. Takeda, M. Nagano, N.S. Dhalla (eds.): *The Hypertrophied Heart.* 2000.
   ISBN 0-7923-7741-9
4. B. Ostadal, M. Nagano, N.S. Dhalla (eds.): *Cardiac Development.* 2002.
   ISBN 1-4020-7052-7
5. P. Singal, I. Dixon, L. Kirshenbaum, N.S. Dhalla (eds.): *Cardiac Remodeling and Failure.* 2002.
   ISBN 1-4020-7177-9
6. N.S. Dhalla, N. Takeda, M. Singh, A. Lukas (eds.): *Myocardial Ischemia and Preconditioning.* 2002.
   ISBN 1-4020-7195-7
7. N.S. Dhalla, L. Hryshko, E. Kardami, P.K. Singal (eds.): *Signal Transduction and Cardiac Hypertrophy.* 2003.
   ISBN 1-4020-7218-X
8. G.N. Pierce, M. Nagano, P. Zahradka, N.S. Dhalla (eds.): *Atherosclerosis, Hypertension and Diabetes.* 2003.
   ISBN 1-4020-7311-9
9. N.S. Dhalla, A. Chockalingam, H.I. Berkowitz, P.K. Singal (eds.): *Frontiers in Cardiovascular Health.* 2003.
   ISBN 1-4020-7451-4

FRONTIERS IN CARDIOVASCULAR HEALTH

Editors

NARANJAN S. DHALLA, PhD, MD (Hon), DSc (Hon)
Distinguished Professor and Director
Institute of Cardiovascular Sciences
St. Boniface General Hospital Research Centre
Faculty of Medicine, University of Manitoba
Winnipeg, Canada

ARUN CHOCKALINGAM, PhD
Assistant Director
Institute of Circulatory & Respiratory Health
Canadian Institutes of Health Research
Vancouver, Canada

H. IVAN BERKOWITZ, MBA
Consultant
Institute of Cardiovascular Sciences
St. Boniface General Hospital Research Centre
Faculty of Medicine, University of Manitoba
Winnipeg, Canada

PAWAN K. SINGAL, PhD, DSc
Professor
Institute of Cardiovascular Sciences
St. Boniface General Hospital Research Centre
Faculty of Medicine, University of Manitoba
Winnipeg, Canada

KLUWER ACADEMIC PUBLISHERS
BOSTON / DORDRECHT / LONDON

Distributors for North, Central and South America:
Kluwer Academic Publishers
101 Philip Drive
Assinippi Park
Norwell, Massachusetts 02061 USA
Telephone (781) 871-6600
Fax (781) 681-9045
E-Mail <kluwer@wkap.com>

Distributors for all other countries:
Kluwer Academic Publishers Group
Post Office Box 322
3300 AH Dordrecht, THE NETHERLANDS
Telephone 31 786 576 000
Fax 31 786 576 254
E-Mail <services@wkap.nl>

Electronic Services <http://www.wkap.nl>

Library of Congress Cataloging-in-Publication Data

Frontiers in cardiovascular health / editors, Naranjan S. Dhalla ...[et al.].
p. ; cm. – (Progress in experimental cardiology ; 9)
Includes bibliographical references and index.
ISBN 1-4020-7451-4 (hardback : alk. paper)
1. Cardiovascular system –Diseases—Prevention. 2. Cardiovascular system—Diseases—Risk factors. I. Dhalla, Naranjan S. II. Series.
[DNLM: 1. Cardiovascular Diseases—etiology. 2. Cardiovascular Diseases—metabolism 3. Cardiovascular Diseases—therapy. 4. Life Style. 5. Risk Factors. WG 120 F9347 2003]
RA645.C34F76 2003
616.1'05—dc21 2003048834

Printed on acid-free paper.
Printed in the United States of America

Contents

A Tribute to Professor Bohuslav Ostadal, DSc, MD

This book is dedicated to Professor Bohuslav Ostadal to recognize his outstanding achievements in the area of Cardiovascular Sciences and Medicine. Prof. Dr. Bohuslav Ostadal D.Sc. is head of the Department of Developmental Cardiology, Institute of Physiology, Academy of Sciences of the Czech Republic in Prague. He studied at the Faculty of Medicine of the Charles University in Prague and received a MUDr (M.D.) in 1963 and completed his Ph.D. thesis in 1968. He started with his scientific career at the Department of Pathological Physiology of the Faculty of Medicine, chaired by one of the founders of modern Czech experimental cardiology Professor O. Poupa. Studies on the onto- and phylogeny of the cardiac muscle for understanding the basis of fetal and neonatal cardiology influenced many young students at that time and became a specialty of the "Prague School" of developmental and comparative cardiology. Prof. Poupa introduced B. Ostadal to the problems of the developing heart, asking him to analyze the relationship between the phylo- and ontogenetic changes of the myocardial blood supply and the development of isoproterenol-induced myocardial necrosis. Their paper on myocardial necrosis in the turtle, showing that the lesions were localized exclusively in the inner spongious, vascularless layer of the cold-blooded heart was published in the American Heart Journal in 1968.

Dr. Ostadal, together with the outstanding Czech embryologist, Dr. Rychter, studied the mechanism of development of coronary vascularization of cardiac muscle and extended this analysis from the ultrastructural point of view during his stay at the Department of Anatomy, University of Wurzburg, Germany in 1969. After he returned to Prague, he encouraged his coworkers in the Institute of Physiology to follow the scientific ideas of Prof. Poupa and to analyze the effects of adaptation to chronic hypoxia on the cardiopulmonary system. This topic was very attractive also for colleagues working in clinical cardiology, particularly Prof. Widimsky and his group; they started a long-lasting cooperation, describing protective and negative signs of adaptation, reversibility of adaptive changes as well as the possible relationship to the human disease and sports medicine. Permanent interest in the developmental approach brought Dr. B. Ostadal in close cooperation with the pediatric cardiologists, particularly with Prof. Samanek and his Kardiocentrum. Together, they demonstrated metabolic adaptation of the atrial and ventricular tissue collected from the hearts of children, operated for congenital cyanotic heart disease. Because of the political situation at the time, all the international contacts were almost completely interrupted and the future was all but promising. In order to compensate for this precarious situation, Dr. Ostadal together with Dr. P. Braveny founded the Czechoslovak Experimental Cardiology Study Group in 1972. The aim of the new society was to acquaint experimental and clinical cardiologists with the newest developments in world cardiology. The Study Group fulfilled this original goal for further 30 years and is still very active.

In November 1989, Dr. Ostadal was elected as director of the Institute of Physiology of the Czechoslovak Academy of Sciences (1990–95) and promoted to full professorship at the Charles University (1992). From 1993 to 1998 he served as a member of the Committee of the International Society for Heart Research and became Secretary General of the XVth World Congress of this Society in Prague in 1995. In 1996, he founded the international journal *Experimental and Clinical Cardiology*, published by the Pulsus Group, Canada, and has since been serving as the editor-in-chief. In 2000 he organized the International Symposium on The Developing Heart in Prague.

As a teacher in the Department of Pathological Physiology of the Faculty of Medicine as well as one of the organizers of the Postgraduate School in Biomedicine at the Charles University, Dr. Ostadal is in close contact with young students. He has been awarded the prize of the Czech Ministry of Health (1995), Czech Medical Association J.E. Purkyne (2000) and has received the Honorary J.E. Purkyne Medal from the Academy of Sciences of the Czech Republic for achievements in biology and medicine (2000). He is an honorary member of the Czech Medical Association, Czech Physiological and Czech Cardiological Society. Dr. Ostadal has published more than 200 full length papers, 2 monographs and edited 3 other monographs. His Department of Developmental Cardiology, a part of Czech Center of Excellence for Experimental Cardiovascular Research, now concentrates on the analysis of the protective mechanisms of adaptation to chronic hypoxia during ontogenetic development, particularly in comparison with another protective phenomenon, ischemic preconditioning. The aim of the whole research team is to help better understand the pathogenetic mechanisms that determine the degree of cardiac tolerance to oxygen deprivation as well as mechanisms responsible for different types of cardiac protection. Over the years, Dr. Ostadal has transformed himself from an avid student to an internationally respected teacher/researcher in Developmental Cardiology.

Naranjan S. Dhalla, PhD, MD (Hon), DSc (Hon)
Arun Chockalingam, PhD
H. Ivan Berkowitz, MBA
Pawan K. Singal, PhD, DSc

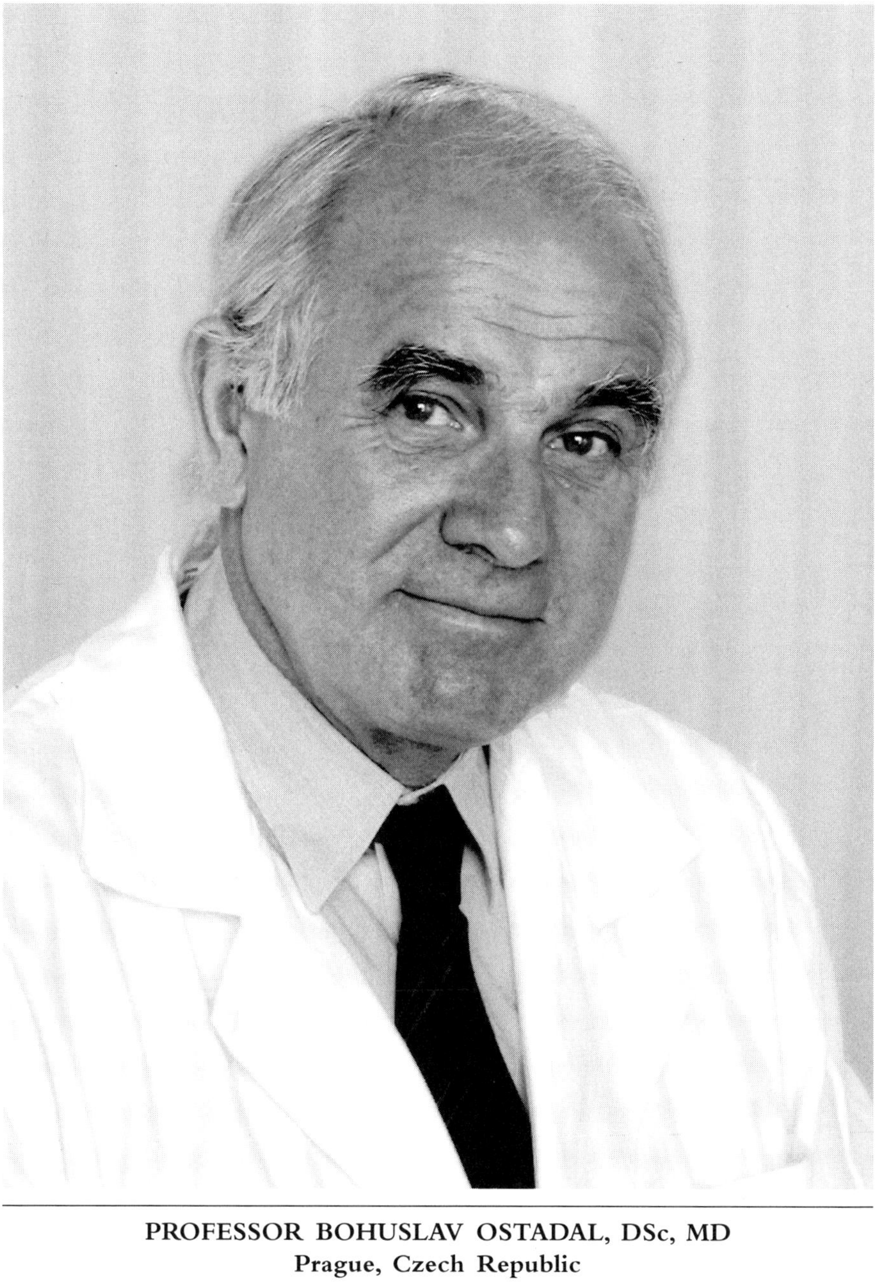

PROFESSOR BOHUSLAV OSTADAL, DSc, MD
Prague, Czech Republic

Preface

The Frontiers in Cardiovascular Health varies between and within nations, depending upon the level at which the battle is fought for better cardiovascular health. According to the 1997 World Health Report, 15 million deaths (i.e. 30% of the total number of deaths) were attributable to cardiovascular diseases and this number is on the rise. The projection for the year 2020 is quite alarming with an expected cardiovascular mortality reaching 50 million. Much of this burden is projected to occur in developing countries, more specifically in the most populous countries of the world, namely China and India. These countries are already burdened with infectious and parasitic diseases and are trying to eradicate such diseases. With increasing life expectancies people all over the world, especially in developing countries, are exposed to degenerative atherosclerosis resulting in increased cardiovascular mortality and morbidity.

In developing countries, resources available for health care are very limited. For example many of the African countries spend less than $10 per person per year on his/her entire health care let alone cardiovascular health. The average health care budget for nearly two thirds of the global population is well below $100 per year, on a per capita basis. Therefore, in developing countries health promotion and primary prevention are the frontiers by necessity. Improving awareness and health education is not only a matter of choice but is an absolute necessity. In developed countries, understanding the pathogenesis at the molecular level and disease prevention are the additional frontiers.

Understanding the pathophysiology, cellular mechanism of disease progression, different risk factors for cardiovascular disease including the traditional and emerging ones, dietary effects on cardiovascular health and cultural differences are as much important as dealing with the economic burden of cardiovascular mortality and morbidity. To conquer this public health enemy number one—cardiovascular disease—the battle must be fought in several fronts. Advancing the research, improving public awareness, people taking control of their health from childhood to advanced ages, and enlightened global health policies are all integral parts of such a strategy.

As we live in a global village the problems of one country are bound to affect another country at a far off distance. Thus, the global cardiovascular research community has the moral responsibility to share the scientific knowledge. The present book, therefore, covers the whole range including risk factors, nutrition and metabolism in cardiovascular health and disease as a global issue. Thus there is urgency in describing the factors that lead to cardiovascular deaths and strategies for their prevention from molecule to population. This book is based on the selected scientific presentations made in the Winnipeg 2001 World Heart Conference. Each chapter is written by authorities in their own domain. The editors gratefully appreciate the readiness of the authors, from every part of the world, to share their research findings and knowledge to create this book.

For an easy reading, the whole book has been divided into three sections. However, an overlap of topics of different papers under these titles is indicative of a one continuum of science that permeates through the book. It is our hope that readers will find the book to be interesting as well as stimulating.

The book is dedicated to Professor Dr. Bohuslav Ostadal for his outstanding contributions in the field of developmental cardiology which have already impacted on our understanding of the cardiovascular disease processes in early life.

This book and the contribution of many of the scientists is only a small step forward in understanding the causes for cardiovascular disease and to improve the cardiovascular health of mankind. Nevertheless, such steps are essential in reaching the frontiers and eventually eradicating cardiovascular diseases.

Naranjan S. Dhalla, PhD, MD (Hon), DSc (Hon)
Arun Chockalingam, PhD
H. Ivan Berkowitz, MBA
Pawan K. Singal, PhD, DSc

Acknowledgments

We are grateful to the following corporations and granting agencies for their generous donations in support of the XVII World Heart Congress of the International Society for Heart Research, the first Public Heart Health Forum as well as publication of this book:

PATRONS:
Western Economic Diversification Canada
Government of Manitoba (Depts. of Industry Trade and Mines; Health; Post-Secondary Education; Culture Heritage and Tourism)
Merck Frosst Canada, Ltd.
Mitsubishi-Tokyo Pharmaceuticals Inc.

PARTNERS:
American Section of the International Society for Heart Research
AstraZeneca
Aventis Pharmaceuticals Inc.
Bayer Canada, Inc.
City of Winnipeg
International Academy of Cardiovascular Sciences
International Society for Heart Research (Kaito Fund, Bayer Yakuhin Fund and Canon Fund)
Kowa Pharmaceuticals
Pfizer Canada
St. Boniface General Hospital Research Foundation

COLLABORATORS:
CanWest Global Foundation
CIHR Institute of Circulatory and Respiratory Health
Eli Lilly
Great-West Life and London Life
Manitoba Liquor Control Commission
Mars Incorporated
Medicure, Inc.

Myles Robinson Memorial Heart Fund
Safeway Food and Drug
University of Manitoba (Faculty of Medicine; Departments of Physiology and Human Anatomy & Cell Science)

BENEFACTORS:
ATL Canada
Beckman Coulter Canada Inc.
Canadian Cardiovascular Society
Canadian Institutes of Health Research
Cardiovascular Solutions, Inc.
Dairy Farmers of Canada
De Fehr Foundation
Faculty of Health Sciences, University of Western Ontario
Heart and Stroke Foundation of Manitoba
Institute of Biodiagnostics, National Research Council of Canada
Japanese Working Group on Cardiac Structure and Metabolism
Manitoba Hydro
Merck KGaA (Germany)
Pulsus Group Inc.
St. Boniface General Hospital Research Centre
Wawanesa Mutual Insurance Company
World Heart Corporation

The collaboration of Ms. Eva Little, Ms. Janet Labarre, Ms. Diane Stowe, Ms. Florence Willerton and Ms. Susan Zettler in coordinating diverse editorial activities associated with this book is gratefully acknowledged. Special thanks are due to Mr. Zachary Rolnik, Ms. Mimi T. Breed, Ms. Melissa Ramondetta and their editorial staff at Kluwer Academic Publishers for their patience, interest and hard work in assembling this volume.

FRONTIERS IN CARDIOVASCULAR HEALTH

I. Risk Factors and Cardiovascular Disease

Frontiers in Cardiovascular Health, edited by
N.S. Dhalla, A. Chockalingam,
H.I. Berkowitz & P.K. Singal
Kluwer Academic Publishers, Boston, 2003

Inflammation and Cardiovascular Disease

James T. Willerson

Texas Heart Institute, St. Luke's Episcopal Hospital, University of Texas Health Science Center at Houston Houston, Texas

Summary. The role of inflammation in initiating and sustaining various cardiovascular problems, including the conversion from stable to unstable coronary heart disease syndromes, vascular aneurysms, and congestive heart failure is reviewed. Various interventions that reduce inflammation in the coronary arteries and hearts in humans, including marked lipid lowering, weight loss, Peroxisome Proliferator Activated Receptors agonists (PPAR), aspirin, and monoclonal antibodies to vascular cell adhesion molecule (VCAM) and intercellular vascular adhesion molecule (ICAM) are identified. Whereas estrogens may promote increases in vascular markers suggesting the presence of inflammation, recent evidence suggests that combined estrogen and progesterone in postmenopausal women may reduce the vascular markers of inflammation. However, the combination of estrogens and progesterone may actually increase the risk of vascular events in menopausal women with cardiovascular disease. Additional work is needed to identify the best ways to prevent and/or modulate vascular and myocardial inflammation with the expectation that from these interventions will come the ability to treat more effectively and perhaps retard the development of atherosclerosis, heart failure and vascular aneurysms.

Inflammation plays a major role in initiating and sustaining cardiovascular problems, including the conversion from stable to unstable coronary heart disease syndromes, the development of vascular aneurysms, and congestive heart failure (1–5). The presence of inflammation also serves as an important predictor of future adverse events following interventional procedures in coronary arteries (6). However, inflammation may also serve to identify the presence of unstable or vulnerable atherosclerotic plaques potentially allowing their treatment prior to their fissuring or ulceration and otherwise causing unstable angina and acute myocardial infarction (7,8). In this chapter, potential mechanisms responsible for vascular and myocar-

Address for Reprints and Correspondence: James T. Willerson, M.D., Cardiology Research, MC 1-191, Texas Heart Institute, P.O. Box 20345, Houston, TX 77225-0345.

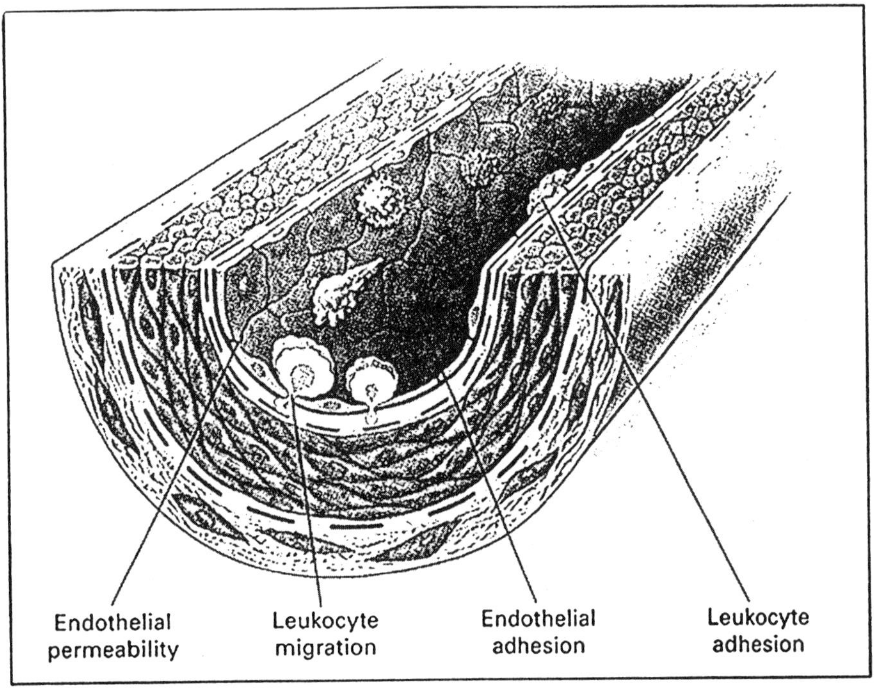

Figure 1. The earliest changes that precede the formation of lesions of atherosclerosis take place in the endothelium. These changes include increased endothelial permeability to lipoproteins and other plasma constituents mediated by nitric oxide, prostacyclin, platelet-derived growth factor, angiotensin I, and endothelin; up-regulation of leukocyte adhesion molecules, including L-selectin, integrins, and platelet-endothelial-cell adhesion molecule 1, and the up-regulation of endothelial adhesion molecules, including E-selectin, P-selectin, intercellular adhesion molecule 1, and vascular-cell adhesion molecule 1; and migration of leukocytes into the artery wall, mediated by oxidized low-density lipoprotein, monocyte chemotactic protein 1, interleukin-8, platelet-derived growth factor, macrophage colony-stimulating factor, and osteopontin. Reproduced from NEJM 1999; 345:117 by permission.

dial inflammation, consequences of such inflammation, systemic markers identifying the presence of inflammation, and potential treatments of cardiovascular inflammation are discussed.

MECHANISMS RESPONSIBLE FOR INFLAMMATION

The response to injury in the vasculature and heart is inflammation. Atherosclerosis occurs as the result of injury of the endothelium (Figure 1). Vascular injuries that lead to inflammation and contribute to atherosclerosis and coronary artery disease are shown in Table 1. It is important to recognize that vascular and myocardial infection from various pathogens results in vascular inflammation and almost certainly contributes to atherosclerosis and the development of acute coronary artery syndromes (9–11). No single infection has yet been identified as playing a major role in vascular injury, inflammation and progression to atherosclerosis; instead, current

Table 1. Pathogenesis of acute coronary artery disease syndromes

1.	Infection—various pathogens
2.	Genetic predisposition resulting from mutations and genetic polymorphisms leading to inflammation, impaired endothelial repair and stability, vascular infection, thrombosis, and/or vasoconstriction
3.	Aging
4.	Oxidized free radicals
5.	Hyperlipidemia
6.	Homocysteine
7.	Diabetes
8.	Smoking
9.	Cocaine
10.	Hypertension
11.	Interventional Injury

evidence favors prior exposure to multiple pathogens as playing a role (12,13). However, there may be a relatively more common infection that plays a major role in vascular infection and atherosclerosis that has not yet been identified.

Genetic predisposition almost certainly leads to inflammation, impaired endothelial vascular repair, vascular infection, thrombosis and vasoconstriction. The aging process itself is associated with altered vascular and myocardial defense mechanisms predisposing some individuals to inflammation. The oxidation of total cholesterol and low density lipoprotein cholesterol (LDL) leads to the production of oxidized radicals that promote vascular inflammation and the recruitment of macrophage-derived monocytes (Figure 2) (14–17). Similarly, interventional injury, including angioplasty and stenting causes endothelial inflammation, thrombosis, and fibroproliferation.

Inflammation causes: 1) smooth muscle cell proliferation and migration; 2) lipid accumulation; and 3) endothelial dysfunction (17,18). Immunologically-mediated cellular injury leads to the activation of T cells; the development of antibodies to heat shock proteins; and antibodies to infectious agents, oxidized LDL, and components of the inflammatory process itself (19,20).

INFLAMMATION AND COMPLEX CORONARY HEART DISEASE LESIONS

Monocyte-derived macrophages and activated T cells play an important role in the development of unstable atherosclerotic plaques (Figure 3) (21,22). Proteases released from macrophages following their entry into the arterial wall degrade collagen in the fibrous atherosclerotic plaque leading to its weakening and fissuring and/or ulceration causing abrupt thrombosis and dynamic vasoconstriction (Figure 3) (21,23,24). Unstable atherosclerotic plaques have thin fibrous caps, numerous inflammatory cells (primarily macrophages but also activated T cells) just beneath the fibrous cap and/or on its surface, and an adjacent lipid pool (Figure 4) (25,26). Thus, the process of inflammation plays a pivotal role in the conversion from stable to unstable coronary heart disease syndromes.

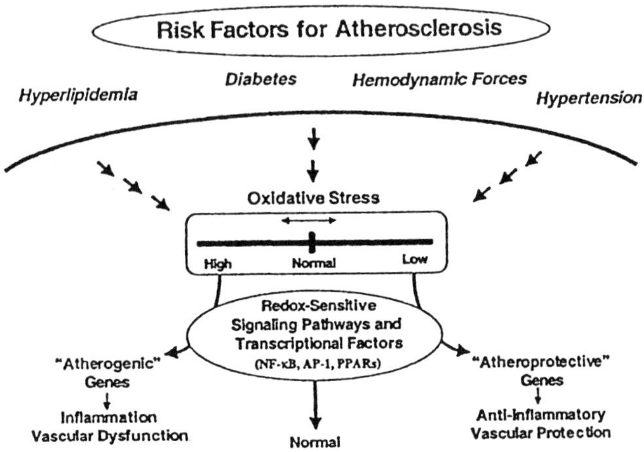

Figure 2. The association of atherosclerotic risk factors, oxidative stress, and redox-sensitive gene expression. Various risk factors for atherosclerosis, including hypertension, hyperlipidemia, diabetes, and vascular hemodynamic stresses (shear stresses), result in intracellular oxidative stress (ROS). The mechanisms by which these risk factors generate oxidative stress are not well characterized and may act synergistically. Various cellular processes are influenced by nutrition and therapeutic interventions may regulate the relative level of intracellular oxidative stress. Relatively high levels of oxidative stress result in the induction of vascular inflammatory ("atherogenic") genes through redox-sensitive signaling pathways and activation of redox-sensitive transcription factors. Relatively lower levels of oxidative stress maintain a noninflammatory or vascular protective effect through induction of "atheroprotective" genes. Thus, ROS produced as a result of an oxidative stress may act as specific regulators in the signal transduction network to relay environmental and physical signals generated at the cell membrane to nuclear regulatory signals, leading to modulation of inflammatory gene expression. Reproduced from Circulation Research 1999; 84:754 by permission.

INFLAMMATION AND PROGRESSIVE CONGESTIVE HEART FAILURE

Considerable evidence has developed indicating that inflammation and the accumulation of selective mediators of inflammation, i.e., tumor necrosis factor α (TNFα) may play a role in the progression of heart failure in experimental animal models and humans (27–30). TNFα is increased in the myocardium of patients with progressive heart failure (29). Transgenic mice over-expressing TNFα develop a dilated cardiomyopathy (5). TNFα has negative inotropic effects on ventricular function (29), and it is probably one of several mediators that accumulate during inflammation contributing to progressive congestive heart failure in selected individuals.

SYSTEMIC MARKERS OF INFLAMMATION

Numerous studies have demonstrated that increases in serum C-reactive protein (CRP) identify individuals at risk for future vascular events, including myocardial infarction, cerebrovascular accidents, and death (6,7,32,33). Elevations in serum C-reactive protein concentration identify patients with unstable angina and non-Q

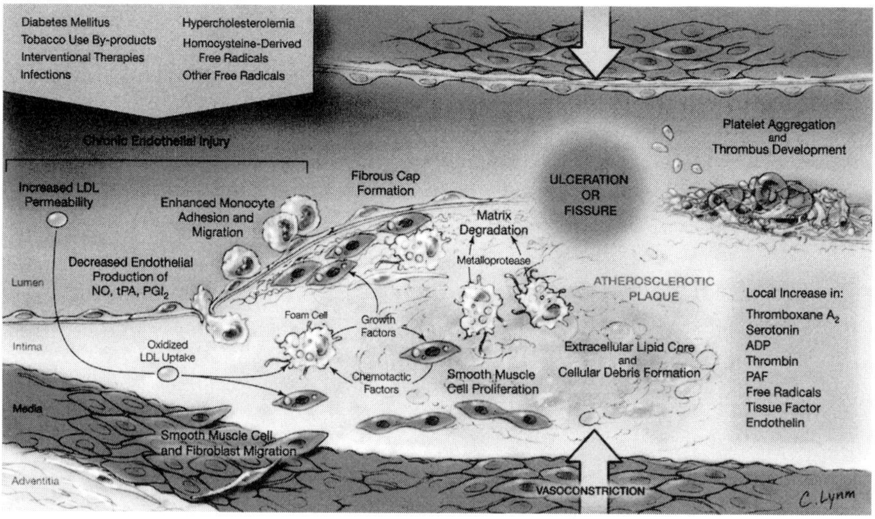

Figure 3a. Chronic endothelial injury, inflammation, and oxidative stress are central to the development of atherosclerosis. Endothelial injury results from a variety of factors including tobacco use, hypercholesterolemia, interventional therapies with angioplasty or coronary stents, and from ulceration or fissuring of atherosclerotic plaques. At sites of endothelial injury, production of endothelial-derived substances (nitric oxide [NO], tissue plasminogen activator [tPA], and prostacyclin [PGI_2]) is decreased, creating a prosthrombotic environment characterized by increased platelet and leukocyte adhesion, increased permeability to plasma lipoproteins, myointimal hyperplasia, and vasoconstriction. Ulceration or fissuring of the atherosclerotic plaque results from degradation of collagent matrix in the fibrous cap by metalloproteases released from macrophages. Exposure of the subendothelium after plaque ulceration or fissuring leads to platelet adhesion and aggregation and local accumulation of largely platelet-derived mediators (thromboxane A_2, serotonin, adenosine diphosphate [ADP], thrombin, platelet activating factor [PAF], oxygen-derived free radicals, tissue factor, and endothelin) that promote thrombus growth, fibroproliferation, and vasoconstriction, LDL indicates low-density lipoprotein. Reproduced from JAMA 2001; 285:583 by permission.

wave myocardial infarction at increased risk for future acute coronary events (33–36). Similarly, elevations in serum CRP predict patients at greater risk of restenosis after interventional procedures (37).

Increases in serum troponin I, serum amyloid-like protein, fibrinogen, and interleukins-1, 2, 6, 8, and 18 concentrations have also been shown to identify patients with unstable angina and non-Q wave myocardial infarction at increased risk for future coronary events (7,36–40). Thus, there are several systemic markers that may be used to identify the presence of inflammation in patients with coronary heart disease that help identify patients at increased risk for future events.

In the case of CRP, more recent evidence has demonstrated that it is not only a marker of inflammation, but it is also a contributor to the development of inflammation. Work from Pasceri et al. and others has demonstrated that CRP amplifies the effects of other activators of inflammation, including endotoxin and causes the

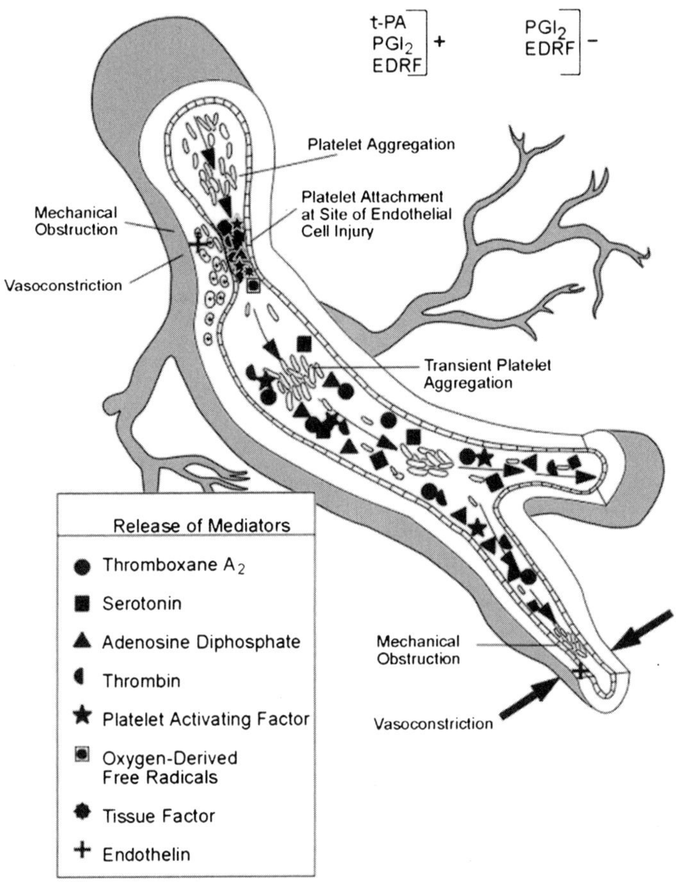

Figure 3b. Schematic diagram suggests probable mechanisms responsible for the conversion from chronic coronary heart disease to acute coronary artery disease syndromes. In this scheme, endothelial injury, generally at sites of atherosclerotic plaques and usually plaque ulceration or fissuring, is associated with platelet adhesion and aggregation and the release and activation of selected mediators, including thromboxane A_2, serotonin, adenosine diphosphate, platelet-activating factor, thrombin, oxygen-derived free radicals, and endothelin. Local accumulation of thromboxane A_2, serotonin, platelet-activating factor, thrombin, adenosine diphosphate, and tissue factor promotes platelet aggregation. Thromboxane A_2, serotonin, thrombin, and platelet activating factor are vasoconstrictors at sites of endothelial injury. Therefore, the conversion from chronic stable to acute unstable coronary heart disease syndromes is usually associated with endothelial injury, platelet aggregation, accumulation of platelet and other cell-derived mediators, further platelet aggregation, and vasoconstriction, with consequent dynamic narrowing of the coronary artery lumen. In addition to atherosclerotic plaque fissuring or ulceration, other reasons for endothelial injury include flow shear stress, hypertension, immune complex deposition and complement activation, infection, and mechanical injury to the endothelium as it occurs with coronary artery angioplasty and after heart transplantation. EDRF, endothelium-deriving relaxing factor; PGI_2, prostaglandin I_2; t-PA, tissue-type plasminogen activator. Reproduced from Willerson JT, Cohn JN: Cardiovascular Medicine. Philadelphia: Churchill Livingstone, 2000.

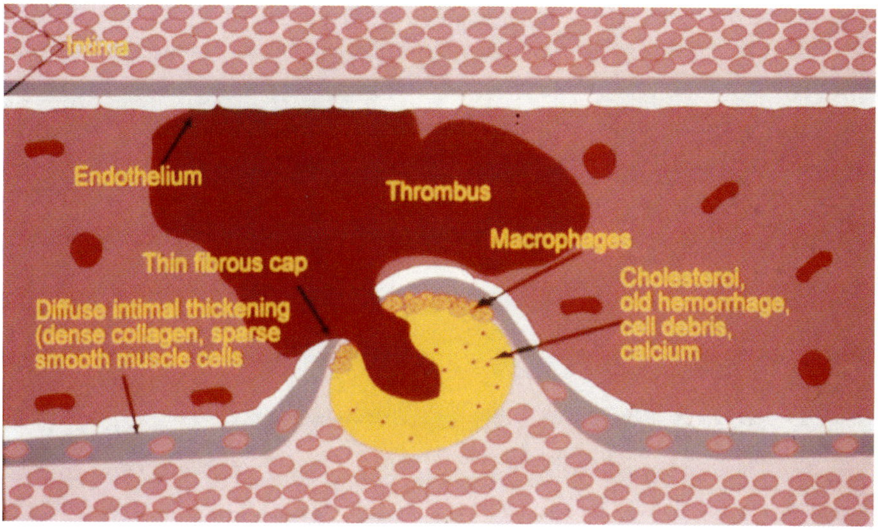

Figure 4. The morphological appearance of the unstable atherosclerotic plaque shows a thin fibrous cap, numerous inflammatory cells underneath and/or on the surface of the atherosclerotic cap, and an adjacent lipid pool.

expression of vascular cell adhesion molecular (VCAM) and intercellular adhesion molecules (ICAM) at physiologically relevant concentrations in cultured vascular cells (41–44). Others have demonstrated that CRP promotes tissue factor production by macrophages in culture and uptake and oxidation of LDL (45).

TREATMENT OPTIONS

Previous studies have shown that marked reduction in total serum cholesterol and LDL concentrations reduces the risk for future coronary events in patients with known coronary atherosclerosis (46–48). More recent evidence from the CARE trial demonstrated that a "statin", such as pravastatin reduces total serum cholesterol, LDL and CRP concentrations (Figure 5) (49). In the CARE study, which was directed at determining the influence of reduction in cholesterol and LDL in reducing future coronary events, the reduction in serum CRP concentrations was identified months to years after the drug was begun (Figure 5). More recent studies have shown that a statin (atorvastatin), that reduces total cholesterol and LDL concentrations also reduces serum CRP concentrations and improves abnormal endothelial function within a few weeks after its administration (50). Thus, marked reduction in total serum cholesterol and LDL cholesterol reduces inflammation and improves endothelial function, although this response requires weeks to months to occur. Similar studies done in experimental animal models have shown that marked

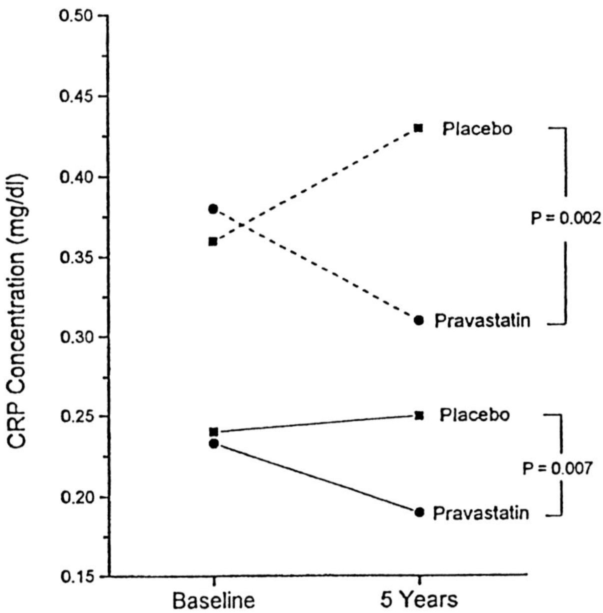

Figure 5. Median (solid lines) and mean (dotted lines) levels of CRP at baseline and at 60 months, according to placebo or pravastatin assignment. Reproduced from Circulation 1999; 100:232 by permission.

reduction in total serum cholesterol and LDL reverses inflammation in atherosclerotic lesions (51).

Ridker et al. have shown that aspirin reduces the risk of myocardial infarction associated with increased serum CRP levels (Figure 6) (52).

Appropriate treatment of an infection also reduces inflammation. Antimicrobial treatment directed at C. pneumoniae has been associated with improvement in endothelial function and reduction in selected serum markers of inflammation, including E-selectin in patients (53).

Weight loss in post-menopausal obese females is associated with reductions in serum CRP concentration (54). Available evidence suggests that estrogens may increase serum CRP concentrations in postmenopausal women (57,58). However, combined estrogen and progesterone therapy decreases serum CRP concentrations and other markers of inflammation (59). This effect, however, has thus far not6 been shown to reduce the risk of vascular events in postmenopausal women with known coronary heart disease. Various drugs and antibodies targeting selected components of the inflammatory process have been investigated or are currently under investigation in acute myocardial ischemia in humans. Pilot studies with methylprednisone in unstable angina (55) and with monoclonal antibodies to the CD18 subunit of the beta2 integrin adhesion receptors in acute myocardial infarction (56) and to tissue factor necrosis did not show the expected benefit.

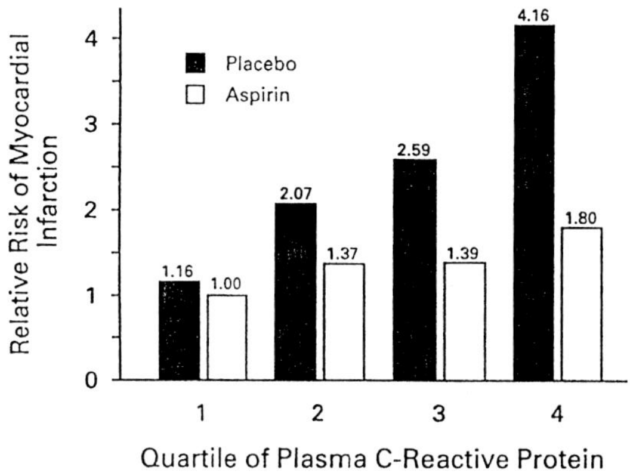

Figure 6. Relative Risk of a First Myocardial Infarction Associated with Base-Line Plasma Concentrations of C-Reactive Protein, Stratified According to Randomized Assignment to Aspirin or Placebo Therapy.

Analyses are limited to events occurring before the unblinding of the aspirin component of the Physicians' Health Study. The reduction in the risk of myocardial infarction associated with the use of aspirin was 13.9 percent in the first (lowest) quartile of C-reactive protein values, 33.4 percent in the second quartile, 46.3 percent in the third quartile, and 55.7 percent in the fourth (highest) quartile. Reproduced by permission from NEJM 1997; 336:978.

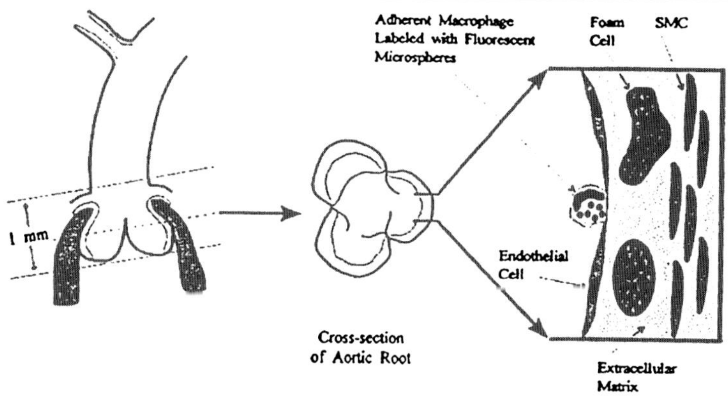

Figure 7. Schematic diagram of the study area depicting a labeled macrophage adhering to the plaque. Reproduced by permission from Circulation 1998; 97:78.

EXPERIMENTAL ANIMAL MODELS

We have developed an experimental model in which macrophages are labeled with fluorescent microspheres and reinjected into Apolipoprotein-E deficient mice where they "home" to atherosclerotic plaques (Figures 7 and 8) (60). We have used this model to demonstrate that monoclonal antibodies directed at VCAM and ICAM markedly diminish macrophage homing and inflammation in atherosclerotic plaques

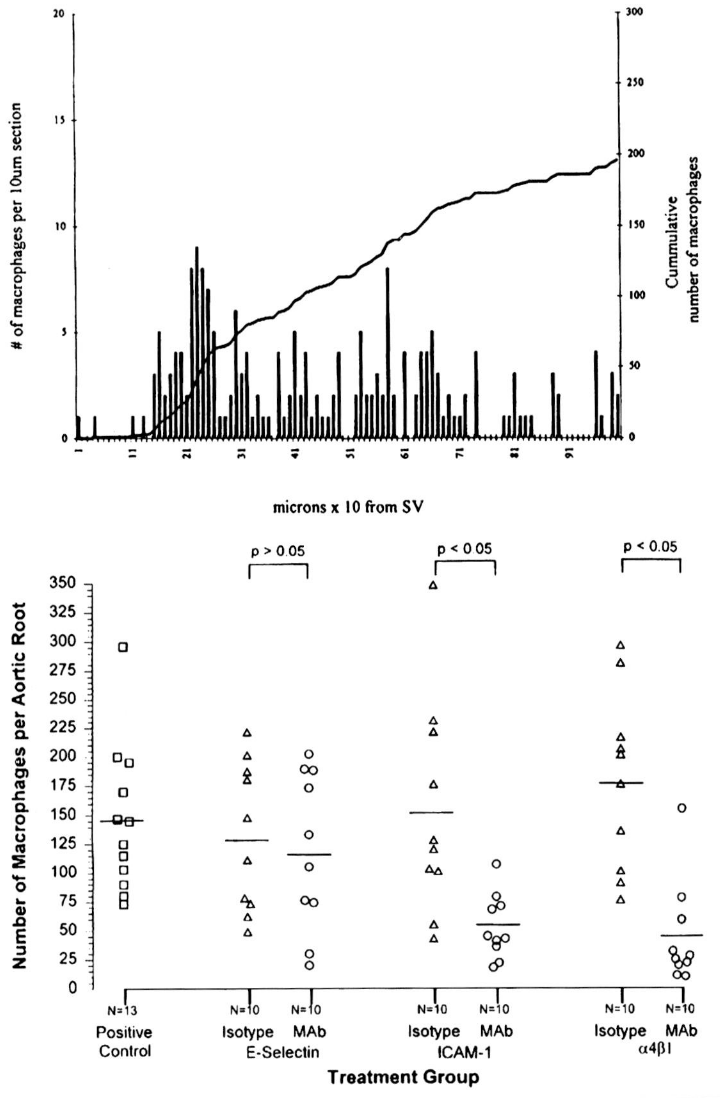

Figure 8. Inhibition of macrophage recruitment by antibodies against α_4 or ICAM-1 but not by anti-E-selectin antibody. The group of mice that were not treated with antibody is labeled as positive control. Appropriate isotype-matched antibodies were used for each specific antibody studied. Mean of each treatment group is indicated by a bar. Comparison of the seven treatment groups was performed with one-way ANOVA followed by Scheffé's test for post hoc pair-wise comparisons. All analyses were done with SAS statistical programs; $P < 0.05$ was considered statistically significant. Reproduced by permission from Circulation 1998; 97:80.

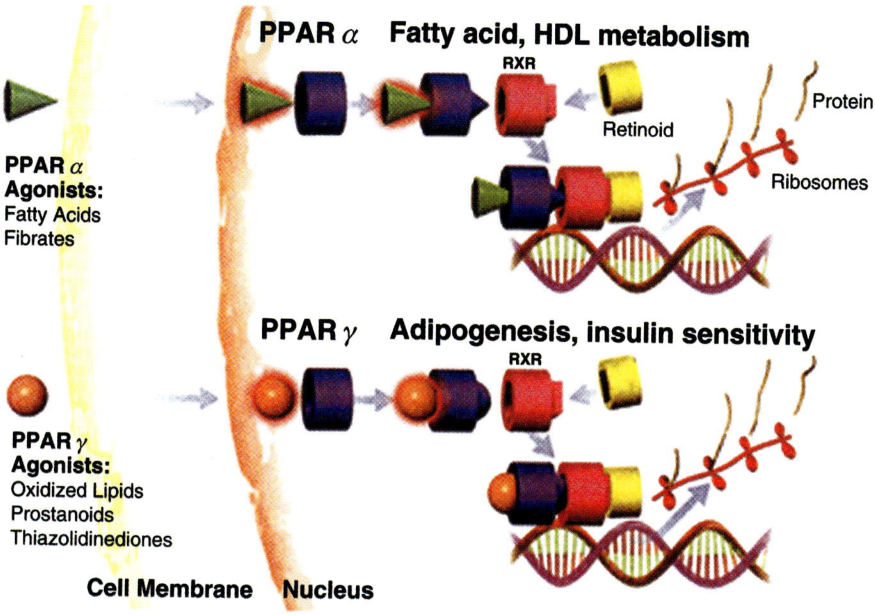

Figure 9. PPAR pathways. Originally recognized as instigator of peroxisomal proliferation unique to rodents. PPARs are nuclear receptors for small lipophilic molecules that freely partition into cells. When these receptors bind their small ligand partner, they pair with another member of nuclear receptor family, retinoid X receptor (RXR). This heterodimeric transcription factor complex then binds to cognate sequences in promoter regions of target genes, altering their transcription. PPAR-α regulates cassette of genes involved in lipoprotein metabolism, raising levels of apolipoprotein A-1, major apolipoprotein of HDL. PPAR-γ regulates expression of genes involved in adipogenesis and insulin sensitivity. Kindreds with mutations that affect function of PPAR-γ develop an insulin resistance syndrome, including hypertension. Reproduced by permission from Circulation 2001; 104:368.

in these mice (60). We have also shown that selected Peroxisome Proliferator Activated Receptor agonists (PPAR) reduce macrophage homing to atherosclerotic plaques, including troglitazone (61). Others have shown that selected PPAR agonists diminish inflammation (62,63). General effects of PPAR agonists are shown in Figure 9.

INFLAMMATION AS A DIRECT PREDICTOR OF UNSTABLE ATHEROSCLEROTIC PLAQUES

Casscells and Willerson hypothesized that inflammation in unstable atherosclerotic plaques results in temperature heterogeneity within the plaque (25). We have shown that temperature heterogeneity exists in human carotid endarterectomy specimens and that the temperature heterogeneity correlates with inflammation (Figure 10). Stefanidis and his colleagues have confirmed these observations and

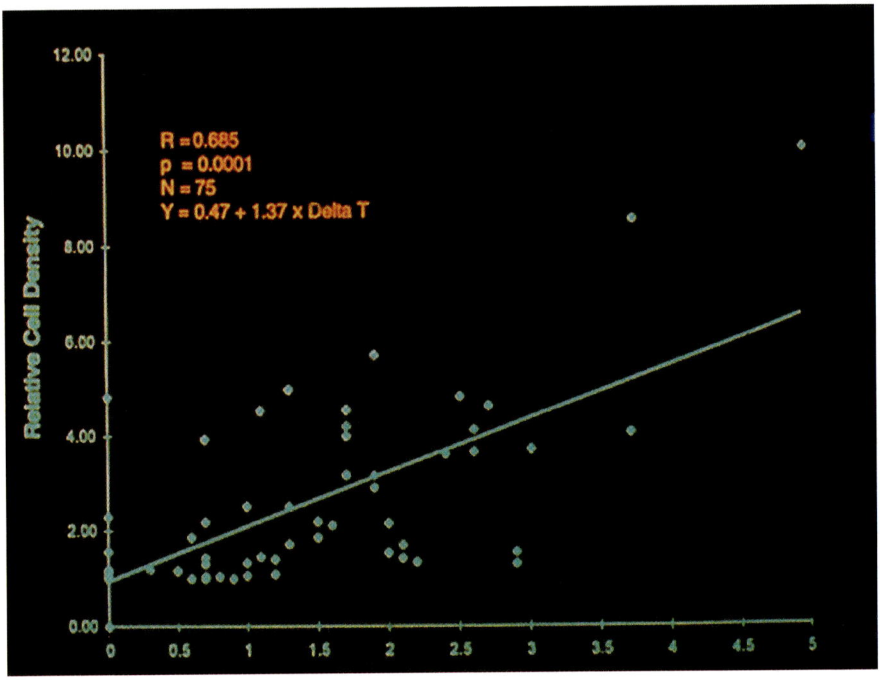

Figure 10. The relationship between inflammation, i.e. relative cell density (vertical axis) and increases in intraplaque temperature in human carotid endarterectomy specimens is shown We have found that approximately 1/3 of human carotid endarterectomy specimens taken from patients with recent transient ischemic attacks or cerebral vascular accidents show temperature heterogeneity between 0.5 degree centigrade and greater. Reproduced by permission from The Lancet 1996; 347:1447–51.

shown in patients with recent unstable angina and acute myocardial infarction temperature heterogeneity in vivo in their coronary arteries (64). Thus, one may also use the presence of inflammation to identify the unstable atherosclerotic plaque(s), hopefully prior to its fissuring or ulceration, although this remains to be proved in additional patient studies. If this proves to be true in humans and systems are developed that allow one to identify vulnerable atherosclerotic plaques prior to their ulceration or fissuring, it may be possible to treat plaques locally with anti-proliferative, anti-inflammatory and anti-thrombotic substances that exert a rapid effect on inflammation and that might subsequently be followed by the administration of statins, aspirin, weight loss, and potentially other modifiers of inflammation with long-term benefit. Such local therapies may well include selected forms of gene therapy and possibly local heating of the unstable plaque itself (65–70).

REFERENCES

1. Ross R. 1999. Atherosclerosis—an inflammatory disease. N Engl J Med 340:115–26.
2. Falk E. 1989. Morphologic features of unstable atherothrombotic plaques underlying acute coronary syndromes. Am J Cardiol 63:114E–120E.
3. Lendon CL, Davies MJ, Born GV, Richardson PD. 1991. Atherosclerotic plaque caps are locally weakened when macrophages density is increased. Atherosclerosis 87:87–90.
4. Goodall S, Crowther M, Hemingway DM, Bell PR, Thompson MM. 2001. Ubiquitous elevation of matrix metalloproteinase-2 expression in the vasculature of patients with abdominal aneurysms. Circulation 104:304–309.
5. Sivasubramanian N, Coker ML, Kurrelmeyer KM, MacLellan WR, DeMayo FJ, Spinale FG, Mann DL. 2001. Left ventricular remodeling in transgenic mice with cardiac restricted overexpression of tumor necrosis factor. Circulation 104:826–831.
6. Chew DP, Bhatt DL, Robbins MA, Penn MS, Schneider JP, Lauer MS, Topol EJ, Ellis SG. 2001. Incremental prognostic value of elevated baseline C-reactive protein among established markers of risk in percutaneous coronary intervention. Circulation 104:992–997.
7. Liuzzo G, Biasucci LM, Gallimore JR, et al. 1994. The prognostic value of C-reactive protein and serum amyloid a protein in severe unstable angina. N Engl J Med 331:417–424.
8. Shah PK, Falk E, Badimon JJ, et al. 1995. Human monocyte-derived macrophages induce collagen breakdown in fibrous caps of atherosclerotic plaques: potential role of matrix-degrading metalloproteinases and implications for plaque rupture. Circulation 92:1565–1569.
9. Muhlestein JB, Horne BD, Carlquist JF, Madsen TE, Bair TL, Pearson RR, Anderson JL. 2000. Cytomegalovirus seropositivity and C-reactive protein have independent and combined predictive value for mortality in patients with angiographically demonstrated coronary artery disease. Circulation 102:1917–1923.
10. Saikku P, Leionen M, Mattila K, et al. 1988. Serological evidence of an association of a novel *Chlamydia*, TWAR, with chronic coronary heart disease and acute myocardial infarction. Lancet 2:983–985.
11. Grayston JT. 1993. Chlamydia in atherosclerosis. Circulation 87:1408–1409.
12. Anderson JL, Carlquist JF, Muhlestein JB, et al. 1998. Evaluation of C-reactive protein, an inflammatory marker, and infectious serology as risk factors for coronary artery disease and myocardial infarction. J Am Coll Cardiol 32:35–41.
13. Ridker PM, Hennekens CH, Stampfer MJ, et al. 1998. Prospective study of herpes simplex virus, cytomegalovirus, and the risk of future myocardial infarction and stroke. Circulation 98:2796–2799.
14. Steinberg D, Parthasarathy S, Carew TE, Khoo JC, Witztum JL. 1989. Beyond cholesterol: modifications of low-density lipoprotein that increase its atherogenicity. N Engl J Med 320:915–920.
15. Marui N, Offermann MK, Swerlick R, Kunsch C, Rosen CA, Ahmad M, Alexander RW, Medford RM. 1993. Vascular cell adhesion molecule-1 (VCAM-1) gene transcription and expression are regulated through an antioxidant-sensitive mechanism in human vascular endothelial cells. J Clin Invest 92:1866–1874.
16. Weber C, Erl W, Pietsch A, Strobel M, Ziegler-Heitbrock HW, Weber PC. 1994. Antioxidants inhibit monocyte adhesion by suppressing nuclear factor-kappa B mobilization and induction of vascular cell adhesion molecule-1 in endothelial cells stimulated to generate radicals. Arterioscler Thromb 14:1665–1673.
17. Lehr HA, Hübner C, Menger MD, et al. 1993. Mechanisms and mediators of leukocyte/endothelium interaction during atherogenesis. Atheroscler Rev 25:49–57.
18. Bhakdi S, Torzewski M, Klouche M, et al. 1999. Complement and atherosclerosis: binding of CRP to degraded, nonoxidized LDL enhances complement activation. Arterioscler Thromb Vasc Biol 19:2384–2354.
19. Serneri GGN, Abbate R, Gori AM, et al. 1992. Transient intermittent lymphocyte activation is responsible for the instability of angina. Circulation 86:790–797.
20. Biasucci LM, Liuzzo G, Fantuzzi G, et al. 1999. Increasing levels of interleukin (IL)-1Ra and IL-6 during the first 2 days of hospitalization in unstable angina are associated with increased risk of in-hospital coronary events. Circulation 99:2079–2084.
21. Libby P, Geng YJ, Aikawa M, Schoenbeck U, Mach F, Clinton SK, Sukhova GK, Lee RT. 1996. Macrophages and atherosclerotic plaque stability. Curr Opin Lipidol 7:330–335.
22. Kockx MK, Knaapen MWM, Martinet W, De Meyer GRY, Verheye S, Herman AG. 2000. Expression of the uncoupling protein UCP-2 in macrophages of unstable human atherosclerotic plaques. Circulation 102:II-12.

23. Hirsh PD, Hillis LD, Campbell WB, Firth BG, Willerson JT. 1981. Release of prostaglandins and thromboxane into the coronary circulation in patients with ischemic heart disease. N Engl J Med 304:685–691.
24. Willerson JT, Golino P, Eidt J, Campbell WB, Buja LM. 1989. Specific platelet mediators and unstable coronary artery lesions. Experimental evidence and potential clinical implications. Circulation 80:198–205.
25. Casscells W, Hathorn B, David M, Krabach T, Vaughn WK, McAllister HA, Bearman G, Willerson JT. 1996. Thermal detection of cellular infiltrates in living atherosclerotic plaques: possible implications for plaque rupture and thrombosis. Lancet 347:1447–1451.
26. Davies MJ, Thomas T. 1981. The pathological basis and microanatomy of occlusive thrombus formation in human coronary arteries. Philos Trans R Soc Lond B Biol Sci 294:225–229.
27. Spinale FG, Coker ML, Krombach SR, et al. 1999. Matrix metalloproteinase inhibition during the development of congestive heart failure: effects on left ventricular dimensions and function. Circ Res 85:364–376.
28. Kapadia S, Lee JR, Torre-Amione G, et al. 1995. Tumor necrosis factor gene and protein expression in adult feline myocardium after endotoxin administration. J Clin Invest 96:1042–1052.
29. Torre-Amione G, Kapadia S, Lee J, et al. 1995. Expression and functional significance of tumor necrosis factor receptors in human myocardium. Circulation 92:1487–1493.
30. Li YY, Feng YQ, Kadokami T, et al. 2000. Myocardial extracellular matrix remodeling in transgenic mice overexpressing tumor necrosis factor alpha can be modulated by anti-tumor necrosis factor alpha therapy. Proc Natl Acad Sci USA 97:12746–12751.
31. Ridker PM, Hennekens CH, Buring JE, et al. 2000. C-reactive protein and other markers of inflammation in the prediction of cardiovascular disease in women. N Engl J Med 342:836–843.
32. Koenig W, Sund M, Froelich M, et al. 1999. C-reactive protein, a sensitive marker of inflammation, predicts future risk of coronary heart disease in initially healthy middle-aged men: results from the MONICA (Monitoring trends and determinants in cardiovascular disease) Augsberg Cohort Study. 1984 to 1992. Circulation 99:237–242.
33. Tracy R, Lemaitre R, Psaty B, et al. 1997. Relationship of C-reactive protein to risk of cardiovascular disease in the elderly: results from the Cardiovascular Health Study and the Rural Health Promotion Project. Arterioscler Thromb Vasc Biol 17:1121–1127.
34. Ridker PM, Glynn RJ, Hennekens CH. 1998. C-reactive protein adds to the predictive value of total and HDL cholesterol in determining risk of first myocardial infarction. Circulation 97: 2007–2011.
35. Maseri A. 1997. Inflammation, atherosclerosis, and ischemic events: exploring the hidden side of the moon. N Engl J Med 336:1014–1016.
36. Haverkate F, Thompson SG, Pyke SDM, Gallimore JR, Pepys MB. 1997. For the European Concerted Action on Thrombosis and Disabilities Angina Pectoris Study Group. Production of C-Reactive protein and risk of coronary events in stable and unstable angina. Lancet 349:462–466.
37. Buffon A, Liuzzo G, Biasucci LM, et al. 1999. Preprocedural serum levels of C-reactive protein predict early complications and late restenosis after coronary angioplasty. J Am Coll Cardiol 34: 1512–1521.
38. Ridker PM, Rifai N, Stampfer MJ, et al. 2000. Plasma concentration of interleukin-6 and the risk of future myocardial infarction among apparently healthy men. Circulation 101:1767–1772.
39. Heeschen C, Hamm CW, Bruemmer J, et al. 2000. Predictive value of C-reactive protein and troponin T in patients with unstable angina: a comparative analysis: CAPTURE Investigators: Chimeric c7E3 Anti-Platelet Therapy in Unstable angina REfractory to standard treatment trial. J Am Coll Cardiol 35:1535–1542.
40. Mallat Z, Corbaz A, Scoazec A, Besnard S, Lesèche G, Chvatchko Y, Tedgui A. 2001. Expression of interleukin-18 in human atherosclerotic plaques and relation to plaque instability. Circulation 104:1598–1603.
41. Pasceri V, Willerson JT, Yeh ETH. 2000. Direct proinflammatory effect of C-reactive protein on human endothelial cells. Circulation 102:2165–2168.
42. Pasceri V, Chang J, Willerson JT, Yeh ETH. 2001. Modulation of C-reactive protein-mediated monocyte chemoattractant protein-1 induction in human endothelial cells by anti-atherosclerosis drugs. Circulation 103(21):2531–2534.
43. Yeh ETH, Anderson HV, Pasceri V, Willerson JT. 2001. C-Reactive protein: Linking inflammation to cardiovascular complications. Editorial. Circulation 104(9):974–975.
44. Theroux P, Willerson JT, Armstrong P. 2000. Acute coronary syndromes. Fifty years of progress. Circulation 102(20 Suppl 4):IV2–IV13.

45. Zwaka TP, Hombach V, Torzewski J. 2001. C-reactive protein-mediated low density lipoprotein uptake by macrophages. Implications for atherosclerosis. Circulation 103:1194–1197.
46. 4S Investigators. 1994. Randomised trial of cholesterol lowering in 4444 patients with coronary heart disease: the Scandinavian Simvastatin Survival Study (4S). Lancet 344:1383–1389.
47. Shepherd J, Cobbe SM, Ford I, Isles CG, Lorimer AR, MacFarlane PW, McKillop JH, Packard CJ. 1995. Prevention of coronary heart disease with pravastatin in men with hypercholesterolemia. N Engl J Med 333:1301–1307.
48. Sacks FM, Pfeffer MA, Moye LA, et al. 1996. The effect of pravastatin on coronary events after myocardial infarction in patients with average cholesterol levels. N Engl J Med 335:1001–1009.
49. Ridker PM, Rifai N, Pfeffer MA, et al. 1999. Long-term effects of pravastatin on plasma concentration of C-reactive protein. Circulation 100:230–235.
50. Dupuis J, Tardif JC, Cernacek P, Theroux P. 1999. Cholesterol reduction rapidly improves endothelial function after acute coronary syndromes: the RECIFE (reduction of cholesterol in ischemia and function of the endothelium) trial. Circulation 99:3227–33.
51. Fukumoto Y, Libby P, Rabkin E, et al. 2001. Statins alter smooth muscle cell accumulation and collagen content in established atheroma of Wantanabe heritable hyperlipidemic rabbits. Circulation 103:993–999.
52. Ridker PM, Cushman M, Stampfer MJ, et al. 1997. Inflammation, aspirin, and the risk of cardiovascular disease in apparently healthy men. N Engl J Med 336:973–797.
53. Anderson JL, Muhlstein JB, Carlquist J, Allen A, Trehan S, Nielson C, Hall Staci, Brady J, Egger M, Horne B, Lim T. 1999. Randomized secondary prevention trial of azithromycin in patients with coronary artery disease and serological evidence for *Chlamydia pneumoniae* infection. The Azithromycin in Coronary Artery Disease: Elimination of Myocardial Infection with Chlamydia (ACADEMIC) Study. Circulation 99:1540–1547.
54. Wakatsuki A, Okatani Y, Ikenoue N, Fukaya T. 2002. Effect of Medroxyprogesterone acetate on vascular inflammatory markers in postmenopausal women receiving estrogen. Circulation In press.
55. Azar RR, Rinfret S, Theroux P, Stone PH, Dakshinamurthy R, Feng YJ, Wu AH, Range G, Waters DD. 2000. A randomized placebo-controlled trial to assess the efficacy of antiinflammatory therapy with methylprednisone in unstable angina (MUNA trial). Eur Heart J 21:2026–2032.
56. Baran KW, Nguyen M, McKendall GR, Lambrew CT, Dykstra G, Palmeri ST, Gibbons RJ, Borzak S, Sobel BE, Gourlay SG, Rundle AC, Gibson CM, Barron HV. 2001. Double-blind, randomized trial of an anti-CD18 antibody in conjunction with recombinant tissue plasminogen activator for acute myocardial infarction: limitation of myocardial infarction following thrombolysis in acute myocardial infarction (LIMIT AMI) study. Circulation 104:2778–2783.
57. Ridker PM, Hennekens CH, Rifai N, Buring JE, Manson JE. 1999. Hormone replacement therapy and increased plasma concentration of C-reactive protein. Circulation 100:713–716.
58. Cushman M, Legault C, Barrett-Connor E, et al. 1999. Effects of postmenopausal hormones on inflammation sensitive proteins: the Postmenopausal Estrogen/Progestin Interventions (PEPI) Study. Circulation 100:717–722.
59. Wakatsuki A, Okatani Y, Ikenoue N, Fukaya T. 2002. Effect of medroxyprogesterone acetate on vascular inflammatory markers in postmenopausal women receiving estrogen. In press, Circulation.
60. Patel SS, Willerson JT, Yeh ET-H. 1998. Inhibition of α_4 integrin and ICAM-1 markedly attenuate macrophage homing to atherosclerotic plaques in ApoE-deficient mice. Circulation 97(1): 75–81.
61. Pasceri V, Wu HD, Willerson JT, Yeh ET-H. 2000. Modulation of vascular inflammation in vitro and in vivo by Peroxisome Proliferator-Activated Receptor-γ activators. Circulation 101:235–238.
62. Marx N, Sukhova GK, Collins T, Libby P, Plutzky J. 1999. PPARα activators inhibit cytokine-induced vascular cell adhesion molecule-1 expression in human endothelial cells. Circulation 99:3125–3131.
63. Marx N, Sukhova G, Murphy C, Libby P, Plutzky J. 1998. Macrophages in human atheroma contain PPARγ: differentiation-dependent PPARγ expression and reduction in MMP-9 activity through PPARγ activation in mononuclear phagocytes. Am J Pathol 153:17–23.
64. Stefanadis C, Toutouzas K, Tsiamis E, Stratos C, Vavuranakis M, Kallikazaros I, Panagiotakos D, Toutouzas P. 2001. Increased local temperature in human coronary atherosclerotic plaques: an independent predictor of clinical outcome in patients undergoing a percutaneous coronary intervention. J Am Coll Cardiol 37:1277–1283.
65. Zoldhelyi P, Chen Z-Q, Shelat HS, McNatt JM, Willerson JT. 2001. Local gene transfer of tissue factor pathway inhibitor regulates intimal hyperplasia in atherosclerotic arteries. Proc Natl Acad Sci USA 98(7):4078–4083.

66. Shyue S-K, Tsai M-J, Liou J-Y, Willerson JT, Wu KK. 2001. Selective augmentation of prostacyclin production by combined prostacyclin synthase and cyclooxygenase-1 gene transfer. Circulation 103(16):2090–2095.
67. Shelat HS, Liu T-J, Hickman-Bick D, Barnhart MK, Vida T, Dillard PM, Willerson JT, Zoldhelyi P. 2001. Growth suppression of human coronary vascular smooth muscle cells by gene transfer of the transcription factor E2F-1. Circulation 103(3):407–414.
68. Zoldhelyi P, Eichstaedt H, Jax T, McNatt JM, Chen Z-Q, Shelat HS, Rose H, Willerson JT. September 1999. The emerging clinical potential of cardiovascular gene therapy. Semin Intervent Cardiol, W.B. Saunders Company LTD, Vol 4:151–165.
69. Zoldhelyi P, McNatt J, Shelat HS, Yamamoto Y, Chen Z-Q, Willerson JT. 2000. Thromboresistance of balloon-injured porcine carotid arteries after local gene transfer of human tissue factor pathway inhibitor. Circulation 101:289–295.
70. Zoldhelyi P, McNatt J, Xu XM, Loose-Mitchell D, Meidell R, Clubb FJ, Buja M, Willerson JT, Wu KK. 1996. Prevention of arterial thrombosis by adenovirus-mediate transfer of cyclooxygenase gene. Circulation 93:10–17.

Frontiers in Cardiovascular Health, edited by
N.S. Dhalla, A. Chockalingam,
H.I. Berkowitz & P.K. Singal
Kluwer Academic Publishers, Boston, 2003

The Role of Inflammation in Cardiac Function and Repair

Mark L. Entman, Keith A. Youker, Venkatesh Lakshminarayanan, Tareck O. Nossuli, Oliver Dewald, C. Wayne Smith, and Nikolaos G. Frangogiannis

Departments of Medicine and Pediatrics and the DeBakey Heart Center Baylor College of Medicine and The Methodist Hospital, Houston, Texas

Summary. Reperfusion of the infarcted myocardium is associated with an intense inflammatory reaction, which may extend ischemic injury, but is also crucial for cardiac repair, improving patient survival. Myocardial necrosis induces complement activation and free radical generation, triggering a cytokine cascade initiated by Tumor Necrosis Factor (TNF)-α release. In addition, chemokine expression is markedly induced in the infarcted myocardium and may have a role in regulating leukocyte infiltration, angiogenesis and granulation tissue formation. Bone marrow-derived stem cells may also be recruited in the infarct thus participating in cardiac repair. Elucidating the complex interactions and regulatory mechanisms responsible for infarct healing may allow us to design effective inflammation-related interventions for the treatment of myocardial infarction.

***Key words*:** chemokines, inflammation, infarction, reperfusion, stem cells.

INTRODUCTION

Modern care of the acute myocardial infarction has demonstrated that prognosis strikingly improved by reperfusion of the infarcted vessel and return of myocardial blood flow (1,2). Substantial evidence suggests that myocardial salvage requires rapid reperfusion in the first 2 to 4 hours after the onset of symptoms which has led to aggressive restructuring of our health system to deliver care as rapidly as possible. In recent years, it has become obvious that optimal healing and repair of the

Address Correspondence to: Mark L. Entman, M.D., Department of Medicine, Section of Cardiovascular Sciences, One Baylor Plaza, Houston, TX 77030-3498. Phone: (713) 798-4188, Fax: (713) 796-0015, E-mail: mentman@bcm.tmc.edu.

myocardial infarction plays an equal role in the long term prognosis of the patient. It has also become clear that reperfusion of the infarcted myocardium promotes effective tissue repair and decreases deleterious ventricular remodeling even under circumstances where reperfusion is effected too late to limit myocardial necrosis (3).

There are striking differences in the cellular response to myocardial infarction in the reperfused myocardium when compared to the permanently obstructed infarct. Reperfusion is associated with an intense inflammatory reaction in which both neutrophils and mononuclear cells rapidly enter the previously ischemic area (4,5). The intensity of this reaction may, under some circumstances, overwhelm normal defenses and actually extend cardiac injury. In our previous work we examined this acute inflammatory response using both in vivo and in vitro techniques (Figure 1). In vitro, we demonstrated neutrophil adhesion to myocardial cells in which ICAM-1 had been induced on the surface the sarcolemma (6). Compartmented transfer of reactive oxygen from the neutrophil to the myocardial cell effected a Mac-1/ICAM-1 dependent injury (7). In vivo, we demonstrated that neutrophils, which migrated from venules into the border zone of the myocardial infarction, were activated so that there was increased Mac-1 on their surface (8). Moreover, we demonstrated the induction of myocyte ICAM-1 in the border zone of the reperfused infarct (9). Finally, the cardiac lymph collected from the reperfused myocardium induced ICAM-1 in isolated cardiac myocytes and activated neutrophils with increased surface expression of Mac-1 (6,10). Antibodies to IL-6 could neutralize ICAM-1

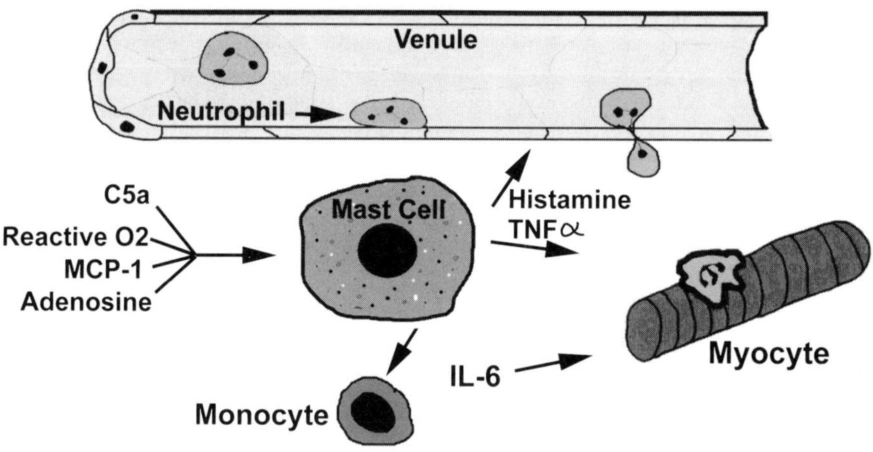

Figure 1. *A diagram of inflammatory cascade leading to cardiac injury*—Neutrophils and monocytes transmigrate from the venule in response to tactic factors; C5a mediates the first several hours. Activation of the neutrophil by C5a upregulates MAC-1 on its surface (not shown). Cardiac mast cells are also activated by C5a before reperfusion, reactive oxygen after reperfusion; MCP-1 and adenosine are also potentially important. Mast cells release histamine which facilitates margination in the venule (via P-selectin—not shown) and TNF-α. The latter stimulates IL-6 production by tissue monocytes. IL-6 upregulates ICAM-1 expression on cardiac myocytes which allows neutrophil-myocyte adhesion via Mac-1/ICAM-1 interaction and resultant injury.

induction by the cardiac lymph and early neutrophil activation in cardiac lymph was attributed to C5a (6,11). In the dog model of myocardial infarction, the origin of early IL-6 production was found to be in monocytes entering reperfused infarct; this induction occurred rapidly and was induced by preformed TNF-α released by cardiac mast cells (12). Finally, the origin of complement activation was shown to be activation of the classic complement pathway through C1q binding to mitochondrial peptides released from infarcted myocardium (13).

Thus, reperfusion of the infarcted myocardium may result in expanded injury but reperfusion appears to be an important factor in efficient cardiac repair. We have resolved this paradox with the assumption that the intensity of early reperfusion-induced inflammation may potentially overwhelm evolved defenses against cell attack but, on the whole, inflammation has evolved as a reaction to injury that is critical in mediating protection and repair. This latter hypothesis is harder to study than the role of inflammation in injury. Studying cardiac injury utilizing both in vivo and in vitro techniques is relatively straightforward and the strategies we developed are useful in evaluating strategies for protecting the tissue against inflammation. However, the complexity of tissue protection and repair belies simple techniques. In our laboratory, we have adopted the experimental approach in which we examine the hypothesis that inflammation is protective by examining potential protective roles for key cellular responses initiated in early reperfusion that have also been linked to injury. In this chapter, we describe potential protective roles of three important mediators in the cell injury response:

I) TNF-α
II) Chemokine induction
III) Cardiac mast cell

Methods of cardiac repair and protection—recent examples

I) *TNF-α*—As described above, TNF-α appears to be the upstream cytokine in the cytokine cascade associated with acute inflammation during reperfusion. In large mammals such as the dog, TNF-α is stored in cardiac mast cells (14) and rapidly released during reperfusion predominantly in the border zone of the myocardial infarction (12). In mice, mast cell number is very low and TNF-α arises during reperfusion as a result of molecular induction potentially effected by reactive oxygen (15). We have demonstrated that the upstream TNF-α is critical to the ultimate initiation of IL-6 production in both monocytes and cardiac myocytes. IL-6 is a critical cytokine in the induction of ICAM-1 in cardiac myocytes in the cardiac infarct border, which renders them vulnerable to inflammatory injury.

These observations led to our studies examining the effect of TNF-α on cardiac injury resulting from myocardial infarction. In collaboration with our colleague, Dr. Douglas L. Mann, we examined the consequence of genetic deletion of either or both of the TNF-α receptors (p55, p75) (16). In our model of mouse myocardial infarction, we demonstrated that there was no apparent difference in cardiovascular structure or function between the wild type animals and the experimental animals. It was demonstrated, however, that deletion of both (but not one) of the TNF-α receptors is associated with a marked *increase* in myocardial infarct size when compared to the other groups. We have subsequently demonstrated that this increase in myocardial infarction size is directly related to an increase in apoptosis in the infarct and border zone areas. Indeed, our studies suggest that myocardial infarction size in the mouse can be reduced by caspase inhibitors, or overexpression of bcl-2 or several other antiapoptotic measures. TNF-α has been demonstrated to be cytoprotective against apoptosis in other cell systems but has also been demonstrated to initiate apoptosis as well. The latter has been linked to activation of the "death domains" and TRADD. Protective effects have not yet been completely elucidated and are currently being studied in our model by our colleagues and us. However, it is noted that both the p55 and p75 pathways activate the TNF-receptor associated factor 2 (TRAF2) which ultimately activates NFκB. The latter has been proposed to be cytoprotective in a variety of mechanisms including induction of manganese superoxide dismutase as well as the cytoprotective mitochondrial protein A20.

II) *Chemokine induction*—Chemokines are rapidly induced in the reperfused myocardial infarction. Peak levels of mRNA for MCP-1 and IL-8 are seen in the first 1 to 3 hours in a dog model; analogous chemokines are found in a mouse model during a similar time course (17,18). In situ hybridization studies have demonstrated that early chemokine induction occurs almost exclusively in the postcapillary venule and induction of these chemokines occurs in vitro in venular endothelium and is easily effected by TNF-α (17,18). In our earlier studies of injury, we ascribed chemokine induction to TNF-α in the myocardial infarction and provided compelling evidence for the role of chemokines in leukocyte trafficking after two hours of reperfusion when C5a levels had dissipated (17). From a functional point of view, this leukocyte trafficking occurring after this time is less likely to be associated with injury and more likely to be associated with cardiac repair. It is important to note that, while chemokines are generally considered to be "leukotactic" agents, they actually function as tactic agents for endothelial cells and for fibroblasts during angiogenesis. This has led to our suggestion that chemokines may play a role in cardiac repair by effecting angiogenesis. Two recent studies speak to this topic.

A) *IP-10*—When studying the cellular response to reperfusion during the first 24 hours, we and others have noted a rapid increase in important factors associated with the initiation of angiogenesis (17,19). VEGF is rapidly induced, fibrin is rapidly deposited extravascularly, and the "angiogenic" chemokines, MCP-1, and IL-8, are rapidly induced in reperfusion (17,18). It was paradoxical, therefore, that we were unable to demonstrate any evidence of angiogenesis during the first 24 hours of reperfusion. An exhaustive examination of the cellular responses to early reperfusion found that the first evidence of angiogenesis to be detected was PCNA expression in venular endothelium and that this response became detectable at 24 hours (20,21).

We hypothesized that a molecular mechanism for suppressing early angiogenesis might exist. In a recent paper, we demonstrated the induction of IP-10 in the venular endothelium of the reperfused infarct (21). IP-10 is a CXC chemokine that is chemotactic for T-lymphocytes of the Th-1 phenotype (22–24). Unlike IL-8, it is a member of a class of chemokines that lack the ELR motif and have been demonstrated to be inhibitory to such angiogenic functions as tubular capillary formation (25) and endothelial proliferation (26). When we compared the regulation of IP-10 in comparison to interleukin-8, we found that they were induced in a similar time course in the venular endothelium in reperfused infarcts. In contrast to IL-8, however, IP-10 mRNA expression actually disappeared by 6 hours of reperfusion and the protein was not detectable by 24 hours. In contrast, mRNA from other chemokines induced in venular endothelium during reperfusion remained elevated for several days. IP-10 is ordinarily induced in monocytes by interferon gamma and this induction is suppressed by the anti-inflammatory cytokine IL-10 which we have demonstrated to be induced in the myocardial infarction over the same time course as the suppression of IP-10 (27). However, endothelial IP-10 induction is effected by TNF-α and could not be suppressed by IL-10 (21); IP-10 induction was specifically suppressed by TGF-beta which we had earlier shown to be active in the reperfused myocardium over the 3 to 6 hour time period (28). Thus, IP-10 induction and suppression in endothelial cells is unique and controlled differently than its induction in monocytes under circumstances where it plays an important lymphotactic role. We postulate that IP-10 induction represents a specific protective mechanism suppressing angiogenesis during early reperfusion to allow proper clearance of infarcted tissue and maturation of the fibrin matrix necessary for efficient angiogenesis.

This elegant control mechanism for angiogenesis is demonstrated in Figure 2.

B) *Reactive oxygen and chemokine induction*—Reactive oxygen has been demonstrated to induce chemokines in a variety of cellular models. The potential role for chemokines in early angiogenesis led us to hypothesize that they might be involved in formation of collateral circulation. Since collateral circulation formation is meant to prevent infarction, we studied chemokine induction in an ischemia and reperfusion model in which there was no myocardial infarction (29). We studied the induction of MCP-1 in this model and found rapid induction of MCP-1 in venular endothelium in the absence of infarction or inflammation. Moreover, the administration of a reactive oxygen scavenger totally prevented the induction of MCP-1. Reactive oxygen dependent induction of MCP-1 was attended by nuclear translocation of NFκB and AP-1 (cJun dimer) in the venular endothelium in which MCP-1 was induced. In vitro, hydrogen peroxide induced MCP-1 in venular endothelium under similar circumstances with activation of NFκB and AP-1 (cJun dimers) (29).

In the mouse model, induction of angiogenic chemokines could also be demonstrated in the venular endothelium in the presence of short periods of ischemia followed by reperfusion. We examined chemokine induction after ischemia-reperfusion

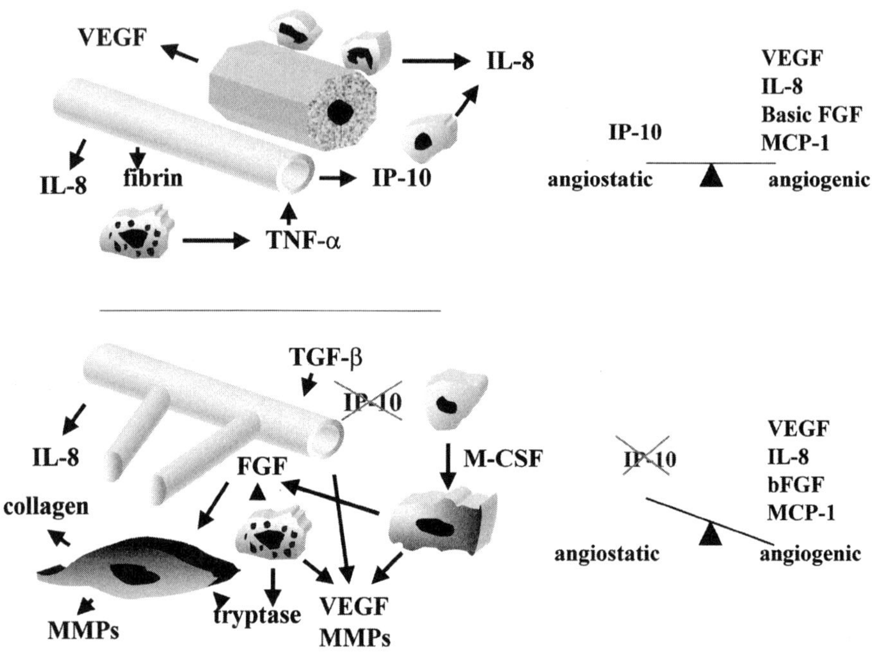

Figure 2. *Angiogenic and angiostatic stimuli in acute myocardial infarction*—angiogenic factors are generated in the extracellular matrix early during ischemia (VEGF, IL-8, and fibrin). Angiogenesis does not begin for 24 hours (see text). We propose this relates to early induction (top panel)of the angiostatic chemokine, IP-10, which suppresses angiogenesis. IP-10 induction is rapidly suppressed by TGF-β released from disintegrating myocytes and is clear by 24 hours. This allows the onset of angiogenesis (bottom panel).

in both wild type animals and animals with genetic deletion of TNF-α receptors (p55/p75—see above). In each case, there was a rapid induction of chemokine in the venular endothelial that could be suppressed by pretreatment with reactive oxygen scavengers and was attended by activation of NFκB and AP-1 as seen in the dog (30).

These observations have lead us to postulate that, during reperfusion, the production of reactive oxygen results in subsequent induction of angiogenic chemokines. This induction of angiogenesis may be of significant importance in development of collateral circulation (Figure 3). It is important to point out, however, that these chemokines are also potentially fibrogenic and, over a long period of time, chemokine induction may also initiate increased fibrosis of the myocardium.

III) *Stem cell factor and bone marrow precursors*—

A) *The Mast Cell*—As described above, we initially studied the mast cell with regard to its function as a source for preformed inflammatory cytokines such as TNF-α which mediate the acute inflammatory process. We demonstrated that TNF-

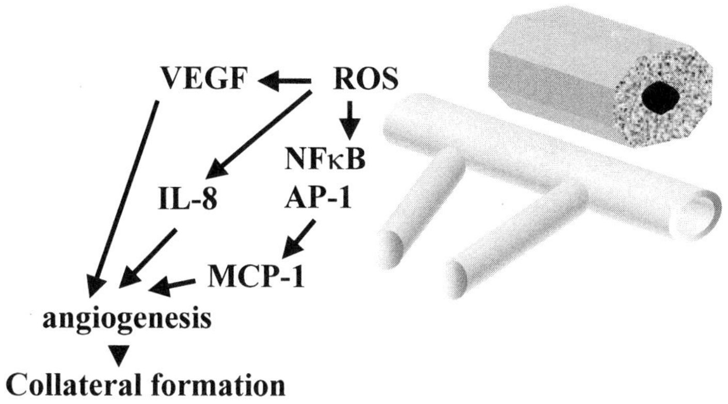

Figure 3. *Angiogenesis during ischemia and reperfusion without infarction*—in the absence of myocardial infarction, angiogenic stimuli are generated by the release of reactive oxygen and activation of transcription factors NFκB and AP1. We propose that this is a primary mechanism of generating collateral flow in a chronically ischemic zone.

α functioned as the "upstream cytokine" in the cytokine cascade leading to induction of IL-6; the latter stimulated production of ICAM-1 in cardiac myocytes on the border of the reperfused myocardial infarction (5).

These observations led to an examination of the potential role for mast cells in cardiac repair. The mast cell is an important source of fibrogenic and angiogenic agents; indeed, the mast cell-specific protease tryptase, is thought to be a potent fibrogenic agent (31). Mast cells also generate VEGF, basic fibroblast growth factor, chemokinetic angiogenic factors, and chymase which is a potential source of conversion of angiotensinogen to angiotensin (32). In our examination of mast cells during the healing phase of a myocardial infarction it became obvious that within the first several days of reperfusion mast cell number increased. In fact, in the newly formed scar areas, mast cell number increased 10 to 12-fold. In these areas, was intense proliferation of endothelial cells and fibroblasts to support a potential role of mast cells in fibrogenesis and angiogenesis. However, there was no evidence of mast cell proliferation in any of the samples (20,33).

In our subsequent experiments, we demonstrated that the increase of mast cell number was associated with an influx of bone marrow derived mast cell precursors which entered from the circulation into the infarcted myocardium. In in vitro studies, the maturation and chemotaxis of mast cell precursors was almost invariably dependent, at least in part, on the presence of stem cell factor. We subsequently demonstrated that monocyte derived macrophages entering into the infarcted area contain stem cell factor mRNA and protein (20). We speculate that this inflammation based flux of bone marrow derived mast cell precursors is an important step in facilitating effective scar formation.

B) *Bone marrow stem cells*—In subsequent experiments, in collaboration with Drs.

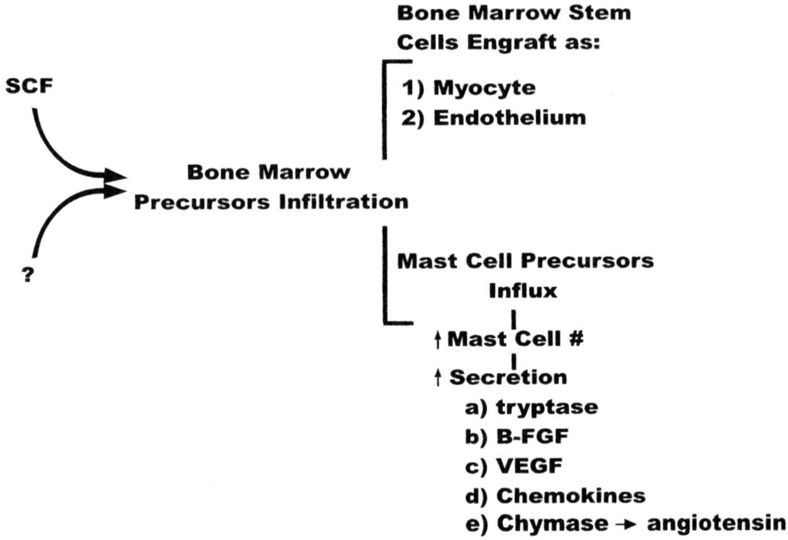

Figure 4. *Bone marrow precursors in the reperfused myocardial infarction*—infiltrating monocytes in the reperfused myocardial infarction begin synthesizing stem cell factor. This is followed by an influx of mast cell precursors so that there is a striking increase in mast cell number and maturation. This results in the increased level and secretion of several angiogenic and fibrogenic factors important in cardiac repair. In addition, evidence suggests that bone marrow derived stem cells also localize in the reperfused myocardial infarction and they have been found to differentiate into cardiac myocytes and venular endothelium. (see text)

Margaret Goodell and Karen Hirschi, we examined the hypothesis of other bone marrow precursors which may participate in the cardiac repair process. Bone marrow stem cells (SP cells) were extracted from c57 BL/6-Rosa mice). This strain of mice has been constructed so that all cells are lac Z-positive. The bone marrow SP cells were then transplanted into congenic wild type c57 BL/6 mouse after irradiation to destroy normal bone marrow. Thus, all bone marrow derived precursors are lac Z-positive. After 12 weeks of transplantation, the mice underwent an infarction and reperfusion protocol previously described in our laboratory. Animals were sacrificed at either 2 or 4 weeks after injury in order to analyze the hearts for incorporation of SP cells or their subsequent progeny in regenerating tissue (34).

Examination of the shams showed no lac Z-positive cells in the heart. In contrast, lac Z-positive cells were seen in the border zone of the myocardial infarction in all of the infarcted animals. Lac Z cardiac myocytes were found primarily in their peri-infarct region at a prevalence of about 0.02% and lac Z-positive endothelial cells were found at a prevalence of about 3.03%. The latter was seen primarily in small venules adjacent to the infarct.

We postulate that engraftment of bone marrow derived stem cells occurs as a compensatory mechanism for tissue loss. The system is obviously a low capacity system which evolved to deal with much lesser injuries than that seen in myocardial infarction. Our laboratory is currently examining potential mechanisms of amplifying this response. Perhaps equally as important is an understanding of the mechanism of the low level loss of cardiac myocytes for which this system evolved to compensate.

Thus, bone marrow precursors and their attraction to an area of injury is of great potential importance to cardiac repair (35) (Figure 4).

REFERENCES

1. ••. 1988. Randomised trial of intravenous streptokinase, oral aspirin, both, or neither among 17,187 cases of suspected acute myocardial infarction: ISIS-2. ISIS-2 (Second International Study of Infarct Survival) Collaborative Group. Lancet 2:349–360.
2. ••. 1993. An international randomized trial comparing four thrombolytic strategies for acute myocardial infarction. The GUSTO investigators. N Engl J Med 329:673–682.
3. ••. 1993. Late Assessment of Thrombolytic Efficacy (LATE) study with alteplase 6–24 hours after onset of acute myocardial infarction. Lancet 342:759–766.
4. Frangogiannis NG, Youker KA, Rossen RD, Gwechenberger M, Lindsey MH, Mendoza LH, Michael LH, Ballantyne CM, Smith CW, Entman ML. 1998. Cytokines and the microcirculation in ischemia and reperfusion. J Mol Cell Cardiol 30:2567–2576.
5. Frangogiannis NG, Smith CW, Entman ML. 2002. The inflammatory response in myocardial infarction. Cardiovasc Res 53:31–47.
6. Youker K, Smith CW, Anderson DC, Miller D, Michael LH, Rossen RD, Entman ML. 1992. Neutrophil adherence to isolated adult cardiac myocytes. Induction by cardiac lymph collected during ischemia and reperfusion. J Clin Invest 89:602–609.
7. Entman ML, Youker K, Shoji T, Kukielka G, Shappell SB, Taylor AA, Smith CW. 1992. Neutrophil induced oxidative injury of cardiac myocytes. A compartmented system requiring CD11b/CD18-ICAM-1 adherence. J Clin Invest 90:1335–1345.
8. Dreyer WJ, Smith CW, Michael LH, Rossen RD, Hughes BJ, Entman ML, Anderson DC. 1989. Canine neutrophil activation by cardiac lymph obtained during reperfusion of ischemic myocardium. Circ Res 65:1751–1762.
9. Youker KA, Hawkins HK, Kukielka GL, Perrard JL, Michael LH, Ballantyne CM, Smith CW, Entman ML. 1994. Molecular evidence for induction of intracellular adhesion molecule-1 in the viable border zone associated with ischemia-reperfusion injury of the dog heart. Circulation 89:2736–2746.
10. Dreyer WJ, Smith CW, Michael LH, Rossen RD, Hughes BJ, Entman ML, Anderson DC. 1989. Canine neutrophil activation by cardiac lymph obtained during reperfusion of ischemic myocardium. Circ Res 65:1751–1762.
11. Dreyer WJ, Michael LH, Nguyen T, Smith CW, Anderson DC, Entman ML, Rossen RD. 1992. Kinetics of C5a release in cardiac lymph of dogs experiencing coronary artery ischemia-reperfusion injury. Circ Res 71:1518–1521.
12. Frangogiannis NG, Lindsey ML, Michael LH, Youker KA, Bressler RB, Mendoza LH, Spengler RN, Smith CW, Entman ML. 1998. Resident cardiac mast cells degranulate and release preformed TNF- alpha, initiating the cytokine cascade in experimental canine myocardial ischemia/reperfusion. Circulation 98:699–710.
13. Kagiyama A, Savage HE, Michael LH, Hanson G, Entman ML, Rossen RD. 1989. Molecular basis of complement activation in ischemic myocardium: identification of specific molecules of mitochondrial origin that bind human C1q and fix complement. Circ Res 64:607–615.
14. Frangogiannis NG, Burns AR, Michael LH, Entman ML. 1999. Histochemical and morphological characteristics of canine cardiac mast cells. Histochem J 31:221–229.
15. Nossuli TO, Lakshminarayanan V, Baumgarten G, Taffet GE, Ballantyne CM, Michael LH, Entman ML. 2000. A chronic mouse model of myocardial ischemia-reperfusion: essential in cytokine studies. Am J Physiol Heart Circ Physiol 278:H1049–H1055.
16. Kurrelmeyer KM, Michael LH, Baumgarten G, Taffet GE, Peschon JJ, Sivasubramanian N, Entman ML, Mann DL. 2000. Endogenous tumor necrosis factor protects the adult cardiac myocyte against ischemic-induced apoptosis in a murine model of acute myocardial infarction. Proc Natl Acad Sci USA 97:5456–5461.

17. Kukielka GL, Smith CW, LaRosa GJ, Manning AM, Mendoza LH, Daly TJ, Hughes BJ, Youker KA, Hawkins HK, Michael LH. 1995. Interleukin-8 gene induction in the myocardium after ischemia and reperfusion in vivo. J Clin Invest 95:89–103.
18. Kumar AG, Ballantyne CM, Michael LH, Kukielka GL, Youker KA, Lindsey ML, Hawkins HK, Birdsall HH, Mackay CR, LaRosa GJ, Rossen RD, Smith CW, Entman ML. 1997. Induction of monocyte chemoattractant protein-1 in the small veins of the ischemic and reperfused canine myocardium. Circulation 95:693–700.
19. Li J, Brown LF, Hibberd MG, Grossman JD, Morgan JP, Simons M. 1996. VEGF, flk-1, and flt-1 expression in a rat myocardial infarction model of angiogenesis. Am J Physiol 270:H1803–H1811.
20. Frangogiannis NG, Perrard JL, Mendoza LH, Burns AR, Lindsey ML, Ballantyne CM, Michael LH, Smith CW, Entman ML. 1998. Stem cell factor induction is associated with mast cell accumulation after canine myocardial ischemia and reperfusion. Circulation 98:687–698.
21. Frangogiannis NG, Mendoza LH, Lewallen M, Michael LH, Smith CW, Entman ML. 2001. Induction and suppression of interferon-inducible protein 10 in reperfused myocardial infarcts may regulate angiogenesis. FASEB J 15:1428–1430.
22. Luster AD, Ravetch JV. 1987. Biochemical characterization of a gamma interferon-inducible cytokine (IP-10). J Exp Med 166:1084–1097.
23. Frangogiannis NG, Mendoza LH, Smith CW, Michael LH, Entman ML. 2000. Induction of the synthesis of the C-X-C chemokine interferon-gamma-inducible protein-10 in experimental canine endotoxemia. Cell Tissue Res 302:365–376.
24. Sallusto F, Lenig D, Mackay CR, Lanzavecchia A. 1998. Flexible programs of chemokine receptor expression on human polarized T helper 1 and 2 lymphocytes. J Exp Med 187:875–883.
25. Angiolillo AL, Sgadari C, Taub DD, Liao F, Farber JM, Maheshwari S, Kleinman HK, Reaman GH, Tosato G. 1995. Human interferon-inducible protein 10 is a potent inhibitor of angiogenesis in vivo. J Exp Med 182:155–162.
26. Luster AD, Greenberg SM, Leder P. 1995. The IP-10 chemokine binds to a specific cell surface heparan sulfate site shared with platelet factor 4 and inhibits endothelial cell proliferation. J Exp Med 182:219–231.
27. Frangogiannis NG, Mendoza LH, Lindsey ML, Ballantyne CM, Michael LH, Smith CW, Entman ML. 2000. IL-10 Is Induced in the Reperfused Myocardium and May Modulate the Reaction to Injury. J Immunol 165:2798–2808.
28. Birdsall HH, Green DM, Trial J, Youker KA, Burns AR, Mackay CR, LaRosa GJ, Hawkins HK, Smith CW, Michael LH, Entman ML, Rossen RD. 1997. Complement C5a, TGF-beta 1, and MCP-1, in sequence, induce migration of monocytes into ischemic canine myocardium within the first one to five hours after reperfusion. Circulation 95:684–692.
29. Lakshminarayanan V, Lewallen M, Frangogiannis NG, Evans AJ, Wedin KE, Michael LH, Entman ML. 2001. Reactive oxygen intermediates induce monocyte chemotactic protein-1 in vascular endothelium after brief ischemia. Am J Pathol 159:1301–1311.
30. Nossuli TO, Frangogiannis NG, Knuefermann P, Lakshminarayanan V, Dewald O, Evans AJ, Peschon J, Mann DL, Michael LH, Entman ML. 2001. Brief murine myocardial I/R induces chemokines in a TNF-alpha-independent manner: role of oxygen radicals. Am J Physiol Heart Circ Physiol 281:H2549–H2558.
31. Ruoss SJ, Hartmann T, Caughey GH. 1991. Mast cell tryptase is a mitogen for cultured fibroblasts. J Clin Invest 88:493–499.
32. Metcalfe DD, Baram D, Mekori YA. 1997. Mast cells. Physiol Rev 77:1033–1079.
33. Frangogiannis NG, Entman ML. 2000. Mast cells in myocardial ischaemia and reperfusion. Academic Press, London. 507–522.
34. Jackson KA, Majka SM, Wang H, Pocius J, Hartley CJ, Majesky MW, Entman ML, Michael LH, Hirschi KK, Goodell MA. 2001. Regeneration of ischemic cardiac muscle and vascular endothelium by adult stem cells. J Clin Invest 107:1395–1402.
35. Orlic D, Kajstura J, Chimenti S, Jakoniuk I, Anderson SM, Li B, Pickel J, McKay R, Nadal-Ginard B, Bodine, DM, Leri A, Anversa P. 2001. Bone marrow cells regenerate infarcted myocardium. Nature 410:701–705.

Frontiers in Cardiovascular Health, edited by
N.S. Dhalla, A. Chockalingam,
H.I. Berkowitz & P.K. Singal
Kluwer Academic Publishers, Boston, 2003

Cardiac Repair Following Infarction

Yao Sun and Karl T. Weber

Divisions of Cardiovascular Diseases
University of Tennessee Health Science Center
Memphis, Tennessee
USA

Summary. Scar tissue that appears following myocardial infarction (MI) consists of persistent, metabolically active and contractile myoFb that reside within its fibrillar collagen scaffolding nourished by a neovascular network. Understanding the evolution and maturation of this tissue, including the architecture of its fibrillar collagen scaffolding and the composition and behavior its vascular network, will be essential if today's interest in rebuilding the infarcted heart is to prove successful. Whether by the grafting of exogenous cardiomyocytes, derived from fetal heart muscle cells or stem cells, or by the homing and transdifferentiation of bone marrow-derived progenitor cells into cardiomyocytes, rebuilt myocardium must ultimately consist of anatomically appropriate, viable and functional myocardial tissue. Such "tissue engineering" will take place in the interstices of the living infarct scar. When and how best to accomplish this goal should prove interesting challenges.

***Key words*:** Myocardial infarction, Vascular network, Collagen, Myofibroblasts.

INTRODUCTION

For over a century, the scar that appears at the site of MI has been considered inert: acellular tissue composed simply of woven fibrillar collagen; its purpose to merely provide tensile strength to the infarct site and thereby resist tissue deformation and

Correspondence: Yao Sun, MD, Ph.D., Division of Cardiovascular Diseases, University of Tennessee Health Science Center, Rm. B310, 956 Court Avenue, Memphis, TN 38163. Tel: (901) 448-4921, Fax: (901) 448-4921, E-mail: yasun@utmem.edu.

prevent myocardial rupture. Despite this simplistic viewpoint, earlier reports recognized that connective tissue continued to accumulate at the infarct site for years after MI and scar tissue was vascularized (1–3). How could this be if there were no fibroblasts present and why perfuse acellular tissue?

Today, the transmural infarct scar is recognized as living tissue (4–5). It is composed of a population of fibroblast-like cells termed myofibroblasts (myoFb) because of their expression of α-smooth muscle actin and resultant contractile behavior. These cells are persistent at the infarct site for years; they do not disappear after the scar has formed (6,5), as is the case in skin where programmed cell death, or apoptosis, accounts for their disappearance (7). Not only are they persistent, but myoFb of the infarct scar continue to turn over type I and III fibrillar collagens long after scar tissue has restored the structural integrity of the infarcted myocardium. In order to carry out these functions, these cells must be nourished. This is accomplished by a neovasculature. Moreover, this structural protein scaffolding is innervated by postganglionic nerve fibers.

MyoFb collagen turnover is regulated by substances they elaborate *de novo*. These include angiotensin (Ang) II and transforming growth factor-β_1 (TGF-β_1). These substances are soluble and therefore able to traverse the heart's common interstitial space, where they can enhance fibroblast collagen synthesis at sites distant to the MI. The resultant fibrosis that appears over time at sites remote to the infarct represents the majority of connective tissue found in ischemic cardiomyopathy. It is considered the major component of the adverse structural remodeling found in the failing human heart of ischemic origin.

Herein we briefly review these various components of the infarct scar that provide for its dynamic nature and define it as living tissue and which will be relevant to "regrowing" myocardial tissue at the infarct site.

TISSUE REPAIR AT THE SITE OF INFARCTION

A highly orchestrated process of tissue repair follows the necrotic loss of cardiomyocytes. It begins with an activation of latent matrix metalloproteinases (MMPs) that degrade the existing extracellular matrix and coronary vasculature (8). This proteolytic activity declines by the end of week 1 postMI coincident with the increased expression of MMP inhibitors, termed tissue inhibitors of MMPs, or TIMPs (9). Circulating inflammatory cells that include neutrophils and monocytes/macrophages arrive at the infarct site soon after MI. They respectively contribute to the proteolytic digestion and phagocytosis of infarcted tissue. These inflammatory cells home to the site of MI drawn there by adhesion molecules and chemoattractant cytokines (or chemokines) expressed by endothelial cells of coronary vasculature that borders on the infarct site. Their migration into the infarct site is facilitated by MMP proteolytic activity while their ability to gain access to the infarct site is determined by the nature of the collateral circulation. Inflammatory cells disappear from the infarct site within weeks following MI, a consequence of their programmed cell death.

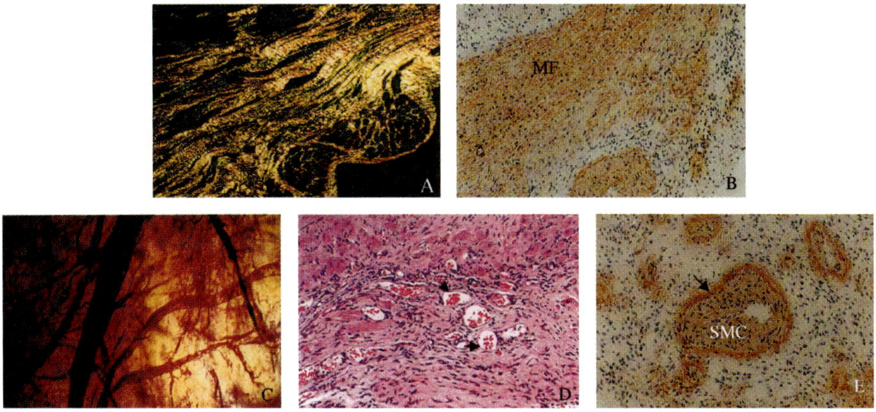

Figure 1. Collagen deposition, myofibroblasts and blood vessels in a four-week-old infarct scar of the infarcted rat heart. Picrosirius red-stained fibrillar collagen, when viewed under polarized light, appears birefringent or yellow in color (panel A). Alpha-smooth muscle actin-positive myofibroblasts (MF) are found within the infarct scar (brown in panel B). A carmine red cast of the neovasculature shows vessels of variable dimensions (panel C). The functionality of these vessels is suggested by the presence of red blood cells (arrowheads) within their lumen (panel D, hematoxylin & eosin stain). Alpha-smooth muscle actin labeling found in the vascular smooth muscle cells (SMC) and myofibroblasts residing in the adventitia (arrow) of vessels that border on the infarct (panel E).

FIBRILLAR COLLAGEN IN SCAR TISSUE

Scar tissue is composed predominantly of type I and III fibrillar collagens. Whittaker et al. (10) have examined the alignment of collagen fibers forming the infarct scar and found them to course in an essentially circumferential direction concordant with the predominant alignment of cardiac muscle fibers (11). Figure 1 (panel A) identifies the dense fibrillar collagen network found in the infarct scar 4 wks after MI in the rat heart.

SCAR MYOFIBROBLASTS

Myofibroblasts are found at the infarct site soon after the arrival of inflammatory cells. Cells which account for the appearance of myoFb are uncertain. They may include: interstitial fibroblasts; adventitial fibroblasts; pericytes, a population of circulating fibroblasts known as fibrocytes; or circulating monocytes or circulating bone marrow-derived progenitor cells that transdifferentiate at the infarct site. It is presumed that TGF-β_1, elaborated by macrophages, governs the appearance of the myoFb phenotype (12).

MyoFb are first found at the infarct site on day 3–4 postMI. They are responsible for formation of the scar via their expression (at mRNA and protein levels) of type I and III fibrillar collagens (5,13). Their growth and the alignment of fibrillar collagen are spatially regulated by their expression of a tissue polarity gene, *frizzled-2*, also found in *Drosophila* and which accounts for planar polarity, such as alignment of limbs and wings during embryonic development (14).

MyoFb remain at the infarct site as is the case in other injured tissues (e.g., skin) which have the capacity to regenerate parenchyma. In postmortem infarcted human heart tissue, myoFb have been found at the infarct site years after MI (6). In the infarcted rodent heart, we have observed myoFb at the infarct site 6 months postMI (5). Figure 1 (panel B) identifies the presence of α-smooth muscle actin-positive myoFb residing in the matrix of the 4-wk-old scar of the infarcted rat heart.

SCAR MYOFIBROBLAST METABOLIC ACTIVITY

Scar myoFb have a diverse portfolio of metabolic activities. *In situ* hybridization, *in vitro* autoradiography and immunohistochemistry have shown that these cells express renin, angiotensin converting enzyme (ACE), and AngII receptors at the infarct site (15–20).

Studied in culture under serum-deprived conditions, which eliminates circulating renin, ACE and AngI, myoFb obtained from the 4-wk-old infarct scar are found to express angiotensinogen, cathepsin D, ACE and AngII receptors (21). In the infarcted rat heart these receptors are found to be predominantly of the AT_1 subtype (15,18,21). In an autocrine manner, AngII regulates myoFb expression of TGF-β_1 and it is this cytokine that regulates myoFb collagen turnover (21,22).

In vivo, AngII-induced expression of TGF-β_1 is also involved in the regulation of fibroblast collagen synthesis at the infarct and remote sites and which is abrogated by AT_1 receptor antagonist (23). The continued expression of ACE and AT_1 receptors and active TGF-β_1 is observed in the infarcted rodent heart months after MI and underscores their persistent metabolic activity.

MORPHOLOGY OF SCAR NEOVASCULATURE

A vascular network begins to form at the infarct site on day 3 postMI. Little is known about its evolution, its ultimate morphologic features and its capacity to deliver and exchange oxygen by conductance and exchange vessels, respectively. Figure 1 (panel C) provides a carmine red "cast" of the scar neovasculature seen at week 4 postMI. Figure 1 (panel D) demonstrates the network as seen by light microscopy. Figure 1 (panel E) identifies α-SMA positive cells found by immunohistochemistry in the neovasculature and which includes vascular smooth muscle cells of arterioles and myoFb present in the perivascular space (or adventitia) of these vessels.

This vascular network is likely derived from several sources: endothelial cell sprouting from neighboring capillaries (angiogenesis); a transdifferentiation of bone marrow progenitor cells into endothelial cells (vasculogenesis); and an enlargement of neighboring collateral vessels (arteriogenesis).

The scar neovasculature nourishes myoFb and provides for their metabolic activity. The capacity of this network to deliver oxygen and nutrients and the oxygen requirements of myoFb have not been investigated. However, they likely are modest given the ability of fibroblasts to withstand hypoxia (24–25) and compared to the native coronary circulation it replaced and which formerly had nourished contractile cardiac myocytes, obligate aerobic cells.

VASOMOTOR REACTIVITY OF SCAR NEOVASCULATURE

The vasomotor reactivity of the coronary circulation found in the infarct rat heart, including the scar vasculature, was examined by Kalkman et al. (26). Using radiolabeled microspheres and an isolated perfused heart preparation, these investigators found total coronary blood flow to be nearly 10 mL/min with flow to 4-wk-old infarct scar to be approximately 1 mL/min. The low perfusion of scar tissue was evident when coronary flow was expressed per unit tissue weight and when compared to viable, contracting myocardium. These investigators further found an impaired vasodilator reserve to nitroprusside and marked vasoconstriction to vasopressin in the vasculature of scar tissue. In response to vasopressin, flow to the scar was barely detectible. Light microscopy revealed thicker walls of resistance arteries found in scar tissue. Whether this hyperreactivity is related to contractile myoFb of the scar and their presence in the scar neovasculature (Figure 1, panel E) has not been addressed.

SCAR INNERVATION

Soon after MI and as part of early proteolytic digestion of infarcted tissue, postganglionic neurons are lost at the infarct site. They are regenerated by week 2 and are formed by nerves sprouting from the surrounding noninfarcted myocardium (27–28). The reinnervation process may even be excessive representing a hyperinervation of the infarct scar (27). Postganglionic nerve fibers with storage granules are entwined within fibrillar collagen that forms the infarct scar (27). Their function remains unknown, but their presence calls into question a potential contribution of catecholamines to scar tissue contraction and arrhythmogenicity.

SCAR CONTRACTILE BEHAVIOR

MyoFb and their α-SMA microfilaments are joined to one another through gap junctions and to the scar's fibrillar collagen network via fibronexi. This creates a contractile scar tissue assembly. The now classic study of Gabbiani et al. (29) demonstrated the contractile behavior of scar tissue. Others have confirmed these findings (30–31). Given the presence of α-SMA in myoFb, present also in vascular smooth muscle cells, it is not surprising that AngII, catecholamines, endothelin-1, serotonin and vasopressin promote scar tissue contraction while papaverine induces its relaxation. As noted earlier, AngII receptors are present in myoFb of the infarct scar (15,18) and one would presume other receptors for these ligands are as well, as is the case for myoFb found in heart valve leaflets (32–35). The contribution of infarct scar tonus to diastolic dysfunction and scar tissue contraction to the appearance of sudden pulmonary edema has been suggested (36), but remains unknown.

REFERENCES

1. Levine SA. 1929. Coronary thrombosis: its various clinical features. Medicine 8:245–418.
2. Mallory GK, White PD, Salcedo-Salgar J. 1939. The speed of healing of myocardial infarction. A study of the pathologic anatomy in seventy-two cases. Am Heart J 18:647–671.
3. Lodge-Patch I. 1951. The ageing of cardiac infarcts, and its influence on cardiac rupture. Br Heart J 13:37–42.
4. Cleutjens JP, Blankesteijn WM, Daemen MJ, Smits JF. 1999. The infarcted myocardium: simply dead tissue, or a lively target for therapeutic interventions. Cardiovasc Res 44:232–241.
5. Sun Y, Weber KT. 2000. Infarct scar: a dynamic tissue. Cardiovasc Res 46:250–256.
6. Willems IEMG, Havenith MG, De Mey JGR, Daemen MJAP. 1994. The α-smooth muscle actin-positive cells in healing human myocardial scars. Am J Pathol 145:868–875.
7. Desmouliére A, Redard M, Darby I, Gabbiani G. 1995. Apoptosis mediates the decrease in cellularity during the transition between granulation tissue and scar. Am J Pathol 146:56–66.
8. Cleutjens JPM, Kandala JC, Guarda E, Guntaka RV, Weber KT. 1995. Regulation of collagen degradation in the rat myocardium after infarction. J Mol Cell Cardiol 27:1281–1292.
9. Sun Y, Zhang JQ, Zhang J, Lamparter S. 2000. Cardiac remodeling by fibrous tissue after infarction in rats. Journal of Laboratory & Clinical Medicine 135:316–323.
10. Whittaker P, Boughner DR, Kloner RA. 1989. Analysis of healing after myocardial infarction using polarized light microscopy. Am J Pathol 134:879–893.
11. Streeter DD, Spotnitz HM, Patel DP, Ross J, Sonnenblick EH. 1969. Fiber orientation in the canine left ventricle during diastole and systole. Circ Res 24:339–347.
12. Desmouliére A, Geinoz A, Gabbiani F, Gabbiani G. 1993. Transforming growth factor-β1 induces α-smooth muscle actin expression in granulation tissue myofibroblasts and in quiescent and growing cultured fibroblasts. J Cell Biol 122:103–111.
13. Cleutjens JPM, Verluyten MJA, Smits JFM, Daemen MJAP. 1995. Collagen remodeling after myocardial infarction in the rat heart. Am J Pathol 147:325–338.
14. Blankesteijn WM, Essers-Janssen YPG, Verluyten MJA, Daemen MJAP, Smits JFM. 1997. A homologue of *Drosophila* tissue polarity gene *frizzled* is expressed in migrating myofibroblasts in the infarcted rat heart. Nat Med 3:541–544.
15. Lefroy DC, Wharton J, Crake T, Knock GA, Rutherford RAD, Suzuki T, Morgan K, Polak JM, Poole-Wilson PA. 1996. Regional changes in angiotensin II receptor density after experimental myocardial infarction. J Mol Cell Cardiol 28:429–440.
16. Passier RC, Smits JF, Verluyten MJ, Daemen MJ. 1996. Expression and localization of renin and angiotensinogen in rat heart after myocardial infarction. Am J Physiol 271:H1040–H1048.
17. Sun Y, Weber KT. 1996. Angiotensin-converting enzyme and wound healing in diverse tissues of the rat. J Lab Clin Med 127:94–101.
18. Sun Y, Weber KT. 1996. Cells expressing angiotensin II receptors in fibrous tissue of rat heart. Cardiovasc Res 31:518–525.
19. Sun Y, Weber KT. 1996. Angiotensin converting enzyme and myofibroblasts during tissue repair in the rat heart. J Mol Cell Cardiol 28:851–858.
20. Sun Y, Zhang J, Zhang JQ, Weber KT. 2001. Renin expression at sites of repair in the infarcted rat heart. J Mol Cell Cardiol 33:995–1003.
21. Katwa LC, Campbell SE, Tyagi SC, Lee SJ, Cicila GT, Weber KT. 1997. Cultured myofibroblasts generate angiotensin peptides *de novo*. J Mol Cell Cardiol 29:1375–1386.
22. Campbell SE, Katwa LC. 1997. Angiotensin II stimulated expression of transforming growth factor-β_1 in cardiac fibroblasts and myofibroblasts. J Mol Cell Cardiol 29:1947–1958.
23. Sun Y, Zhang JQ, Zhang J, Ramires FJA. 1998. Angiotensin II, transforming growth factor-β_1 and repair in the infarcted heart. J Mol Cell Cardiol 30:1559–1569.
24. Packer L, Fuehr K. 1977. Low oxygen concentration extends the lifespan of cultured human diploid cells. Nature 267:423–425.
25. Zhang S, Azhar G, Nagano K, Wei JY. 2001. Differential vulnerability to oxidative stress in rat cardiac myocytes versus fibroblasts. J Am Coll Cardiol 38:2055–2062.
26. Kalkman EA, van Haren P, Saxena PR, Schoemaker RG. 1997. Regionally different vascular response to vasoactive substances in the remodelled infarcted rat heart; aberrant vasculature in the infarct scar. J Mol Cell Cardiol 29:1487–1497.
27. Vracko R, Thorning D, Frederickson RG. 1990. Fate of nerve fibers in necrotic, healing, and healed rat myocardium. Lab Invest 63:490–501.

28. Chen PS, Chen LS, Cao JM, Sharifi B, Karagueuzian HS, Fishbein MC. 2001. Sympathetic nerve sprouting, electrical remodeling and the mechanisms of sudden cardiac death. Cardiovasc Res 50: 409–416.
29. Gabbiani G, Hirschel BJ, Ryan GB, Statkov PR, Majno G. 1972. Granulation tissue as a contractile organ. A study of structure and function. J Exp Med 135:719–734.
30. Appleton I, Tomlinson A, Chander CL, Willoughby DA. 1992. Effect of endothelin-1 on croton oil-induced granulation tissue in the rat. A pharmacologic and immunohistochemical study. Lab Invest 67:703–710.
31. Gabbiani G. 1998. Evolution and clinical implications of the myofibroblast concept. Cardiovasc Res 38:545–548.
32. Pinto JE, Viglione P, Saavedra JM. 1991. Autoradiographic localization and quantification of rat heart angiotensin converting enzyme. Am J Hypertens 4:321–326.
33. Yamada H, Fabris B, Allen AM, Jackson B, Johnston CI, Mendelsohn FAO. 1991. Localization of angiotensin converting enzyme in rat heart. Circ Res 68:141–149.
34. Sun Y, Diaz-Arias AA, Weber KT. 1994. Angiotensin-converting enzyme, bradykinin and angiotensin II receptor binding in rat skin, tendon and heart valves: an in vitro quantitative autoradiographic study. J Lab Clin Med 123:372–377.
35. Chester AH, Misfeld M, Yacoub MH. 2000. Receptor-mediated contraction of aortic valve leaflets. J Heart Valve Dis 9:250–254.
36. Weber KT. 1997. Extracellular matrix remodeling in heart failure. A role for de novo angiotensin II generation. Circulation 96:4065–4082.

Frontiers in Cardiovascular Health, edited by
N.S. Dhalla, A. Chockalingam,
H.I. Berkowitz & P.K. Singal
Kluwer Academic Publishers, Boston, 2003

Protein and Phospholipids Composition of Human Myocardium in Children with Congenital Heart Disease

Václav Pelouch,[1,6] Marie Milerová,[2,6] Bohumil Hučín,[3] Michaela Adamcová,[4] Blanka Panušková,[5] and Jan Škovránek[3]

[1] *Department of Medical Chemistry and Biochemistry, Charles University, 2nd Faculty of Medicine, Prague*
[2] *Institute of Physiology, Czech Acad. Sciences, Prague*
[3] *Kardiocentrum, Faculty Hospital Motol, 2nd Faculty of Medicine, Prague*
[4] *Department of Physiology, Charles University, Faculty of Medicine, Hradec Králové*
[5] *Department of Animal Physiology, Charles University, Faculty of Sciences, Prague*
[6] *Centre for Experimental Cardiovascular Research, Prague, Czech Republic*

Summary. Congenital heart disease is caused by abnormalities in the first 6–8 weeks of fetal life; incidence of heart malformations is approximately eight out of 1000; they resulted from aberrant organogenesis due to dysfunction of genes and the encoded proteins. We, therefore, analyzed *protein and phospholipids profiles of human myocardium* (tissue samples were obtained during surgery of children with normoxemic and hypoxemic congenital heart disease). Protein profile of the atrial and ventricular myocardium differs significantly; higher concentration of *non-collagenous proteins* due to contractile ones and lower concentration of *extracellular matrix proteins* (ECM) due to pepsin-insoluble collagenous proteins were in ventricles. Furthermore, there were significant differences in activities of metabolic enzymes from both glycolytic and oxidative pathways; it correlated with higher amount of cardiolipin in ventricle (mitochondrial phospholipids). Moreover, electrophoretic pattern of both heavy and light chains of myosin in ventricular and atrial musculature of damage myocardium were different; however, hypoxemia decreased ATPase activity of myosin in ventricle only. Compartmentation of troponin T between myofibrillar and cytosolic pools was not affected by hypoxemia. Synthesis of newly formed collagenous proteins depend on balance between synthetic and degradation processes; they are mediated by metaloproteinases (major band in atria and ventricle has mol. .weight of 95kDa). Hypoxemia induced in atria both higher amount of collagen (predominantly collagen III) and activation of metaloproteinases. Significantly

Supported by grants: NA/6350-3, NA/6496-3 Grant agency—Ministery of Heath, Czech Republic.
Corresponding author: Prof. RNDr. Václav Pelouch, CSc., Tel.: 420 2 57210345, Fax: 420 2 57210995, E-mail: vaclav.pelouch@lfmotol.cuni.cz.

higher concentration of *phospholipids* was in ventricles; hypoxemia did not affected this atrio/ventricular difference. However, composition of phospholipids species in both parts of diseased myocardium did not differ (phosphatidylcholine and phosphatidylethanolamine occupied about 70% from all phosholipids). Surgeons, who are reconstructing cardiac anatomy, should be aware that they are dealing with biochemical abnormal tissue and they should respect atrio/ventricular differences.

***Key words*:** congenital heart disease, biochemical composition, contractile proteins, collagenous proteins, phospholipids.

INTRODUCTION

Congenital cardiovascular malformations remain the single largest cause of infant morbidity and mortality; their primary prevention is still impossible due to multifactor etiology. Despite the significant progress in understanding of molecular mechanisms of different diseases, relative little is known about congenital heart disease. It is due to complicated prenatal development of cardiac muscle: wrapped tube is stepwise changed to four-chambered heart; individual compartments have specific morphological, biochemical and functional characteristics. Right atrium, consisted of two portions derived from different segments of embryonic heart tube; it is a relatively prominent chamber in intrauterine life. On the other hand, structure of ventricles is different: right ventricle has ellipsoidal shape, left ventricle has cylindrical shape. The myocardium undergoes many changes in its structure and function during fetal and newborn periods even in healthy men. How these changes are interrelated and controlled remain in large part, to be resolved. Congenital heart disease is caused by developmental abnormalities in the first six to eight weeks of fetal life; the period when the fetal cardiovascular system being formed. The incidence of heart malformations is approximately eight/ 1000 live births (for review see 1–6). However, distribution of congenital heart disease between boys and girls is not equally: predominance of one sex was found in 13 from 18 categories of those diseases in live-born children. Similar conclusion followed from cohort of children who died prior to introduction of cardiac surgery; individual reports have, however, different results (6).

Congenital heart disease may be grouped into two main groups:

1) *normoxemic* (acyanotic) heart diseases with either increased (e.g. atrial septal defect -ASD, ventricular septal defect -VSD) or normal pulmonary circulation (e.g. pulmonary stenosis, aortic arch malformations); they have *left to right cardiac shunt* (arterial blood to venous)
2) *hypoxemic* (cyanotic) heart diseases with either increased (e.g. complete transposition of great arteries, double outlet of RV) or both normal and decreased pulmonary circulation (e.g. Tetralogy of Fallot, hypoplastic RV with ASD); they have *right to left cardiac shunt* (venous blood to arterial)

All human congenital heart defects have, however, hypertrophied myocardium as a consequence. Whereas in normoxemic disease the prime impulse is volume overloaded, in hypoxemic defects this is predominantly pressure load (7–8). There were common practice to wait with palliative or definitive surgical procedures until the early stages of myocardial decompensation were reached. Recently, as a result of common effort of surgeons, epidemiologists, basic scientists and pediatric cardiologists, the major shift in surgery is to operate earlier—before child status can deteriorate. Furthermore, in the Centre of prenatal cardiology of the Kardiocentrum, University Hospital Motol many thousands women in the 17th–41st week of pregnancy were examined by echocardiography; special ECHO was indicated in particular by geneticists and gynecologists. The most frequently found anomaly was a hypoplastic left heart and complete detect of AV septum; prenatal incidence of these serious anomalies is substantially higher than in postnatal life (9–10).

Because congenital cardiovascular disease resulted from aberrant organogenesis, it seems obvious that dysfunction of genes and the encoded proteins (mutation of contractile, mitochondrial and structural proteins or energy-producing enzymes) are main candidates (11–14). We, therefore, analyzed *biochemical profile* of human myocardium (atrial and ventricular samples). In short survey we would like to *summarized data of both protein and phospholipids composition of myocardium in different congenital heart disease* (15–25).

Statistical analyses

All results are expressed as means and their standard errors of the means (S.E.M.) The statistical significance of differences was determined by one way ANOVA by Bonferroni t-test ($p < 0.05$), with corresponding values for atrial musculature.

PROTEIN COMPOSITION OF ATRIAL AND VENTRICULAR MUSCULATURE

a) Protein interactions in cardiac filaments; ontogenetic aspects

Contractility of myocardium is brought about by complex interactions of *non-collagenous proteins* (formed by both contractile and metabolic proteins of myocardium). Moreover, calcium ions act as activator of these molecular interventions. The impulses for contraction of fetal or newborn cardiac muscle differ from mature myocardium: whereas in adults, calcium ions are released from and removed to cytosolic compartment by *sarcoplasmic reticulum*, this sequestration in immature cardiac muscle is undeveloped; here Na/Ca exchanger, together with calcium influx across the sarcolemma play dominant roles (26–27). Muscle filaments of myocardium are build up from *contractile proteins*. There are two major contractile proteins: *actin and myosin* (about 70%) and several minor contractile proteins: *regulatory* (20%) and *modulatory proteins* (10%). The energy for contraction-relaxation is derived by *metabolic proteins*—enzymes of metabolic pathways—localized in different compartments of cardiac muscle.

There are characteristic structural changes of contractile proteins during ontogeny of myocardium. Myosin (localized in A zone of myofibrils) is composed from two monomers of heavy chains (HC); each one has two light chains (LC_1, LC_2). Their molecular weights are in order of 200 and 20 kDa (for HC and LC, respectively). The electrophoretic pattern of rat cardiac myosin has revealed three types of HC dimers (two homodimers: $\alpha - \alpha = V_1$ myosin HC isoform with highest ATPase activity, $\beta - \beta = V_3$ HC isoform with lowest ATPase activity and one HC heterodimer $\alpha - \beta$ = V2—medium ATPase activity). Embryonic or newborn rat myocardium has V_3 only, then, during early postnatal development, this isoenzyme of myosin slowly disappears and V_1 is stepwise synthesizes; around weaning period, when ATPase activity is maximal, reached 100%. On the other hand, cardiac myosin from ventricle of healthy adult rats has lower ATPase activity due to presence of V_3 isoform. However, V_1 is still dominant one in adult rat myocardium. Furthermore, structure of atrial myosin, its ATPase activity as well as mobility of rat atrial HC dimers are different. Moreover, ontogenetic changes of LC of cardiac muscle were detected in both atrial and ventricular musculature of different species; however, situation in human myocardium—both atrial and ventricular musculatures are still a matter of speculations (28–33).

Regulatory proteins (tropomyosin-troponin) of cardiac muscle of filaments (I zone) are responsible for both transducing the effect of calcium ions on the contractile machinery and modulation of molecular interactions between myosin and actin filaments; proteins of tropomyosin-troponin complex display multiple isoforms which are encoded by distinct genes. Their expression correlated with ATPase activity of myofibrilles. There are many factors which affected composition of regulatory proteins in cardiac muscle, however, ontogenetic development and phosphorylation states via protein kinases C or A could be taken into consideration. Much less is known about modulatory proteins; they both participate in fine structure of myofibrils and transfer chemical energy derived by metabolic to contractile proteins via proteins localized in M zones of cardiac filaments (34–38).

Moreover, structure of individual proteins of myofibrils is affected by the complex of *extracellular matrix* (ECM) *proteins.* This protein fraction of cardiac muscle is very heterogeneous: composed from arrays of different types of collagens, elastin, proteoglycans and glycoproteins; all items are decorated by sugar moiety—glycosaminoglycans. All these components (they occupied about two thirds of all cells of myocardium) serve a variety of functions important to tissue integrity, efficiency of muscular both systolic and diastolic pumps and, therefore, play also significant role in both contraction and relaxation phases of cardiac cycles. Developmental changes of ECM proteins during fetal cardiac development included formation of three-dimension collagen I and collagen III network; it could be detected in cardiac jelly at very early stages of embryonic development. Furthermore, changes of ECM proteins are predominantly characterized by remodelation of collagen I /collagen III ratio and/or by proportion of ECM proteins to the contractile proteins (39–43). Moreover, ECM proteins affected the deposition of individual contractile proteins either during perinatal development of myofilaments or during remodelation of cardiac muscle under different pathological situations (44).

b) Isolation of protein fractions from myocardium of children with congenital heart disease

Samples of cardiac tissue (right atrial -RA or right ventricular musculature -RV) were obtained during surgery of children with congenital heart disease; tissue were derived from both *normoxemic* (VSD, ASD—saturation of oxygen around 94%) and *hypoxemic patients* (Tetralogy of Fallot, saturation around 77%); they were rapidly transferred into precooled test tubes and frozen (−80°C). Later, they were thawed and treated with different buffers to isolated two fractions of *non-collagenous proteins* (metabolic and contractile proteins). After removal non-collagenous proteins, rest of tissue was used for isolation of two fractions of *collagenous proteins* (all extracellular matrix proteins); treatment was done by using pepsin in 0.5 M acetic acid (pepsin was held in ratio 1:10 −100 with proteins)—incubation under mild shaking 24 h at 4°C. Then supernatant was removed by centrifugation—fraction of *soluble collagenous proteins* (predominantly newly synthesized collagens) and pellet was solved in 1.1 mol/l NaOH and heated twice 10 min at 105°C; this procedure derived the fragments of *insoluble collagenous proteins*. Protein and hydroxyproline fraction were estimated in all four fractions; purity of each fraction was done by PAGE ELPHO (different concentration) and standards of molecular weight were used for determination of molecular weights of individual bands (45–46). Furthermore, for qualitative characterization of individual fractions—electrophoresis (for contractile and soluble collagenous proteins) and zymography (for metalloproteinase's) were used.

c) Protein profile of atrial and ventricular musculature in congenital heart disease; effect of hypoxemia

It was demonstrated that concentration of total protein of atrial and ventricular musculature in normoxemic patients is different; higher concentration was in atrial musculature. This atrio-ventricular difference disappears in hypoxemic patients (Figure 1).

The concentration of contractile proteins was significantly higher in RV. On the other hand, concentration total extracellular matrix proteins was higher in RA due to higher amount of insoluble collagenous proteins in RA (Table 1). Furthermore, concentration of both metabolic and pepsin-soluble collagenous proteins in normoxemic patients were neither different nor affected by hypoxemia. Moreover, hypoxemia induced remodelation of non-collagenous proteins (proportion of metabolic and contractile proteins was 1.88 versus 1.68, $p < 0.05$, for normoxemic and hypoxemic RA respectively, however, 1.51 versus 1.49, NS, for normoxemic and hypoxemic RV). Therefore, significant difference, therefore, was observed in fraction of non-collagenous protein of hypoxemic patients (Table 1).

d) Qualitative parameters of protein fractions; effect of hypoxemia

1) Characterization non-collagenous proteins

The concentration of metabolic proteins in both atrial and ventricular musculature does not differ (see Table 1). On the other hand, there are differences in *activities of metabolic enzymes of RA and RV* (Table 2) Whereas hexokinase (glucose phoshorylating enzyme) exhibits higher activity in RA, the other metabolic enzymes (typical for both glycolytic pathway and oxidative pathways in mitochondrial matrix) have higher activities in RV of children patients (Table 2). This result is in good agree-

Table 1. Protein composition of right atrial (RA) and right ventricular (RV) parts of myocardium in children with normoxemic and hypoxemic congenital heart disease. Concentration of proteins in different *non-collagenous* (total non-collagenous proteins are formed by metabolic and contractile proteins) and *total extracellular proteins* (total extracellular proteins are formed by proteins in pepsin soluble and pepsin insoluble fractions of collagenous proteins)

	Normoxemia		Hypoxemia	
Fraction	RA	RV	RA	RV
Metabolic	44.14 ± 1.82	42.08 ± 1.96	38.94 ± 2.08	40.21 ± 2.10
Contractile	23.42 ± 1.01	27.85 ± 1.90[a]	23.09 ± 1.80	26.86 ± 1.42[a]
Total non-collagenous	67.90 ± 1.94	70.11 ± 2.00	62.92 ± 1.58	67.41 ± 1.84[a]
Soluble-collagenous	16.21 ± 1.02	18.14 ± 1.31	16.52 ± 1.04	18.95 ± 1.21
Insoluble-collagenous	25.90 ± 2.82	12.40 ± 0.98[a]	20.98 ± 3.00	12.09 ± 0.96[a]
Total extracell. matrix	42.85 ± 1.99	31.45 ± 2.10[a]	38.11 ± 2.11	30.41 ± 2.30[a]

Data are given in mg/g wet weight as means ± S.E.M.
Significance: [a]$p < 0.05$ versus respective value of RA.

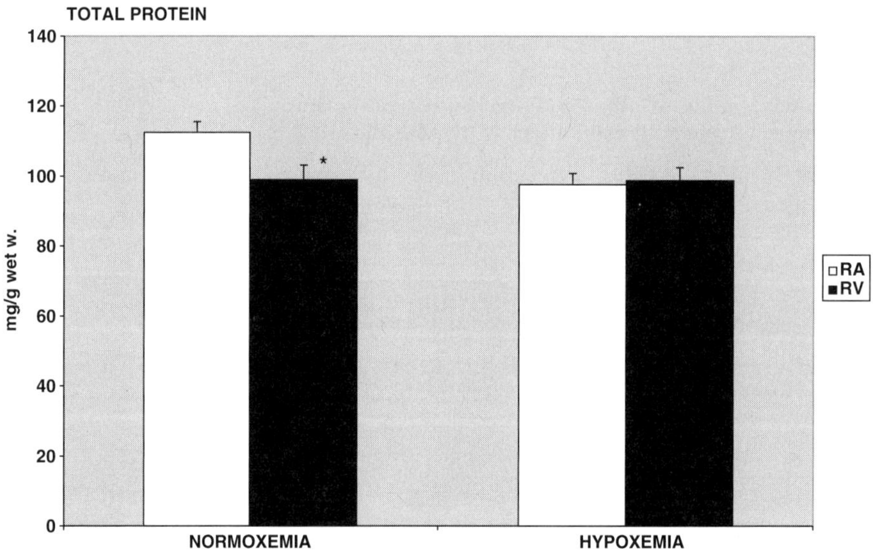

Figure 1. Concentration total protein in myocardium (right atrium—RA and right ventricle—RV) of normoxemic and hypoxemic patients with congenital heart disease.
Values are means ± S.E.M (expressed as mg per g of wet weight).
Significance *$p < 0.05$ versus RA.

ment with our observation that content of mitochondria (as judged from estimation of *cardiolipin*—typical phospholipid of mitochondrial membrane) is significantly higher in RV as compared with RA (Figure 2).

Hypoxemia lowered capacity of oxidative enzymes in both cardiac parts (citrate synthase—CS, malate dehydrogenase—MDH, 3-hydroxyacyl-CoA dehydrogenase-

Table 2. Activity of energy supplying enzymes in right atrial and right ventricular musculature of myocardium of children with congenital heart disease; short characteristics of individual enzymes

Enzymes	Atrium	Ventricle	Characteristics
HK	higher	lower	glukose metabolism
TPDH, GPDH	lower	higher	glycolytic enzymes
CS, MDH	lower	higher	Krebs cycle
HODH	lower	higher	fatty acids metabolism

HK —hexokinase (glycolytic enzyme).
TPDH, GPDH—triosephosphate dehydrogenase, glycerol-3 phosphate dehydrogenase (glycolytic enzymes).
CS, MDH —citrate synthase, malate dehydrogenase (enzymes of Krebs cycle).
HODH —hydroxyacyl coezym A dehydrogenase (degradation of fatty acid).

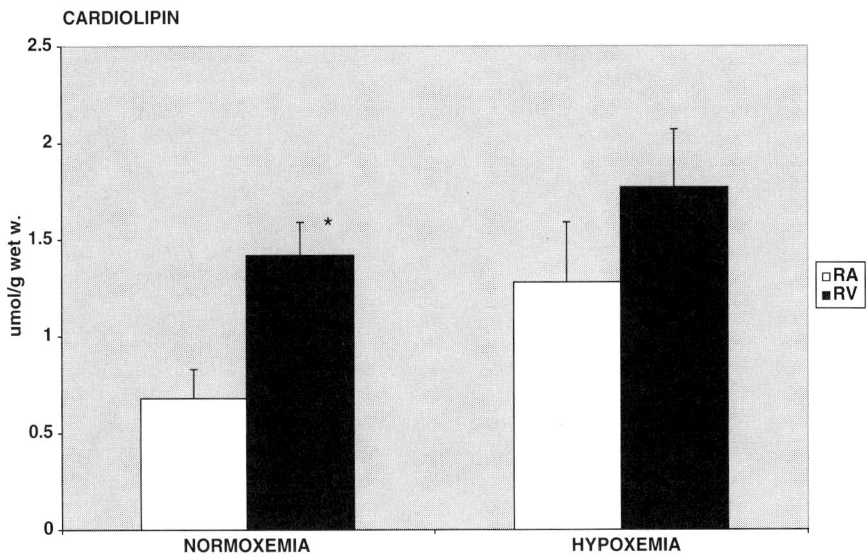

Figure 2. Concentration cardiolipin (typical phospholipids of mitochondrial membranes) in myocardium (right atrium—RA and right ventricle—RV) of normoxemic and hypoxemic patients with congenital heart disease.
Values are means ± S.E.M (expressed as μmol P_i per g of wet weight).
Significance *$p < 0.05$ versus RA.

HODH—enzyme typical for oxidation of fatty acids); the changes were more pronounced in RA of hypoxemic patients (where, in addition to Krebs cycle enzymes, activity of triosophoshate dehydrogenase—TPDH and glycerol-3-phosphate dehydrogenase- GPDH were significantly decreased (15,47). Furthermore, hypoxemia has tendency to elevate concentration of cardiolipin in both parts of cardiac muscle; however, this increase did not reach significant value. (Figure 2). It is, probably, a

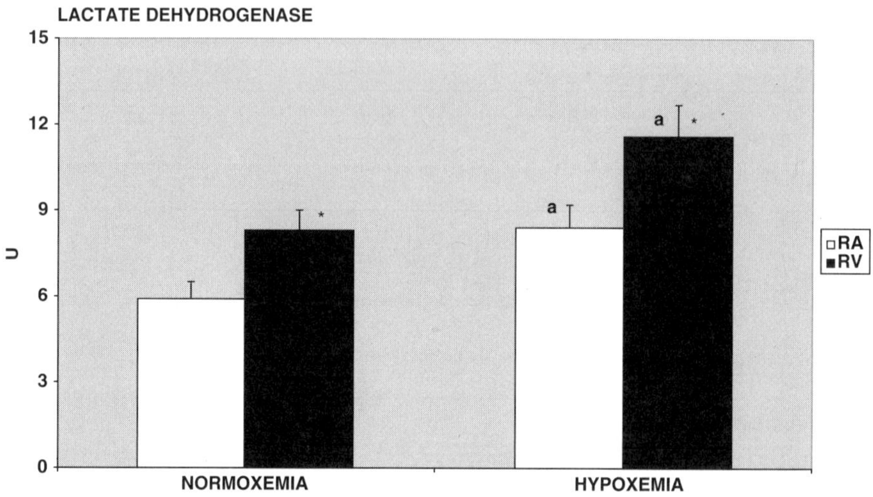

Figure 3. Activity of lactate dehydrogenase in myocardium (right atrium—RA and right ventricle—RV) of normoxemic and hypoxemic patients with congenital heart disease.
Values are means ± S.E.M (expressed as U per 50 mg of wet weight).
Significance *$p < 0.05$ versus RA.
[a]$p < 0.05$ versus respective value of normoxemia.

consequence of lowered activity of enzymes responsible for aerobic oxidation of substrate in hypoxemia. Moreover, the activity of *lactate dehydrogenase* (LDH)—enzyme responsible for proportion of pyruvate /lactate, is significantly higher in samples of RV (Figure 3). Hypoxemia elevated activity of this enzyme in both part of myocardium; atrio-ventricular difference, however, persisted.

This result is in good agreement with observation (48) that human pediatric cardiomyocytes, derived from ventricle of tissue biopsy specimens of pediatric patients (held in chronic hypoxia: P_{o2} = 40 mm Hg for 7 days—model to study the effect of cyanosis) have significantly higher both lactate production and lactate to pyruvate ratio. On the other hand, concentration of pyruvate and activities of both pyruvate dehydrogenase and mitochondrial membrane enzymes (responsible for oxidative phosphorylation) were in those patients significantly lower (48–49). Furthermore, newborns, who needed an operation for congenital heart disease within first month of life, had lowest both blood pH and blood base excess; they were in metabolic acidosis (50). Moreover, chronic hypoxia modulated nitric oxide formation via two types of nitric oxide synthases (NOS); however, inducible NOS activity was higher and endothelial NOS activity was reduced in samples of RA of cyanotic patients. It may represent an alternative mechanism to counteract the effect of hypoxemia in cardiovascular system (52–54) via the cyclic nucleotides (cGMP and cAMP).

Electrophoresis of contractile protein fraction—derived from both types of musculatures (data are not shown—see 17, 50) has reveal all items of contractile proteins: HC

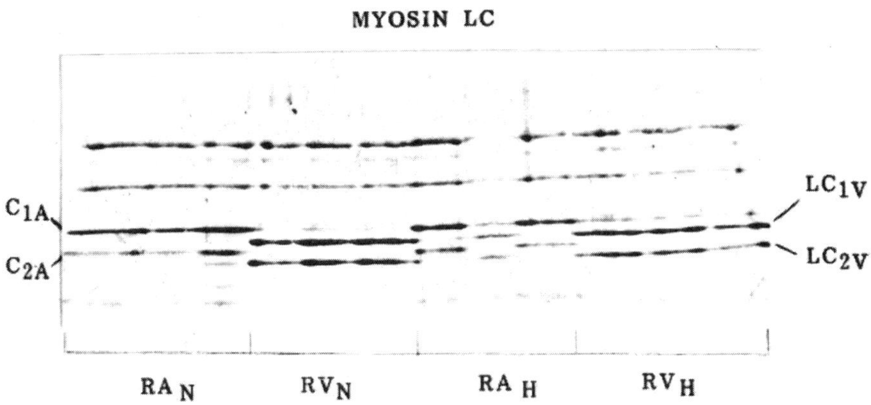

Figure 4. Electrophoretic profile of light chains (LC) of cardiac myosin (right atrium—RA and right ventricle—RV) of normoxemic (N) and hypoxemic patients (H) with congenital heart disease. Mobility of ventricle LC (LC_{1v} and LC_{2V}) were compared with mobility of atrial LC (C_{1A} and C_{2a})

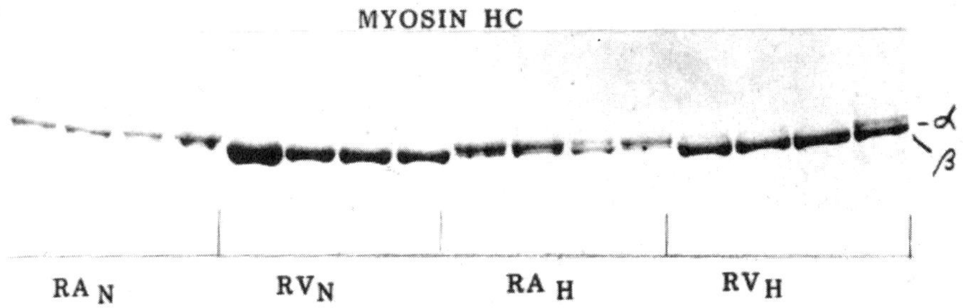

Figure 5. Electrophoretic profile of heavy chains (HC) of cardiac myosin (right atrium—RA and right ventricle—RV) of normoxemic (N) and hypoxemic patients (H) with congenital heart disease. Mobility of ventricle HC were compared with mobility of atrial HC (α, β).

and LC of myosin, actin, regulatory and modulatory proteins. Discontinuous electrophoresis was, however, not able to separate different isoform of HC as well as different LC of cardiac myosin from RA and RV. It was, therefore, a reason why these samples were analyze by another electrophoretic techniques (Figures 4, 5). *Electrophoretic pattern of LC* was not identical: mobility's of LC for atrial and ventricular myosin derived from children myocardium are different (Figure 4). Moreover, samples of ventricle myosin (beside LC_{1v} and LC_{2v}—ventricular myosin origin) were contaminated by atrial light chains (C_{1A} and C_{2A}—atrial myosin origin) and vice versa; higher amount of contamination was in samples derived from hypoxemic patients.

High molecular weight electrophoretic bands -*myosin HC* were separated by using of PAGE in sacharose gradient. There are different mobility of atrial and ventricu-

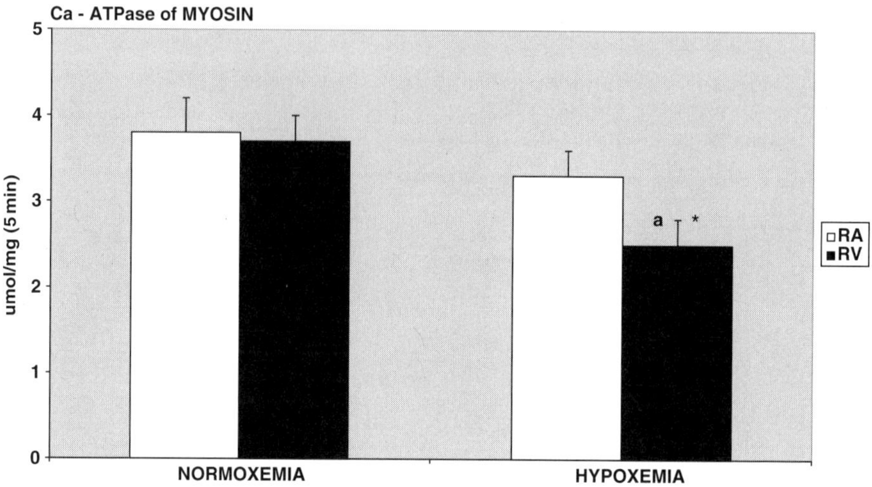

Figure 6. Activity of cardiac myosin Ca^{++}-ATPase activity (right atrium—RA and right ventricle—RV) of normoxemic and hypoxemic patients with congenital heart disease.
Values are means ± S.E.M (expressed as U per 50 mg of wet weight).
Significance *$p < 0.05$ versus RA.
[a]$p < 0.05$ versus normoxemic RV.

lar myosin HC: typical band for human atria is α chain, β chain of HC is typical for ventricle of human myocardium of children patients. Hypoxemia does not affect this dominancy, however, second weak band, however, appeared in both myosin (α and β for ventricle and atria, respectively).

Enzyme activity of cardiac myosin (Ca—ATPase) from RA and RV of normoxemic patients is not different (Figure 6). However, hypoxemia decreased this one in RV only and, therefore, atrio-ventricular difference appeared (Figure 6).

We are not able to correlate this finding with structural remodelation of LC and HC (Figures 4, 5). It is due to that the role of both HC and LC derived from myosin in neonates and infants suffering from congenital heart disease is still under questions: in the cases with pressure overloaded RA the amount of beta HC was found to be 1,6 times higher than in the cases with normal pressure. On the other hand, presence of ventricular LC in atria did not correlate with pressure or volume overload (50, 51); genes from myosin HC and LC are not expressed coordinately. It seems important to conserve during surgery interventions as much as possible samples of cardiac myosin for these structural and enzymatic analysis.

In recent years, there has been a trend towards earlier repair of congenital heart defects. Furthermore, it was concluded (18,22) that cardiac troponins are very specific markers of myocardial injury in pediatric cardiac surgery. For this purpose we did fractionation of tissue samples and then *intracellular compartmentation of troponin T* (Figure 7). The cytosolic pool of cTnT represents about 12.5%, the myofibrillar

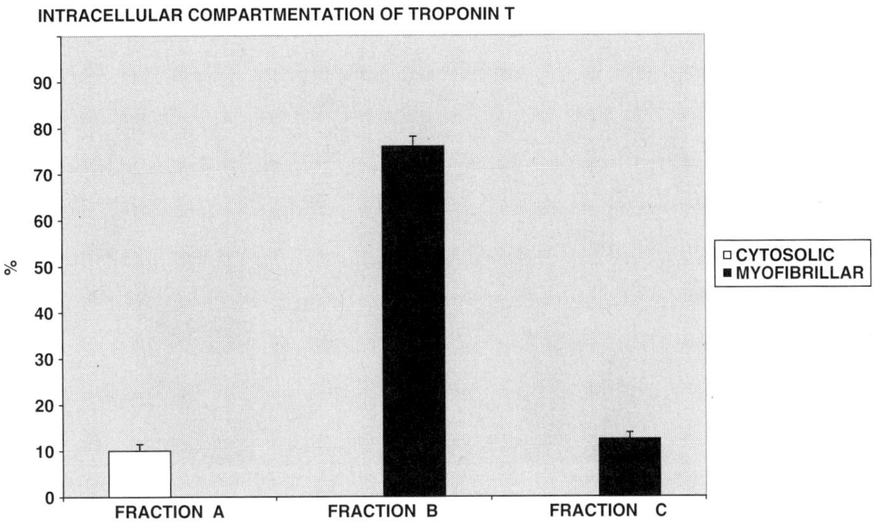

Figure 7. Intracellular compartmentation of cardiac troponin T (cTnT). Samples of cardiac tissue were treated with different buffers to isolate three fractions: A—cytosolic fraction (white column), B and C myofibrillar fractions (black columns); pool of cTnT was measured by commercial kit Elecsys Troponin T Immunoassay Roche (for details see (35) Adamcova and Pelouch, 2001).

pool was about 87.5%; hypoxemia did not affect this proportion. Moreover, this proportion in RV and RA was not significantly different.

2) Characterization of collagenous proteins

ECM cardiac proteins were characterized by estimation of either total amount of those proteins (see Table 1) or by concentration of hydroxyproline—a typical amino acid for collagen (Figure 8). Furthermore, the concentration of both protein and hydroxyproline in pepsin-soluble and pepsin-insoluble fractions of collagenous proteins were analyzed (Tables 1, 3). *Total amount of collagen* was higher in RA both normoxemic and hypoxemic patients; hypoxemia did not elevated total concentration of collagen in either parts of children myocardium (Figure 8).

Higher amount of collagen in RA was due to higher concentration of HYP in fraction of pepsin insoluble (highly maturated collagen) ECM proteins; it was not affected by hypoxemia (Table 3).

It was rather surprising that hypoxemia did not elevate total amount of cardiac collagen but only remodelated proportion HYP in both collagenous fractions. However, hypoxemia elevated concentration of HYP in pepsin-soluble fraction of collagenous proteins (newly formed collagen) in RA only. Concentration of HYP in pepsin-soluble collagenous proteins in RA of hypoxemic patients was about twice higher in comparison with that in RA of normoxemic patients (it represented 22% from total amount of HYP in RA_H—compare with 12% which is typical for RA_N).

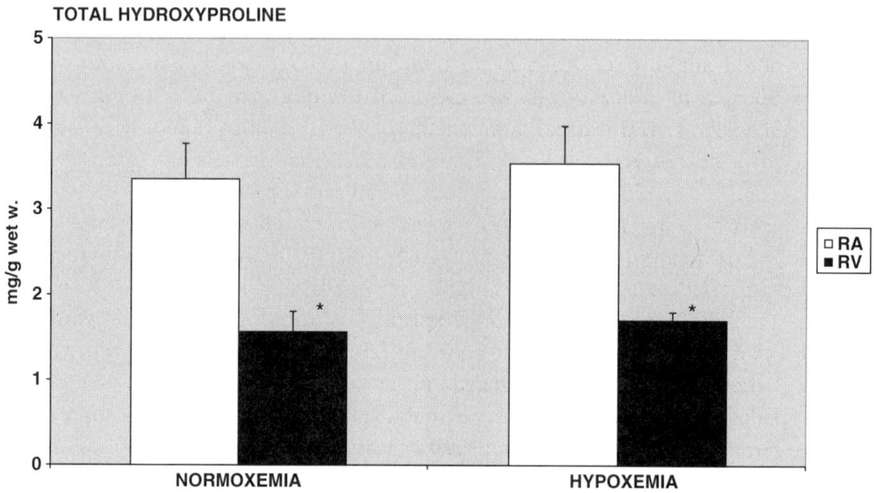

Figure 8. Concentration of total hydroxyproline (typical amino acid for collagen) in myocardium (right atrium—RA and right ventricle—RV) of normoxemic and hypoxemic patients with congenital heart disease.
Values are means ± S.E.M (expressed as mg per g of wet weight).
Significance *p < 0.05 versus RA.

Table 3. Concentration hydroxyproline in pepsin-soluble collagenous fraction (soluble-collagen.), pepsin-insoluble collagenous fraction (insoluble-collagen.) and total collagenous proteins of myocardium (right atrium-RA and right ventricle-RV) in normoxemic and hypoxemic patients with congenital heart disease. Values are means ± S.E.M (expressed as mg per g of wet weight)

	Normoxemia		Hypoxemia	
Fraction	RA	RV	RA	RV
Soluble-collagen.	0.43 ± 0.02	0.42 ± 0.03	0.79 ± 0.11	0.44 ± 0.02[a]
Insoluble-collagen.	3.16 ± 0.21	1.24 ± 0.21[a]	2.98 ± 0.31	1.23 ± 0.22[a]
Total collagenous	3.60 ± 0.24	1.66 ± 0.11[a]	3.77 ± 0.35	1.69 ± 0.16[a]

Significance [a]p < 0.05 or less versus RA in respective group.

On the other hand, about 25% from total amount occupied HYP in the same fraction of both RV_N and RV_H. It could be mentioned that, in rats after administration of nitrofen on day 9.5 of gestation (model for congenital heart disease), the fetuses have also significantly reduced expression of ECM proteins in cardiac muscle (49). We, therefore, concluded that *hypoxemia predominantly remodelate proportion of different fractions of cardiac collagen.* Furthermore, quantitative characteristic of ECM proteins resulted from both synthetic and degradative pathways; higher activity of metaloproteinases (enzymes responsible for degradation of ECM proteins) was in RA. Their activation was induced by hypoxemia, again predominantly in RA; however, the impulse for this elevation could be a smaller fragments of collagen found in eletrophoretic pattern of pepsin-soluble fraction of this proteins (data are not shown here—see, 17, 23).

PHOSPHOLIPIDS COMPOSITION OF ATRIAL AND VENTRICULAR MUSCULATURE

a) Isolation of phospholipids fractions from myocardium of children with congenital heart disease

Tissue samples, obtained during surgery of children with congenital hearts, were frozen (−80°C) and kept at this temperature until the next isolation. Later, they were thawed and both samples of RA and RV were pulverized and homogenized. Phospholipids (from about 100 mg wet tissue) were extracted in three steps according to the modified method of Folch et al. (55). The first extraction was performed in three portions (0.25 ml each) of the chloroform- methanol mixture (1:3, 2:1 and 2:1) in the precooled mortar. Subsequent extractions were performed in a mixture 2:1 (0.6 ml each) 0.9% NaCl in water (20% volume of extract) was added. After a vigorous shaking the lower lipid layer was dried at 40°C under a stream of nitrogen.

Individual *phospholipids classes* were separated by two dimensional thin layer chromatography (Silica Gel H-Merck as slurry of 22.5 g in 62 ml water containing 2.5 g of magnon-Merck was spread in 0.25 mm layer with a spreader—Desaga on glass plates (20 × 20 cm). Solvent mixtures were used according to the method of Rouser et al. (56). The *phospholipids spots* were visualized by iodine vapors, scraped out and analyzed for *phosphorus* (55,57); major components are phosphatidylcholine (PC) and phosphatidyldiethanolamine (PE), minor components are phosphatidylserine (PS) and phosphatidylinositol (PI). Furthermore, diphoshatidylglycerol (DPG—[cardiolipin] -major lipid of mitochondrial membranes) was detected as phospholipids spots as well (57).

b) Phospholipids profile of atrial and ventricular musculature in congenital heart disease; effect of hypoxemia

Quantitative difference of phospholipids was observed already in normoxemic patients (Figure 9). The lower concentration of total phospholipids was in RA. Neither elevation of phospholipids nor atrio-ventricular difference were affected by hypoxemia. Qualitative analysis have shown that about 70% from total composition in both cardiac parts is formed by PC and PE (40 and 30% respectively). This proportion of major phospholipids items was not affected by hypoxemia (58) in neither part of myocardium (Figure 9).

In this paper we summarized some of both our data and other available information dealing with protein and phospholipids composition of the structurally changes of myocardium in children suffer from congenital heart disease. It could be concluded that atrial and ventricular musculature have different qualitative and quantitative compositions of both *myofibrillar and extracellular matrix proteins.* Atrio-

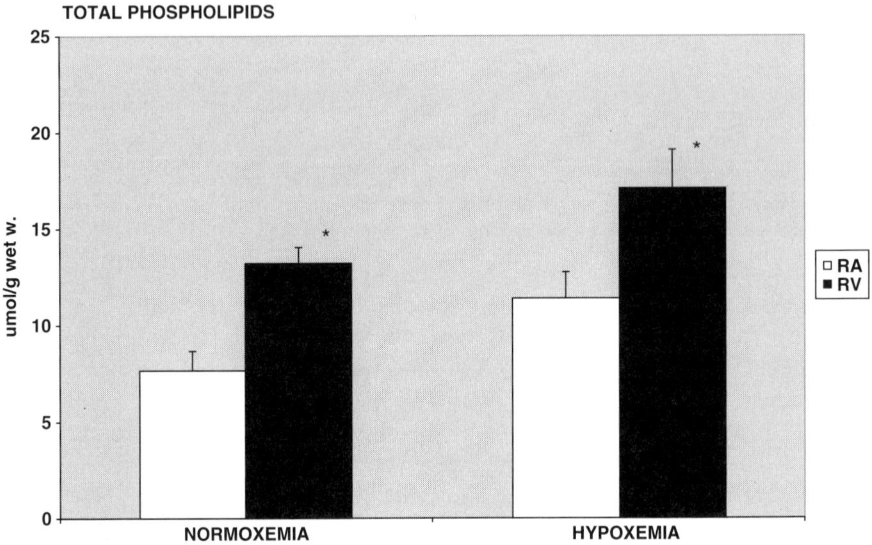

Figure 9. Concentration of total phospholipids in myocardium (right atrium—RA and right ventricle—RV) of normoxemic and hypoxemic patients with congenital heart disease.
Values are means ± S.E.M (expressed as μmol P_i per g of wet weight).
Significance *$p < 0.05$ versus RA (data from (58)).

ventricular differences were observed even in the level of phospholipids; however, proportion of major phospholipids did not differ. Moreover, qualitative and quantitative parameters of both proteins and phospholipids *were not dramatically affected by low blood oxygen saturation* in hypoxemic patients. Surgeons who are reconstructing cardiac anatomy should be aware that they are dealing: a) with biochemically abnormal tissue, b) they should respect atrio/ventricular differences, c) morphologically, biochemically and structurally affected tissue might be a one of reason explained the failures or late problems in children who had surgery for congenital heart disease

REFERENCES

1. Developmental Mechanisms of Heart Disease. Ed. Clark EB, Markwald RR, Takao A. 1995. Futura Publishing company, Inc. Armonk, New York 10504.
2. The Developing Heart. Ed. B Ošt'ádal, Nagano M, Takeda N, Dhalla NS. 1997. Lippincott-Raven Publishers, Philadelphia, PA 19106–3780.
3. Gittenberg-de Groot AC, Bartelings MM, Poelman RE. 1995. Overview: Cardiac Morphogenesis. In: Developmental Mechanisms of Heart Disease. Ed. Clark EB, Markwald RR, Takao A, 157–168.
4. Markwald RR. 1995. Overview: Formation and Early Morphogenesis of the Primary Heart Tube. In: Developmental Mechanisms of Heart Disease. Ed. Clark EB, Markwald RR, Takao A, 149–155.
5. Pexieder T, Blanc O, Pelouch V, Ošt'ádalová I, Milerová M, Ošt'ádal B. 1995. Late Fetal Development of Retinoic Acid-Induced Transposition of Great Arteries: *Morphology, Physiology, and Biochemistry.* In: Developmental Mechanisms of Heart Disease. Ed. Clark EB, Markwald RR, Takao A, 297–307.

6. Šamánek M. 1994. Boy: girl ratio in children born withdifferent forms of cardiac malformation: A population-based study. Pediatr Cardiol 15:53–57.
7. Morgan HF, Baker KM. 1991. Cardiac hypertrophy: mechanical, neural and endocrine dependence. Circulation 83:13–25.
8. Burn J. 1995. Overview: Heart malformation—the human model. In: Developmental mechanisms of heart disease. Mount Kisco. NY: Futura Publishing. Ed. Clark EB, Markward RR, Takao A, 489–504.
9. Škovranek J, Marek J, Povýšilová V. 1997. Prenatal Cardiology. Cs Pediat 52:332–338.
10. Hučín B. 1999. Outline of the history of Czech cardiac surgery. Extl Clin Cardiol 4:85–88.
11. Strauss AW, Johnson MC. 1996. The genetic basis of pediatric cardiovascular diseases. Seminars in Perinatology 20:564–576.
12. Olson EN, Srivastava D. 1996. Molecular pathways controlling heart development. Science 272:671–676.
13. Srivastava D, Olson EN. 2000. A genetic blueprint for cardiac development. Nature 407:221–226.
14. Payne RM, Johnson MC, Grant JW, Strauss AW. 1995. Toward a molecular understanding of congenital heart disease. Circulation 91:494–504.
15. Bass A, Šamánek M, Ošt'ádal B, Hučín B, Stejskalová M, Pelouch V. 1988. Differences between atrial and ventricular energy supplying enzymes in children. J Applied Cardiology 3:397–405.
16. Pelouch V, Milerová M, Oštádal B, Šamánek M, Hučín B. 1993. Protein profiling of human atrial and ventricular musculature: The effect of normoxaemia and hypoxaemia in congenital heart diseases. Physiol Res 42:235–242.
17. Pelouch V, Milerová M, Ošt'ádal B, Hučín B, Šamánek M. 1995. Differences between atrial and ventricular protein profiling in children with congenital heart disease. Mol Cell Biochem 147:43–49.
18. Adamcová M, Pelouch V. 1999. Isoforms of troponin in normal and diseased myocardium. Physiol Res 48:235–247.
19. Pelouch V, Dixon IMC, Golfman L, Beamish RE, Dhalla NS. 1994. Role of extracellular matrix proteins in heart function. Mol Cel Biochem 129:101–120.
20. Pexieder T, Blank O, Pelouch V, Oštádalova I, Milerová M, Oštádal B. Late fetal development of retinoid acid-induced transposition great arteries; morphology, physiology and biochemistry. In: Developmental mechanisms of heart disease. Mount Kisco. NY: Futura Publishing. Ed. Clark EB, Markward RR, Takao A, 297–308.
21. Pelouch V, Pexieder T, Milerová M, Ošt'ádal B, Šamánek M. 1997. Protein Remodeling of Malformed Human and Mouse Heart. In: The Developing Heart. Ed. Ošt'ádal B, Nagano M, Takeda A, Dhalla NS, 357–372.
22. Adamcova M, Pelouch V. 1999. Isolation of cardiac troponin T in human atrial and ventricular musculature Acta Medica 44:43–44.
23. Pelouch V, Milerová M, Hučín B, Škovránek J, Oštádal B. 2000. Biochemical composition of contractile and collagenous proteins of atrial and ventricular musculature: the effect of normoxemia and hypoxemia. Exptl Clin Cardiol 5:441.
24. Adamcová M, Pelouch V, Kukačka J. 2001. Regulatory proteins in cardiac muscle of children with congenital heart diseases. J Mol Cell Cardiol 33, A1.
25. Pelouch V, Milerova M, Škovránek J, Hučín B, Adamcová M. 2001. Protein profile of myocardium in children with congenital heart disease. J Mol Cell Cardiol 33:A92.
26. Černohorsky J, Kolař F, Pelouch V, Korecký B, Vetter R. 1998. Thyroid control of sarcolemmal Na/Ca -ATPase in developing rat heart. Am J Physiol 275:H264–H273.
27. Boerth SR, Coetzee WA, Artman M. 1995. Expression and Functional Activity of the Cardiac Sarcolemmal Na^+–Ca^{2+} Exchanger During Perinatal Development. In: Developmental Mechanisms of Heart Disease. Ed. Clark EB, Markwald RR, Takao A, 441–448.
28. Swynghedauw B. 1986. Developmental and functional adaptation of contractile proteins in cardiac and skeletal muscles. Physiol Rev 66:710–771.
29. Hoh JFY, McGrath PA, Hale PT. 1978. Electrophoretic analysis of multiple forms of rat cardiac myosin: effect of hypophysectomy and thyroxine replacement. J Mol Cell Cardiol 10:1053–1076.
30. Pelouch V. 1995. Molecular aspects of regulation of cardiac contraction. Physiol Res 44:53–60.
31. Bandman E. 1985. Myosin isoenzyme transitions in muscle development, maturation and disease. Int Rev Cytol 97:97–131.
32. Hirzel HO, Tuchschmid CR, Schneider J, Krayenbuehl HP, Schaub MC. 1985. Relationship between myosin isoenzyme composition, hemodynamics and myocardial structure in various forms of human cardiac hypertrophy. Circ Res 57:729–740.

33. Schaub MC, Hefti MA, Zuelling RA, Morano I. 1998. Modulation of contractility in human cardiac hypertrophy by myosin essential light chain isoforms. Cardiovasc Res 37:381–404.
34. Malhotra A. 1994. Role of regulatory proteins (troponin-tropomyosin) in pathological states. Mol Cell Biochem 135:43–50.
35. Adamcova M, Pelouch V. Regulatory protein of myocardium with congenital heart disease. Acta Medica, 44:13–17, Suppl., 2001.
36. Morano I, Hadicke K, Grom S, Koch A, Erdmann E, Krause E-G. 1994. Titin, myosin light chains in the developing and failing human heart. J Mol Cell Cardiol 26:261–368.
37. Sabry MA, Dhoot GK. 1989. Identification of and changes in the expression of troponin T isoforms in developing avian and mammalian heart. J Mol Cell Cardiol 21:85–91.
38. Solaro RJ. 1995. Troponin C-troponin I interactions and molecular signalling in cardiac myofilaments. Adv Exp Med Biol 382:109–115.
39. Borg TK, Nakagawa M, Carver W, Terracio L. 1995. Overview: Extracellular Matrix, Receptors, and Heart Development. In: Developmental Mechanisms of Heart Disease. Ed. Clark EB, Markwald RR, Takao A, 175–184.
40. Pelouch V, Dixon IMC, Golfman L, Beamish RE, Dhalla NS. 1993. Role of extracellular matrix proteins in heart function. Mol Cell Biochem 129:101–120.
41. Weber ET. 2001. Cardioreparation in hypertensive heart disease. Hypertension 38:588–591.
42. Bulew BS, Weber KT. 2000. Connective tissue and the heart. Functional significance and regulatory mechanisms. Cardiol Clin 18:435–42.
43. Lamparter S, Sun Y, Weber KT. 1999. Angiotensin II receptor blockade during gestation attenuates collagen formation in the developing rat heart. Cardiovasc Res 43:165–172.
44. Fisher SA, Periasamy M. 1994. Collagen synthesis inhibitors disrupt embryonic cardiocyte myofibrillogenesis and alter the expression of cardiac specific genes in vivo. J Mol Cell Cardiol 26: 721–731.
45. Pelouch V, Kolář F, Khuchua ZA, Elizarova GV, Milerová M, Oštádal B, Saks VA. 1996 A cardiac phoshocreatine deficiency induced by GPA during postnatal development in rat. Mol Cell Biochem 163/164:67–76.
46. Pelouch V, Kolář F, Milerová M, Ošt'ádal B. 1997. Effect of preweaning nutritional state on the cardiac protein profile and functional performance of the rat heart. Mol Cell Biochem 177:221–228.
47. Šamánek M, Bass A, Oštádal B, Hučín B, Stejskalová M. 1989. Effect of hypoxemia on enzymes supplying myocardial energy in children with congenital heart disease. Int J Cardiol 25:265–270.
48. Merante F, Mickle DAG, Weisel RD, LI R, Tumiati LC, RAo V, Williams WG, Robinson BH. 1998. Myocardial aerobic metabolism is impaired in a cell culture as a model of cyanotic heart disease. Am J Physiol 275:H 1673–H 1681.
49. Guarino N, Shima H, Puri P. 2001. Structural immaturity of heart in congenital diaphragmatic hernia in rats. J Pediatr Surg 36:770–773.
50. Verheijen PM, Lisowski LA, Stoutennbeek P, Hitchcock JF, Brenner JI, Copel JA, Kleinman CS, Meijboom EJ, Bennink GB. 2001. Prenatal diagnosis of congenital heart disease affects preoperative acidosis in the newborn patients. J Thorac Cardiovasc Surg 121:798–803.
51. Shi QW, Danilczyk U, Wang JX, See YP, Williams WG, Trusler GA, Beaulieu R, Rose V, Jackowki G. 1991. Expression of ventricular myosin subunits in atria of children with congenital heart disease. Circ Res 69:1601–1607.
52. Ferreiro CR, Chagas AC, Carvalho MH, Dantas AP, Jatene MB, Bento De Souza LC, Lemos Da Luz P. 2001. Infuence of hypoxia on nitric oxide synthase activity and gene expression in children with congenital heart disease: a novel pathophysiological adaptive mechanism. Circulation 103:2272–2276.
53. Šamánek M, Hučín B, Klenerová V, Hynie S. 1997. Effects of Hypoxia on Adenylyl Cyclase Activity in Developing Human Heart. In: The Developing Heart. Ed. Ošt'ádal B, Nagano M, Takeda A, Dhalla NS, 385–391.
54. Rimensberger PC, Sparh-Schopfer I, Berner M, Jaeggi E, Kalandros A, Friedli B, Bergetti M. 2001. Inhaled nitric oxide versus iloprost in secondary pulmonary hypertension in children with congenital heart disease: vasodilator capacity and cellular mechanism. Circulation 103:544–548.
55. Folch J, Lees M, Sloane-Stanlez GH. 1957. A simple method for isolation and purification of total lipids from animal tissue. J Biol Chem 226:497–509.
56. Rouser G, Flrischner SF, Yamamoto A. 1970. Two dimensional thin layer chromatographic separation of polar lipids and determination of phospholipids by phosphorus analysis of spots. Lipids 5:494–496.

57. Mrnka L, Novákova O, Pelouch V, Novák F. 1996. Phospholipids composition in the rat heart exposed to pressure overload from birth. Physiol Res 45:83–85.
58. Hamplova B, Pelouch V, Nováková O, Škovránek J, Hučin B, Novák F. 2003. Phospholipid composition of human myocardium in children with normoxemic and hypoxemic congenital heart disease. Physiol Res 52.

Frontiers in Cardiovascular Health, edited by
N.S. Dhalla, A. Chockalingam,
H.I. Berkowitz & P.K. Singal
Kluwer Academic Publishers, Boston, 2003

Human Atherosclerosis: New Participants?

Yu. A. Romanov,[1] E.L. Soboleva,[1] V.N. Smirnov,[1] and, A. Bobik[2]

[1] *Cardiology Research Center, Moscow, Russia*
[2] *Alfred Baker Medical Unit, Baker Medical Research Institute & Alfred Hospital, Melbourne, Australia*

Summary. Human atherosclerosis is multi-factorial disease involving several physiological and pathological mechanisms related to remodeling of vascular wall in response to various inflammatory, immune-autoimmune, hormonal, and other disturbances. In spite of such causal complexity, the list of cellular participants is limited to a few vascular and blood-borne cells. Here we demonstrate that human atherosclerosis, although chronic disease, causes same central response as does acute tissue injury, i.e. mobilization of bone marrow stem/progenitor cells into peripheral blood, gradual stem cell accumulation in the injury site followed by tissue remodeling. Driven by chemical signaling from inflammatory foci on vasculature lining, colony-forming units (CFUs) for hemopoietic lineages and pluripotent mesenchymal cells leave bone marrow and start to circulate in blood. A percentage of hemopoietic CFUs as well as of stromal CFUs become resident in aortic intima forming loci of ectopic hemopoiesis. On the other hand, stromal differentiation in vascular intima initiated by putative risk factors (including high LDL) results in fibrosis, formation of osteoid and chondroid matrices, calcification and appearance of osteoclasts and adipocytes. It is this sequence of events rather than migration and proliferation of smooth muscle cells form cellular basis of human atherosclerosis. From this point of view, human atherosclerosis is just natural cell therapy of vascular wall exerted via basic mechanism for tissue regeneration, i.e. mobilization of bone marrow stem/progenitor cells and their transport to injury location. Vascular stenosis is viewed as undesirable and unpredictable consequence of physiological cell therapy of vascular inflammation. The type of a particular plaque (fibrotic, ossified, adipocyte-rich, etc.) is determined by microenvironment where clonogenic bone marrow stem cell comes to.

Correspondence: Vladimir N. Smirnov, Director, Institute of Experimental Cardiology, National Cardiology Research Center, 3-rd Cherepkovskaya Str, 15-A, Moscow 121552, Russian Federation.

Key words: atherosclerosis, bone marrow, endothelium, colony-forming units, mesenchymal stem cells, extracellular matrix, hypercholesterolemia.

INTRODUCTION

It is now generally accepted that atherosclerosis is multi-factorial disease involving many physiological and pathological mechanisms. They include abnormalities in genes or interactions between apparently "normal" genes, variations in hemodynamic forces in different regions of vasculature, immune disturbances including autoimmune diseases, viral infections, etc, together with important risk-factors, such as hypercholesterolemia, arterial hypertension and diabetes (1–7). Because of this complexity, in particular, interactions between the different mechanisms and frequently involving the local environment (e.g. smoking), it has been difficult to identify any single factor/mechanism as being mostly responsible for the progression of atherosclerosis. Numerous hypotheses have been developed to explain why the disease develops in humans. As early as 1852, von Rokitansky suggested that the fibrin which deposits in injured areas of the vascular wall may be responsible for the formation of atherosclerotic lesions (8). In the middle of the 19th century Virchow indicated that the accumulation of lipids in the vascular intima promotes the proliferation of cells and the development of atherosclerosis (9). Subsequently, Anitschkov et al. (10) developed a cholesterol-induced model of atherosclerosis in rabbits. He defined atherosclerosis as a chronic disease characterized by the *primary* deposition of lipids in the arterial wall; *secondary* was reactive proliferation of connective tissue, resulting in the formation of sclerotic thickenings, or plaques. Subsequently, other hypotheses were developed, of which the most popular was that put forward by Ross (11,12). He implied that atherosclerosis is the result of injury to the endothelium and was accompanied by adhesion of platelets. Platelet activation on an endothelium-denuded subendothelial surface was followed by migration of monocytes into intima. Consequently, foam cells of macrophage origin develop, and there is migration and proliferation of smooth muscle cells (SMCs); a large extracellular matrix also develops resulting in tissue fibrosis. Unfortunately, studies utilizing human atherosclerotic and normal large arteries could not confirm the absence of endothelium in regions known to be susceptible to atherosclerosis; rather the endothelium always appeared intact (13–15). Ross than modified his hypothesis to include "endothelial injury" where, rather that implying endothelial cell (EC) denudation, a complex set of yet to be fully defined intracellular changes/abnormalities were proposed to occur in ECs, resulting in dysfunctional endothelium (16–19). The term "endothelial dysfunction" now includes any alterations in endothelial barrier function (20), disturbances in endothelium-dependent vascular tone regulation (21), changes in fibrinolytic activity (22), the activation of ECs by the immune system and proinflammatory cytokines, etc. (7,23,24). "Endothelial dysfunction" can alter vascular reactivity and contribute to vasospasm, the adhesion, transmigration and accumulation of cells of hematopoietic lineage in vascular intima, disturbances in proliferative and secretory ability of vascular SMCs, as well as changes in the ability of ECs to regenerate.

ATHEROSCLEROSIS: AN INFLAMMATORY DISEASE

Recently there has been a strong emphasis on understanding how inflammatory phenomena in the vascular wall contribute to the pathogenesis of atherosclerosis (25–28). Immune based vascular pathologies such as vasculitis, graft rejection and even ischemia-reperfusion injury exhibit features in common with atherosclerosis. The adhesion of circulating blood cells to the endothelium and their transmigration into subendothelial intima is an obligatory component of many acute and chronic inflammatory reactions and one of the earliest events of atherogenesis (27,29,30). An example of the physiological role of migrating blood-borne cells into the vascular wall and underlying tissues is the involvement of leukocytes in various defense mechanisms. Neutrophyls are the first to appear in response to a local infection/lesioned region to neutralize pathogen/pathogenic stimulus. Subsequently, lymphocytes invade the affected area providing a local immune response and stimulating immunity. Usually, the combined effects of a number of different cell types are required to remove a pathogen and facilitate reparation of injured tissue.

Blood-borne cells can also exert effects that may be detrimental to tissues, by altering the balance of important metabolic processes in vascular wall. Such "negative" effects within the vessel's intima is frequently the consequence of their high synthetic and secretory activity (31). Even when interacting with the endothelium, such blood-borne cells are already partly activated (32,33). Their final fate and functions are determined by vessel's microenvironment, by at least two factors: the extracellular matrix and the cocktail of cytokines produced by blood-borne cells themselves, the endothelium, and the smooth muscle cells.

ENDOTHELIAL ACTIVATION—PREREQUISITE FOR INITIATION OF ATHEROSCLEROSIS

Events that lead to atherosclerosis in the intima can only occur if the arterial wall possesses regions of functionally changed or activated ECs that express specific cell surface receptors necessary for the recruitment of inflammatory cells into the intima. That this occurs during the early stages of atherogenesis is supported by a number of studies demonstrating that various classes of cellular adhesion molecules (CAMs) expressed by endothelium can be localized to atherosclerosis-prone regions of vessels, in both animals with experimental atherosclerosis and in humans, using immunohistochemistry (34–37). Simultaneously, in the subendothelium, clusters of cells of hematopoietic origin (macrophages, lymphocytes) can be frequently observed. Such complexity makes it difficult to precisely determine the primary and most important change in EC properties necessary for atherogenesis. On the one hand, hematopoietic cells infiltrating the intima of an artery can induce CAM expression by endothelium, by secreting either proinflammatory cytokines and/or growth factors. On the other hand, the ability of these cells to enter subendothelial space is highly dependent of their migration through the endothelial barrier. It is most likely that an elevation in CAM expression by the endothelium in specific regions of vasculature is the primary event in the development of atherogenesis.

Viruses are among the many factor/systems that are able to both directly or indirectly affect the expression of various classes of CAMs by ECs and participate in the initiation of inflammatory changes in vascular wall. They include those of herpes virus family, such as the two most ubiquitous viruses in humans: herpes simplex type I virus (HSV-1) and cytomegalovirus (CMV) (38–41). Both viruses can infect ECs and SMCs to induce a number of vascular structural and functional changes. Infection by these viruses can be latent and followed by periods of reactivation. It is during periods of reactivation that complications may arise due to infection, including vascular complications, particularly in patients on immunosuppressive therapy. One of the mechanisms underlying the inflammatory reaction in HSV-1-infected ECs is the induction by this virus of P-selectin expression (38). Our studies (42) indicate that E-selectin also participates in initiating EC-leukocyte interaction. Consequently, peripheral blood leukocytes adhere avidly to HSV-1-infected ECs, even in the absence of other known additional stimuli (43). Leukocytes activated by contact with infected ECs secrete a cocktail of cytokines and interferons to further augment the progression of inflammation in the vascular wall (44).

To date the most prominent virus linked to the progression of atherosclerosis and transplant-atherosclerosis, where similar cellular mechanisms are operative, is the CMV (39–41). Like HSV-1, primary CMV infection of vascular wall or reactivation of latent virus are the triggers in the chain of pathological events that participate in atherosclerosis. The highest number of ECs and intimal SMCs possessing a viral genome or displaying signs of virus reactivation, occur in the areas where there is evidence for early stage developing atherosclerosis (45).

ENDOTHELIAL HETEROGENEITY—MORPHOLOGICAL BASIS OF ATHEROSCLEROSIS IN HUMANS

Morphological heterogeneity of endothelium in large vessels, defined by cell size, protein content and ploidy is one of the most pronounced features which differentiates the human endothelial lining from the endothelium of experimental animals (Figure 1A). Such EC heterogeneity was studied most intensively during the 1970's and 80's when it was thought to be relevant to atherogenesis. The elevation in proportion of giant multinucleated, so-called "variant" ECs, in arteries with atherosclerotic lesions, together with strong correlations with age of the human subjects, suggested a hitherto previously unknown morphological change in ECs that appeared fundamental to the genesis of atherosclerosis (46–49). Nevertheless, despite extensive studies of these cells, their metabolic profiles seems similar to other ECs and their precise role in atherosclerosis remains to be defined (50–52).

Another interesting and probably important characteristic of ECs in large human arteries is their ability to form clusters, composed of cells of similar size and shape (Figure 1B). The consistency, with which clusterized endothelium occurs in atherosclerosis-prone areas and zones surrounding already existing atherosclerotic plaques, supports the proposal that this form of heterogeneity is relevant in atherogenesis (53–55). It has been suggested that this clusterization of ECs may originate from the clonal growth of so-called "cambial" ECs which maintain a high prolifer-

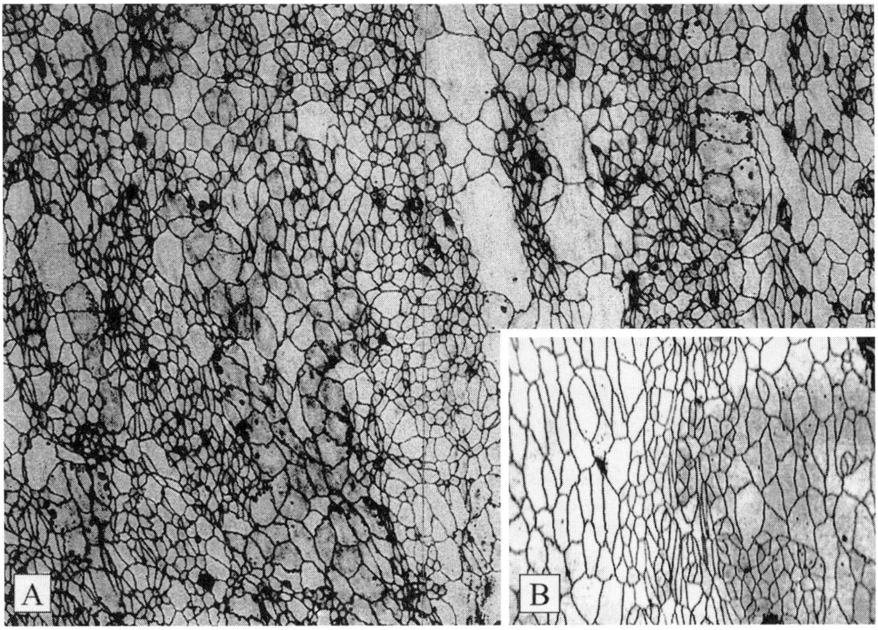

Figure 1. Morphological heterogeneity of the human vascular endothelium in situ.
A—Fragment ($2.4\,mm^2$) of endothelial lining in area without visible signs of atherosclerosis of adult human aorta. Silver nitrate staining; ×150.
B—Fragment of clustered endothelium formed by three neighboring distinct cell populations. Silver nitrate staining; ×400.

ative potential, although it is well known that the ability of the endothelium to regenerate decreases with age (55,56). In cell culture, these ECs are able to form discrete colonies and can be differentiated from other cell types by both morphological and functional parameters. For example, confluent clonal EC populations obtained from individual cambial cells can be differentiated on the basis of their ability to express E-selectin, ICAM-1 and VCAM-1 during exposure to cytokines (55). It is likely that such polymorphism exists in ECs of individual cell clusters in situ. If present, the vascular endothelium lining relatively large areas of arteries would consist of populations with varying levels of expression of proinflammatory parameters and differ in their capability to attract different populations of blood-borne mononuclear cells, i.e. initiate atherogenesis. The attraction of this proposal is that it can at least in part explain locality as well as predominant topography of atherosclerotic lesions in human vessels.

BONE MARROW ORIGIN OF HEMATOPOIETIC PROGENITORS IN INTIMA

The main source of hematopoietic and mesenchymal stem cells in vertebrates, including humans, is bone marrow (57 and ref.). Nevertheless, peripheral blood,

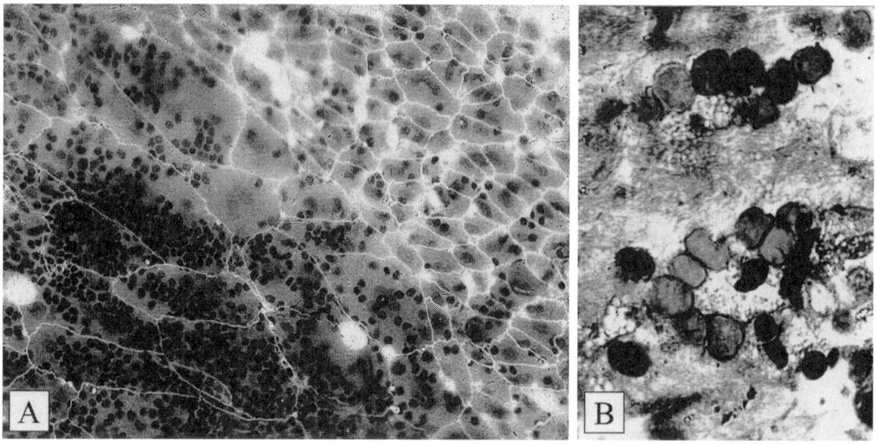

Figure 2. The composition of leukocyte infiltrates in human aortic intima.
A—Subendothelial clusters of blood-borne cells. Silver nitrate and propidium iodide double staining of the total intima preparation; ×800.
B—Cluster of low-differentiated blast-like mononuclear cells. Semi-thin section was made parallel to luminal surface of the vessel. Toluidine blue staining; ×1000.

even under normal physiological conditions, contains very low number of $CD34^+$ mononuclear cells (58). Hematopoietic stem cells (HPCs) can interact with the endothelium by mechanisms similar to those of mature leukocytes (59–61), and their interaction with activated endothelium in atherosclerosis-prone areas of vasculature can lead to their transmigration into the subendothelial space.

Our studies during the 1980's were the first to demonstrate the presence in human aortic intima of hematopoietic and stromal stem/progenitor cells of bone marrow origin (54,62–67), in addition to other commonly found cell types. Stromal stem cells were also found in the peripheral blood of patients with hyperlipidemia and coronary sclerosis (63,64,68).

An accumulation of lymphocyte-like cells can be frequently observed within a thin layer of lipid infiltrated subendothelial intima, as well as in non-involved zones (Figure 2A). Significant regions of these clusters are composed of blast-like cells which exhibit high nuclear area : cytoplasmic area ratio as well as uncondensed chromatin (Figure 2B). Some cells are in various stages of mitosis and differentiation (64,65).

The presence of HPCs in the intima can be confirmed using a variety of methods that include the detection of the HPC marker CD34 antigen, and by the ability of such cells to form hematopoietic colonies in semi-solid cultures (colony-forming units, CFUs). Our preliminary data (Soboleva E.L., unpublished observation) indicates that a significant number of CD34-positive cells can be isolated following mild enzymatic digestion of prefibrotic vascular intima lesions.

Evidence supporting the presence of low-differentiated cells of hematopoietic lineage in the intima includes the following: after placing into cell culture human

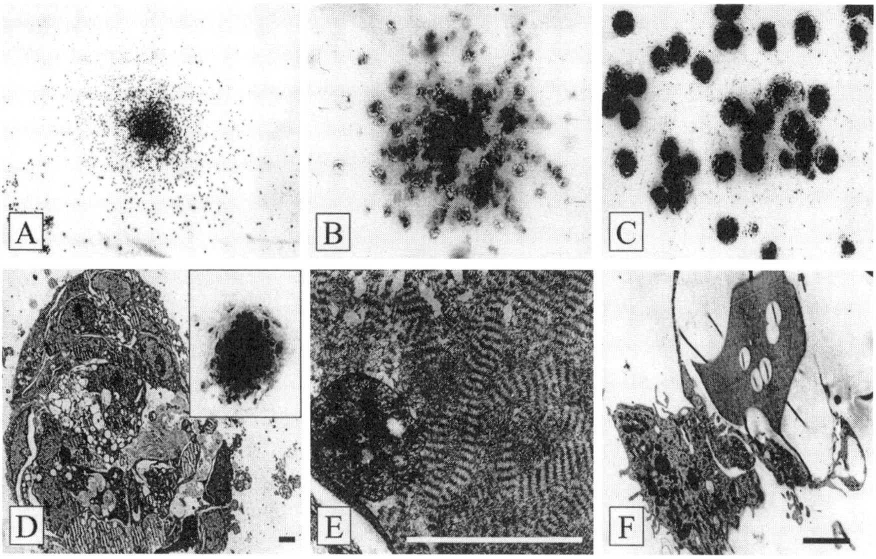

Figure 3. Hemopoietic and stromal colonies in culture of intimal cells from human aorta.
A—mixed granulocyte-macrophage colony. Giemsa staining; ×40;
B—monocyte-macrophage colony. Staining for nonspecific esterase; ×160;
C—basophyl/mast cell colony. Toluidine blue staining; ×400.
D—Stromal (dense) colony. TEM, bar equals to 2 μm. Insert, phase contrast, ×40.
E—Fragment of dense colony shown on D at higher magnification. Bar represents 2 μm.
F—bone-like extracellular matrix surrounded by osteoblast-like cell. Bar represents 2 μm.

aortic intimal cells from regions of arteries with differing levels of atherosclerosis severity, the presence of CFUs for various hematopoietic lineages can be clearly demonstrated. By several criteria including growth characteristics, morphology, ultrastructural features, activity of several enzymes plus a number of other characteristics, these cells were shown to be CFU-M (monocyte), CFU-GM (granulocyte/macrophage) and CFU-BM (basophyl/mast cell) (Figure 3). Greatest number of hematopoietic progenitors are present in early lipid intimal lesions. In the case of CFU-GM, frequency is 5.8 ± 2.1 per 10^5 nucleated cells, whereas it is 1.3 ± 0.3 and 0.078 ± 0.68 from non-lesioned areas and lipo-fibrous plaques, respectively. In contrast, cultures of intimal cells derived from fibrous plaques contain no such hematopoietic colonies (54,63–66).

The presence of HPCs in subendothelial intima may explain the paradox concerning observations on proliferating intimal cells in large human arteries. The increase in macrophage numbers is usually explained not only by migration of monocytes across the endothelium and differentiation to macrophages but also by their proliferation within intima (69–72). However, it is well known that monocytes and macrophages are cells in the terminal stages of differentiation of hematopoietic lineage and not capable of proliferation. The only feasible explanation is for the proliferating cells to be either stem, or progenitor, cells. Such cells also need to be considered when considering the role of SMC proliferation in the genesis of atherosclerotic plaque (see later).

Thus, current evidence indicates that HPCs not only migrate into vascular intima but also localize within the intimal micromilieu in regions where they can actively proliferate and differentiate. These processes within the intima are dependent on the presence of specific growth factors and the nature and characteristics of extracellular matrix (preferably, osteoid and/or calcified).

HEMATOPOIETIC MICROENVIRONMENT IN INTIMA

The microenvironmental condition within the intima must be favorable for HPCs to survive, replicate and differentiate. This is often realized in the human intima: a large variety of growth factors/cytokines required by HPCs can be produced by local resident cells, the ECs, SMCs and the generally smaller populations of blood-born cells within the intima, monocytes-macrophages and lymphocytes. Other cell participants can include pericytes and/or myofibroblasts, or bone marrow (CFU-F / stromal precursor cells / mesenchymal stem cells), supporting homing and local hematopoiesis by producing hematopoietic growth factors (73,74). As far as mesenchymal stem cells (MSCs) are concerned, it is known that under certain conditions they are also able, like HPCs, leave the bone marrow and circulate in blood (75–78). Being multipotential, MSCs possess the capability of differentiating into many cell types depending on the tissue they ultimately invade. The ability of bone marrow stromal cells (CFU-F) to differentiate in vitro into cell types of different tissues, e.g. fibroblasts, adipocytes, chondrocytes, and osteoblasts, rather than hematopoietic cells was first demonstrated more than 30 years ago (79–81). Later, it was shown that these cells could transdifferentiate into even more cell types, ECs and SMCs, hepatocytes, neurons, neuroglia, etc. (77,82–86). Whilst the physiological role of bone marrow pluripotential mesenchymal progenitors and the factors/mechanisms that enhance their ability to leave the "central depot" and circulate in peripheral blood are yet to be elucidated, there is a large body of data to supports the concept that mobilization of mesenchymal bone marrow stem cells may be a general mechanism for tissue regeneration or remodeling after injury (87–89). If true, this method of peripheral tissue reparation involving bone marrow MSCs should also apply to vascular wall regeneration and/or remodeling after injury.

As mentioned above, the increase in cell number within the vascular intima during the course of atherosclerosis progression cannot be explained by the proliferation of SMCs or their migration from media, as suggested by some investigators. The development of atherosclerotic plaques has now been shown not to be by associated with increase in the number of cells which possess the ultrastructural phenotype of SMCs (Figure 4); rather there is hypersecretion of extracellular matrix by the SMCs and possibly other cell types (90). There is however, a significant number of proliferating (PCNA-positive) fibroblast-like cells (myofibroblasts, "modified"

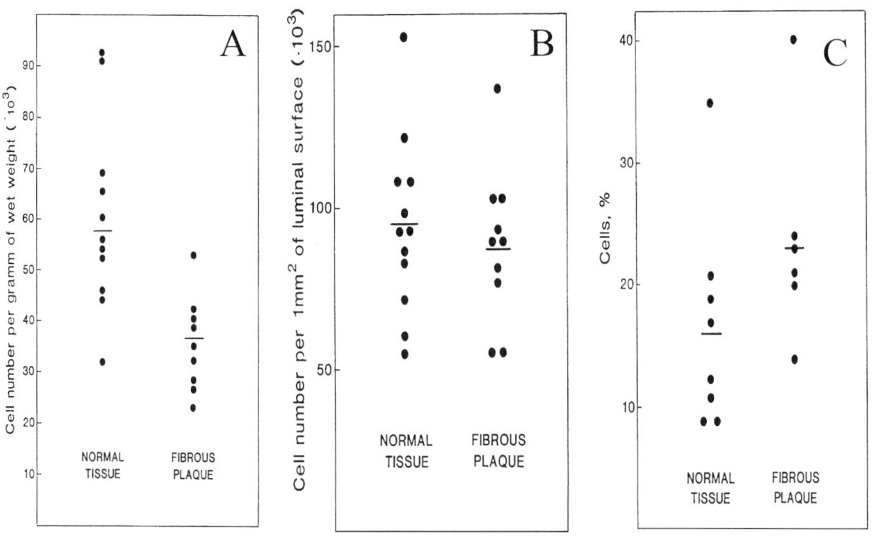

Figure 4. Smooth muscle cell content in normal intima *vs* fibrous atherosclerotic plaque of adult human aorta.
A—per unit of volume; B—per unit of luminal surface; C—proportion of synthetically active SMCs. Relative SMC content was determined after alkaline dissociation of the intima.

SMCs) in the intima that do not resemble well known SMC phenotype. These cells do not express markers characteristic of SMCs (70), further indicating that the increase in intima cellularity during the progression of atherosclerotic plaque is unlikely to be the consequence of SMC proliferation (71). The theory of "clonal" origin of cells forming atherosclerotic plaque also implies SMC proliferation (91,92), although their precise origin has not been demonstrated. Finally the lesion characteristics/structure, such differences in calcification, the presence of elements of bone, chondrocytic or fatty tissue cannot be explained by simply implicating the "classical" types of resident intimal cells. Our observations suggest that the origin of these cells lies outside vascular system.

There are now many studies that indicate that cells of bone marrow are critically important in the remodeling of various tissues under physiological and/or pathological conditions. For example, the development of transplant atherosclerosis (also referred to as chronic vascular rejection or graft vascular disease), is linked to repopulation of the vascular intima by recipient cells rather than being due to migration and proliferation of cells from the media of the donor (93–95). The observations by Quaini et al. indicate that in transplanted hearts, within few days after transplantation, a significant proportion of cells present are those from the recipient, though their origin was not established (96). Bone marrow derived endothelial precursor cells can actively participate in both reendothelialization of vascular grafts and revascularization of ischemic myocardium (97–101). It has been suggested that these processes might be significantly accelerated/enhanced by increasing progenitor cell content in peripheral blood (97,98,102).

On the basis of the above data, indicating that bone marrow MSCs participate in the reparation of many injured tissues, it is not unreasonable to hypothesize that these cells can also repopulate vascular intima in response of inflammation. In essence one would expect these cells to be present in detectable numbers among other cellular elements in the intima.

Using experimental approach, described above for intimal cells in semi-solid or "attached to glass" cultures, we demonstrated that, in addition to hematopoietic CFUs, low-differentiated progenitors of stromal lineage are also present in vascular intima (54,64,66). In cell culture, these progenitors form so-called "dense" colonies consisting of fibroblast-like cells that produce a collagenous and sometimes osteoid matrix (Figure 3 D-F). Because of their ability to proliferate and differentiate into stroma-forming cellular elements of chondroid and osseous tissues, MSCs can fulfill the role of cells, forming the bone-like microenvironment in vascular intima, there by providing second requirement necessary for proliferation of hematopoietic cells.

We have been unable to isolate or culture MSCs from peripheral blood of healthy donors (Table 1), probably due to the very low numbers of these cells in blood. Data by other studies are not unambiguous (57,75). It is possible that bone marrow mesenchymal cells enter the blood stream only during a brief yet to be defined period, largely in response to the presence of inflammatory foci or some other signal which initiates their participation in a tissue response (87,89,103). Also, the failure to culture such cells to date makes it difficult to rule out the existence in vascular wall of a certain number of reserved "resident" mesenchymal progenitors, as has been reported in other tissues (83,101,104). Further studies are clearly required to clarify these aspects.

HYPERCHOLESTEROLEMIA, BONE MARROW AND ATHEROSCLEROSIS

Hypercholesterolemia is unquestionably the most important of the known risk factors for atherosclerosis. The pathophysiological importance of hypercholesterolemia for atherosclerosis may be explained by the direct effect of high lipid concentrations, especially of modified and/or partially oxidized lipids, on the function of cells in the arterial wall, initially the endothelium. ECs respond to high lipid concentrations by making cardinal changes in their metabolic profile, resulting in proinflammatory activation. Subsequent well described events include the adhesion of specific blood-borne cells to the endothelium and migration into intima of blood cells, followed by formation of intimal infiltrates, etc. It is very likely that hypercholesterolemia is the factor that enhances the rate of tissue injury as well as its reparation by mechanism involving bone marrow mesenchymal cells.

Such an involvement is supported by measurements of MSCs numbers in the peripheral blood of patients with high plasma LDL levels (hypercholesterolemia IIa and IIb types) (66,68,105,106). When peripheral blood mononuclear cells from

Table 1. Stromal growth in agar seeded with blood mononuclears from donors and coronary patients with primary hyperlypoproneinemia IIa/IIb types

No	Patients/Donors			Ratio of stromal colonies to total number of colonies	Stromal colonies, per cent of total number of colonies
	Sex	Age	Type of HLP		
1	M	48	HLP II b	29/34	85
2	M	47	HLP II b	9/12	75
3	F	43	HLP II b	18/25	72
4	F	53	HLP II a	34/77	44
5	F	37	HLP II b	52/67	78
6	F	43	HLP II b	44/69	64
7	M	45	HLP II b	58/75	77
8	M	41	HLP II b	40/54	74
9	M	46	HLP II b	17/34	50
10	F	16	HLP II b	31/33	91
11	F	42	HLP II a	11/18	61
12	F	52	HLP II a	12/20	60
13	F	54	HLP II b	7/11	64
14	F	42	HLP II a	4/5	80
15	M	49	HLP II a	14/20	72
16	M	36	HLP II a	9/13	70
17	F	16	HLP II b	6/11	55
18	F	6	HLP II a	21/49	43
19	F	30	HLP II a	13/34	38
20	F	30	HLP II b	12/72	17
21	M	30	Donor	0/39	0
22	F	28	Donor	0/48	0
23	M	29	Donor	0/43	0
24	M	26	Donor	0/46	0
25	F	32	Donor	0/73	0
26	M	45	Donor	0/14	0
27	M	33	Donor	0/28	0
28	F	36	Donor	0/26	0

	Patients:	Donors:
Total cholesterol (mM/L)	7.2–18.9	<6.2
CH LDL (mM/L)	4.9–9.8	<4.1
CH HDL (mM/L)	0.7–0.9	1.05–1.86
Triglycerides (mM/L)	2.0–6.6	<2.0

patients with high plasma LDL or a suspension of intimal cells are grown in culture, we find a high frequency of stromal colonies when compared to cultures from healthy donors with normal plasma LDL levels (Table 1). Such colonies contain fibroblast-like cells surrounded by extracellular matrix with different levels of structural organization, osteoblast forming bone-like lamellas, osteoclasts (Figure 5), and cells with phenotype of myofibroblasts, adipocytes and endothelial cells (66). An essentially similar situation is likely to occur in a variety of pathological conditions caused by cytotoxic agent accumulation in the circulation components and characterized by peripheral lesions, for example, in diabetes.

Simultaneously, the response to hypercholesterolemia may not be limited to effect in the arterial wall. Hypercholesterolemia may also affect other tissues, for example,

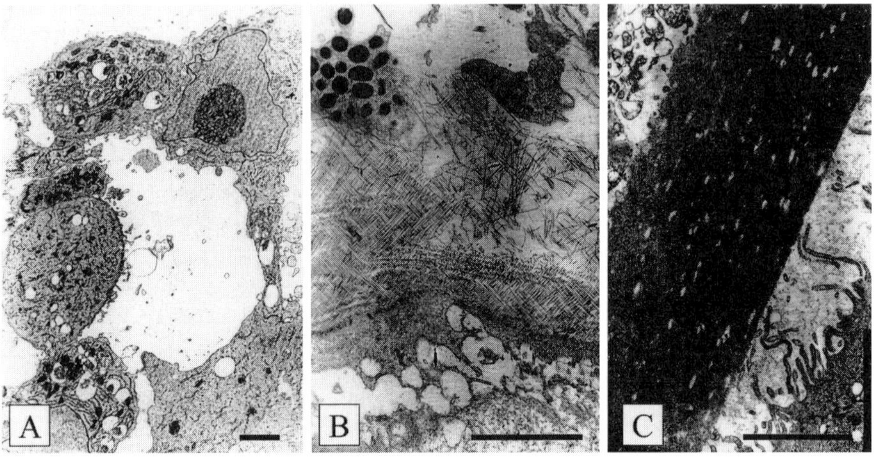

Figure 5. TEM-fragments of stromal colonies in culture of PBMC from the blood of patients with hypercholesterolemia IIA/IIB types.
A—fibroblast-like cells with immature irregular reticular matrix;
B—fibrillar extracellular matrix;
C—osteoid matrix with bone lamella in the middle and fragment of osteoclast with numerous processes of plasma membrane. Bars represent 2 μm.

the bone marrow itself, which is rich in blood vessels. Under such conditions injury to the bone marrow can be direct as well as indirect, the consequence of direct cytotoxicity by high concentrations of LDLs and their derivatives, and injury of the bone marrow's microvasculature and impairing its function. This is supported by recent studies on bone marrow biopsy specimens taken from patients with familial hypercholesterolemia and coronary sclerosis (105,106) where the aplasia of myeloid tissue and focal sclerosis of various degrees was readily demonstrated (Figure 6).

Although bone marrow may be irreversibly changed by such mechanisms, the individual still needs blood cells and the processes important for tissue regeneration still require large number of mesenchymal progenitor cells. Hence, the question arises: where are these cells produced, besides bone marrow? Can the ectopic hematopoiesis mechanism which functions so reliably in embryogenesis contribute under such conditions? If the answer is yes, then the question becomes where? The vascular wall could theoretically fulfill such a need. Formation of intimal micromilieu for hematopoiesis is provided by circulating MSCs which are able to enter vascular intima. The luminal vascular surface area is enormous (in adults about 70 m^2). Also, the mass of ECs, one of the putative candidates capable of supporting hematopoiesis is more than 1 kg (107). To enter the blood stream cells generated via vascular hematopoiesis only need to migrate across the thin endothelial barrier. Under these conditions, the foci of ectopic hematopoiesis located in the large and peripheral vessels may only provide a rather limited assistance to the impaired bone marrow because of the absence of the lacunas present in bone marrow. This is at

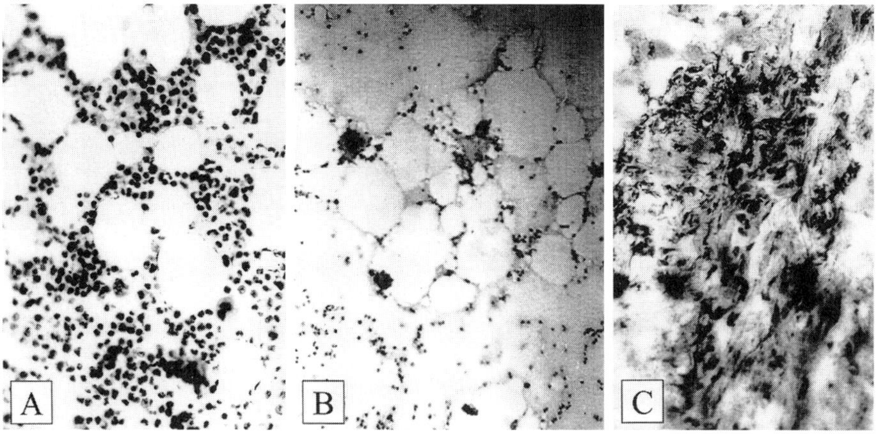

Figure 6. The morphology of bone marrow in healthy donors and patients with familial hypercholesterolemia IIa/IIb-type.
A—"normal" bone marrow (sternal punction biopsy) with an approximately equal fat-myeloid tissue ratio and high cellularity;
B—hypoplastic "empty" bone marrow with prevalence of fatty tissue;
C—foci of fibroblast-like cells surrounded by fibrous tissue. Giemsa staining; ×400.

least in part compensated for by the growth of new capillaries from the adventitial side of the vessels (108,109). It is through such newly formed capillaries that the cellular elements might "quietly" leave the vessel wall and move into the slow general capillary circulation. Because remodeling of the vascular wall occurs much more slowly than the proliferation of hematopoietic progenitors, the size of plaques can exceed a "critical mass". Then the thin fibrous cap can be ruptured by the enormous and persistent mechanical forces of flowing blood, leading to the unfortunate and well known effects of tissue infarction.

CONCLUDING REMARKS

The sequence of the events described above is probably a relatively frequent occurrence. It is likely that bone marrow participates not only in formation of so-called "complex" atherosclerotic plaques, which are mostly responsible for myocardial infarction and stroke, but is also involved in reparation of affected tissues, such as the heart and brain. In other words, both the remodeling of infarcted tissue and neovascularization of injured tissue requires the direct participation of circulating bone marrow progenitor cells (110). Can one utilize this reparative ability of bone marrow therapeutically to treat tissues detrimentally affected by ruptured lesions, if not to prevent atherosclerosis? A number of investigators have now commenced to address this question (97–100,111,112). The results obtained thus far in experimental animal model systems, together with some clinical observations suggest that bone marrow is likely to be useful to treat detrimentally affected cardiac and brain tissue.

ACKNOWLEDGEMENTS

This publication is the part of collaborative effort in cardiology between Russian Federation and Australia supported by their respective Ministry's of Health.

REFERENCES

1. Wick J, Perschinka H, Millonig G. 2001. Atherosclerosis as an autoimmune disease: an update. Trends Immunol, 22:665–669.
2. Najemnick C, Sinzinger H, Kritz H. 1999. Endothelial dysfunction, atherosclerosis and diabetes. Acta Med Austriaca, 26:148–153.
3. Landmesser U, Hornig B, Drexler H. 2000. Endothelial dysfunction in hypercholesterolemia: mechanisms, pathophysiological importance, and therapeutic interventions. Semin Thromb Hemost, 26:529–537.
4. Benitez RM. 1999. Atherosclerosis: an infectious disease? Hosp Pract, 34:79–82, 85–86.
5. LaRosa JC. 1998. Atherogenesis and its relationship to coronary risk factors. Clin Cornerstone, 1:3–14.
6. Gimbrone MA Jr. 1999. Endothelial dysfunction, hemodynamic forces, and atherosclerosis. Thromb Haemostas, 82:722–726.
7. Libbi P, Hansson GK. 1991. Involvement of immune system in human atherogenesis: current knowledge and unanswered questions. Lab Invest, 64:5–15.
8. Rokitansky K. 1855. The organs of circulation. In: A manual of pathological anatomy, Blanchard & Lea, Philadelphia, pp. 201–208.
9. Virchow R. 1858. Cellular pathology, John Churchill, London.
10. Anitschkov N. 1913. Uber die veranderungen der kaninchenaorta bei experimenteller cholesterinsteatose. Beitr Pathol Anat Allgem Pathol, 56:379–405.
11. Ross R, Glomset JA. 1976. The pathogenesis of atherosclerosis. N Engl J Med, 295:469–377.
12. Ross R. 1986. The pathogenesis of atherosclerosis: an update. N Engl J Med, 314:488–500.
13. Schwenke DC, Carew TE. 1989. Initiation of atherosclerotic lesions in cholesterol-fed rabbits: I. Focal increases in arterial LDL precede development of fatty streak lesion. Arteriosclerosis, 9:895–907.
14. Witztum JL. 1990. The role of monocytes and oxidized LDL in atherosclerosis. Atherosclerosis Reviews, 21:59–69.
15. Simionescu N, Simionescu M. 1993. Proatherosclerotic events: pathobiochemical changes occurring in the arterial wall before monocyte migration. FASEB J, 7:1359–1366.
16. Ross R. 1992. Endothelial dysfunction and atherosclerosis. In: Endothelial cell dysfunction (Simionescu N, Simionescu M, Eds.), Plenum Press, NY, pp. 295–307.
17. Gimbrone MA Jr, Topper JN, Nagel T, Anderson KR, Garcia-Cardena G. 2000. Endothelial dysfunction, hemodynamic forces, and atherogenesis. Ann NY Acad Sci, 902:230–240.
18. Toborek M, Kaiser S. 1999. Endothelial cell functions. Relation to atherogenesis. Basic Res Cardiol, 94:295–314.
19. Shimokawa H. 1999. Primary endothelial dysfunction: Atherosclerosis. J Mol Cell Cardiol, 31:23–37.
20. Lum H, Malik AB. 1994. Regulation of vascular endothelial barrier function. Amer J Physiol, 267:L223–L241.
21. Vanhoutte PM, Mombouli JV. 1996. Vascular endothelium: vasoactive mediators. Progr Cardiovasc Dis, 39:229–238.
22. Mann KG. 1997. Thrombosis: theoretical considerations. Amer J Clin Nutr, 65 (suppl. 5): 1657S–1664S.
23. Hill GE, Whitten CW. 1997. The role of the vascular endothelium in inflammatory syndromes, atherogenesis, and the propagation of disease. J Cardiothorac Vasc Anesth, 11:316–321.
24. Gown AM, Tsukada T, Ross R. 1986. Human atherosclerosis. II. Immunocytochemical analysis of the cellular composition of human atherosclerotic lesions. Amer J Pathol, 125:191–207.
25. Plutzky J. 2001. Inflammatory pathways in atherosclerosis and acute coronary syndromes. Amer J Cardiol, 88:10K–15K.
26. Koenig W. 2001. Inflammation and coronary heart disease: an overview. Cardiol Rev, 9:31–35.
27. Ross R. 1999. Atherosclerosis: an inflammatory disease. N Engl J Med, 340:115–126.
28. Robbie L, LibbY P. 2001. Inflammation and atherothrombosis. Ann NY Acad Sci, 947:167–180.

29. Faggiotto A, Ross R, Harker L. 1984. Studies of hypercholesterolemia in the nonhuman primate. I. Changes that lead to fatty streak formation. Arteriosclerosis, 4:323–340.
30. Munro JM, Cotran RS. 1988. The pathogenesis of atherosclerosis: Atherogenesis and inflammation. Lab Invest, 58:249–261.
31. Cassatella MA. 1995. The production of cytokines by polymorphonuclear neutrophyls. Immunol Today, 16:21–33.
32. Zimmerman GA, Prescott SM, McIntyre TM. 1992. Endothelial cell interaction with granulocytes: tethering and signaling molecules. Immunol Today, 13:93–100.
33. Lorant DE, Patel KD, McIntyre TM, McEver RP, Prescott SM, Zimmerman GA. 1991. Coexpression of GMP-140 and PAF by endothelium stimulated by histamine or thrombin: a juxtacrine system for adhesion and activation of neutrophyls. J Cell Biol, 115:223–234.
34. Cybulsky MI, Gimbrone MA Jr. 1991. Endothelial expression of mononuclear leukocyte adhesion molecule during atherogenesis. Science, 251:788–791.
35. Poston RN, Haskard DO, Coucher JR, Gall NP, Johnson-Tidey RR. 1992. Expression of intercellular adhesion molecule-1 in atherosclerotic plaque. Amer J Pathol, 140:665–673.
36. O'Brien KD, Allen MD, McDonald TO, Chait A, Harlan JM, Fishbein D, McCarty J, Ferguson M, Hudkins K, Benjamin CD, Lobb R, Alpers CE. 1993. Vascular cell adhesion molecule-1 is expressed in human coronary atherosclerotic plaques. Implication for the mode of progression of advanced coronary atherosclerosis. J Clin Invest, 92:945–951.
37. Wood KM, Cadogan MD, Ramshaw AL, Parums DV. 1993. The distribution of adhesion molecules in human atherosclerosis. Histopathology, 22:437–444.
38. Hajjar DP. 1991. Viral pathogenesis of atherosclerosis. Impact of molecular mimicry and viral genes. Amer J Pathol, 139:1195–1211.
39. Persoons MCJ, Daemen MJAP, Bruning JH, Bruggeman CA. 1994. Active cytomegalovirus infection of arterial smooth muscle cells in immunocompromised rats. A clue to herpesvirus-associated atherogenesis. Circ Res, 75:214–220.
40. Melnick JL, Adam E, Debakey ME. 1993. Cytomegalovirus and atherosclerosis. Eur Heart J, 14:30–38.
41. Childs B, Emanuel D. 1993. Cytomegalovirus infection and compromise. Exp Hematol, 21: 198–200.
42. Scheglovitova ON, Romanov YuA, Maksianina EV, Kabaeva NV. 2001. Herpes simplex type I virus infection of cultured human vascular endothelial cells: expression of cell adhesion molecules and induction of interferon and cytokine production by blood mononuclear cells. Russian J Immunol, 6:367–376.
43. Bevilacqua MP. 1993. Endothelial-leukocyte adhesion molecules. Annu Rev Immunol, 11:767–804.
44. Scheglovitova ON, Romanov YuA, Maksianina EV, Svintsitskaya VA, Pronin AG. 2002. Herpes simplex type I virus infected human vascular endothelial cells induce the production of anti-viral and proinflammatory factors by peripheral blood leukocytes in vitro. Russian J Immunol, in press.
45. Pampou SYu, Gnedoy SN, Bystrevskaya VB, Smirnov VN, Chazov EI, Melnick JL, DeBakey ME. 2000. Cytomegalovirus genome and the immediate-early antigen in cells of different layers of human aorta. Virchows Arch, 436:539–552.
46. Antonov AS, Nikolaeva MA, Klueva TS, Romanov YuA, Babaev VR, Bystrevskaya VB, Perov NA, Repin VS, Smirnov VN. 1986. Primary culture of endothelial cells from atherosclerotic human aorta. I. Identification, morphological and ultrastructural characteristics of two endothelial subpopulations. Atherosclerosis, 59:1–19.
47. Tokunaga O, Fan J, Watanabe T. 1989. Atherosclerosis- and age-related multinucleated variant endothelial cells in primary culture from human aorta. Amer J Pathol, 135:967–976.
48. Smirnov VN, Repin VS, Tkachuk VA, Chazov EI. 1988. Vascular endothelium in atherosclerosis a multidisciplinary approach. In: Endothelial cells (Ryan US, Ed.) 3:139–215.
49. Watanabe T, Tokunaga O. 1990. Multinucleated variant endothelial cell. Its characteristics and relation to atherosclerosis. Ann NY Acad Sci, 598:217–222.
50. Wu L, Satoh T, Tokunaga O. 1999. Formation of multinucleated variant endothelial cells in vitro and investigation of MVECs' features. Fukuoka Igaku Zasshi, 90:377–391.
51. Satoh T, Sasatomi E, Yamasaki F, Ishida H, Wu L, Tokunaga O. 1998. Multinucleated variant endothelial cells (MVECs) of human aorta: expression of tumor suppressor gene p53 and relation to atherosclerosis and aging. Endothelium, 6:123–132.
52. Tokunaga O, Satoh T, Yamasaki F, Wu L. 1998. Multinucleated variant endothelial cells (MVECs) in human aorta: chromosomal aneuploidy and elevated uptake of LDL. Semin Thromb Hemost, 24:279–284.

53. Romanov YuA, Antonov AS. 1991. Morphological and functional features of human aortic endothelium. I. Two variants of endothelial organization in atherosclerosis. Cytologiya, 33:7–15 (in Russian).
54. Romanov YuA, Balyasnikova IV, Bystrevskaya VB, Byzova TV, Ilyinskaya OP, Krushinsky AV, Latsis RV, Soboleva EL, Tararak EM, Smirnov VN. 1995. Endothelial heterogeneity and intimal blood-borne cells. Relation to human atherosclerosis. Ann NY Acad Sci, 748:12–37.
55. Romanov YuA, Khodakova TG, Kabaeva NV, Dormeneva EV, Pronin AG. 1999. Clustering of human aortic endothelium: possible involvement in atherogenesis. Angiol Vasc Surg, 5 (suppl): 166–180.
56. Romanov YuA, Kabaeva NV, Dormeneva EV. 1998. Morphological and functional features of human aortic endothelium. III. Growth in culture and formation of colonies at low seeding density. Cytologiya, 40:127–132 (in Russian).
57. Huss R. 2000. Isolation of primary and immortalized CD34-hematopoietic and mesenchymal stem cells from various sources. Stem Cells, 18:1–9.
58. Bender JG, Unverzagt K, Walker DE, Lee W, Smith S, Williams S, Van Epps DE. 1994. Phenotypic analysis and characterization of CD34+ cells from normal human bone marrow, cord blood, peripheral blood, and mobilized peripheral blood from patients undergoing autologous stem cell transplantation. Clin Immunol Immunopathol, 70:10–18.
59. Levesque JP, Leavesley DI, Niutta S, Vadas M, Simmons PJ. 1995. Cytokines increase human hemopoietic cells adhesiveness by activation of very late antigen (VLA)-4 and VLA-5 integrins. J Exp Med, 181:1805–1815.
60. Voermans C, Rood PML, Hordijk PL, Gerritsen WR, van der Schoot CE. 2000. Adhesion molecules involved in transendothelial migration of human hematopoietic progenitor cells. Stem Cells, 18:435–443.
61. Whetton AD, Graham GJ. 1999. Homing and mobilization in the stem cell niche. Trends Cell Biol, 9:233–238.
62. Chazov EI, Repin VS, Orekhov AN, Antonov AS, Preobrazhensky SN, Soboleva EL, Smirnov VN. 1986. What has been learned studying human arteries. Atherosclerosis Reviews, Raven Press, 14:7–60.
63. Soboleva EL, Popkova VM. 1989. Hemopoietic progenitor cells (CFU-GM) in the intima of human atheromatous aorta. Bull Exp Biol Med, 5:600–604 (in Russian).
64. Soboleva EL, Smirnov VN. 1995. Local hemo- and stromopoiesis in human vascular wall. Lectures of XIII-th Meeting of the International Society of Haematology, pp. 134–139.
65. Soboleva EL, Popkova VM, Saburova OS, Tararak EM, Tvorogova MG, Smirnov VN. 1995. Colony forming units and atherosclerosis. In: Atherosclerosis X, Elsevier Science, pp. 919–925.
66. Soboleva EL, Saburova OS, Rozhkova TA, Tvorogova MG. 1999. Stem cells of hemopoietic and stromal differentiation lineages and human atherosclerosis. Angiol Vasc Surg, 5 (suppl):190–203.
67. Smirnov VN, Antonov AS, Bystrevskaya VB, Voyno-Yasenetskaya TA, Kabaeva NV, Romanov YuA, Sukhova GA, Soboleva EL, Tkachuk VA, Tararak EM. 1992. Cellular polymorphism in human aortic intima. Atherosclerosis IX, Proc. IX-th Int. Symp. on Atherosclerosis, pp. 295–298.
68. Soboleva EL, Shindler EM, Saburova OS, Tvorogova MG, Smirnov VN. 1994. Colony-forming units for fibroblasts (CFU-f) in the peripheral blood of patients with primary hypercholesterolemia. In: New pathogenic aspects of atherosclerosis. Nordrhein-Westfalische Academie der Wissenschaffen, Westdeutscher Verlag, pp. 79–93.
69. Ross R. 1993. The pathogenesis of atherosclerosis: a perspective for the 1990s. Nature, 362: 801–808.
70. Gordon D, Reidy MA, Benditt EP, Schwartz SM. 1990. Cell proliferation in coronary arteries. Proc Natl Acad Sci USA, 87:4600–4604.
71. Schwartz SM, O'Brien ERM. 1995. Absence of replication of vascular smooth muscle. Atherosclerosis X, Elsevier Science, pp. 704–720.
72. Stary HC. 1993. The evolution of human atherosclerotic lesions. Merck & Co., Inc West Point.
73. Deans RJ, Moseley AB. 2000. Mesenchymal stem cells: biology and potential clinical uses. Exp Hematol, 28:875–884.
74. Minguell JJ. 2000. Biology and clinical utilization of mesenchymal progenitor cells. Braz J Med Biol Res, 33:881–887.
75. Huss R, Lange C, Weissinger EM, Kolb H-J, Thalmeier K. 2000. Evidence of peripheral blood-derived, plastic-adherent $CD34^{-/low}$ hematopoietic stem cell clones with mesenchymal stem cell characteristics. Stem Cells, 18:252–260.
76. Kuznetsov SA, Mankani MH, Gronthos SG, Satomura K, Bianco P, Robey PG. 2001. Circulating skeletal stem cells. J Cell Biol, 153:1133–1139.

77. Rafii S. 2000. Circulating endothelial precursors: mystery, reality, and promise. J Clin Invest, 105: 17–19.
78. Zvaifler NJ, Marinova-Mutafchieva L, Adams G, Edwards CJ, Moss J, Burger JA, Maini RN. 2000. Mesenchymal precursor cells in the blood of normal individuals. Arthr Res, 2:477–488.
79. Friedenstein AJ, Chailakhjan RK, Lalykina KS. 1970. The development of fibroblast colonies in monolayer cultures of guinea-pig bone marrow and spleen cells. Cell Tissue Kinet, 3:393–403.
80. Friedenstein AJ, Deriglasova UF, Kulagina NN, Panasuk AF, Rudakova SF, Luria EA, Rudakov IA. 1974. Precursors for fibroblasts in different populations of hematopoietic cells as detected by the in vitro colony assay method. Exp Hematol, 2:83–92.
81. Friedenstein AJ. 1990. Osteogenic stem cells in the bone marrow. Bone and Mineral Research, 7:243–272.
82. Pittenger MF, Maccay AM. 2000. Multipotential human mesenchymal stem cells. Graft, 3:288–294.
83. Toma C, Pittenger MF, Cahill KS, Byrne BJ, Kessler PD. 2002. Human mesenchymal stem cells differentiate to a cardiomyocyte phenotype in the adult murine heart. Circulation, 105:93–98.
84. Sanchez-Ramos J, Song S, Cardozo-Pelaez F, Hazzi C, Stedeford T, Willing A, Freeman TB, Saporta S, Janssen W, Patel N, Cooper DR, Sanberg PR. 2000. Adult bone marrow stromal cells differentiate into neural cells in vitro. Exp Neurol, 164:247–256.
85. Clarke D, Frisen J. 2001. Differentiation potential of adult stem cells. Curr Opin Gen Devel, 11:575–580.
86. Makino S, Fukuda K, Miyoshi S, Konishi F, Kodama H, Pan J, Sano M, Takahashi T, Hori S, Abe H, Hata J, Umezawa A, Ogawa S. 1999. Cardiomyocytes can be generated from marrow stromal cells in vitro. J Clin Invest, 103:697–705.
87. Springer ML, Brazelton TR, Blau HM. 2001. Not the usual suspects: the unexpected sources of tissue regeneration. J Clin Invest, 107:1355–1356.
88. Mackenzie TC, Flake AW. 2001. Human mesenchymal stem cell persist, demonstrate site-specific multipotential differentiation, and are present in sites of wound healing and tissue regeneration after transplantation into fetal sheep. Blood Cell Mol Dis, 27:601–604.
89. Gill M, Dias S, Hattori K, Rivera ML, Hioklin D, Witte L, Girardi L, Yurt R, Himel H, Rafii S. 2001. Vascular trauma induces rapid but transient mobilization of VEGFR2(+)AC133(+) endothelial precursor cells. Circ Res, 88:167–174.
90. Krushinsky AV, Nestaiko GV. 1987. Morphology of smooth muscle cells from normal and atherosclerotic human aorta. Soc Med Rev A Cardiol, 1:35–73.
91. Benditt EP, Benditt JM. 1973. Evidence for a monoclonal origin of human atherosclerotic plaques. Proc Natl Acad Sci USA, 70:1753–1756.
92. Pearson TA, Dillman JM, Heptinstall RH. 1987. Clonal mapping of the human aorta. Relationship of monoclonal characteristics, lesion thickness, and age in normal intima and atherosclerotic lesions. Am J Pathol, 126:33–39.
93. Hillebrands JL, Klatter FA, van den Hurk BM, Popa ER, Nieuwenhuis P, Rosing J. 2001. Origin of neointimal endothelium and alpha-actin-positive smooth muscle cells in transplant arteriosclerosis. J Clin Invest, 107:1411–1422.
94. Brazelton TR, Adams B, Shorthouse R, Morris RE. 1999. Chronic rejection: the result of uncontrolled remodeling of graft tissue by recipient mesenchymal cells? Data from two rodent models and the effects of immunosuppressive therapies. Inflamm Res, 48 (suppl. 2):S134–S135.
95. Grimm PC, Nickerson P, Jeffery J, Savani RC, Gough J, McKenna RM, Stern E, Rush DN. 2001. Neointimal and tubulointersticial infiltration by recipient mesenchymal cells in chronic renal-allograft rejection. N Engl J Med, 345:93–97.
96. Quaini F, Urbanek K, Beltrami AP, Finato N, Beltrami CA, Nadal-Ginard B, Kajstura J, Leri A, Anversa P. 2002. Chimerism of the transplanted heart. N Engl J Med, 346:5–15.
97. Orlic D, Kajstura J, Chimenti S, Jakoniuk I, Anderson SM, Li B, Pickel J, McKay R, Nadal-Ginard B, Bodine DM, Leri A, Anversa P. 2001. Bone marrow cells regenerate infarcted myocardium. Nature, 410:701–705.
98. Orlic D, Kajstura J, Chimenti S, Limana F, Jakoniuk I, Quaini F, Nadal-Ginard B, Bodine DM, Leri A, Anversa P. 2001a. Mobilized bone marrow cells repair the infarcted heart, improving function and survival. PNAS, 98:10344–10349.
99. Kamihata H, Matsubara H, Nishiue T, Fujiyama S, Tsutsumi Y, Ozono R, Masaki H, Mori Y, Iba O, Tateishi E, Kosaki A, Shintani S, Murohara T. 2001. Implantation of bone marrow mononuclear cells into ischemic myocardium enhances collateral perfusion and regional function via side supply of angioblasts, angiogenic ligands, and cytokines. Circulation, 104:1046–1052.

100. Jackson KA, Majka SM, Wang H, Pocius J, Hartley CJ, Majesky MW, Entman ML, Michael LH, Hirschi KK, Goodell MA. 2001. Regeneration of ischemic cardiac muscle and vascular endothelium by adult stem cells. J Clin Invest, 107:1395–1402.
101. Asakura A, Komaki M, Rudnichki M. 2001. Muscle satellite cells are multipotential stem cells that exhibit myogenic, osteogenic, and adipogenic differentiation. Differentiation, 68:245–253.
102. Bhattacharya V, McSweeney PA, Shi Q, Bruno B, Ishida A, Nash R, Storb RF, Sauvage LR, Hammond WP, Wu MH. 2000. Enhanced endothelialization and microvessel formation in polyester grafts seeded with CD34+ bone marrow cells. Blood, 95:581–585.
103. Campbell JH, Efendy Jl, Han C, Girjes AA, Campbell GR. 2000. Haemopoietic origin of myofibroblasts formed in the peritoneal cavity in response to a foreign body. J Vasc Res, 37:364–371.
104. Zuk PA, Zhu M, Mizuno H, Huang J, Futrell JW, Katz AJ, Benhaim P, Lorenz HP, Hedrick MH. 2001. Multilineage cells from human adipose tissue: implication for cell-based therapies. Tissue Eng, 7:211–228.
105. Soboleva EL, Kukharchuk VV, Akchurin RS, Smirnov VN. 1997. Bone marrow colony-forming units for fibroblasts in the blood of patients with primary hyperlipidemia. Atherosclerosis, 134:302.
106. Smirnov VN, Soboleva EL, Rogova EM, Akchurin RS, Chazov EI. 1998. Bone marrow response to hypercholesterolemia (HCL) in coronary patients. Atherosclerosis, 136 (suppl):63.
107. Bassenge E. 1996. Endothelial function in different organs. Prog Cardiovasc Dis, 39:209–228.
108. Pels K, Labinaz M, O'Brien ER. 1997. Arterial wall neovascularization—potential role in atherosclerosis and restenosis. Jpn Circ J, 61:893–904.
109. Moulton KS. 2001. Plaque angiogenesis and atherosclerosis. Curr Atheroscler Rep, 3:225–233.
110. Freedman SB, Isner JM. 2001. Therapeutic angiogenesis for ischemic cardiovascular disease. J Mol Cell Cardiol, 33:379–393.
111. Tomita S, Li R-K, Weisel RD, Mickle DAD, Kim E-J, Sakai T, Jia Z-Q. 1999. Autologous transplantation of bone marrow cells improves damaged heart function. Circulation, 100 (suppl. II): 247–256.
112. Strauer BE, Brehm M, Zeus T, Gattermann N, Hernandez A, Sorg RV, Kogler G, Wernet P. 2001. Intrakoronare, humane autologe stannzelltransplantation zur myokardregeneration nach herzinfarkt. Dtsch Med Wschr, 126:932–938.

Frontiers in Cardiovascular Health, edited by
N.S. Dhalla, A. Chockalingam,
H.I. Berkowitz & P.K. Singal
Kluwer Academic Publishers, Boston, 2003

Aging and Dietary Lipids Modulate Ca^{2+}-Dependent Mitochondrial Function in the Post-Ischemic Heart

Salvatore Pepe

Cardiac Surgical Research Unit, Baker Heart Research Institute
Monash University Faculty of Medicine, Melbourne, Australia

Summary. A key feature of advanced age is a reduced threshold for excess Ca^{2+} loading during events that stimulate increased Ca^{2+} entry, such as augmented cardiac work, oxidative stress or post-ischemic reflow. Remodeling of myocardial cell membranes is a major factor underlying the relative Ca^{2+} intolerance in senescence and greater vulnerability to ischemic injury. In addition to cell death, surviving myocytes increase in size and exhibit altered gene expression of key effector proteins, including those that sustain Ca^{2+} homeostasis. Age-associated membrane changes, that may also be influenced by diet, include increases in membrane rigidity, cholesterol, phosphatidylcholine, omega-6 polyunsaturated fatty acids (PUFA), 4-hydroxy-2-nonenal, and decreases in omega-3 PUFA, cardiolipin. These alterations have profound consequences on the efficacy of membrane proteins involved with ion homeostasis, signal transduction, redox reactions and oxidative phosphorylation. However, some of the age-related detrimental adaptations may be beneficially modified by dietary strategy. Diet rich in omega-3 PUFA reverses the age-associated membrane omega-3 : omega-6 PUFA imbalance, and dysfunctional Ca^{2+} metabolism, facilitating increased efficiency of mitochondrial energy production and improved tolerance of ischemia and reperfusion.

Key words: omega-3 polyunsaturated fatty acids, cardiolipin, mitochondria, calcium.

Correspondence: Dr S. Pepe, Cardiac Surgical Research Unit, Baker Heart Research Institute, POB 6492 St Kilda Rd. Central, Melbourne, VIC 8008, Australia. Tel: +61-3-85321310, Fax: +61-3-85321314, E-mail: spepe@baker.edu.au.

INTRODUCTION

The senescent myocardium has numerous structural, physiological and biochemical features that involve a reduction in the number of myocytes, cell enlargement and alteration of metabolic, ionic and electrical properties of myocytes, compared to hearts from young adults (1–7). In addition, mechanisms to detoxify or minimize production of reactive oxygen species (ROS) appear impaired in advanced age. The consequence of this cumulative cellular remodeling is predominantly an age-associated reduction in the capacity to recover from ischemia-reperfusion injury.

During each cycle of cardiac myocyte excitation and contraction, Ca^{2+} influx occurs and triggers Ca^{2+} release from the sarcoplasmic reticulum via Ca^{2+} release channels (5). Ca^{2+} induced- Ca^{2+} release results in a transient rise of cytosolic Ca^{2+} (Ca_i) and triggers activation of contractile proteins until Ca^{2+} is returned to the sarcoplasmic reticulum by Ca^{2+}-ATPase pumps or extruded from the cell by Na^+-Ca^{2+} exchangers (8,9). With increased age, a Ca^{2+}-dependent increase in diastolic relaxation time occurs partly due to a reduced removal of cytosolic Ca^{2+} by the sarcoplasmic reticulum pump and Na^+/Ca^{2+} exchanger (8,10–13), and thus contribute to the augmentation and prolongation of the Ca_i transient (5). Conditions that demand increased cardiac output trigger catecholamine release from neurons ending in the heart to stimulate increased Ca^{2+} influx, oxygen consumption, ATP synthesis and a greater force of contraction. With the rise in intracellular Ca^{2+}, increased mitochondrial Ca^{2+} (Ca_M) uptake and activation of Ca^{2+}-dependent pyruvate dehydrogenase occurs to drive the maintenance of $NADH/NAD^+$, proton motive force (the H^+ electrochemical gradient, $\Delta\mu H$), and membrane potential ($\Delta\psi_m$), across the inner mitochondrial membrane respiratory chain, and stimulates a greater rate of ATP synthesis (14,15).

As the energy requirement of myocardial excitation-contraction coupling during cardiac work is predominantly supported by mitochondria, they play a key role in the onset of age-associated changes in Ca^{2+}-dependent processes supporting heart metabolism and contractile function. The aim of this brief review is to describe how specific changes to cardiac mitochondrial membranes can influence crucial Ca^{2+}-dependent metabolic processes that are perturbed particularly during myocardial ischemia and reperfusion. Notably, mitochondrial membrane phospholipid composition is altered by aging or diet, and such modification can modulate mitochondrial Ca^{2+} homeostasis and myocardial capacity to recover from ischemia-reperfusion stress.

THE EFFECT OF AGE ON POST-ISCHEMIC LOSS OF CA^{2+} HOMEOSTASIS

A common feature of cardiac ischemia and reperfusion during advanced age is increased vulnerability to the perturbation of Ca^{2+}-management systems resulting in highly elevated intracellular Ca^{2+} that precipitates systolic and diastolic contractile dysfunction (16). Although brief ischemia perturbs Ca^{2+} homeostasis, Ca_M buffering reserve permits normal function which is only breached by sustained ischemia and calcium "overload" at supra-micromolar levels, particularly upon reperfusion (17,18).

This breach has consequences for a variety of related mitochondrial effects, many of which are facilitated and enhanced by advanced age: reduced efficiency of Ca_M handling, increased permeability of the inner mitochondrial membrane to solutes occurs causing mitochondrial swelling, "proton leak", decreased ADP-induced oxygen consumption, prolonged conversion of ADP to ATP, reduced oxidative phosphorylation rates and a degree of uncoupling between respiration and ATP synthesis (19–23). Such uncoupling causes reduced efficiency of oxygen utilisation and augmented free radical production (23–30). Besides Ca^{2+}-overload, post-ischemic appearance of markers predictive of irreversible cell injury include: increased acidosis and P_i; decreased superoxide dismutase activity; accumulation of free radicals; activation of phospholipases; accumulation of long-chain acyl CoA and toxic products of membrane lipid peroxidation; and formation of protein adducts (19–23,31–36). At this end-stage, diminished ATP supply results in complete loss of intracellular Ca^{2+} homeostasis, which may result in ventricular fibrillation (5,19). At such excessive levels of Ca_M, the mitochondrial membrane permeability transition (MPT) is more likely occur.

AGE-ASSSOCIATED INCIDENCE IN POTENTIAL TRIGGERS OF MPT

Ca_M-dependent cyclophilin-D binding to adenine nucleotide translocase facilitates conformational changes that cause adenine nucleotide translocase to form a non-specific pore (21). The "MPT pore" is presently considered to be a multi-protein complex that includes a voltage dependent anion channel. Cyclophilin-D binding is increased following augmented oxidative stress (and/or thiol agents from lipid peroxidation products) that sensitize the MPT to Ca^{2+}. Mitochondrial matrix adenine nucleotide binding to adenine nucleotide translocase decreases the sensitivity of the MPT to Ca^{2+}. However, this substrate-dependent reduction in Ca^{2+} sensitivity may be diminished by products of lipid peroxidation that modify specific thiol groups on adenine nucleotide translocase, to the extent that $\Delta\psi_m$ may be attenuated, ATP synthesis fails and MPT is enhanced (21). In addition to Ca_M, P_i, long-chain acyl CoA, adenine nucleotides, the redox state of specific protein thiols, and ROS also stimulate opening of the MPT pore which depolarises the mitochondrion and dissipates $\Delta\psi_m$ preventing oxidative phosphorylation (21,32). Following the collapse of $\Delta\psi_m$, opening of the MPT pore results in the release of mitochondrial contents, including cytochrome c. Released cytochrome c interacts with Apaf-1 and procaspase-9 to activate caspase-3, initiating a cascade of events leading to cell death via apoptosis and/or necrosis (21,33).

Polyunsaturated fatty acids (PUFA) released from membrane phospholipids by ischemia and reperfusion undergo lipid peroxidation by reacting with ROS to produce various aldehydes, alkenals, and alkenes (31). The highly reactive hydroxyalkenal, 4-hydroxy-2-nonenal (HNE), is formed by superoxide reactions with membrane ω-6 PUFA (31). HNE reacts with protein sulfhydryl and thiol groups consequently altering protein conformation that interferes with numerous enzyme and ion exchange systems (31,34,35). Such HNE reactions that form protein adducts may adversely modify adenine nucleotide translocase and cyclophilin-D to interfere with $\Delta\psi_m$ and ultimately contribute to MPT.

Notably, mitochondrial ROS in the heart has been reported to increase with age (24–27,34). A number of endogenous mitochondrial antioxidant defenses may also diminish with age and thus reduce the capacity for efficient management of ROS (1,26–28). Oxidative stress occurs due to an imbalance between the formation of ROS and antioxidant defenses. This imbalance may augment the amount of membrane bilayer PUFAs that are converted to lipid hydroperoxides. The reactive products generated in this process permeate through to other intracellular membranes and may act as toxic second messengers in addition to other ROS-induced signal transduction reactions (31). As the mitochondrial respiratory chain represents a major subcellular source of ROS species during reperfusion of ischemic myocardium (29,30,34), and ischemic/reperfusion has been associated with decreased rates of NADH-linked state 3 (ADP-dependent) respiration (24,29,37–39), mitochondria are therefore primary targets of lipid peroxidation and HNE-mediated dysfunction. Perfusate levels of HNE are increased in the reperfused post-ischemic myocardium (36), and recent studies show that exposure of intact cardiac mitochondria to HNE results in a decline of NADH-linked respiration (39). Thus, the status of Ca_i, pH, $\Delta\psi_m$, membrane lipid and protein reactivity of mitochondria and the ambient level of oxidative stress influence the propensity of mitochondria to undergo MPT and cell death, particularly in aging where these factors are modified.

MODIFICATION OF LIPID COMPOSITION ALTERS MEMBRANE PROTEIN FUNCTION

The function of proteins that regulate membrane influx and efflux of Ca^{2+} between intracellular Ca^{2+} storage sites, the cytosol and outside the cell, depends upon their conformation and position within these membranes, both of which are partly determined by the membrane phospholipid composition. In particular, the PUFA composition of membrane phospholipids has been shown to affect membrane ion permeability. Dietary ω-3 PUFA content, which increases ω-3 : ω-6 PUFA content in membrane phospholipids, auspiciously modifies the relative activity of Ca^{2+}-Mg^{2+}-ATPase, Ca^{2+} uptake into the SR, and Na^+/Ca^{2+} exchanger activity (40–42). A decrease in ATP-dependent Ca^{2+} uptake has been observed in cardiac SR membranes from rats fed ω-3 PUFA-rich fish oil-supplemented diet compared with those fed a corn oil-supplemented diet (42).

However, the sensitivity of functional membrane proteins to the acute effects of PUFA has also been reported. In a conscious dog model of infarction, experimentally induced acute VF can be prevented by the prior intravenous infusion of a ω-3 PUFA-rich emulsion (43). In isolated ventricular myocytes, the acute addition of ω-3 PUFA to the bathing medium protects against Ca^{2+} overload induced by ouabain or BAYK8644 (44). PUFA acutely delivered to isolated cardiac myocytes have been shown to modify L-type Ca^{2+}, K^+, Na^+ channels and Ca^{2+}-spark activities via a direct action on functional protein properties (45–48).

Recently it has been reported (49), that following a diet-induced increase in the ratio of ω-3 to ω-6 PUFA in myocardial membrane phospholipids, the erythrocyte-perfused isolated working rat heart preparation has a reduced rate of oxygen consumption without decline in cardiac output or external work, even at high left ventricular filling pressures. Notably, hearts with augmented ω-3 : ω-6 PUFA had greater capacity to recover contractile function after ischemia and reperfusion and did so with greater efficiency of oxygen utilisation per unit work performed, compared to hearts with a low ω-3 : ω-6 PUFA. These effects have been attributed to membrane-dependent modulation of mitochondrial respiration (22,49,50). In addition, hearts with high ω-3 : ω-6 PUFA content elicited a high ventricular fibrillation threshold and low incidence of reperfusion arrhythmias compared to ω-6 PUFA-enriched hearts (49,51,52).

AGE-ASSOCIATED REDUCTION IN MITOCHONDRIAL ω-3 : ω-6 PUFA AND CARDIOLIPIN

An increase in sarcolemmal and mitochondrial membrane content of arachidonic acid (20 : 4 ω-6 PUFA) and a reduction in docosahexaenoic acid (22 : 6 ω-3 PUFA) occur in the heart with aging (22,51–53). The protective effects of ω-3 PUFAs against Ca^{2+} overload and fatal arrhythmia have been demonstrated both in the hearts of old animals and in younger animals even after long term diet rich in ω-6 PUFA (22,49,51–53). Thus, the decline in the content of cardiac cell membrane ω-3 PUFAs (low ω-3 : ω-6 PUFA) with aging may result in an increased vulnerability to Ca^{2+} overload induced by high work states, ischemia and reperfusion or oxidative stress itself.

These age-associated qualitative changes to membrane PUFAs can be reversed or exaggerated by dietary manipulation with ω-3 PUFA or ω-6 PUFA–rich diet (Figure 1). The effect of ω-3 PUFA or ω-6 PUFA–rich diet on cardiac mitochondrial membranes after six weeks was examined in young and senescent Wistar rats (6 and 24 month old) (22). Diet rich in ω-3 PUFA prevented the age-associated decline in ω-3 PUFAs and increase in ω-6 PUFAs measured in cardiac mitochondrial membranes. In these same experiments, ω-3 PUFA-rich diet restored the inner mitochondrial membrane-specific phospholipid, cardiolipin (diphospatidylglycerol) in 24 mo rat hearts to the higher levels measured in 6 mo hearts and prevented the age-linked increase in phosphatidylcholine. In contrast, ω-6 PUFA–rich diet augmented the age-associated increase in ω-6 PUFAs, phosphatidylcholine and the decline in omega-3 PUFAs and cardiolipin.

Cardiolipin is a crucial mitochondrial membrane phospholipid specifically required for the functional activity of cytochrome *c* oxidase and adenine nucleotide translocase (54–56). The capacity to influence cardiolipin levels by dietary manipulation of ω-3 : ω-6 PUFA has profound potential consequences to adenine nucleotide translocase and cytochrome c oxidase activity with regard to triggering MPT (54).

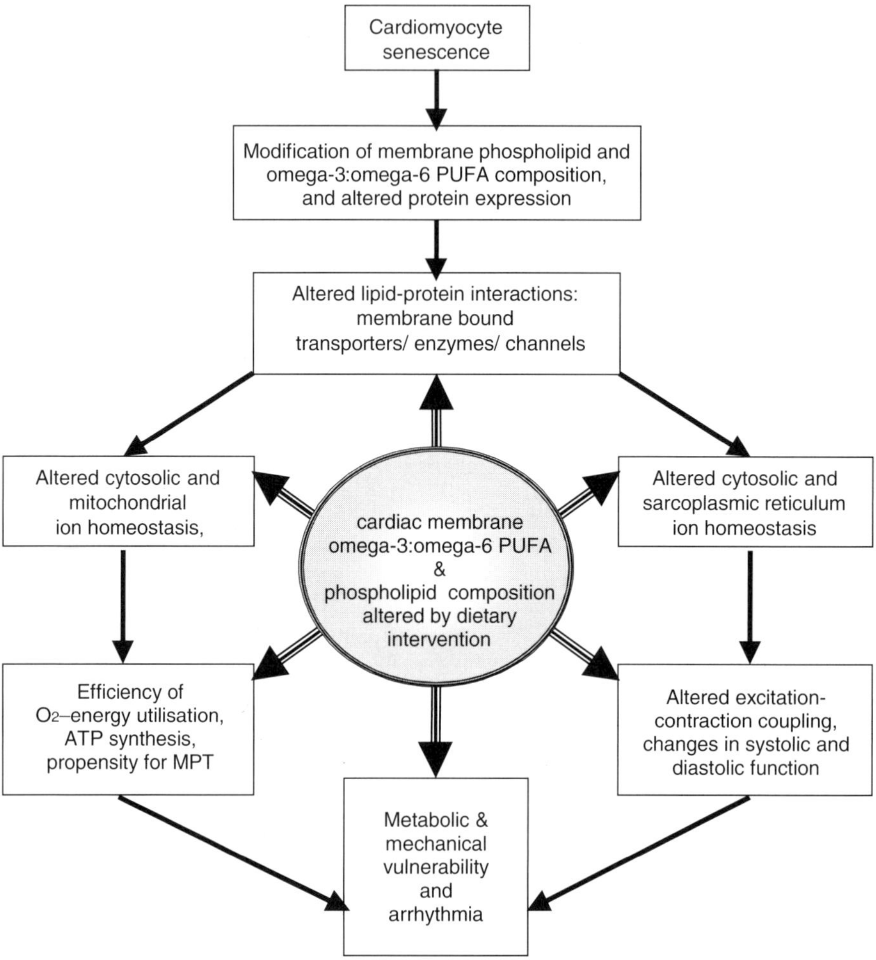

Figure 1. A scheme linking the age-associated changes in cardiac membrane phospholipids and PUFA to cellular mechanisms of altered mitochondrial metabolism and excitation-contraction coupling that ultimately confer cellular vulnerability to the metabolic challenges of high energy demand, ischemia, reperfusion and oxidative stress. The central sphere indicates the potential modulation of cellular function induced by dietary PUFA intervention that modifies the ratio of ω-3 to ω-6 PUFA in membrane phospholipids. With advancing age, the ω-3 : ω-6 PUFA is greatly reduced and has substantial detrimental impact on cardiovascular function, particularly at the level of intracellular Ca^{2+} homeostasis, reducing the cellular capacity to tolerate and adapt to ischemic stress. Although these effects can be augmented further by diets rich in ω-6 PUFA (i.e., animal fats), ω-3 PUFA-rich diet (i.e., marine oils) attenuates these effects via specific modification of membrane phospholipid composition.

ω-3 PUFA ATTENUATES REPERFUSION-INDUCED CA^{2+} PERTURBATION

Significant effects of age and diet on total Ca_M become apparent after ischemia and reperfusion (I/R) in isolated rat myocardium following dietary lipid-induced manipulation of ω-3:ω-6 PUFA content in the phospholipids of mitochondrial membranes (22). Total Ca_M after I/R was markedly greater in the ω-6 PUFA-rich hearts (low ω-3:ω-6 PUFA) than in the ω-3 PUFA-rich hearts (high ω-3:ω-6 PUFA). In senescent (24-mo) ω-6 PUFA hearts there was a greater increase in total Ca_M values after I/R compared to young adult (6-mo) ω-6 PUFA hearts. Compared to the ω-6 PUFA groups, total Ca_M values in 6- and 24-mo ω-3 PUFA groups did not differ, and both showed a lower net uptake of Ca^{2+} than 6- and 24-mo ω-6 PUFA hearts. After I/R, group differences due to age and diet, with regard to the proportion of activated pyruvate dehydrogenase (PDH_A) mirrored those seen for total Ca_M. Despite greater Ca_M and PDH_A in 24-mo ω-6 PUFA hearts, these exhibited the least post-ischemic recovery of systolic function while ω-3 PUFA hearts had the highest values of ventricular systolic pressure during reperfusion. When all groups were treated with 3.4 μM ruthenium red to block mitochondrial uniporter uptake of Ca^{2+} (57) (and the Ca^{2+}-dependent activation of PDH), the effects of age and dietary PUFA on Ca_M and PDH_A during reperfusion were abolished and post-ischemic contractile recovery was increased in all groups (22). Thus, the ω-3 to ω-6 PUFA ratio and cardiolipin content of mitochondrial membranes may be crucial factors that influence efficient Ca^{2+} homeostasis, oxygen consumption, energy metabolism and demand-matched contractile performance particularly during post-ischemic reflow.

CONCLUSIONS

The numerous constitutive changes that occur in heart cells with increased age markedly reduce the cellular capacity to tolerate and adapt to ischemic stress. A distinct decrease in the ratio of mitochondrial membrane ω-3 to ω-6 PUFA, and a decrease in the mitochondrial phospholipid, cardiolipin, occurs in aged rat hearts. Together with altered Ca^{2+} homeostasis, raised Ca_M levels, increased activation of mitochondrial dehydrogenases, perturbations in efficient electron transport, overproduction of ROS (and the inability to scavenge this excess), and toxic lipid peroxidation products are linked to inefficient post-ischemic mitochondrial function in aging hearts. Moreover, the age-associated increase in ω-6 PUFA, the preferred target of ROS-induced peroxidation that leads to the formation of HNE (31), may be a mechanism for increased HNE-induced modification of key mitochondrial proteins (35,38,39), following post-ischemic reflow, attenuation of oxidative phosphorylation and increased likelihood of inducing MPT.

These factors contribute to reduced tolerance of reperfusion injury, as seen in limited recovery of contractile function, and potentially to mitochondria-dependent cell death. A diet rich in ω-3 PUFA increases the ratio of membrane ω-3 to ω-6 PUFA and cardiolipin content may prove a potent strategy in attenuating major age-associated changes to membranes ultimately altering Ca^{2+}-dependent processes (Figure 1).

REFERENCES

1. Hansford R. 1983. Bioenergetics in aging. Biochim Biophys Acta 726:41–80.
2. Anversa P, Palackal T, Sonnenblick EH, Olivetti G, Meggs LG, Capasso JM. 1990. Myocyte cell loss and myocyte cellular hyperplasia in the hypertrophied aging rat heart. Circ Res 67:871–885.
3. Olivetti G, Melissari M, Capasso JM, Anversa P. 1991. Cardiomyopathy of the aging human heart. Myocyte loss and reactive cellular hypertrophy. Circ Res 68:1560–1568.
4. Walker K, Lakatta E, Houser S. 1993. Age-associated changes in membrane currents in rat ventriculuar myocytes. Cardiovasc Res 27:1968–1977.
5. Lakatta EG. 1992. Functional implications of spontaneous sarcoplasmic reticulum Ca^{2+} release in the heart. Cardiovasc Res 26:193–214.
6. Lakatta EG. 1993. Cardiovascular regulatory mechanisms in advanced age. Physiol Rev 73:413–467.
7. Lakatta EG. 1998. Cardiovascular aging: Perspectives from humans to rodents. Am J Geriat Cardiol 7:32–45.
8. Froehlich J, Lakatta E, Beard E, Spurgeon H, Weisfeldt M, Gerstenblith G. 1978. Studies of sarcoplasmic reticulum function and contraction duration in young adult and aged rat myocardium. J Mol Cell Cardiol 10:427–438.
9. Schmidt U, delMonte F, Miyamoto M, Matsui T, Gwathmey J, Rosenzweig A, Hajjar R. 1999. Restoration of diastolic function in senescent rat hearts through adenoviral gene transfer of sarcoplasmic reticulum Ca^{2+}-ATPase. Circulation 101:790–796.
10. Narayanan N. 1981. Differential alterations in ATP-supported calcium transport activities of sarcoplasmic reticulum and sarcolemma of aging myocardium. Biochim Biophys Acta 678:442–459.
11. Heyliger C, Prakash A, McNeill J. 1988. Alterations in membrane Na^{+} -Ca^{2+} exchange in the aging myocardium. Age 11:1–6.
12. Heyliger C, Prakash A, McNeill J. 1989. Effect of calmodulin on sarcoplasmic reticular Ca^{2+} transport in the aging heart. Mol Cell Biochem 85:75–79.
13. Josephson R, Silverman H, Lakatta E, Stern M, Zweier J. 1991. Study of the mechanisms of hydrogen peroxide and hydroxyl free radical-induced cellular injury and calcium overload in cardiac myocytes. J Biol Chem 266:2354–2361.
14. Gunter TE, Pffeifer DR. 1990. Mechanisms by which mitochondria transport calcium. Am J Physiol 258:C755–C786.
15. Hansford R. 1994. Physiological role of mitochondrial calcium transport. J Bioenerg Biomemb 26:495–508.
16. Hano O, Bogdanov K, Sakai M, Danziger R, Spurgeon H, Lakatta E. 1995. Reduced threshold for myocardial cell calcium intolerance in the rat heart with aging. Am J Physiol 269:H1607–H1612.
17. Miyata H, Lakatta E, Stern M, Silverman H. 1992. Relation of mitochondrial and cytosolic free calcium to cardiac myocyte recovery after exposure to anoxia. Circ Res 71:605–613.
18. Miyata H, Silverman H, Sollott S, Lakatta E, Stern M, Hansford R. 1991. Measurement of mitochondrial free Ca^{2+} concentration in living single rat cardiac myocytes. Am J Physiol 261:H1123–H1134.
19. Ferrari R. 1996. The role of mitochondria in ischemic heart disease. J Cardiovasc Pharmacol 28(suplement 1):S1–S10.
20. DiLisa F, Menabo R, Canton M, Petronilli V. 1998. The role of mitochondria in the salvage and injury of the ischemic myocardium. Biochim Biophys Acta 1366:69–78.
21. Halestrap A, Kerr P, Javador S, Woodfield K. 1998. Elucidationg the mechanism of the permeability transition pore and its role in reperfusion injury in the heart. Biochim Biophys Acta 1366:79–94.
22. Pepe S, Tsuchiya N, Lakatta E, Hansford R. 1999. PUFA and aging modulate cardiac mitochondrial membrane lipid composition and Ca^{2+} activation of PDH. Am J Physiol 276:H149–H158.
23. Jahangir A, Ozcan C, Holmuhamedov EL, Terzic A. 2001. Increased calcium vulnerability of senescent cardiac mitochondria: protective role for a mitochondrial potassium channel opener. Mech Ageing Dev 122:1073–1086.
24. Nohl H, Breuninger V, Hegner D. 1978. Influence of mitochondrial radical formation on energy linked respiration. Eur J Biochem 90:385–390.
25. Sawada M, Carlson J. 1987. Changes in superoxide radical and lipid peroxide formation in the brain, heart and liver during the lifetime of the rat. Mech Aging Dev 41:125–137.
26. Sohal R, Arnold L, Sohal B. 1990. Age-related changes in antioxidant enzymes and prooxidant generation in tissues of the rat with special reference to parameters in two insect species. Free Rad Biol Med 10:495–500.

27. Papa S. 1996. Mitochondrial oxidative phosphorylation changes in the life span. Molecular aspects and physiopathological implications. Biochim Biophys Acta 1276:87–105.
28. Rosenfeldt FL, Pepe S, Ou R, Mariani JA, Rowland MA, Nagley P, Linanne AW. 1999. Coenzyme Q_{10} improves the tolerance of senescent myocardium to aerobic and ischemic stress: studies in rats and human atrial tissue. Biofactors 9:291–299.
29. Ambrosio G, Zweier J, Duilio C, Kuppusamy P, Santoro G, Elia P, Tritto I, Cirillo P, Condorelli. 1993. Evidence that mitochondrial respiration is a source of potentially toxic oxygen free readicals in intact rabbit hearts subjected to ischemia and reflow. J Biol Chem 268:18532–18541.
30. McCord JM. 1985. Oxygen derived free radicals in post ischemic tissue injury. New Engl J Med 312:159–163.
31. Esterbauer H, Schaur R, Zollner H. 1991. Chemistry and biochemistry of 4-hydroxynonenal, malonaldehyde and related aldehydes. Free Rad Biol Med 11:81–128.
32. Lapidus RG, Sokolov PM. 1994. The mitochondrial permeability transition. Interactions of spermine, ADP and inorganic phosphate. J Biol Chem 269:18931–18936.
33. Lenaz G. 1998. Role of mitochondria in oxidative stress and ageing. Biochim Biophys Acta 1366:53–68.
34. Lucas D, Szweda L. 1998. Cardiac reperfusion injury: Aging, lipid peroxidation, and mitochondrial dysfunction. Proc Natl Acad Sci U.S.A. 95:510–514.
35. Lucas D, Szweda L. 1999. Declines in mitochondrial respiration during cardiac reperfusion: age-dependent inactivation of α-ketoglutarate dehydrogenase. Proc Natl Acad Sci, U.S.A. 96:6689–6693.
36. Blasig I, Grune T, Schonheit K, Rohde E, Jakstadt M, Haseloff R, Siems W. 1995. 4-Hydroxynonenal, a novel indicator of lipid peroxidation for reperfusion. Am J Physiol 268:H14–H22.
37. Das D, George A, Liu X, Rao P. 1989. Detection of the hydroxyl radical in the mitochondria of ischemic-reperfused myocardium by trapping salicylate. Biochem Biophys Res Commun 165:1004–1009.
38. Humphries K, Szweda L. 1998. Selective inactivation of α-ketoglutarate dehydrogenase and pyruvate dehydrogenase: reaction of lipoic acid with 4-hydroxy-2-nonenal. Biochemistry (USA) 37:15835–15841.
39. Humphries K, Yoo Y, Szweda L. 1998. Inhibition of NADH-linked mitochondrial respiration by 4-hydroxy-2-nonenal. Biochemistry (USA) 37:552–557.
40. Phillipson R, Ward R. 1985. Effects of fatty acids on Na^{2+}/Ca^{2+} exchange and calcium permeability of cardiac sarcoplasmic reticulum vesicles. J Biol Chem 260:9666–9671.
41. Swanson J, Likesh B, Kinsella J. 1989. Ca^{2+}/Mg^{2+}ATPase of mouse cardiac sarcoplasmic reticulum is affected by membrane *n*-6 and *n*-3 polyunsaturated fatty acid content. J Nutr 119:364–372.
42. Taffet G, Pharm T, Bick D, Entma M, Pownall H, Bick R. 1993. The calcium uptake of the rat heart sarcoplasmic reticulum is altered by dietary lipid. J Memb Biol 131:35–42.
43. Billman G, Hallaq H, Leaf A. 1994. Prevention of ischemia-induced ventricular fibrillation by omega 3 fatty acids. Proc Nat Acad Sci U.S.A. 91:4427–4430.
44. Hallaq H, Smith T, Leaf A. 1992. Modulation of dihydropyridine-sensitive calcium channels in heart cells by fish oil fatty acids. Proc Nat Acad Sci USA 89:1760–1764.
45. Pepe S, Bogdanov K, Hallaq H, Spurgeon H, Leaf A, Lakatta E. 1994. ω-3 Polyunsaturated fatty acid modulates dihydropyridine effects on L-type Ca^{2+} channels, cytosolic Ca^{2+}, and contraction in adult rat cardiac myocytes. Proc Nat Acad Sci U.S.A. 91:8832–8836.
46. Bogdanov K, Spurgeon H, Vinogradova T, Lakatta E. 1998. Modulation of the transient outward current in adult rat ventricular myocytes by polyunsaturated fatty acids. Am J Physiol 274: H571–H579.
47. Xiao YF, Kang JX, Morgan JP, Leaf A. 1995. Blocking effects of polyunsaturated fatty acids on Na^{+} channels of neonatal rat ventricular myocytes. Proc Natl Acad Sci USA 21;92:11000–11004.
48. Xiao YF, Gomez AM, Morgan JP, Lederer WJ, Leaf A. 1997. Suppression of voltage-gated L-type Ca^{2+} currents by polyunsaturated fatty acids in adult and neonatal rat ventricular myocytes. Proc Natl Acad Sci USA 94:4182–4187.
49. Pepe S, McLennan P. 2002. Increased ventricular fibrillation threshold and reduced incidence of cardiac arrhythmias after polyunsaturated fish oil dietary supplementation. Circulation 105:2303–2308.
50. Demaison L, Sergiel JP, Moreau D, Grynberg A. 1994. Influence of the phospholipid n-3/n-6 PUFA ratio on mitochondrial oxidative metabolism before and after myocardial ischemia. Biochim Biophys Acta 1227:53–59.

51. Pepe S, McLennan P. 1996. Increased ventricular fibrillation threshold and reduced incidence of cardiac arrhythmias after polyunsaturated fish oil dietary supplementation. J Nutr 126:34–42.
52. McLennan P, Abeywardena M, Charnock J. 1990. Reversal of the arrhythmogenic effects of long-term saturated fatty acid intake by dietary *n*-3 and *n*-6 polyunsaturated fatty acids. Am J Clin Nutr 51:53–58.
53. McLennan P, Abeywardena M, Charnock J. 1989. The influence of age and dietary fat in animal model of sudden cardiac death. Aus NZ J Med 19:1–5.
54. Beyer K, Klingenberg M. 1985. ADP/ATP carrier protein from beef heart mitochondria has high amounts of tightly bound cardiolipin, as revealed by ^{31}P nuclear magnetic resonance. Biochemistry 24:3821–3826.
55. Noel H, Pande SV. 1986. An essential requirement of cardiolipin for mitochondrial acetylcarnitine translocase activity. Eur J Biochem 155:99–102.
56. Paradies G, Petrosillo G, Pistolese M, Ruggiero F. 2000. The effect of reactive oxygen species generated from the mitochondrial electron transport chain on the cytochrome *c* oxidase activity and on the cardiolipin content in bovine heart submitochondrial particles. FEBS Letters 466:323–326.
57. Matlib MA, Zhou Z, Knight S, Ahmed S, Choi KM, Krause-Bauer J, Phillips R, Altschuld R, Katsube Y, Sperelakis N, Bers DM. 1998. Oxygen-bridged dinuclear ruthenium amine complex specifically inhibits Ca^{2+} uptake into mitochondria in vitro and in situ in single cardiac myocytes. J Biol Chem 273:10223–10231.

Frontiers in Cardiovascular Health, edited by
N.S. Dhalla, A. Chockalingam,
H.I. Berkowitz & P.K. Singal
Kluwer Academic Publishers, Boston, 2003

The Role of Nuclear Receptors in HDL Formation

Gordon A. Francis

*CIHR Group on Molecular and Cell Biology of Lipids
and Departments of Medicine and Biochemistry,
328 HMRC, University of Alberta, Edmonton, AB, Canada T6G 2S2*

Summary. HDL levels are stronger predictors of an individuals risk for ischemic vascular disease than are LDL levels, yet our ability to raise HDL clinically has lagged far behind our ability to lower LDL. A dramatic increase in our understanding of the mechanisms of HDL formation at the cellular and nuclear receptor level in recent years has provided promising new targets to utilize for the raising of HDL levels. This review summarizes our current knowledge of the role of nuclear receptors in enhancing the various mechanisms of HDL formation.

Key words: HDL, nuclear receptors, atherosclerosis, apolipoproteins, ABCA1.

INTRODUCTION

Despite advances in their prevention and treatment in the Western world, diseases resulting from atherosclerosis remain the leading cause of death in both the developed and developing world (1). The strikingly increased risk of ischemic vascular disease associated with low levels of high density lipoprotein (HDL) cholesterol has been demonstrated in numerous epidemiologic studies worldwide [reviewed in (2)]. HDL levels have in fact been found to be stronger predictors of risk for ischemic vascular disease than are LDL levels (2). The lag in development of HDL-raising therapies compared to LDL-lowering therapies for the treatment and prevention of

Corresponding Author: Gordon A. Francis, 328 HMRC, University of Alberta, Edmonton, AB T6G 2S2, Canada. Tel: 780-492-9193, Fax: 780-492-3383, E-mail: gordon.francis@ualberta.ca.

atherosclerosis has been due in large part to a lack of understanding of the mechanisms of HDL formation in vivo. Recent discoveries at the nuclear and cellular levels have provided promising new targets to utilize to raise HDL clinically.

HDL is thought to be protective for numerous reasons (3), the chief among these being stimulation of the return of cholesterol to the liver for excretion in bile, or "reverse" cholesterol transport (4). Numerous transgenic animal models, while not identifying the major protective action of HDL, have demonstrated the protective effects of overexpressing human apolipoprotein A-I (apoA-I) and raising HDL levels in decreasing the formation of atherosclerotic lesions (5–8). Infusion of a pro-apoA-I liposome complex into hypercholesterolemic human patients was found to increase fecal steroid excretion, indicating that raising HDL levels does indeed increase total reverse cholesterol transport and cholesterol excretion (9).

HDL are formed through three principal mechanisms: 1) the synthesis of de-lipidated or poorly lipidated HDL proteins (apolipoproteins, apos) by the liver and intestine; 2) the delivery of surface lipid and protein components to HDL from very low density lipoproteins (VLDL) and chylomicrons; and 3) the removal of cellular cholesterol and phospholipids by apoA-I, the principal protein of HDL, in the first step of reverse cholesterol transport. This latter pathway represents the major route for return of cellular cholesterol to the liver for excretion in bile, the only effective means of cholesterol removal from the body. HDL levels may therefore be raised by increasing the synthesis of HDL proteins, enhancing the hydrolysis of triglyceride-rich lipoproteins, or increasing the delivery of cellular lipids to lipid-poor HDL proteins. Nuclear receptors are involved in regulating the genes involved in all of these three mechanisms, and this review will focus on the role of nuclear receptors in these pathways.

NUCLEAR RECEPTORS

General concepts

Nuclear receptors (NRs) are one of the largest group of transcription factors, with 48 distinct members now identified in the human genome (10,11). These factors bind to DNA in the nucleus to activate the transcription of genes following binding of small molecular ligands such as fatty acids, cholesterol metabolites (oxysterols), or synthetic ligands such as the fibric acid class of drugs to the NR. Several of these receptors were characterized prior to their ligands being identified, and because of this were designated "orphan" receptors. As their natural and synthetic ligands have become known, many of these orphans have now been "adopted" (12).

Most NRs are active as dimers—either homodimers or heterodimers with the retinoid X receptor (RXR, NR2B1)—although a subset of them can bind and stimulate transcription as monomers. These dimers bind to nuclear receptor response elements in the promoter regions of their target genes (e.g., the gene for the major HDL apolipoprotein, apoA-I) following activation of one or the other, or both, of the dimer partners by their ligands (13). The NRs controlling HDL formation, including the peroxisome proliferator activated receptors (PPARs) and liver X receptors (LXRs), all form obligate heterodimers with RXR, and ligand binding to one or the other partner stabilizes the heterodimer association (13). Unlike some other RXR heterodimer partners, the PPARs and LXR may be activated permissively by binding of RXR ligands ("rexinoids") alone to the heterodimer (14–17), but are synergistically activated by simultaneous binding of ligands for both dimer partners (13,18). The activity of the NR heterodimers is also controlled by the binding of corepressors, which inhibit their transcriptional activation, or coactivators, that enhance their ability to activate their target genes. The activities of these cofactors range from chromatin remodeling and modifications of core histones (acetylation, phosphorylation, and methylation status) that allow transcription to occur, to recruitment of the basic transcriptional machinery (19). Cofactor recruitment is therefore an integral part of NR signaling pathways (20).

Nuclear receptors regulating HDL formation

PPARs and LXR are the nuclear receptors that are currently known to have the greatest impact on HDL formation. The PPAR class of receptors was actually discovered in the course of development of lipid-lowering drugs, the fibric acid derivatives or fibrates. Clofibrate, the first of this class to be developed, was noted to have the effect of inducing proliferation of the cell organelles peroxisomes in rodents (21,22). The receptor activated by clofibrate and several other "peroxisome proliferators" was subsequently cloned and given the name peroxisome proliferator activated receptor alpha (PPARα) (23). PPARβ/δ and PPARγ were subsequently identified as structural homologs of PPARα that control expression of other metabolic genes, but do not induce peroxisome proliferation (24–26).

The PPAR subfamily of nuclear receptors all bind as heterodimers with RXR to peroxisome proliferator response elements (PPRE) in the target gene, preferentially consisting of a direct repeat of the hormone receptor response element half site spaced by 1 nucleotide (DR-1) (13). PPARα (NR1C1) is expressed in several metabolically active tissues including liver, kidney, heart, and skeletal muscle (27,28), and is also present in monocytes as well as vascular endothelial and smooth muscle cells (29–31). Fatty acids are the main natural ligands of PPARα (32–35), and the fibrate class of drugs are the main synthetic ligands for PPARα currently in use. PPARβ/δ (NR1C2) was the second PPAR cloned, and is expressed ubiquitously but with highest levels found in brain, adipose tissue and skin (27, 36). It is mentioned here mainly because synthetic ligands for this isoform have recently been found to increase expression of ABCA1 and raise HDL levels in an animal model (37). PPARγ is expressed in highest levels in adipose tissue, large intestine and hematopoietic cells, with lower amounts in several other tissues including smooth muscle cells and macrophages (28,38–40). PPARγ is critically important for adipocyte differentiation and uptake of fats by adipocytes. Through these and other actions synthetic PPARγ ligands such as the thiazolidinediones (41,42) are effective in increasing free fatty acid uptake by adipocytes and decreasing insulin resistance in type 2 diabetes. PPARγ ligands have also been found to increase the expression of ABCA1 indirectly via upregulation of LXR (43).

The LXR or "liver X receptor" is another class of orphan nuclear receptors that increase HDL levels and are activated by oxysterols, oxidized derivatives of cholesterol generated in cells in response to elevated cell cholesterol content (44,45). Two different LXR genes have been described, LXRα (RLD-1 or NR1H3) and LXRβ (NER, UR, OR-1 or NR1H2). LXRα is expressed to a high extent in liver with lower levels being present in intestine, kidney, spleen and adipose tissue (28,46). LXRβ is more ubiquitously expressed, however, less is known about its function. Both LXR isoforms bind preferentially as heterodimers with RXR to DR4 response elements in the genes they activate (46–49). Synthetic non-steroidal agonists of LXR are now being developed as potential therapeutic agents to raise HDL clinically.

NUCLEAR RECEPTOR CONTROL OF HDL FORMATION AND REVERSE CHOLESTEROL TRANSPORT

Nuclear receptors control HDL formation both at the level of the liver and non-hepatic ("peripheral") cells. This control occurs through activation of genes involved in HDL apolipoprotein formation, provision of surface components for HDL formation from triglyceride (TG)-rich lipoproteins, and the stimulation of lipid delivery to free HDL apoproteins for new HDL particle formation. In addition, nuclear receptors regulate genes involved in further steps of the reverse cholesterol transport pathway that modulate HDL structure and thereby influence circulating HDL levels.

A. Enhancement of apo A-I and apo A-II synthesis by PPARα

Synthesis of apo A-I and apo A-II, the two major proteins of HDL, by the liver and intestine is the first step in HDL particle formation. Increased apo A-I and apo A-II synthesis by the liver occurs in response to fibrate-induced PPARα activation of the human apolipoprotein A-I and A-II genes (50–53). A recent study showed rabbits expressing the human apo A-I transgene along with its PPAR response elements showed an increase in human apo A-I mRNA and mass in response to fenofibrate treatment in the absence of any peroxisome proliferative effect of the fibrate (54).

B. Delivery of redundant surface components of triglyceride-rich lipoproteins to HDL

The second mechanism for increasing HDL-cholesterol concentrations in plasma is the delivery of redundant surface phospholipid and apolipoprotein components of VLDL and chylomicrons onto HDL during hydrolysis of TG-rich particles by lipoprotein lipase (LPL) (55–57). The action of lipoprotein lipase—most active in the vascular endothelium overlying the major sites of energy usage and storage, skeletal muscle and adipocytes—is inhibited by another apolipoprotein in plasma, apoC-III. PPARα has been reported to inhibit expression of apoc-III (58,59), a protein that inhibits both the TG-hydrolyzing action of lipoprotein lipase and the uptake of TG-rich lipoprotein remnants (60,61). PPARα and γ agonists have also been found to increase LPL expression in the liver (PPARα) (62), adipocytes (62), and skeletal muscle (63) (PPARγ), and macrophages (PPARα and γ) (64,65). The combined effects of PPAR ligands on lowering apoC-III and increasing LPL increase overall hydrolysis of TG-rich lipoproteins and therefore provide additional surface components for donation to HDL particles, raising HDL levels in plasma. The overall contribution of this mechanism of HDL formation to total HDL cholesterol levels is currently unknown.

Hypertriglyceridemia of any cause can also lead to lowering of HDL cholesterol due to cholesteryl ester transfer protein (CETP)-mediated transfer of TG to HDL from TG-rich particles and displacement of HDL cholesterol (66). Another major effect of PPARα is to stimulate the β-oxidation of fatty acids in the liver (32,33,35). Increased diversion of fatty acids into β-oxidation decreases the availability of fatty-acyl CoA substrates for triglyceride synthesis, and therefore very low density lipoprotein (VLDL) secretion by the liver. The overall reduction of VLDL particle secretion into plasma induced by PPARα agonists thereby decreases the availability of TG-rich particles for CETP to transfer TG to HDL. This therefore represents another, but indirect, way that PPARα raises HDL cholesterol levels.

C. Apolipoprotein-mediated cellular lipid efflux and ABCA1

The third and rate-limiting mechanism of HDL formation is the removal of cellular phospholipids and cholesterol by lipid-free or lipid-poor HDL apolipoproteins (67). The importance of this pathway was highlighted by the discovery that, despite normal synthesis of HDL apolipoproteins (68,69), cultured cells isolated from patients with the low HDL syndrome Tangier disease failed to release both phospholipids and cholesterol to apo A-I (70,71). The extremely low HDL levels in Tangier disease suggested that apolipoprotein-mediated cellular lipid efflux, as opposed to apolipoprotein synthesis, retrieval of redundant TG-rich lipoprotein components, or passive cholesterol efflux from cells (72), was the most critical determinant of HDL particle formation. The subsequent discovery of the gene defect in Tangier disease and familial HDL deficiency—mutations in the ATP-binding cassette transporter AI (ABCA1) (73–78)—and the discovery of the regulation of ABCA1 by nuclear receptors has now generated a huge interest in the study of nuclear-receptor dependent mechanisms to raise HDL levels for the treatment of atherosclerosis.

1) Cellular location and proposed function of ABCA1

Members of the ABC transporter superfamily are involved in transmembrane transport of a large variety of substrates. They couple the energy provided by ATP hydrolysis to the transport of substrates across membranes. The ABCA1 transporter is localized to the plasma membrane, early and late endosomal, lysosomal and possibly Golgi compartments of cells (76,79,80), and is thought to actively mediate either phospholipid alone (81–83) or both phospholipid and cholesterol delivery (76,84,85) from cells to apoA-I from both intracellular and plasma membrane lipid sources (86). The widespread expression of human ABCA1 in numerous tissues (87,88), including the liver and even the vascular endothelium (89), strongly suggests the likelihood that apoA-I-mediated lipid efflux via ABCA1 occurs in numerous tissues in addition to macrophages. We have recently found that apoA-I mediates the depletion of cholesterol and phospholipids from cultured primary hepatocytes, generating HDL particles and decreasing the secretion of VLDL (G. Francis and R. Lehner, unpublished observations). These results suggest, that in addition to "peripheral" (non-hepatic) cells, the liver itself is a source of lipids for HDL formation that may then be redirected back to the liver for excretion in the "reverse" cholesterol transport pathway. The upregulation of ABCA1 for HDL formation by nuclear receptors regardless of the main tissue supplying these lipids, is therefore a promising direction to pursue in the development of new anti-atherosclerotic therapies.

2) Enhancement of ABCA1 expression by nuclear receptors

The expression of ABCA1 is tightly regulated by the cellular content of cholesterol, through oxysterol-dependent activation of LXR (90–93). An LXR response element has been identified in the human ABCA1 promoter that binds both LXRα and LXRβ and mediates transcriptional induction of this promoter by both LXR and (its heterodimer partner) RXR ligands (90,91). LXR/RXR-stimulated cholesterol efflux from macrophages, mediated through the induction of ABCA1 expression, was therefore invoked to be responsible for the dramatic reduction in atherosclerosis observed in apo$E^{-/-}$ mice treated with RXR ligands (94). Other nuclear receptor agonists, including those for PPARα and PPARγ, activate ABCA1 expression indirectly via enhanced transcription of LXRα (43,95). These in vivo data underscore the potential usefulness of synthetic LXR, PPAR or RXR agonists in raising HDL, levels for the prevention or treatment of atherosclerosis. Recently, a selective PPARβ/δ agonist has also been reported that enhances expression of ABCA1, raises HDL and improves other lipid parameters in insulin-resistant monkeys (37).

Consistent with a potential beneficial effect of pharmacological activation of LXR/RXR is the fact that the ABCA1 promoter is only suboptimally activated by oxysterols that are relatively abundant in foam cells (91). In addition, ABCA1 expression is downregulated rapidly upon HDL or apoA-I-mediated removal of lipids from cultured cells (76,87). Synthetic LXR agonists are being developed that may have the ability to increase ABCA1-dependent lipid mobilization to apoA-I and increase HDL levels clinically, and supercede the need for high cell oxysterol content to turn on ABCA1 (96–99). One concern about LXR agonists has been their propensity to increase triglyceride levels through activation of SREBP-1c (92,96) and induction of fatty acid synthase (99,100). To date, the mouse models of atherosclerosis used have shown an ability of LXR and other nuclear receptors agonists to increase ABCA1 expression and decrease atherosclerosis, but consistent effects on HDL and triglyceride levels have not been found (94) (98). Overexpression of the human ABCA1 transgene in normal mice led to an increase in HDL and decrease in atherosclerosis (101), providing further promise that enhancement of ABCA1 expression is a useful route to pursue in the development of anti-atherosclerotic therapies.

Nuclear receptor agonists that specifically enhance ABCA1 expression without inducing hypertriglyceridemia are currently being pursued. Other mechanisms of enhancing ABCA1 expression, such as the use of cyclic AMP-dependent pathways (102,103), may also prove useful as novel means to raise HDL.

D. Additional nuclear receptor effects on reverse cholesterol transport

In addition to enhancing ABCA1 expression, nuclear receptors have also been implicated in the expression of other proteins in the reverse cholesterol transport pathway that facilitate the transport of tissue-derived cholesterol back to the liver for excretion in bile. Following the delivery of phospholipids and probably some cholesterol to apoA-I via ABCA1, the nascent HDL particle dissociates from ABCA1 (104) and circulates in plasma where it is converted into larger HDL particles by deriving additional lipids from cells via passive cholesterol efflux (105), the LPL-dependent hydrolysis of TG-rich lipoproteins, and transfer of lipids from TG-rich lipoproteins via phospholipid transfer protein (PLTP) and cholesteryl ester transfer protein (CETP). It has been reported that another nuclear receptor, the farnesoid X receptor or FXR, activated by bile acids, induces the PLTP gene through FXR/RXR heterodimer binding to the PTLP gene FXR response element (106). PLTP may also be activated by PPARα, and this may explain a portion of the HDL-raising effects of fibric acid derivatives (107). CETP mediates the transfer of HDL cholesteryl esters to apoB-containing particles for return to the liver, and in exchange receives triglycerides from these particles (108). This modification of HDL by CETP makes the HDL more susceptible to hydrolysis by hepatic lipase at the hepatocyte surface, an important component of the regeneration of small HDL particles and free apoA-I that can then recirculate in the reverse cholesterol transport pathway. In this way, CETP likely represents an anti-atherogenic protein. The CETP gene has been shown to be upregulated in response to hypercholesterolemia (109). Luo et al. showed that both LXRα and LXRβ transactivate the CETP promoter in a sterol-dependent manner (110), and hence coordinately regulate the CETP-mediated delivery of HDL cholesterol esters to the liver.

The final uptake of cholesterol carried on HDL by the liver is mediated through the concerted actions of scavenger receptor B-I (SR-BI) and hepatic lipase. Whether these players in reverse cholesterol transport are activated by nuclear receptors at the hepatic level is not yet known. Although the role of SR-BI in mediating cholesterol efflux to HDL from peripheral cells remains controversial, some evidence suggests SR-BI is expressed in atherosclerotic tissue macrophages and is increased in cultured macrophages in response to both PPARα and PPARγ ligands (111).

CONCLUSIONS

The raising of HDL cholesterol levels is a major and keenly pursued target for enhancing our ability to treat and prevent vascular disease caused by atherosclerosis. The remarkable increase in our understanding of the mechanisms of HDL formation at both the cellular and subcellular levels in recent years promises to uncover several novel paths to pursue in achieving this important goal.

ACKNOWLEDGMENTS

This work was supported in part by an operating grant from the Canadian Institutes of Health Research and a Visiting Scientist Award from the Heart and Stroke Foundation of Canada. GAF is a Scholar of the Alberta Heritage Foundation for Medical Research.

REFERENCES

1. Murray CJ, Lopez AD. 1997. Mortality by cause for eight regions of the world: Global Burden of Disease Study. Lancet 349:1269–1276.
2. Rubins HB, Robins SJ, Iwane MK, Boden WE, Elam MB, Fye CL, Gordon DJ, Schaefer EJ, Schectman G, Wittes JT. 1993. Rationale and design of the Department of Veterans Affairs high density lipoprotein intervention trial (HIT) for secondary prevention of coronary artery disease in men with low high density lipoprotein cholesterol and desirable low density lipoprotein cholesterol. American Journal of Cardiology 71:45–52.
3. Francis GA, Perry RJ. 1999. Targeting HDL-mediated cellular cholesterol efflux for the treatment and prevention of atherosclerosis. Clin Chim Acta 286:219–230.
4. Fielding CJ, Fielding PE. 1995. Molecular physiology of reverse cholesterol transport. J Lipid Res 36:211–228.
5. Rubin EM, Krauss RM, Spangler EA, Verstuyft JG, Clift SM. 1991. Inhibition of early atherogenesis in transgenic mice by human apolipoprotein AI. Nature 353:265–267.
6. Plump AS, Scott CJ, Breslow JL. 1994. Human apolipoprotein A-I gene expression increases high density lipoprotein and suppresses atherosclerosis in the apolipoprotein E-deficient mouse. Proc Natl Acad Sci USA 91:9607–9611.
7. Paszty C, Maeda N, Verstuyft J, Rubin EM. 1994. Apolipoprotein AI transgene mice corrects apolipoprotein E deficiency-induced atherosclerosis in mice. J Clin Invest 94:899–903.
8. Duverger N, Kruth H, Emmanuel F, Caillaud JM, Viglietta C, Castro G, Tailleux A, Fievet C, Fruchart JC, Houdebine LM, Denefle P. 1996. Inhibition of atherosclerosis development in cholesterol-fed human apolipoprotein AI-transgenic rabbits. Circulation 94:713–717.
9. Eriksson M, Carlson LA, Miettinen TA, Angelin B. 1999. Stimulation of fecal steroid excretion after infusion of recombinant proapolipoprotein A-I: Potential reverse cholesterol transport in humans. Circulation 1000:594–598.
10. Maglich JM, Sluder A, Guan X, Shi Y, McKee DD, Carrick K, Kamdar K, Willson TM, Moore JT. 2001. Comparison of complete nuclear receptor sets from the human, Caenorhabditis elegans and Drosophila genomes. Genome Biol 2: RESEARCH0029.0021–0029.0027.
11. Robinson-Rechavi M, Carpentier AS, Duffraisse M, Laudet V. 2001. How many nuclear receptors are there in the human genome? Trends in Genetics 17:554–556.
12. Chawla A, Repa JJ, Evans RM, Mangelsdorf DJ. 2001. Nuclear receptors and lipid physiology: opening the X-files. Science 294:1866–1870.
13. Mangelsdorf DJ, Evans RM. 1995. The RXR heterodimers and orphan receptors. Cell 83:841–850.
14. Blumberg B, Evans RM. 1998. Orphan nuclear receptors—new ligands and new possibilities. Genes Dev 12:3149–3155.
15. Kliewer SA, Moore JT, Wade L, Staudinger JL, Watson MA, Jones SA, McKee DD, Oliver BB, Willson TM, Zetterstrom RH, Perlmann T, Lehmann JM. 1998. An orphan nuclear receptor activated by pregnanes defines a novel steroid signalling pathway. Cell 92:73–82.
16. Willy PJ, Mangelsdorf DJ. 1996. Unique requirements for retinoid-dependent transcriptional activation by the orphan receptor LXR. Genes & Dev 12:289–298.
17. Wiebel FF, Gustafsson J-A. 1997. Heterodimeric interaction between retinoid X receptor a and orphan receptor OR-1 reveals dimerization induced activation as a novel mechanism of nuclear receptor activation. Mol Cell Biol 17:3977–3986.
18. Aranda A, Pascual A. 2001. Nuclear hormone receptors and gene expression. Physiol Rev 81: 1269–1304.
19. Glass CK, Rosenfeld MG. 2000. The coregulator exchange in transcriptional functions of nuclear receptors. Genes Dev 14:121–141.
20. Nolte RT, Wisely GB, Westin S, Cobb JE, Lambert MH, Kurokawa R, Rosenfeld MG, Willson TM, Glass CK, Milburn MV. 1998. Ligand binding and co-activator assembly of the peroxisome proliferator-activated receptor g. Nature 395:137–143.

21. Thorp JM, Waring WS. 1962. Modification of metabolism and distribution of lipids by ethyl chlorophenoxyisobutyrate. Nature 194:948–949.
22. Hess R, Staubli W, Riess W. 1965. Nature of the hepatomegalic effect produced by ethyl chlorophenoxyisobutyrate in the rat. Nature 208:856–858.
23. Isseman I, Green S. 1990. Activation of a member of the steroid hormone receptor superfamily by peroxisome proliferators. Nature 347:645–650.
24. Graves RA, Tontonoz P, Spiegelman BM. 1992. Analysis of a tissue-specific enhancer: ARF6 regulates adipogenic gene expression. Mol Cell Biol 12:1202–1208.
25. Dreyer C, Krey G, Keller H, Givel F, Helftenbein G, Wahli W. 1992. Control of the peroxisomal b-oxidation pathway by a novel family of nuclear hormone receptors. Cell 68:879–887.
26. Schmidt A, Endo N, Rutledge SJ, Vogel R, Shinar D, Rodan GA. 1992. Identification of a new member of the steroid hormone receptor superfamily that is activated by a peroxisome proliferator and fatty acids. Mol Endocrinol 6:1634–1641.
27. Braissant O, Foufelle F, Scotto C, Dauca M, Wahli W. 1995. Differential expression of peroxisome proliferator-activated receptors (PPARs): Tissue distribution of PPAR-a, -b, and g in the adult rat. Endocrinology 137:354–366.
28. Auboeuf D, Rieusset J, Fajas L, Vallier P, Frering V, Riou JP, Laville M, Staels B, Auwerx J, Vidal H. 1997. Tissue distribution and quantification of the expression of PPARs and LXRa in humans: no alterations in adipose tissue of obese and NIDDM patients. Diabetes 46:1319–1327.
29. Chinetti G, Griglio S, Antonucci M, Torra IP, Delerive P, Majid Z, Fruchart JC, Chapman J, Najib J, Staels B. 1998. Activation of peroxisome proliferator-activated receptors alpha and gamma induces apoptosis of human monocyte-derived macrophages. J Biol Chem 273:25573–25580.
30. Inoue I, Shino K, Noji S, Awata T, Katayama S. 1998. Expression of peroxisome proliferator-activated receptor alpha (PPARa) in primary cultures of human vascular endothelial cells. Biochem Biophys Res Commun 246:370–374.
31. Staels B, Koenig W, Habib A, Merval R, Lebret M, Torra IP, Delerive P, Fadel A, Chinetti G, Fruchart JC, Najib J, Maclouf J, Tedgui A. 1998. Activation of human aortic smooth-muscle cells is inhibited by PPARalpha but not by PPARgamma activators. Nature 393:790–793.
32. Isseman I, Prince RA, Tugwood JD, Green S. 1993. The peroxisome proliferator-activated receptor: retinoic X receptor heterodimer is activated by fatty acids and fibrate hypolipidaemic drugs. Journal of Molecular Endocrinology 11:37–47.
33. Keller H, Dreyer C, Medin J, Mahfoudi A, Ozato K, Wahli W. 1993. Fatty acids and retinoids control lipid metabolism through activation of peroxisome proliferator-activated receptor-retinoid X receptor heterodimers. Proc Natl Acad Sci USA 90:2160–2164.
34. Kliewer SA, Forman BM, Blumberg B, Ong ES, Borgmeyer U, Mangelsdorf DJ, Umesono K, Evans RM. 1994. Differential expression and activation of a family of murine peroxisome proliferator-activated receptors. Proc Natl Acad Sci USA 91:7355–7359.
35. Forman BM, Chen J, Evans RM. 1997. Hypolipidemic drugs, polyunsaturated fatty acids, and eicosanoids are ligands for peroxisome proliferator-activated receptors a and d. Proc Natl Acad Sci USA 94:4312–4317.
36. Amri E-Z, Bonino F, Ailhaud G, Abumrad NA, Grimaldi PA. 1995. Cloning of a protein that mediates transcriptional effects of fatty acids in preadipocytes. J Biol Chem 270:2367–2371.
37. Oliver WR, Jr., Shenk JL, Snaith MR, Russell CS, Plunket KD, Bodkin NL, Lewis MC, Winegar DA, Sznaidman ML, Lambert MH, Xu HE, Sternbach DD, Kliewer SA, Hansen BC, Willson TM. 2001. A selective peroxisome proliferator-activated receptor delta agonist promotes reverse cholesterol transport. Proc Natl Acad Sci U S A 98:5306–5311.
38. Ijima K, Yoshizumi M, Ako J, Eto M, Kim S, Hashimoto M. 1998. Expression of peroxisome proliferator activated receptor g (PPARg) in rat smooth muscle cells. Biochem Biophys Res Commun 247:353–356.
39. Loviscach M, Rehman N, Carter L, Mudaliar S, Mohadeen P, Ciaraldi TP, Veerkamp JH, Henry RR. 2000. Distribution of peroxisome proliferator-activated receptors (PPARs) in human skeletal muscle and adipose tissue: relation to insulin action [In Process Citation]. Diabetologia 43:304–311.
40. Dubois M, Pattou F, Kerr-Conte J, Gmyr V, Vandewalle B, Desreumaux P, Auwerx J, Schoonjans K, Lefebvre J. 2000. Expression of peroxisome proliferator-activated receptor gamma (PPARgamma) in normal human pancreatic islet cells. Diabetologia 43:1165–1169.
41. Lehmann JM, Moore LB, Smith-Oliver TA, Wilkison WO, Willson TM, Kliewer SA. 1995. An antidiabetic thiazolidinedione is a high affinity ligand for Peroxisome Proliferator-Activated Receptor g (PPARg). J Biol Chem 270:12953–12956.

42. Forman BM, Tontonoz P, Chen J, Brun RP, Spiegelman BM, Evans RM. 1995. 15-Deoxy-D12,14 prostaglandin J2 is a ligand for the adipocyte determination factor PPARg. Cell 83:803–812.
43. Chawla A, Boisvert WA, Lee CH, Laffitte BA, Barak Y, Joseph SB, Liao D, Nagy L, Edwards PA, Curtiss LK, Evans RM, Tontonoz P. 2001. A PPAR gamma-LXR-ABCA1 pathway in macrophages is involved in cholesterol efflux and atherogenesis. Mol Cell 7:161–171.
44. Janowski BA, Willy PJ, Devi TR, Falck JR, Mangelsdorf DJ. 1996. An oxysterol signalling pathway mediated by the nuclear receptor LXRa. Nature 383:728–731.
45. Lehmann JM, Kliewer SA, Moore LB, Smith-Oliver TA, Oliver BB, Su JL, Sundseth SS, Winegar DA, Blanchard DE, Spencer TA, Willson TM. 1997. Activation of the nuclear receptor LXR by oxysterols defines a new hormone response pathway. J Biol Chem 272: 3137–3140.
46. Willy PJ, Umesono K, Ong ES, Evans RM, Heyman RA, Mangelsdorf DJ. 1995. LXR, a nuclear receptor that defines a distinct retinoid response pathway. Genes & Dev 9:1033–1045.
47. Apfel R, Benbrook D, Lernhardt E, Ortiz MA, Salbert G, Pfahl M. 1994. A novel orphan receptor specific for a subset of thyroid hormone-responsive elements and its interaction with the retinoid/thyroid hormone receptor subfamily. Mol Cell Biol 14:7025–7035.
48. Song C, Kokontis JM, Hiipakka RA, Liao S. 1994. Ubiquitous receptor: a receptor that modulates gene activation by retinoic acid and thyroid hormone receptors. Proc Natl Acad Sci USA 91: 10809–10813.
49. Teboul M, Enmark E, Li Q, Wikström AC, Pelto-Huikko M, Gustafsson J-A. 1995. OR-1, a member of the nuclear receptor superfamily that interacts with the 9-cis-retinoic acid receptor. Proc Natl Acad Sci USA 92:2096–2100.
50. Vu-Dac N, Schoonjans K, Laine B, Fruchart JC, Auwerx J, Staels B. 1994. Negative regulation of the human apolipoprotein A-I promoter by fibrates can be attenuated by the interaction of the peroxisome proliferator-activated receptor with its response element. J Biol Chem 269: 31012–31018.
51. Vu-Dac N, Schoonjans K, Kosykh V, Dallongeville J, Fruchart J-C, Staels B, Auwerx J. 1995. Fibrates increase human apolipoprotein A-II expression through activation of the peroxisome proliferator-activated receptor. J Clin Invest 96:741–750.
52. Vu-Dac N, Schoonjans K, Kosykh V, Dallongeville J, Heyman RA, Staels B, Auwerx J. 1996. Retinoids increase human apolipoprotein A-II expression through activation of the retinoid X receptor but not the retinoic acid receptor. Mol Cell Biol 16:3350–3360.
53. Vu-Dac N, Chopin-Delannoy S, Gervois P, Bonnelye E, Martin G, Fruchart JC, Laudet V, Staels B. 1998. The nuclear receptors peroxisome proliferator-activated receptor alpha and Rev-erbalpha mediate the species-specific regulation of apolipoprotein A-I expression by fibrates. J Biol Chem 273:25713–25720.
54. Hennuyer N, Poulain P, Madsen L, Berge RK, Houdebine LM, Branellec D, Fruchart JC, Fievet C, Duverger N, Staels B. 1999. Beneficial effects of fibrates on apolipoprotein A-I metabolism occur independently of any peroxisome proliferative response. Circulation 99:2445–2451.
55. Tall AR, Green PH, Glickman RM, Riley JW. 1979. Metabolic fate of chylomicron phospholipids and apoproteins in the rat. J Clin Invest 64:977–989.
56. Havel RJ, Kane JP. 1995. Structure and metabolism of plasma lipoproteins. In *The Metabolic and Molecular Bases of Inherited Disease*, ed. CR Scriver, Beaudet, A.L., Sly, W.S., and Valle, D., pp. 1841–1852. New York: McGraw Hill Inc.
57. Bisgaier CL, Essenburg AD, Barnett BC, Auerbach BJ, Haubenwallner S, Leff T, White AD, Creger P, Pape ME, Rea TJ, Newton RS. 1998. A novel compound that elevates high density lipoprotein and activates the peroxisome proliferator activated receptor. J Lipid Res 39:17–30.
58. Staels B, Vu-Dac N, Kosykh V, Saladin R, Fruchart JC, Dallongeville J, Auwerx J. 1995. Fibrates down-regulate apolipoprotein C-III expression independent of induction of peroxisomal Acyl Co-enzyme A Oxidase. J Clin Invest 95:705–712.
59. Haubenwallner S, Essenburg AD, Barnett BC, Pape ME, DeMattos RB, Krause BR, Minton LL, Auerbach BJ, Newton RS, Leff T, Bisgaier CL. 1995. Hypolipidemic activity of select fibrates correlates to changes in hepatic apolipoprotein C-III expression: a potential physiologic basis for their mode of action. J Lipid Res 36:2541–2551.
60. Wang CS, McConathy WJ, Kloer HU, Alaupovic P. 1985. Modulation of lipoprotein lipase activity by apolipoproteins. Effect of apolipoprotein C-III. J Clin Invest 75:384–390.
61. Shachter NS. 2001. Apolipoproteins C-I and C-III as important modulators of lipoprotein metabolism. Curr Opin Lipidol 12:297–304.

62. Schoonjans K, Peinado-Onsurbe J, Lefebvre AM, Heyman R, Briggs M, Deeb S, Staels B, Auwerx J. 1996. PPARa and PPARg activators direct a tissue-specific transcriptional response via a PPRE in the lipoprotein lipase gene. EMBO J 15:5336–5348.
63. Lapsys NM, Kriketos AD, Lim-Fraser M, Poynten AM, Lowy A, Furler SM, Chisholm DJ, Cooney GJ. 2000. Expression of genes involved in lipid metabolism correlate with peroxisome proliferator-activated receptor gamma expression in human skeletal muscle. J Clin Endocrinol Metab 85: 4293–4297.
64. Michaud SE, Renier G. 2001. Direct regulatory effect of fatty acids on macrophage lipoprotein lipase: potential role of PPARs. Diabetes 50:660–666.
65. Akiyama TE, Sakai S, Lambert G, Nicol CJ, Matsusue K, Pimprale S, Lee YH, Ricote M, Glass CK, Brewer HB, Jr., Gonzalez FJ. 2002. Conditional disruption of the peroxisome proliferator-activated receptor gamma gene in mice results in lowered expression of ABCA1, ABCG1, and apoE in macrophages and reduced cholesterol efflux. Mol Cell Biol 22:2607–2619.
66. Bruce C, Chouinard RA, Jr., Tall AR. 1998. Plasma lipid transfer proteins, high-density lipoproteins, and reverse cholesterol transport. Annu Rev Nutr 18:297–330.
67. Oram JF, Yokoyama S. 1996. Apolipoprotein-mediated removal of cellular cholesterol and phospholipids. J Lipid Res 37:2473–2491.
68. Makrides SC, Ruiz-Opazo N, Hayden M, Nussbaum AL, Breslow JL, Zannis VI. 1988. Sequence and expression of Tangier apoA-I gene. Eur J Biochem 173:465–471.
69. Kay LL, Ronan R, Schaefer EJ, Brewer HB, Jr. 1982. Tangier disease: a structural defect in apolipoprotein A-I (apoA-I Tangier). Proc Natl Acad Sci U S A 79:2485–2489.
70. Francis GA, Knopp RH, Oram JF. 1995. Defective removal of cellular cholesterol and phospholipids by apolipoprotein A-I in Tangier Disease. J Clin Invest 96:78–87.
71. Remaley AT, Schumacher UK, Stonik JA, Farsi BD, Nazih H, Brewer HB, Jr. 1997. Decreased reverse cholesterol transport from Tangier disease fibroblasts. Acceptor specificity and effect of brefeldin on lipid efflux. Arterioscler Thromb Vasc Biol 17:1813–1821.
72. Phillips MC, Gillotte KL, Haynes MP, Johnson WJ, Lund-Katz S, Rothblat GH. 1998. Mechanisms of high density lipoprotein-mediated efflux of cholesterol from cell plasma membranes. Atherosclerosis 137 Suppl: S13–S17.
73. Brooks-Wilson A, Marcil M, Clee SM, Zhang LH, Roomp K, van Dam M, Yu L, Brewer C, Collins JA, Molhuizen HO, Loubser O, Ouelette BF, Fichter K, Ashbourne-Excoffon KJ, Sensen CW, Scherer S, Mott S, Denis M, Martindale D, Frohlich J, Morgan K, Koop B, Pimstone S, Kastelein JJ, Hayden MR. 1999. Mutations in ABC1 in Tangier disease and familial high-density lipoprotein deficiency. Nat Genet 22:336–345.
74. Bodzioch M, Orso E, Klucken J, Langmann T, Bottcher A, Diederich W, Drobnik W, Barlage S, Buchler C, Porsch-Ozcurumez M, Kaminski WE, Hahmann HW, Oette K, Rothe G, Aslanidis C, Lackner KJ, Schmitz G. 1999. The gene encoding ATP-binding cassette transporter 1 is mutated in Tangier disease. Nat Genet 22:347–351.
75. Rust S, Rosier M, Funke H, Real J, Amoura Z, Piette JC, Deleuze JF, Brewer HB, Duverger N, Denefle P, Assmann G. 1999. Tangier disease is caused by mutations in the gene encoding ATP-binding cassette transporter 1. Nat Genet 22:352–355.
76. Lawn RM, Wade DP, Garvin MR, Wang X, Schwartz K, Porter JG, Seilhamer JJ, Vaughan AM, Oram JF. 1999. The Tangier disease gene product ABC1 controls the cellular apolipoprotein-mediated lipid removal pathway. J Clin Invest 104:R25–R31.
77. Marcil M, Brooks-Wilson A, Clee SM, Roomp K, Zhang LH, Yu L, Collins JA, van Dam M, Molhuizen HO, Loubster O, Ouellette BF, Sensen CW, Fichter K, Mott S, Denis M, Boucher B, Pimstone S, Genest J, Jr., Kastelein JJ, Hayden MR. 1999. Mutations in the ABC1 gene in familial HDL deficiency with defective cholesterol efflux. Lancet 354:1341–1346.
78. Brousseau ME, Eberhart GP, Dupuis J, Asztalos BF, Goldkamp AL, Schaefer EJ, Freeman MW. 2000. Cellular cholesterol efflux in heterozygotes for tangier disease is markedly reduced and correlates with high density lipoprotein cholesterol concentration and particle size. J Lipid Res 41:1125–1135.
79. Neufeld EB, Remaley AT, Demosky SJ, Stonik JA, Cooney AM, Comly M, Dwyer NK, Zhang M, Blanchette-Mackie J, Santamarina-Fojo S, Brewer HB, Jr. 2001. Cellular localization and trafficking of the human ABCA1 transporter. J Biol Chem 276:27584–27590.
80. Orso E, Broccardo C, Kaminski WE, Bottcher A, Liebisch G, Drobnik W, Gotz A, Chambenoit O, Diederich W, Langmann T, Spruss T, Luciani MF, Rothe G, Lackner KJ, Chimini G, Schmitz G. 2000. Transport of lipids from golgi to plasma membrane is defective in tangier disease patients and Abc1-deficient mice. Nat Genet 24:192–196.

81. Hamon Y, Broccardo C, Chambenoit O, Luciani MF, Toti F, Chaslin S, Freyssinet JM, Devaux PF, McNeish J, Marguet D, Chimini G. 2000. ABC1 promotes engulfment of apoptotic cells and transbilayer redistribution of phosphatidylserine. Nat Cell Biol 2:399–406.
82. Fielding PE, Nagao K, Hakamata H, Chimini G, Fielding CJ. 2000. A two-step mechanism for free cholesterol and phospholipid efflux from human vascular cells to apolipoprotein A-1. Biochemistry 39:14113–14120.
83. Wang N, Silver DL, Thiele C, Tall AR. 2001. ATP-binding cassette transporter A1 (ABCA1) functions as a cholesterol efflux regulatory protein. J Biol Chem 276:23742–23747.
84. Mendez AJ, Lin G, Wade DP, Lawn RM, Oram JF. 2001. Membrane lipid domains distinct from cholesterol/sphingomyelin-rich rafts are involved in the ABCA1-mediated lipid secretory pathway. J Biol Chem 276:3158–3166.
85. Oram JF, Lawn RM. 2001. ABCA1. The gatekeeper for eliminating excess tissue cholesterol. J Lipid Res 42:1173–1179.
86. Chen W, Silver DL, Smith JD, Tall AR. 2000. Scavenger receptor-BI inhibits ATP-binding cassette transporter 1- mediated cholesterol efflux in macrophages. J Biol Chem 275:30794–30800.
87. Langmann T, Klucken J, Reil M, Liebisch G, Luciani MF, Chimini G, Kaminski WE, Schmitz G. 1999. Molecular cloning of the human ATP-binding cassette transporter 1 (hABC1): evidence for sterol-dependent regulation in macrophages. Biochem Biophys Res Commun 257:29–33.
88. Lawn RM, Wade DP, Couse TL, Wilcox JN. 2001. Localization of human ATP-binding cassette transporter 1 (ABC1) in normal and atherosclerotic tissues. Arterioscler Thromb Vasc Biol 21:378–385.
89. Liao H, Langmann T, Schmitz G, Zhu Y. 2002. Native LDL upregulation of ATP-binding cassette transporter-1 in human vascular endothelial cells. Arterioscler Thromb Vasc Biol 22:127–132.
90. Schwartz K, Lawn R, Wade DP. 2000. ABC1 gene expression and apoA-I-mediated cholesterol efflux are regulated by LXR. Biochem Biophys Res Commun 274:794–802.
91. Costet P, Luo Y, Wang N, Tall AR. 2000. Sterol-dependent transactivation of the human ABC1 promoter by liver X receptor/retinoid X receptor. J Biol Chem 275:28240–28245.
92. Repa JJ, Liang G, Ou J, Bashmakov Y, Lobaccaro JM, Shimomura I, Shan B, Brown MS, Goldstein JL, Mangelsdorf DJ. 2000. Regulation of mouse sterol regulatory element-binding protein-1c gene (SREBP-1c) by oxysterol receptors, LXRalpha and LXRbeta. Genes Dev 14:2819–2830.
93. Venkateswaran A, Laffitte BA, Joseph SB, Mak PA, Wilpitz DC, Edwards PA, Tontonoz P. 2000. Control of cellular cholesterol efflux by the nuclear oxysterol receptor LXR alpha. Proc Natl Acad Sci U S A 97:12097–12102.
94. Claudel T, Leibowitz MD, Fievet C, Tailleux A, Wagner B, Repa JJ, Torpier G, Lobaccaro JM, Paterniti JR, Mangelsdorf DJ, Heyman RA, Auwerx J. 2001. Reduction of atherosclerosis in apolipoprotein E knockout mice by activation of the retinoid X receptor. Proc Natl Acad Sci USA 98:2610–2615.
95. Chinetti G, Lestavel S, Bocher V, Remaley AT, Neve B, Torra IP, Teissier E, Minnich A, Jaye M, Duverger N, Brewer HB, Fruchart JC, Clavey V, Staels B. 2001. PPAR-alpha and PPAR-gamma activators induce cholesterol removal from human macrophage foam cells through stimulation of the ABCA1 pathway. Nat Med 7:53–58.
96. Schultz JR, Tu H, Luk A, Repa JJ, Medina JC, Li L, Schwendner S, Wang S, Thoolen M, Mangelsdorf DJ, Lustig KD, Shan B. 2000. Role of LXRs in control of lipogenesis. Genes Dev 14:2831–2838.
97. Song C, Hiipakka RA, Liao S. 2000. Selective activation of liver X receptor alpha by 6alpha-hydroxy bile acids and analogs. Steroids 65:423–427.
98. Sparrow CP, Baffic J, Lam MH, Lund EG, Adams AD, Fu X, Hayes N, Jones AB, Macnaul KL, Ondeyka J, Singh S, Wang J, Zhou G, Moller DE, Wright SD, Menke JG. 2002. A potent synthetic LXR agonist is more effective than cholesterol loading at inducing ABCA1 mRNA and stimulating cholesterol efflux. J Biol Chem 277:10021–10027.
99. Joseph SB, Laffitte BA, Patel PH, Watson MA, Matsukuma KE, Walczak R, Collins JL, Osborne TF, Tontonoz P. 2002. Direct and indirect mechanisms for regulation of fatty acid synthase gene expression by liver X receptors. J Biol Chem 277:11019–11025.
100. Liang G, Yang J, Horton JD, Hammer RE, Goldstein JL, Brown MS. 2002. Diminished hepatic response to fasting/refeeding and liver X receptor agonists in mice with selective deficiency of sterol regulatory element-binding protein-1c. J Biol Chem 277:9520–9528.
101. Joyce CW, Amar MJ, Lambert G, Vaisman BL, Paigen B, Najib-Fruchart J, Hoyt RF, Jr., Neufeld ED, Remaley AT, Fredrickson DS, Brewer HB, Jr., Santamarina-Fojo S. 2002. The ATP binding

cassette transporter A1 (ABCA1) modulates the development of aortic atherosclerosis in C57BL/6 and apoE-knockout mice. Proc Natl Acad Sci USA 99:407–412.

102. Oram JF, Lawn RM, Garvin MR, Wade DP. 2000. ABCA1 is the cAMP-inducible apolipoprotein receptor that mediates cholesterol secretion from macrophages. J Biol Chem 275:34508–34511.
103. Takahashi Y, Miyata M, Zheng P, Imazato T, Horwitz A, Smith JD. 2000. Identification of cAMP analogue inducible genes in RAW264 macrophages. Biochim Biophys Acta 1492:385–394.
104. Wang N, Silver DL, Costet P, Tall AR. 2000. Specific Binding of ApoA-I, Enhanced Cholesterol Efflux, and Altered Plasma Membrane Morphology in Cells Expressing ABC1. J Biol Chem 275:33053–33058.
105. Rothblatt GH, Mahlberg FH, Johnson WJ, Phillips MC. 1992. Apolipoprotein, membrane cholesterol domains and the regulation of cholesterol efflux. J Lipid Res 33:1091–1097.
106. Urizar NL, Dowhan DH, Moore DD. 2000. The farnesoid X-activated receptor mediates bile acid activation of phospholipid transfer protein gene expression. J Biol Chem 275:39313–39317.
107. Bouly M, Masson D, Gross B, Jiang XC, Fievet C, Castro G, Tall AR, Fruchart JC, Staels B, Lagrost L, Luc G. 2001. Induction of the phospholipid transfer protein gene accounts for the high density lipoprotein enlargement in mice treated with fenofibrate. J Biol Chem 276:25841–25847.
108. Tall A. 1993. Plasma cholesteryl ester transfer protein. J Lipid Res 34:1255–1274.
109. Jiang XC, Agellon LB, Walsh A, Breslow JL, Tall A. 1992. Dietary cholesterol increases transcription of the human cholesteryl ester transfer protein gene in transgenic mice. Dependence on natural flanking sequences. J Clin Invest 90:1290–1295.
110. Luo Y, Tall AR. 2000. Sterol upregulation of human CETP expression in vitro and in transgenic mice by an LXR element. J Clin Invest 105:513–520.
111. Chinetti G, Gbaguidi FG, Griglio S, Mallat Z, Antonucci M, Poulain P, Chapman J, Fruchart JC, Tedgui A, Najib-Fruchart J, Staels B. 2000. CLA-1/SR-BI is expressed in atherosclerotic lesion macrophages and regulated by activators of peroxisome proliferator-activated receptors. Circulation 101:2411–2417.

Frontiers in Cardiovascular Health, edited by
N.S. Dhalla, A. Chockalingam,
H.I. Berkowitz & P.K. Singal
Kluwer Academic Publishers, Boston, 2003

Vascular Complications in Diabetes: Risk Factors and Pathogenic Correlates

Punam K. Chohan, Thomas Netticadan, and Naranjan S. Dhalla

Institute of Cardiovascular Sciences
St. Boniface General Hospital Research Centre
& Department of Physiology, Faculty of Medicine
University of Manitoba, Winnipeg, Canada

Summary. Vascular complications due to diabetes are a major cause of morbidity and mortality in the developing and the developed countries. The advent of insulin and oral hypoglycemic drugs has helped gain a better glycemic control thereby improving the quality of life and life expectancy; however, it has become necessary to gain a better insight into the various pathogenic mechanisms of different cardiovascular complications in diabetes in order to devise better and effective therapeutic tools. Although emerging and existing risk factors need to be studies and new therapeutic targets remain to be identified, hyperglycemia seems to play a major role as the initiator of various cardiovascular complications such as hypertension, atherosclerosis and insulin resistance in diabetes mellitus. It appears that oxidative stress, activation of protein kinase C and glycation of several proteins are involved in the genesis of diabetes-induced vascular complications.

***Key words*:** Hyperglycemia, protein kinase C, advanced glycation end products, reactive oxygen species, hyperlipidemia

INTRODUCTION

Diabetes mellitus (DM) is one of the most common endocrine diseases which include a group of metabolic disorders sharing the common biochemical marker of hyperglycemia. There are different types of DM that are caused by the complex

Address for Correspondence: Naranjan S. Dhalla, Institute of Cardiovascular Sciences, St. Boniface General Hospital Research Centre, 351 Tache Avenue, Winnipeg, Manitoba R2H 2A6 Canada. Tel: (204) 235-3417, Fax: (204) 233-6723, E-mail: nsdhalla@sbrc.ca.

Table 1. Classification of diabetes mellitus based on etiology

1. **Type 1 diabetes** (caused by pancreatic beta cell destruction by autoimmunity or other unknown causes, leading to absolute insulin deficiency).
2. **Type 2 diabetes** (caused by end organ receptor defect leading to insulin resistance and hyperinsulinemia). This is the more commonly encountered types of diabetes in clinical practice. It is estimated that 80–85% of diabetics have type II diabetes.
3. **Other types of diabetes caused by:**
   - Genetic defect of beta cell function and it includes maturity onset diabetes of young (MODY)
   - Genetic defect in insulin action
   - Disease pathologies affecting exocrine and endocrine pancreas
   - Adverse effects of chemicals and drugs on pancreas
   - Autoimmunity against insulin receptors
   - Diabetes associated with genetic syndromes (Down's syndrome)
4. **Maternal diabetes mellitus** (seen in pregnant women)

interaction of hereditary and environmental factors as well as lifestyle choices (Table 1). The causative factors leading to hyperglycemia are different in different types of DM and may include reduced insulin secretion from the pancreas, decreased utilization of glucose by the end organs and increased hepatic glucose production. Hyperglycemia and related biochemical abnormalities in lipid and lipoprotein metabolism produce widespread hostile environment in the body because almost every system in the body pays a heavy penalty due to this metabolic derangement. With the advent of insulin and oral hypoglycemic drugs life quality and life expectancy of diabetic patients have been improved and acute complications such as diabetic ketoacidosis and nonketotic hyperosmolar coma do not remain life threatening. But the chronic complications such as retinopathy, neuropathy, nephropathy, cardiomyopathy and vascular disease still represent a major cause of mortality and morbidity in diabetic patients. The Framingham study showed that diabetes increases the relative risk of coronary heart disease (CHD) by 66% in men and 203% in women during a period of 20 years (1). Surveys like the Diabetes Control and Complications Trials (DCCT) and United Kingdom Prospective Diabetes Study (UKPDS) have demonstrated that hyperglycemia play an important part in the pathogenesis of vascular complications (2). In this article, an attempt has been made to emphasize that hyperglycemia is the initiator of a sequence of events that manifest in multiple organ damage. Furthermore, appropriate information has been provided to show how hyperglycemia produces a diverse range of pathologies.

A. Cardiovascular risk factors in DM:

1. Hypertension

Hypertension is twice as common in diabetics (mainly type II DM) than in non-diabetics (3). It contributes to the heightened risk of cardiovascular, stroke, renal and retinal diseases and accelerates other complications of DM (4–6). Factor et al. (7) have confirmed that hypertensive diabetics suffer increased myocellular damage which may account for the higher mortality rate than seen in non diabetics. Etiologically it has been linked to insulin resistance. Increased endogenous insulin may lead to increased sodium by stimulating proximal tubular reabsorbtion, sympathetic nervous system activation and vascular hypertrophy, which may causes increased vasoconstriction and consequently lead to rise in blood pressure (8). Rigid control of hypertension results in significant reduction in morbidity and mortality from DM. This fact was confirmed in UKPDS, which showed that early treatment of even minor increase in blood pressure profoundly reduced cardiovascular complications in patients with type II diabetes, independent of the glycemic control (9). Antihypertension management should first emphasize on lifestyle modifications such as gradual weight loss, exercise, stress therapy and limiting salt intake. Antihypertensive agents should be selected based on the advantage and disadvantage of the therapeutic agent in the context of individual patients' risk profile. Commonly used antihypertensive drugs in DM are angiotensin converting enzyme inhibitors (ACEI), alpha-adrenergic blockers, calcium channel blockers (CCB), beta-blockers, thiazide diuretics, central adrenergic antagonists and vasodilators.

2. Dyslipidemia

Individuals with DM may have several forms of dyslipidemias but the most frequent pattern of altered lipid profile is modest elevation of plasma triglycerides and reduced high-density lipoproteins (HDL) levels as compared with general population. The factors that can contribute to lipid disturbances in diabetic subjects are insulin deficiency, insulin resistance, obesity, aging, high-fat diet, certain drugs or associated renal disease (10–13). Under the conditions of reduced or impaired insulin action, there is stimulation of triglyceride lipase which leads to an increase in adipose tissue lipolysis. Subsequently greater amounts of free fatty acids (FFA) are transported to liver, to augment hepatic triglyceride synthesis and to increase the production of VLDL particles. Additionally there is defective clearance of triglyceride rich lipoproteins (VLDL and chylomicron) due to the altered activity of endothelium bound lipoprotein lipase. This enzyme require the presence of insulin for its activity and is responsible for initial clearance and subsequent catabolism of lipoproteins (14). This expanded circulating VLDL-riglyceride pool drives bi-directional exchange reaction between lipoproteins to enrich LDL and HDL with triglyceride, in return for their cholesteryl ester. These triglyceride-enriched LDL and HDL particles undergo hydrolysis by hepatic lipase, which is hyperactive in type 2 DM and results in the formation of small dense LDL particles (15). These small LDL particles have increased atherogenic potential because they are easily glycated and susceptible to peroxidation (16). This may enhance their uptake by macrophages, thereby releasing specific cytokines and contributing to foam cell formation which may cause endothelial and smooth muscle cell damage (17).

3. Insulin resistance and hyperinsulinemia

Insulin resistance seen mainly in type II diabetes is characterized by reduced sensitivity of the tissues to the action of insulin. When insulin resistance exists, the body attempts to overcome this by secreting more insulin from pancreas to maintain the euglucemic status. This results in a compensatory state of hyperinsulinemia, a marker for this syndrome, and an accepted risk indicator for cardiovascular disease (CVD). It has been shown that the cardiovascular effect of hyperinsulinemia is mainly attributable to the cluster of risk factors that represent components of the metabolic or the insulin resistance syndrome [hyperinsulinemia, hypertension, dyslipidemia, central obesity, elevated levels of plasminogen activator inhibitor (PAI) and type II DM] (18,19). Two recent studies have shown that endothelial function is compromised in diabetes and inverse correlation occurs between insulin resistance and endothelial function (20,21). Whether insulin resistance is a cause or consequence of endothelial function remains to be clarified. The data showing that insulin therapy in type II diabetes can improve the forearm blood response to endothelium dependent vasodilation indicate the impact of insulin therapy on endothelial function in type II diabetes (22). Subjects with insulin resistance are at a higher risk for CVD than those with impaired β-cell secretory function (23). This was confirmed by the Funagata Diabetes Study of the Japanese population indicating that the possible clinical counterpart of insulin resistance i.e. impaired glucose tolerance (IGT) is associated with increased cardiovascular mortality as compared with a defect in the insulin secretion (24).

B. Pathogenesis of diabetic complications:

Multiple hypothesis have been put forth to explain various complications of DM. Chronic hyperglycemia acts as an initiator and accelerator of the upstream of vascular events eventually manifesting as microvascular complications such as retinopathy, neuropathy and nephropathy as well as macrovascular complications such as coronary artery disease, peripheral vascular disease and cerebrovascular disease. The deleterious effects of hyperglycemia are characteristically seen in those tissues that are not dependent on insulin for glucose entry into the cells. Increased extracellular glucose concentration causes upregulation of glucose transporters (GLUT1 and GLUT4), as a result of which the intracellular glucose concentrations also rises. This consequent increase in glycolytic flux inside the cells leads to the progression of various diabetic complications (25). Tissue injury then results from acute changes in protein structure and function and chronic changes in gene expression. The pathogenic effects induced in different tissues by these mechanisms are specific for each particular complication. Different pathways (Table 2) are proposed to overlap with one another and work in an interrelated manner. Evidence for their roles comes from the use of specific inhibitors and their beneficial effects for reducing diabetic complications.

1. Activation of protein kinase C (PKC)

Phosphorylation and dephosphorylation reactions regulate numerous biological processes such as function of contractile proteins, ion transport across the cell membrane, energy metabolism and modulation of gene expression. These reactions are

Table 2. Pathogenetic pathways involved in diabetes-induced abnormalities

1.	Activation of protein kinase C isoforms
2.	Glycation
3.	Oxidative stress
4.	Activation of polyol pathway and metabolic pseudohypoxia

catalyzed by protein kinases (that transfer phosphate group to substrate) and phosphatases (that hydrolyze protein-bound phosphate group). PKC is a calcium-phospholipid dependent kinase that phosphorylates proteins at serine/threonine residues. It was first identified two decades ago in rat brain (26). 12 isoforms of PKC have been cloned and characterized so far, of which PKC β and α appear to be activated in the aorta and heart of diabetic rats using immunoblotting approach (27,28). Increased de novo synthesis of diacylglycerol (DAG) from phosphatidic acid as a result of intracellular hyperglycemia (in the cells that use glucose independently of insulin), is the primary step leading to activation and translocation of the inactive form of PKC from cytosol to sarcolemma and thus activating it (29). A recent study has shown that diabetes induced increase in non-esterified fatty acids (NEFA), play an important role in modulating PKC in vascular cells independently of de novo DAG synthesis (30). The interaction between AGE (advanced glycation end products) and their cell surface receptors (RAGE) could also lead to activation of $PKC\beta_{II}$ (31). Activation of one or more isoforms of PKC leads to an array of biochemical changes in cellular signaling mechanisms involving cell surface receptors, enzyme systems and second messengers. The activation of PKC has been implicated as a strong candidate in the pathophysiology of diabetic micro- and macroangiopathic alterations. Such effects are caused by a wide range of unfavourable impacts on endothelial integrity, ion handling and substrate metabolism, vascular permeability, gene expression and smooth muscle growth. The in vivo administration of specific PKC inhibitors like LY290181 or LY333531 prevents glucose induced increase in endothelial permeability and corresponding microvascular blood flow in diabetic rat (38,39). Vitamin E can also ameliorate hyperglycemia induced DAG-PKC activation by activating DAG kinase, which increases the metabolism of DAG (40,41). PKC therefore may be a potential target for vascular complications and cardiomyopathy in diabetes.

2. Glycation

Reducing sugars such as glucose or fructose, react nonenzymatically with amino groups in proteins, lipids and nucleic acids to form reversible early glycosylation products termed Schiff's bases which then rearrange to form the more stable Amabori products. These undergo a slow and complex series of chemical rearrangements to form irreversible AGE which are a complex and heterogeneous group of compounds that have widespread pathological implications. Although glycation is the salient feature of physiological metabolism, rate of glycation may be increased or renal clearance is decreased in certain pathophysiological states such as in diabetes or aging. The chemical outcome of AGE reaction is the formation of covalent cross-links between stable and long lived proteins such as collagen. This is one of the central underlying processes by which they cause damage and contribute to the development of chronic vascular complication of diabetes and many other disease pathologies (42).

Several features of AGE actions have direct influence on the pathogenesis of atherosclerosis. By activating redox sensitive transcription factors NFαβ, AGEs have been shown to upregulate VCAM-I expression which mediates the adhesion of monocytes to the endothelial surface, followed by migration into the intima. This is considered to be one of the primary steps in atherogenesis. AGEs bound to lipids has prolonged half-life which contributes to the oxidation and glycoxidation and the subsequent formation of modified LDL (oxLDL) and VLDL. The modified LDL is not recognized by LDL receptors, instead it is taken up by macrophage scavenger receptor (MSR), leading to the formation of foam cells and promotion of atherosclerotic process. Using immunohistochemistry AGEs accumulation has been found on the extracellular matrix proteins and foam cells. The pathological cross-links induced by AGE on the vessel wall matrix, trap the lipoproteins and slow down the movement of cholesterol from the arterial wall towards the circulation. This results in lipoprotein accumulation and accelerates the development of atherosclerosis. By increasing vascular permeability and exerting negative influence on coagulation and fibronolytic systems, AGEs promote procoagulant state and favour atherothrombosis (50,51). Both animal studies and recently reported phase-III trials using aminoguanidine, which cleaves AGE induced chemical cross links, have shown some promise in limiting the progression of a number of diabetic complications like retinopathy, neuropathy and nephropathy (52,53).

3. Oxidative stress

Increased formation of reactive intermediates of oxygen reduction termed as reactive oxygen species (ROS) such as superoxide anions, hydrogen peroxide H_2O_2 and hydroxyl radicals in diabetes may cause oxidative damage to proteins, lipids and nucleotides. It has been shown that free radicals and the resultant oxidative stress make a significant contribution in the pathophysiology of diabetic vascular complications mainly seen in the form of dysfunctional endothelium (54–56). Several researchers have provided evidence that high glucose concentrations in endothelial and smooth muscle cells can directly lead to the formation of ROS (57,58). The molecular mechanism of biological oxidation by glucose was first identified in 1912 by Maillard (59) and is referred to as Maillard's reaction. It involves the formation of irreversible glycoxidation products of proteins and glucose termed as AGE. The most direct link of hyperglycemia to oxidative stress includes autoxidation of glucose to yield radical anions, which further reduce molecular oxygen to form superoxide anions (60). This may result in oxidation of lipids or activation of platelets (61,62).

The established association between atherosclerosis and lipid peroxidation in plasma has already been outlined. Alteration in sorbitol pathway activity, changes in the levels of inflammatory mediators and imbalance resulting from increased generation of free radicals and gradual depletion of tissue's antioxidant defense system, can also lead to the state of oxidative stress in diabetes. Very recently it has been shown that increased formation of peroxide can occur form mitochondria due to uncoupling of electron flux from the ATP synthesis in hyperglycemic condition (63). The pathogenic concept of elevated free radicals and antioxidant depletion can be indirectly inferred from the beneficial effect of vitamin E and other antioxidants in increasing the antioxidants levels, preventing the oxidation of lipids and proteins, improving endothelial functions, and increasing the efficiency of insulin (64–67).

4. Activation of polyol pathway and hyperglycemic pseudohypoxia

The polyol pathway is the biochemical pathway that converts glucose to polyol(a group of sugars including sorbitol). At physiological glucose concentrations, this pathway operates by converting aldehydes to alcohol (68). But in hyperglycemic states like DM, there is an activation of polyol pathway, which is possibly a biochemical attempt to reduce the high concentration of glucose especially in non-insulin dependent tissues like retina, lens, kidney, red blood cells, nerve tissue and endothelium (69,70). Aldose reductase (AR) is the first and the rate-limiting enzyme of this pathway that reduces glucose to sorbitol. An increased amount of sorbitol is formed which is unable to cross the cell membrane and accumulates intracellularily to produces osmotic stress. This could possibly result in cataract formation and nervous system complications (69,70). Long term effects of aldose reductase inhibitor, ponalrestat, has been shown to prevent some of the diabetic complications in rats (71). The sorbitol formation is also coupled to depletion of hydrogen donating cofactor, NADPH, essential in the regeneration of antioxidant molecules such as reduced glutathione, ascorbate and tocopherol from oxidized forms. The activity of the polyol pathway may also contribute to increase in cytosolic ratio of free $NADH^+/NAD^+$ coupled with the oxidaton of sorbitol to fructose catalyzed by sorbitol dehydrogenase (SDH). This redox state has been referred to as hyperglycemic pseudohypoxia because it causes very similar effects as produced by true hypoxia on vascular and neural function and is a feature of poorly controlled DM (68). The ratio of free NADH to NAD^+ influence the activity of various enzyme systems, therefore any increase in this ratio can drive biological reactions to form those precursors that can ultimately lead to AGE formation, PKC activation and oxidative stress. Several parameters of cellular functions are adversely affected by this redox imbalance, such as electrophysiology, contractility, hemodynamics and vascular permeability (72).

CONCLUSION

Although much progress has been made in the field of diabetes-induced vascular disease, the possible interactions between the various hyperglycemic, metabolic and biochemical pathways have not been systematically and thoroughly evaluated. Different mechanisms play a dominant role at a different stage or in different cell types and target tissues in DM. Moreover the mechanisms leading to diabetic complications in vasculature are not fully understood and no single theory has emerged that can explain all the pathologic changes. Use of specific inhibitors have largely failed to reproduce animals results. Therefore to devise an effective tool for the prevention and treatment of vascular complications in diabetes, a great understanding of the pathogenic pattern is required. Along with the tight glycemic control, which remain the cornerstone of interventions, rigorous research and treatment of independent risk factors should be pursued.

ACKNOWLEDGEMENTS

The work reported in this article was supported by the Canadian Institutes of Health Research (CIHR) Group in Experimental Cardiology. NSD holds CIHR/ Pharmaceutical Research and Development Chair in Cardiovascular Research supported by Merck Frosst of Canada.

REFERENCES

1. Kannel WB, McGee DL. 1979. Diabetes and cardiovascular risk factors: the Framingham study. Circulation 59:8–13.
2. UK Prospective Diabetes Study (UKPDS) Group. 1998. Intensive blood-glucose control with sulphonylureas or insulin compared with conventional treatment and risk of complications in patients with type 2 diabetes (UKPDS 33). Lancet 352:837–853.
3. Christlieb AR, Warram JH, Krolewski AS, Busick EJ, Ganda OP, Asmal AC, Soeldner JS, Bradley RF. 1981. Hypertension: the major risk factor in juvenile-onset insulin-dependent diabetics. Diabetes 30(Suppl 2):90–96.
4. Rosenstock J, Raskin P. 1986. Early diabetic nephropathy: assessment and potential therapeutic interventions. Diabetes Care 9:529–545.
5. Knowler WC, Bennett PH, Ballintine EJ. 1980. Increased incidence of retinopathy in diabetics with elevated blood pressure. A six-year follow-up study in Pima Indians. N Engl J Med 302:645–650.
6. MacMahon S, Peto R, Cutler J, Collins R, Sorlie P, Neaton J, Abbott R, Godwin J, Dyer A, Stamler J. 1990. Blood pressure, stroke, and coronary heart disease. Part 1. Prolonged differences in blood pressure: prospective observational studies corrected for the regression dilution bias. Lancet 335:765–774.
7. Factor SM, Borczuk A, Charron MJ, Fein FS, van Hoeven KH, Sonnenblick EH. 1996. Myocardial alterations in diabetes and hypertension. Diabetes Res Clin Pract 31(Suppl):S133–S142.
8. Semplicini A, Ceolotto G, Massimino M, Valle R, Serena L, De Toni R, Pessina AC, Dal Palu C. 1994. Interactions between insulin and sodium homeostasis in essential hypertension. Am J Med Sci 307(Suppl 1):S43–S46.
9. UK Prospective Diabetes Study Group. 1998. Tight blood pressure control and risk of macrovascular and microvascular complications in type 2 diabetes: UKPDS 38. Brit Med J 317:703–713.
10. Reaven GM, Greenfield MS. 1981. Diabetic hypertriglyceridemia: evidence for three clinical syndromes. Diabetes 30(Suppl 2):66–75.
11. Malmstrom R, Packard CJ, Caslake M, Bedford D, Stewart P, Yki-Jarvinen H, Shepherd J, Taskinen MR. 1997. Defective regulation of triglyceride metabolism by insulin in the liver in NIDDM. Diabetologia 40:454–462.
12. Pfeifer MA, Brunzell JD, Best JD, Judzewitsch RG, Halter JB, Porte D Jr. 1983. The response of plasma triglyceride, cholesterol, and lipoprotein lipase to treatment in non-insulin-dependent diabetic subjects without familial hypertriglyceridemia. Diabetes 32:525–531.
13. Lewis GF, Uffelman KD, Szeto LW, Weller B, Steiner G. 1995. Interaction between free fatty acids and insulin in the acute control of very low density lipoprotein production in humans. J Clin Invest 95:158–166.

14. De Man FH, Cabezas MC, Van Barlingen HH, Erkelens DW, de Bruin TW. 1996. Triglyceride-rich lipoproteins in non-insulin-dependent diabetes mellitus: post-prandial metabolism and relation to premature atherosclerosis. Eur J Clin Invest 26:89–108.
15. NCEP Expert Panel. 1993. Summary of the second report of the national Cholesterol Education Program (NECP) expert panel on detection, evaluation and treatment of high blood cholesterol (Adult treatment panel II). JAMA 209:3015.
16. Sattar N, Petrie JR, Jaap AJ. 1998. The atherogenic lipoprotein phenotype and vascular endothelial dysfunction. Atherosclerosis 138:229–235.
17. Heinecke JW. 1998. Oxidants and antioxidants in the pathogenesis of atherosclerosis: implications for the oxidized low density lipoprotein hypothesis. Atherosclerosis 141:1–15.
18. Lehto S, Ronnemaa T, Pyorala K, Laakso M. 2000. Cardiovascular risk factors clustering with endogenous hyperinsulinaemia predict death from coronary heart disease in patients with Type II diabetes. Diabetologia 43:148–155.
19. Pyorala M, Miettinen H, Halonen P, Laakso M, Pyorala K. 2000. Insulin resistance syndrome predicts the risk of coronary heart disease and stroke in healthy middle-aged men: the 22-year follow-up results of the Helsinki Policemen Study. Arterioscler Thromb Vasc Biol 20:538–544.
20. Laight DW, Carrier MJ, Anggard EE. 2000. Antioxidants, diabetes and endothelial dysfunction. Cardiovasc Res 47:457–464.
21. Cullen P. 2000. Evidence that triglycerides are an independent coronary heart disease risk factor. Am J Cardiol 86:943–949.
22. Vehkavaara S, Makimattila S, Schlenzka A, Vakkilainen J, Westerbacka J, Yki-Jarinen H. 2000. Insulin therapy improves endothelial function in type 2 diabetes. Arterioscler Thromb Vasc Biol 20:545–550.
23. Tominaga M, Eguchi H, Manaka H, Igarashi K, Kato T, Sekikawa A. 1999. Impaired glucose tolerance is a risk factor for cardiovascular disease, but not impaired fasting glucose. The Funagata Diabetes Study. Diabetes Care 22:920–924.
24. Haffner SM, Mykkanen L, Festa A, Burke JP, Stern MP. 2000. Insulin-resistant prediabetic subjects have more atherogenic risk factors than insulin-sensitive prediabetic subjects: implications for preventing coronary heart disease during the prediabetic state. Circulation 101:975–980.
25. Kaiser N, Sasson S, Feener EP, Boukobza-Vardi N, Higashi S, Moller DE, Davidheiser S, Przybylski RJ, King GL. 1993. Differential regulation of glucose transport and transporters by glucose in vascular endothelial and smooth muscle cells. Diabetes 42:80–89.
26. Inoue M, Kishimoto A, Takai Y, Nishizuka Y. 1977. Studies on a cyclic nucleotide-independent protein kinase and its proenzyme in mammalian tissues. II. Proenzyme and its activation by calcium-dependent protease from rat brain. J Biol Chem 252:7610–7616.
27. Inoguchi T, Battan R, Handler E, Sportsman JR, Heath W, King GL. 1992. Preferential elevation of protein kinase C isoform beta II and diacylglycerol levels in the aorta and heart of diabetic rats: differential reversibility to glycemic control by islet cell transplantation. Proc Natl Acad Sci USA 89:11059–11063.
28. Kunisaki M, Bursell SE, Umeda F, Nawata H, King GL. 1994. Normalization of diacylglycerol-protein kinase C activation by vitamin E in aorta of diabetic rats and cultured rat smooth muscle cells exposed to elevated glucose levels. Diabetes 43:1372–1377.
29. Xia P, Inoguchi T, Kern TS, Engerman RL, Oates PJ, King GL. 1994. Characterization of the mechanism for the chronic activation of diacylglycerol-protein kinase C pathway in diabetes and hypergalactosemia. Diabetes 43:1122–1129.
30. Lu X, Yang XY, Howard RL, Walsh JP. 2000. Fatty acids modulate protein kinase C activation in porcine vascular smooth muscle cells independently of their effect on de novo diacylglycerol synthesis. Diabetologia 43:1136–1144.
31. Scivittaro V, Ganz MB, Weiss MF. 2000. AGEs induce oxidative stress and activate protein kinase C-beta(II) in neonatal mesangial cells. Am J Physiol Renal Physiol 278:F676–F683.
32. Park JY, Takahara N, Gabriele A, Chou E, Naruse K, Suzuma K, Yamauchi T, Ha SW, Meier M, Rhodes CJ, King GL. 2000. Induction of endothelin-1 expression by glucose: an effect of protein kinase C activation. Diabetes 49:1239–1248.
33. Ikeda U, Takahashi M, Shimada K. 1998. Monocyte-endothelial cell interaction in atherogenesis and thrombosis. Clin Cardiol 21:11–14.
34. Kreuzer J, Denger S, Schmidts A, Jahn L, Merten M, von Hodenberg E. 1996. Fibrinogen promotes monocyte adhesion via a protein kinase C dependent mechanism. J Mol Med 74:161–165.
35. Williams B. 1995. Glucose-induced vascular smooth muscle dysfunction: the role of protein kinase C. J Hypertens 13:477–486.

36. Liu X, Wang J, Takeda N, Binaglia L, Panagia V, Dhalla NS. 1999. Changes in cardiac protein kinase C activities and isozymes in streptozotocin-induced diabetes. Am J Physiol 277:E798–E804.
37. Stasek JE Jr, Patterson CE, Garcia JG. 1992. Protein kinase C phosphorylates caldesmon77 and vimentin and enhances albumin permeability across cultured bovine pulmonary artery endothelial cell monolayers. J Cell Physiol 153:62–75.
38. Birch KA, Heath WF, Hermeling RN, Johnston CM, Stramm L, Dell C, Smith C, Williamson JR, Reifel-Miller. 1996. ALY290181, an inhibitor of diabetes-induced vascular dysfunction, blocks protein kinase C-stimulated transcriptional activation through inhibition of transcription factor binding to a phorbol response element. Diabetes 45:642–650.
39. Ishii H, Koya D, King GL. 1998. Protein kinase C activation and its role in the development of vascular complications in diabetes mellitus. J Mol Med 76:21–31.
40. Tran K, Proulx PR, Chan AC. 1994. Vitamin E suppresses diacylglycerol (DAG) level in thrombin-stimulated endothelial cells through an increase of DAG kinase activity. Biochim Biophys Acta 1212:193–202.
41. Lee IK, Koya D, Ishi H, Kanoh H, King GL. 1999. d-Alpha-tocopherol prevents the hyperglycemia induced activation of diacylglycerol (DAG)-protein kinase C (PKC) pathway in vascular smooth muscle cell by an increase of DAG kinase activity. Diabetes Res Clin Pract 45:183–190.
42. Bucala R. 1997. Lipid and lipoprotein modification by advanced glycosylation end-products: role in atherosclerosis. Exp Physiol 1997; 82:327–337.
43. Kunt T, Forst T, Wilhelm A, Tritschler H, Pfuetzner A, Harzer O, Engelbach M, Zschaebitz A, Stofft E, Beyer J. 1999. Alpha-lipoic acid reduces expression of vascular cell adhesion molecule-1 and endothelial adhesion of human monocytes after stimulation with advanced glycation end products. Clin Sci (Lond) 96:75–82.
44. Hoff HF, Whitaker TE, O'Neil J. 1992. Oxidation of low-density lipoprotein leads to particle aggregation and altered macrophage recognition. J Biol Chem 267:602–609.
45. Mamo JC, Szeto L, Steiner G. 1990. Glycation of very low-density lipoprotein from rat plasma impairs its catabolism. Diabetologia 33:339–345.
46. Sobal G, Sinzinger H, Menzel EJ. 1999. Binding of long-term glycated low-density lipoprotein and AGE-albumin by peripheral monocytes and endothelial cells. J Recept Signal Transduct Res 19: 267–281.
47. Stitt AW, He C, Friedman S, Scher L, Rossi P, Ong L, Founds H, Li YM, Bucala R, Vlassara H. 1997. Elevated AGE-modified ApoB in sera of euglycemic, normolipidemic patients with atherosclerosis: relationship to tissue AGEs. Mol Med 3:617–627.
48. Bierhaus A, Hofmann MA, Ziegler R, Nawroth PP. 1998. AGEs and their interaction with AGE-receptors in vascular disease and diabetes mellitus. I. The AGE concept. Cardiovasc Res 37:586–600.
49. Chappey O, Dosquet C, Wautier MP, Wautier JL. 1997. Advanced glycation end products, oxidant stress and vascular lesions. Eur J Clin Invest 27:97–108.
50. Dahl-Jorgenson K. 1998. Biochemical markers of diabetic microangiopatthy. Past, present and future. Horm Res 50(Suppl):12–16.
51. Steano A, Davi G, Patrono C. 1991. In vivo platelet activation in diabetes mellitus. Semin Thromb Hemost 17:422–425.
52. Vlassara H. 1996. Advanced glycation end products and atherosclerosis. Ann Med 28:419–426.
53. Ulrich P, Zhang X. 1997. Pharmacological reversal of advanced glycation end-product-mediated protein crosslinking. Diabetologia 40(Suppl 2):S157-S159.
54. Giugliano D, Cerrello A. 1996. Oxidative stress and diabetic vascular complications. Diabetes Care 19:257–267.
55. Tesfamarium B. 1994. Free radicals in diabetic endothelial cell dysfunction. Free Radic Biol Med 16:383–391.
56. Pieper GM, Gross GJ. 1998. Oxygen free radicals abolish endothelium dependent relaxation in diabetic rat aorta. Am J Physiol 255:H825–H833.
57. Dux L, Stockklauser-Farber K, Rosen P. 1999. Generation of reactive oxygen intermediates, activation of NFKappaB, and induction if apoptosis in human endothelial cells by glucose: Role of nitric oxide synthase? Free Rad Med Biol 27:752–763.
58. Graier WF, Simecek S, Kukuvetz WR, Kostner GM. 1996. High-glucose induced changes in endothelial Ca^{2+}/EDRF signalling are due to generation of superoxide anions. Diabetes 45: 1386–1395.
59. Maillard LC. 1912. Acton des adices amines sur les sucres: formation des melanoidines par voie methodique. CR Hebd Seances Acad Sci 154:66–68.

60. Wolff SP, Dean RT. 1987. Glucose autoxidation and protein modification. The potential role of "autoxidative glycosylation" in diabetes. Biochem J 245:243–250.
61. Keaney Jr JF. 1994. Antioxidant protection of low-density lipoprotein and its role in the prevention of atherosclerotic vascular disease. In: Natural Antioxidant in Human Health and Disease, Academic Press, San Diego, pp. 303–352.
62. Salvemini D, de Nucci G, Sneddon JM, Vane JR. 1989. Superoxide anions enhance platelet adhesion and aggregation. Br J Pharmacol 97:1145–1150.
63. Nishikawa T, Edelstein D, Du XL, Yamagishi S, Matsumura T, Kaneda Y, Yorek MA, Beebe D, Oates PJ, Hammes HP, Giardino I, Brownlee M. 2000. Normalizing mitochondrial superoxide production blocks three pathways of hyperglycaemic damage. Nature 404:787–790.
64. Douillet C, Chancerelle Y, Cruz C, Maroncles C, Kergonou JF, Renaud S, Ciavatti M. 1993. High dosage vitamin E effect on oxidative status and serum lipids distribution in streptozotocin-induced diabetic rats. Biochem Med Metab Biol 50:265–276.
65. Paolisso G, D'Amore A, Giugliano D, Ceriello A, Varricchio M, D'Onofrio F. 1993. Pharmacologic doses of vitamin E improve insulin action in healthy subjects and non-insulin-dependent diabetic patients. Am J Clin Nutr 57:650–656.
66. Ting HH, Timimi FK, Boles KS, Creager SJ, Ganz P, Creager MA. 1996. Vitamin C improves endothelium-dependent vasodilation in patients with non-insulin-dependent diabetes mellitus. J Clin Invest 97:22–28.
67. Bierhaus A, Chevion S, Chevion M, Hofmann M, Quehenberger P, Illmer T, Luther T, Berentshtein E, Tritschler H, Muller M, Wahl P, Ziegler R, Nawroth PP. 1997. Advanced glycation end product-induced activation of NF-kappaB is suppressed by alpha-lipoic acid in cultured endothelial cells. Diabetes 46:1481–1490.
68. Williamson JR, Chang K, Frangos M, Hasan KS, Ido Y, Kawamura T, Nyengaard JR, van den Enden M, Kilo C, Tilton RG. 1993. Hyperglycemic pseudohypoxia and diabetic complications. Diabetes 42:801–813.
69. Wyngaarden JB (ed.). 1985. Cecil's Textbook of Medicine, 17th ed. WB Saunders, Philadelphia.
70. Thomas JH, Gillhab B (eds). 1989. Will's Biochemical Basis of Medicine, 2nd ed. Kent, Butterworth & Co Ltd.
71. Sima AA, Prashar A, Zhang WX, Chakrabarti S, Greene DA. 1990. Preventive effects of long term aldose reductase inhibitor (ponalrestol) on nerve conduction, several nerve structures in the spontaneously diabetic Bio-Breeding rat. J Clin Invest 85:1410–1420.
72. Pugliese G, Tilton RG, Williamson JR. 1991. Glucose-induced metabolic imbalances in the pathogenesis of diabetic vascular disease. Diabetes Metab Rev 7:35–59.

Frontiers in Cardiovascular Health, edited by
N.S. Dhalla, A. Chockalingam,
H.I. Berkowitz & P.K. Singal
Kluwer Academic Publishers, Boston, 2003

Hypercholesterolemia and Cardiovascular Risk in Diabetic Patients

Chiara Bolego,[1,2] Andrea Poli,[1] and Rodolfo Paoletti[2]

[1] *Nutrition Foundation of Italy, Via S Pietro all'Orto, 17, 20121 Milan, Italy*
[2] *Department of Pharmacological Sciences, Via Balzaretti, 9, 20133 Milan, Italy*

Summary. The present paper will emphasize the relative importance of cardiovascular disease (CVD) incidence and treatment in diabetic patients. As a result from epidemiological and intervention studies, diabetics have been included in the highest risk category for the development of cardiovascular diseases, which represent also the major cause of death for these patients. The relatively slight reduction of cardiovascular morbidity and mortality in diabetic patients achieved by pharmacological control of blood glucose levels stresses the relevance of other risk factors such as LDL- and HDL-cholesterol levels for the occurrence of CVD in diabetes. According to the Third Report of the National Cholesterol Education Program, the maintenance of LDL cholesterol levels within the target level of 100 mg/dL by both life-style modifications and the use of lipid-lowering agents will further improve CVD morbidity and mortality in diabetic patients.

***Key words*:** diabetes, cardiovascular heart disease, atherosclerosis, risk factors, guidelines.

INTRODUCTION

Diabetes represents an independent risk factor for the development of atherosclerotic disease. Cardiovascular diseases, which include coronary heart disease (CHD), cerebrovascular disease and peripheral vascular disease, also occur with higher than normal frequency in diabetes and are the major cause of morbidity and death in diabetic patients. Endothelial damage and vascular dysfunction represent the initial

Author for correspondence: Prof. Rodolfo Paoletti, Department of Pharmacological Sciences, University of Milan, Via Balzaretti, 9, 20133 Milan, Italy. Phone: ++39 2 5031838, Fax: ++39 2 50318266, E-mail: rodolfo.paoletti@unimi.it.

steps of the formation of atherosclerotic lesions in diabetes. The most important factors involved in the onset and progression of diabetic vascular dysfunction are: a) excessive production of triglyceride-rich lipoproteins, which are associated with a higher risk of coronary artery disease (1); b) presence of small, dense LDL particles, which are cytotoxic for endothelial cells and exert a higher susceptibility to oxidation (2,3); c) increased oxidative stress linked to hyperglycaemia and the formation of AGEs (advanced glycosylation end-products) (4,5); d) decrease of serum HDL, which exhibits an antiatherogenic and antioxidant potential (6). Oxidative stress is also responsible for enhanced NO inactivation, further interfering with the maintenance of a functional endothelium (7).

Cardiovascular risk in diabetic patients is likely to be multifactorial in origin and the modified lipid and lipoprotein profile along with glucose intolerance represent the most relevant factors called into question to predict and prevent CHD in diabetes (8–10).

Results from several observational studies clearly indicate the relevance of cardiovascular morbidity and mortality associated with atherosclerosis in diabetes, which is decreased less than expected by achieving an intensive blood-glucose control by either insulin or sulphanylureas (11).

On the other hand, treatment of diabetic patients with either high or average cholesterol levels with hypolipidemic agents, such as statins, significantly reduces the frequency of coronary events (12,13).

Accordingly, the Third Report of the National Cholesterol Education Program (ATP III) outlines the relevance of cardiovascular disease prevention in diabetic patients, who are included in the high-risk patients, with a suggested LDL-cholesterol goal of ≤100 mg/dl to be achieved first with lifestyle changes and then with LDL-lowering therapy (14).

CORONARY HEART DISEASE IN DIABETES: OBSERVATIONAL STUDIES

In diabetics, cardiovascular disease mortality greatly exceeds mortality for all other causes. In the USA, where diabetes is the fourth most common cause of death, cardiovascular diseases, and CHD in particular, account for as much as 75% of all mortality in type 2 diabetes, and only 10% to 12% of deaths are related to specific complications of diabetes (15). Results from the Framingham study indicate that the relative risk to develop CHD is greater for diabetic women with respect to diabetic men, thus fading the difference in CHD incidence observed between men and premenopausal women (16). This may be related to the loss of estrogen protection in terms of cardiovascular morbidity and mortality, which is observed in premenopausal non-diabetic women with respect to men (17). In particular, the incidence of cardiovascular disease among diabetic men was roughly twice that observed among the non-diabetic counterparts. Among diabetic women, the incidence of coronary events was almost three times as high as that among non-diabetic women.

More recent data from the Strong Heart Study performed in a native US population further confirm that diabetics have an increased risk for CVD morbidity and mortality when compared to non-diabetic subjects, irrespective of gender. Moreover, this study showed that lethality is greater in diabetics with CVD than in non diabetic patients affected by the same disease (10).

In a small population study from Finland, diabetic patients without previous myocardial infarction were shown to have a similar risk of all-cause mortality to non-diabetic patients with previous myocardial infarction in a 7-years follow-up (18). Moreover, diabetic patients with a history of myocardial infarction at baseline had the worst prognosis and 50% of these patients at the end of the follow-up period were dead (18). Similar data have been recently obtained in a large cohort study of US male physicians. These data indicate that diabetes is associated with a substantial increase in all-cause and CHD mortality. For all-cause mortality, the magnitude of excess risk conferred by diabetes is similar to that conferred by a history of CHD; for mortality from CHD, a history of CHD is a more potent predictor of death. However, the presence of both diabetes and CHD identifies a particular high-risk group (19).

The high cardiovascular mortality reported in Haffner's and Lotufo's studies for diabetic patients with previous CHD is in accordance with results from other observational studies. Indeed, it has been widely reported that diabetic patients who have experienced CHD have a poorer long-term prognosis than non-diabetic patients with CHD. For both men and women with CHD, diabetes is associated with a significant higher risk of cardiovascular death (20).

Therefore, current clinical evidence provides a rationale for treating cardiovascular risk factors in diabetic patients as aggressively as in non-diabetic patients with prior myocardial infarction. In particular, the high mortality rate in diabetics after the first myocardial infarction further confirms the importance of a primary prevention treatment in these population group.

Interestingly, by comparing heart disease mortality trends in the US population, a smaller decline in mortality for diabetic patients with respect to patients without diabetes has been observed. Indeed, during the period 1971–1993, non-diabetic men experienced a 36% decline in age-adjusted heart disease mortality compared with a 13% decline for diabetic men. Moreover, heart disease mortality declined by 27% in non-diabetic women but increased by 23% in diabetic women (21). One could expect that the improvement of medical strategies to prevent and treat coronary disease in diabetes could have a beneficial impact in reducing CHD mortality also in diabetics.

CORONARY HEART DISEASE IN DIABETES: INTERVENTION STUDIES

The efficacy of pharmacological therapies for the treatment and prevention of CHD in diabetes has been evaluated in several controlled studies. The UK Prospective Diabetes Study (UKPDS) analyzed the effect of intensive blood-glucose control with either sulphanylurea or insulin on the risk of microvascular and macrovascular complications in patients with type 2 diabetes. Overall, glycemic control substantially decreased the risk of microvascular complications. There was evidence, albeit inconclusive, of a small risk reduction also for fatal and non-fatal myocardial infarction, but diabetes-related mortality and all-cause mortality were not modified by controlling blood glucose levels (11). These data suggest that the pharmacological control of other predictors of CHD impaired by diabetes, such as the blood pressure and the lipid profile, may improve the prognosis and outcome of diabetic patients.

Type 2 diabetic patients show frequent lipid abnormalities characterized by increased triglycerides and decreased HDL-cholesterol levels as well as by qualitative and metabolic abnormalities of all lipoprotein classes (22).

The prevalence of dyslipidemia in insulin-dependent type-1 diabetic patients is similar to that observed in the non-diabetic population. However, the excess risk conferred by dyslipidemia in diabetics is higher than in non-diabetic patients, thus encouraging a vigorous control of the lipid profile in diabetes (23).

The Strong Heart Study evaluated the role of lipid levels as a risk factor for the development of cardiovascular disease in diabetes. In this analysis both LDL and HDL cholesterol were strong independent predictors of CHD in a diabetic population. There was a linear correlation between the LDL cholesterol levels and the increase in CVD risk. In particular, the incidence rate for CVD in diabetic men and women was higher in those with LDL cholesterol level >100 mg/dL compared with those with levels <100 mg/dL. HDL cholesterol had a strong inverse effect, with a 10-mg/dL decrease in HDL cholesterol associated with a 22% increase in CVD risk (10).

Statins are efficacious and potent hypolipidemic drugs with a pharmacological profile which could well counteract diabetes-associated lipid abnormalities, thus likely reducing the number of cardiovascular events and improving the life expectancy of diabetic patients.

Results from intervention studies in diabetic patients treated with statins are promising. The efficacy of a hypocholesterolemic treatment with simvastatin has been evaluated in a post-hoc subgroup analysis on diabetic patients participating in the Scandinavian Simvastatin Survival Study (4S). A significant decrease was found in the incidence of major CHD events (CHD death or nonfatal myocardial infarction) between diabetic patients on simvastatin treatment (20 or 40 mg/die) with respect to placebo-treated patients (Relative Risk, RR = 0.45, $p < 0.002$). As for all-cause mortality, the difference between simvastatin- and placebo-treated patients did not reach statistical significance, probably because of the relatively small number of patients enrolled in the study (n = 200) (RR = 0.57, $p < 0.09$). However, it is worth mentioning that the absolute clinical benefit achieved by cholesterol lowering may be greater in diabetic than in non-diabetic patients with CHD because diabetic patients have a higher absolute risk of recurrent CHD events and other atherosclerotic events. In particular, remarkable differences in relative risks between diabetic and non-diabetic patients treated with simvastatin were observed for cerebrovascular events (RRs 0.8 and 0.4 for non-diabetics and diabetics, respectively) and for major coronary events (RRs 0.65 and 0.45 for non-diabetics and diabetics, respectively) (12).

The Cholesterol and Recurrent Events trial (CARE) evaluated the effect of a lipid lowering therapy with pravastatin versus placebo in about 600 patients with clinical diagnosis of diabetes and average cholesterol levels (136 mg/dL). Pravastatin tretament (40 mg/die) reduced the absolute risk of coronary events for diabetic and non-diabetic patients by 8% and 5% and the relative risk by 25% ($p = 0.05$) and 23% ($p < 0.001$), respectively. Thus, even though the predominant lipid abnormality in diabetic patients is the combination of high triglycerides and low HDL, a therapeutic strategy aimed at lowering LDL cholesterol has major benefit. (13).

In the recent Heart Protection study with a 5-year follow-up period, about 20,000 high risk patients have been enrolled and randomized to simvastatin 40 mg/die or placebo treatment. In diabetic patients free of previuos CHD randomized to active treatment, a significant reduction of major cardiovascular end-points observed (RR = 0.8) (24). This data have shown for the first time in a large cohort study the efficacy of statin treatment in diabetic patients in primary prevention.

Several clinical studies, which further evaluate the effects of lipid lowering therapies in diabetic patients, are still ongoing. The Collaborative Atorvastatin Diabetes Study (CARDS) and the Atorvastatin Study for Prevention of Coronary Heart Disease Endpoints in NIDDM (ASPEN) will assess the efficacy of atorvastatin treatment on the reduction of cardiovascular events in diabetes.

Moreover, the potential beneficial effect of pravastatin treatment in older diabetic patients is currently under evaluation in the Antihypertensive and Lipid Lowering Treatment to Prevent Heart Attack Trial (24).

Results from all these studies will provide important information on which therapy could be the best and most efficacious for the management of diabetes.

CHOLESTEROL CONTROL IN DIABETES: PROPOSAL OF THE NATIONAL CHOLESTEROL EDUCATION PROGRAM IN USA (ATP III)

As previously mentioned, the Third Report of The Expert Panel on Detection, Evaluation, and Treatment of Cholesterol (Adult Treatment Panel III or ATP III), which constitutes the National Cholesterol Education Program's USA guidelines for cholesterol management, has been recently published (14).

ATP III updated the recommendation for use of an hypocholesterolemic therapy (25), accordingly to novel evidences from recent clinical trials.

ATP III basic principle for prevention is that the intensity of risk-reduction therapies (both dietetic and pharmacological) should be adjusted to a person's absolute risk to develop cardiovascular diseases.

Indeed, the major new features of ATP III are the focus on primary prevention in subjects with multiple risk factors and the proposal for more aggressive LDL-lowering therapy, previously adopted in secondary prevention, in certain group of patients considered at high cardiovascular risk (e.g. diabetics). Risk determinants in addition to LDL cholesterol levels and major cardiovascular risk factors (hypertension, smoking, abdominal obesity) include the presence or absence of CHD and other clinical forms of atherosclerotic disease. Table 1 reports total, LDL and HDL cholesterol considered to be optimal according to the ATP III guidelines.

Table 1. ATP III classification of LDL, total and HDL cholesterol (mg/dL)

LDL Cholesterol	
<100	Optimal
100–129	Near or above optimal
130–159	Borderline high
160–189	High
≥190	Very high
Total Cholesterol	
<200	Desiderable
200–239	Borderline high
≥240	High
HDL Cholesterol	
<40	Low
≥60	High

Table 2. Optimal values of LDL- and HDL-cholesterol in relation to coronary risk

Risk Category	LDL Cholesterol (mg/dL)	Non-HDL Cholesterol (mg/dL)
CHD or CHD risk equivalents (es. DIABETES)	<100	<130
≥2 Risk factors*	<130	<160
0–1 Risk factors	<160	<190

* smoking, blood pressure >140/190 mmHg, HDL-C <40 mg/dL, familial history of CHD, age.

ATP III identifies 3 categories of risk that modify the goals and modalities of LDL-lowering therapy (Table 2). The category at highest risk consists of persons who already experienced CHD, CVD, peripheral vascular disease, aortic aneurism or carry a 10-years risk to develop CHD >20% (more than 20 of 100 such individuals will develop CHD or have a recurrent CHD event within 10 years).

Accordingly to previously described observational and intervention trials, diabetic patients have been included in the highest risk category and a more intensive prevention strategy has been warrented for these patients. LDL cholesterol goals vary in relation to the CHD risk categories (the higher is the risk to develop CHD, the lower is the LDL cholesterol goal, see Table 2). Indeed ATP III established that for diabetics, similar to patients in secondary prevention, the lowest LDL cholesterol goal is <100 mg/dL.

Besides and in addition to an LDL-lowering therapy, ATP III recommends a multifaceted lifestyle approach, in relation to LDL-cholesterol levels at baseline for each risk-category described (Table 3). In particular, diabetic patients with LDL-cholesterol levels ≥130 mg/dL are encouraged to start hypocholesterolemic therapy, whereas for LDL-cholesterol ≥100 mg/dl a therapeutic lifestyle modification (diet,

Table 3. LDL cholesterol and cutpoints for therapeutic lifestyle changes and drug therapy in different risk categories

	LDL Goal (mg/dL)	LDL level at which to initiate therapeutic lifestyle changes (mg/dL)*	LDL level at which to consider drug therapy (mg/dL)
CHD or CHD risk equivalents (es. DIABETES)	<100	≥100	≥130 (100–129: drug optional)
≥2 Risk factors	<130	≥130	130–160
0–1 Risk factors	<160	≥160	≥190

*reduced intakes with diet of saturated fats and cholesterol; therapeutic options for enhancing LDL lowering such as plant sterols, stanols and viscous fiber; increased physical activity; weight reduction.

physical activity, etc.) could be considered before or in association with an hypocholesterolemic therapy.

As for diabetic patients with hypertriglyceridemia, ATP III guidelines suggest to take as a target non-HDL cholesterol levels, which are calculated by the difference between total and HDL choleterol values. The goal for non-HDL cholesterol in diabetics with high serum trygligerides can be set at 30 mg/dL higher than that for LDL-cholesterol (Table 2). Since ATP III has fixed LDL goal for diabetics at 100 mg/dL, an accepatable triglyceride value should be considered 150 mg/dL. According to Friedewald's equation, triglycerides (as VLDL-cholesterol) contribute to cholesterol calculation for 30 mg/dL.

CONCLUSIONS

Results from observational studies clearly indicate that cardiovascular disease represents the major cause of morbidity and death among diabetic patients. Furthermore, clinically manifest CHD has a worse prognosis in diabetic than in non-diabetic subjects.

LDL and HDL-cholesterol levels, more than plasma glucose levels, may be taken as a marker for coronary events in diabetes.

According to results from available clinical studies, new guidelines for cholesterol management and control (ATP III) include diabetics in the group of high-risk patients and set the optimal LDL cholesterol value for these subjects at 100 mg/dL. Therefore, along with life-style modifications, HMG-CoA reductase inhibitors may represent a first choice class of drugs to treat diabetic patients in order to prevent cardiovascular diseases.

Data from ongoing intervention trials with statins will shed light on the clinical relevance of extending statin use in diabetes, by assessing the impact of cholesterol control on cardiovascular morbidity and mortality in this pathological condition.

REFERENCES

1. Hennig B, Chung BH, Watkins BA, Alvarado A. 1992. Disruption of endothelial barrier function by lypolitic remnants of triglyceride-rich lipoproteins. Atherosclerosis 95:235–247.
2. Tan KC, Ai VH, Chow WS, Chau MT, Leong L, Lam KS. 1999. Influence of low density lipoprotein (LDL) subfraction profile and LDL oxidation on endothelium-dependent and independent vasodilation in patients with type 2 diabetes. J Clin Endocrinol Metab 84:3212–3216.
3. Vakkilainen J, Makimattila S, Seppala-Lindroos A, Vehkavaara S, Lahdenpera S, Groop PH, Taskinen MR, Yki-Jarvinen H. 2000. Endothelial dysfunction in men with small LDL particles. Circulation 102(7):716–21.
4. Giuliano D, Coppola L. 1997. Stress ossidativo e complicanze diabetiche: un possibile nesso patogenetico. Giornale Italiano Diabetologia 17:11–123.
5. Williams SB, Goldfine AB, Timimi FK, Ting HH, Roddy MA, Simonson DC, Creager MA. 1998. Acute hyperglycemia attenuates endothelium-dependent vasodilation in humans in vivo. Circulation 97:1695–701.
6. Syvanne M, Taskinen MR. 1997. Lipids and lipoprotein as coronary risk factors in non-insulin dependent diabetes mellitus. Lancet 350(1):20–23.
7. Honig MLH, Morrison PJ, Banga JD, Stroes ESG, Rabelink TJ. 1998. Nitric oxide availability in diabetes mellitus. Diabetes Met Rev 14:241–249.
8. Fontbonne AM, Eschwege EM. 1991. Insulin and cardiovascular disease. Paris Prospective Study. Diabetes Care 14:461–469.
9. McNeill KL, Fontana L, Russell-Jones DL, Rajman I, Ritter JM, Chowienczyk PJ. 2000. Inhibitory effects of low-density lipoproteins from men with type II diabetes on endothelium-dependent relaxation. J Am Coll Cardiol 35:1622–1627.
10. Howard BV, Robbins DC, Sievers ML, Lee ET, Rhoades D, Devereux RB, Cowan LD, Gray RS, Welty TK, Go OT, Howard WJ. 2000. LDL cholesterol as a strong predictor of coronary heart disease in diabetic individuals with insulin resistance and low LDL. The Strong Heart Study. Arterioscler Thromb Vasc Biol 20:830–835.
11. UKPDS Group. (UKPDS 33). 1998. UK Prospective Diabetes Study. Lancet 352:837–865.
12. Pyörälä K, Pedersen TR, Kjeksus J, Faergeman O, Olsson AG, Thorgeirsson G. 1997. Cholesterol lowering with simvastatin improves prognosis of diabetic patients with coronary heart disease: a subgroup analysis of the Scandinavian Simvastatin Survival Study (4S). Diabetes Care 20:614–620.
13. Goldberg RB, Mellies MJ, Sacks FM, Moye LA, Howard BV, Howard WJ, Davis BR, Cole TG, Pfeffer MA, Braunwald E. 1998. Cardiovascular events and their reduction with pravastatin in diabetic and glucose-intolerant myocardial infarction survivors with average cholesterol levels: subgroup analyses in the cholesterol and recurrent events (CARE) trial. The Care Investigators. Circulation 98:2513–2519.
14. Adult Treatment Panel III. 2001. Executive summary of the third report of the national cholesterol education program (NCEP) expert panel on detection, evaluation and treatment of high blood cholesterol in adults. JAMA 285: 2486–2493.
15. Nathan DM, Meigs J, Singer DE. 1997. The epidemiology of cardiovascular disease in type 2 diabetes mellitus: how sweet it is . . . or is it? Lancet 350(1):S14–S19.
16. Kannel WB, Wilson PW. 1995. Risk factors that attenuate the female coronary disease advantage. Arch Intern Med 155:57–61.
17. Kannel WB, McGee DL. 1979. Diabetes and cardiovascular risk factors: the Framingham study. Circulation 59:8–13.
18. Haffner SM, Lehto S, Ronnemaa T, Pyörälä K, Laakso M. 1998. Mortality from coronary heart disease in subjects with type 2 diabetes and in nondiabetic subjects with and without prior myocardial infarction. N Engl J Med 339:229–234.
19. Lotufo PA, Gaziano M, Chae CU, Ajani UA, Moreno-John G, Buring JE, Manson JE. 2001. Diabetes and all-cause and coronary heart disease mortality among US male physicians. Arch Intern Med 161:242–247.
20. Sprafka JM, Burke GL, Folsom AR, McGovern PG, Hahn LP. 1991. Trends in prevalence of diabetes mellitus in patients with myocardial infarction and effect of diabetes on survival. The Minnesota Heart Survey. Diabetes Care 4:537–543.
21. Gu K, Cowie CC, Harris MI. 1999. Diabetes and decline in heart disease mortality in US adults. JAMA 281:1291–1297.
22. Verges B. 2001. Statins and diabetic hyperlipidimia. Ann Endocrinol (Paris) 62:128–132.

23. Assmann G, Schulte H, von Eckardstein A. 1996. Hyperglyceridemia and elevated levels of lipoprotein (a) are risk factors for major coronary events in middle-aged men. Am J Cardiol 77:1179–1184.
24. Heart Protection Study Collaborative Group. 2002. MRC/BHF Heart Protection Study of Cholesterol Lowering with Simvastetin in 20536 high-risk individuals: a randomized placebo-controlled trial. Leucet 360:7–22.
25. Adult Treatment Panel II. 1993. Summary of the second report of the National Cholesterol Education Program (NCEP) Expert Panel on Detection, Evaluation, and Treatment of High Blood Cholesterol in Adults (Adult Treatment Panel II). JAMA. 269:3015–23.

Frontiers in Cardiovascular Health, edited by
N.S. Dhalla, A. Chockalingam,
H.I. Berkowitz & P.K. Singal
Kluwer Academic Publishers, Boston, 2003

Altered Substrate Utilization in the Diabetic Heart: Role of Lipoprotein Lipase

Thomas Chacko Pulinilkunnil, Nandakumar Sambandam, and Brian Rodrigues

Division of Pharmacology and Toxicology, Faculty of Pharmaceutical Sciences
The University of British Columbia, 2146 East Mall
Vancouver, British Columbia
Canada V6T 1Z3

Summary. The heart has a limited potential to synthesize FFA and therefore FFA is supplied to cardiac cells from several sources: through lipolysis of endogenous cardiac triglyceride (TG) stores, or from exogenous sources in the blood. Lipoprotein lipase (LPL), a gate-keeping enzyme synthesized in cardiomyocytes, catalyzes the breakdown of the TG component of lipoproteins (very low density lipoproteins or VLDL, and chylomicrons) to provide FFA to the heart. It is the vascular endothelial-bound LPL that determines the rate of plasma TG clearance and hence, it is also called heparin-releasable "functional" LPL. Functional LPL is regulated by numerous dietary and hormonal factors, and is sensitive to pathophysiological alterations like those observed during diabetes. In this condition, lack of insulin impairs cardiac glucose transport and oxidation, resulting in FFA becoming the preferred means of energy supply. To make available this increased requirement of the heart for FFA, diabetic heart upregulates its luminal LPL activity. Chronically elevated cardiac LPL during diabetes can result in abnormal FFA supply and utilization by the heart tissue that could potentially initiate and sustain cardiac dysfunction during diabetes. As effective blood glucose control is difficult during Type 1 diabetes, it is conceivable that a parallel increase in functional cardiac LPL activity in insulin-treated diabetic individuals may predispose them to premature death from cardiac disease. By gaining more insight into the initial metabolic processes in the diabetic heart, we can attempt to piece together a part of the cascade of events leading to diabetic cardiomyopathy. Therefore understanding both the role and the mechanism(s) of dysregulation of cardiac LPL activity in the overall disease process could attenuate cardiovascular complications associated with diabetes.

***Key words*:** Diabetes, STZ, LPL, and FFA.

Author for Correspondence: Dr. B. Rodrigues, Division of Pharmacology and Toxicology, Faculty of Pharmaceutical Sciences, The University of British Columbia, 2146 East Mall, Vancouver, BC, Canada V6T 1Z3. Tel: (604)822-4758, Fax: (604)822-3035, E-mail: rodrigue@unixg.ubc.ca.

GENERAL OVERVIEW

Clinical and experimental studies have established that a cardiomyopathy occurs during diabetes (1,2). Although a number of factors have been implicated in the development of this disease state (3), increasing evidence suggests that a metabolic derangement in fuel supply and utilization by cardiac myocytes could be a primary biochemical lesion in the pathogenesis of diabetic cardiomyopathy. Under normal aerobic conditions, cellular energy in the form of ATP is obtained via the oxidation of various substrates, with free fatty acids (FFA) being the preferred energy substrate utilized by the heart muscle (4). In diabetes, energy production is almost entirely via β-oxidation of FFA, a process that may have deleterious effects on myocardial function. This results from the abnormally high requirement for oxygen during FFA metabolism, an intracellular accumulation of potentially toxic intermediates, and a FFA-induced inhibition of glucose oxidation (5). A consequence of these effects is an aberrant intracellular handling of Ca^{2+} that leads to Ca^{2+} overload, cell death, and eventual cardiac dysfunction (6).

The heart has a limited potential to synthesize FFA. Hence, FFA are supplied to cardiac cells from several sources: through lipolysis of endogenous cardiac triglyceride (TG) stores, or from exogenous sources in the blood (as free acid bound to albumin or as TG in lipoproteins). Lipoprotein lipase (LPL) is the enzyme that catalyzes the breakdown of the TG component of lipoproteins (very low density lipoproteins or VLDL, and chylomicrons). Vascular endothelial-bound LPL determines the rate of plasma TG clearance and partially regulates FFA supply to the tissues; hence, it is also called heparin-releasable "functional" LPL (7). Since endothelial cells cannot synthesize LPL, the enzyme is synthesized by the parenchymal cells of a variety of extrahepatic tissues, including adipose, heart, skeletal muscle, brain, and ovary. In the adult heart, LPL is synthesized and processed in myocytes and is translocated onto heparan sulfate proteoglycan (HSPGs) binding sites on the luminal surface of endothelial cells (8) where it actively metabolizes lipoproteins. CHYL and VLDL bind transiently to endothelium binding lipolysis sites where heparin-releasable endothelial LPL hydrolyzes the TG core to FFA and 2-monoacylglycerol (9), which are then transported into the heart for numerous metabolic and structural tasks.

The approximate contribution of FFA from exogenous or endogenous sources towards β-oxidation in the diabetic heart is not known. In an insulin-deficient state, adipose tissue lipolysis is enhanced, resulting in an elevated circulating FFA (10). In addition, an increased activity of myocardial enzymes that catalyze the synthesis of TG, together with a rise in CoA levels, promotes the production of TG during diabetes (11). Subsequent hydrolysis of this augmented TG store could also lead to high tissue FFA levels (12,13). These processes serve to guarantee FFA supply to the diabetic heart to compensate for the diminished contribution of glucose as an energy source. Considering these mechanisms that enhance cardiac FFA levels, the relative contribution of cardiac LPL activity to the delivery of FFA to the diabetic heart is unknown. An additional caveat is that available information on the influence of diabetes on heart LPL is inconclusive. Thus, LPL immunoreactive protein or activity has been reported to be unchanged (14–16) increased (17–20) or decreased (21–25) in the diabetic rat heart. In part, this variability between different studies could be due to the diversity in the rat strains used, the dosage of streptozotocin (STZ) used to induce diabetes, and the duration of the diabetic state. In addition, many of the above investigations utilized procedures which did not distinguish between the heparin-releasable component (localized on capillary endothelial cells that is implicated in the hydrolysis of circulating TG) and cellular (i.e., non-heparin-releasable pool that represents a storage form of the enzyme) pools of cardiac LPL as cellular LPL activity or protein levels have largely been obtained using whole heart homogenates. Hence, an understanding of the regulation of LPL in the heart is paramount to elucidate the etiology of diabetic cardiomyopathy.

LIPOPROTEIN LIPASE

Synthesis, activation and translocation

LPL, present on the luminal surface of the capillary endothelium, hydrolyzes the TG component of circulating lipoproteins like CHYL and VLDL, and releases FFA, which are subsequently utilized by tissues for various metabolic tasks. In this way, LPL plays a rate limiting role in the clearance of TG-rich lipoproteins from the circulation and in the supply of TG derived FFA to various tissues. LPL biosynthesis has been extensively studied in cell cultures. 3T3-L1 adipocytes (26), Ob-17 preadipocytes, and Chinese hamster ovarian (CHO) cell cultures (27) were some of the cell lines used to delineate biosynthetic pathways for LPL. LPL is synthesized as an inactive, monomeric proenzyme in the rough endoplasmic reticulum (ER) and activated somewhere between the ER and Golgi apparatus. The active enzyme is a dimer with asparagine (Asn) linked glycosylation. Glycosylation of the N-terminal domain at the Asn residue of LPL is required for its catalytic activity.

Glycosyl moieties are added co-translationally to Asn residues on nascent LPL polypeptide by a dolichol (a lipid)-linked oligosaccharide [Glc_3-$Man_9(GlcNAc)_2$] (23). This glycoprotein with mannose rich glycosyl residues in the ER is endo-β-N-acetylglucosaminidase H (endo-H) sensitive. Indeed, N-linked oligosaccharide undergoes a series of modifications: 1) terminal glucose residues are removed by glucosidase I and II in ER, 2) one mannose residue is then removed by α-mannosidase giving rise to high mannose peptide [Man_8-$(GlcNAc)_2$-protein] which is then transferred to cis-Golgi, a receiving center of the Golgi complex. Although the exact location of Golgi processing enzymes is not clear, three mannose residues are removed by mannosidase I in cis-Golgi. 3) As the glycoprotein moves through medial-Golgi, GlcNAc is added and two more mannose residues are removed by mannosidase II resulting in the formation of [GlcNAc-$Man_3(GlcNAc)_2$]-protein. 4) In the trans-Golgi, this protein is further modified by a series of transferases, which add GlcNAc, galactose and sialic acid residues to give rise to a endo-H resistant glycoprotein (Figure 1, 23). Vannier and Alihaud (28) proposed that LPL exists as an inactive monomer within the ER and the activation of LPL occurs only after

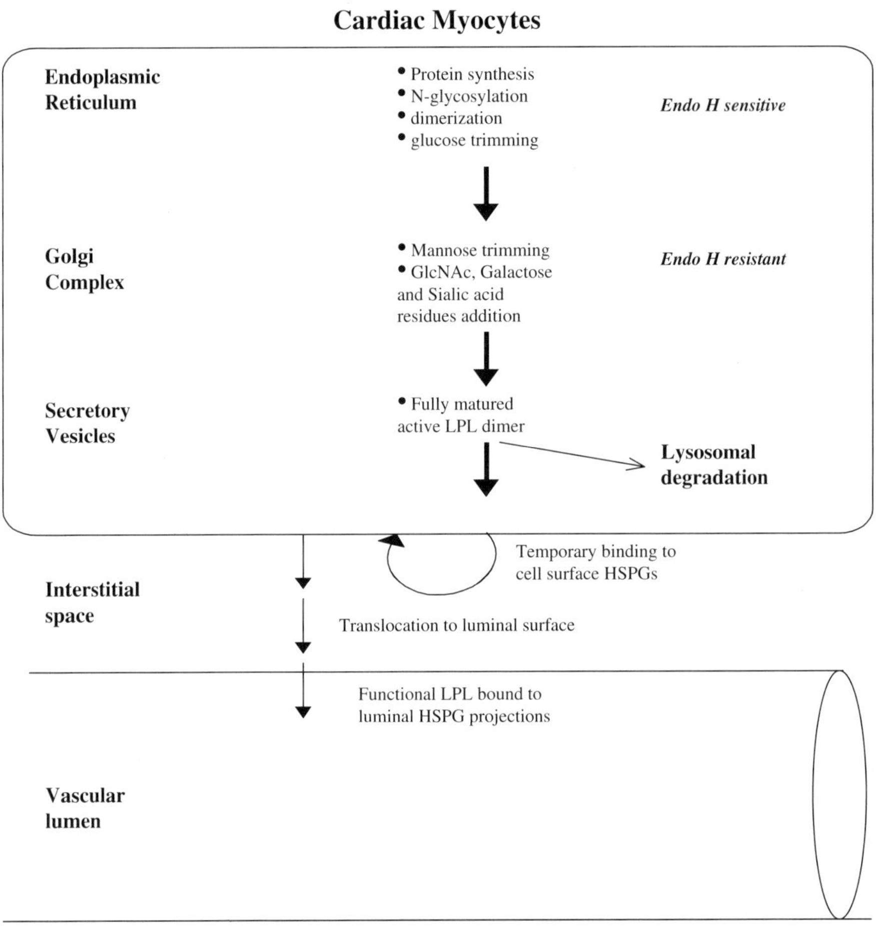

Figure 1. Schematic diagram of LPL synthesis, activation and secretion from cardiac myocytes.

translocation to the cis/medial-Golgi. However, Ben-Zeev et al. (27) demonstrated that translocation of LPL from ER to cis-Golgi is not required for full expression of enzyme activity. Various approaches like brefeldin A treatment (to disassemble the cis/medial-Golgi complex), incubation at 16°C (to prevent the movement of proteins from ER to Golgi), and tagging with KDEL (a specific ER retention signal) caused retention of fully active LPL in its high mannose form within the ER, blocking secretion into the medium. Also, it was shown that mannose trimming was not necessary for the activation and secretion of LPL (27). However, a significant reduction in LPL specific activity and secretion occurred when glucosidase inhibitors like castanospermin and N-methyl-deoxynojirimycin inhibited glucose trimming of LPL oligosaccharides. Therefore, the authors concluded that while glucose trimming is essential for activation and secretion of LPL, further oligosaccharide processing or translocation to the cis-Golgi is not required for full expression of lipolytic activity (27). Liu et al. (29), utilizing metabolic labeling of perfused guinea pig hearts, demonstrated that LPL is assembled into dimers in the ER and that the processing of oligosaccharide chains occurs after dimerization. Recently, Scow et al. (30), using the cld/cld mouse model showed that glycosylation and dimerization alone do not produce active LPL but transport of LPL out of the ER is essential for the secretion of active enzyme. LPL accumulates in the trans-Golgi in its fully active form with a half time of approximately one hour (7).

LPL secretion

LPL, like other proteins, reaches the plasma membrane from the ER through a vesicular transport system. In general, vesicles are sculpted from the ER with the help of ER coat proteins like COP I/COP II (31). These coat proteins are then removed to allow the fusion of the vesicle to the target membranes like Golgi and plasma membranes. The specific proteins called SNAP receptors (SNARE) bring about the docking of the vesicles to the target membrane. SNAREs (present on vesicles, v-SNAREs) bind to specific t-SNAREs (present on the target membranes) to dock the vesicle to appropriate target membranes. NSF (N-ethylmaleimide-sensitive fusion protein) and SNAP (soluble NSF attachment protein) then bind to the SNARE complex and initiate an energy dependent fusion process. NSF mediated ATP hydrolysis produces energy required in this process. The target specific vesicular transport is dictated by the intrinsic signal from the protein being transported. In the LPL molecule, a signal peptide of 17–27 amino acids and oligosaccharides were proposed to be involved in the directional transport of the protein (7,23), but the details of the transport process remain to be elucidated.

LPL is secreted by the parenchymal cells as an active enzyme in its homodimeric form by constitutive and regulated mechanisms (23). The constitutive release of LPL occurs spontaneously and the rate of release matches the rate of synthesis. The regulated release occurs in response to a secretogogue (e.g. heparin). For regulated release to occur, the enzyme has to be packaged and stored in secretory vesicles until it is released. All cell types that produce LPL exhibit constitutive release while some cells exhibit both constitutive and regulated release (for example Ob-17, 3T3-L1 adipocytes, cardiac myocytes and mesenchymal cells). Heparin is a major secretogogue, acts by releasing LPL from its cell surface binding sites and therby stimulates secretion of additional enzyme from within the cells (7). Release of LPL from cells is also possibly controlled by metabolic demand (32). Addition of increasing concentrations of oleic acid prevented the release of LPL by cultured endothelial cells (33). Recently, Anderson et al. (34) demonstrated that FFA inhibited LPL secretion by isolated cardiac myocytes suggesting a feed-back inhibition of LPL secretion by the lipolytic products.

LPL translocation

LPL, after being secreted, binds to parenchymal cells transiently before it is translocated to the endothelial surface in the vascular lumen. Translocation of LPL from its site of synthesis (myocytes/adipocytes) to the endothelial cell surface in the vascular lumen is not clearly understood. The subendothelial basement membranes are proposed to sequester and stabilize the LPL secreted by non-endothelial cells (35). Extracellular matrix (ECM) in the subendothelial space is composed of collagens (type I, III, and IV), fibronectin, laminin and glycosaminoglycans (GAG) like heparan sulfate-, dermatan sulfate-, chondroitin sulfate-proteoglycans of which LPL binds mainly to the heparan sulfate proteoglycans (HSPG). It was first proposed that LPL could move along bridges of HSPG molecules that connect parenchymal cells with capillary endothelial cells (36). In fact, binding of LPL to HSPG at the basolateral surface of the endothelium was shown to be necessary for an efficient transport to the apical surface (37). The removal of HSPGs by heparinase digestion suppressed this transport process (37). However, co-localization of HSPG and LPL within the transport vesicles was not required for the secretion of active LPL as shown in HSPG deficient Chinese hamster ovarian (CHO) cells (38). Nevertheless, LPL produced by wild type CHO cells (which express HSPG) was found to be more stable than LPL produced by the mutant cells. Stins et al. (33) further proved that the movement of LPL across the endothelial cells was polarized towards the apical (also known as luminal) surface. Transport of LPL was therefore appreciably greater from the basolateral (also known as abluminal) to the apical surface than in the opposite direction. Recently, fragments of HSPG, heparan sulfate (HS) oligosaccharides have been shown to act like extracellular chaperones for LPL and enable the transport of the enzyme in its active form across the endothelial cells (39). Endothelial cells release a heparanase-like enzyme during the lipolytic encounter of LPL with VLDL in the co-cultures of endothelial cells and adipocytes. This heparanase-like enzyme then cleaves surface bound HSPGs to release HS-oligosaccharides (39). HS-oligosaccharides bind non-covalently to LPL molecules and escort them to the apical surface of endothelial cells and probably prevent LPL degradation in interstitial fluid. Moreover, HS-oligosaccharides have also been shown to enhance transport of LPL across endothelial cells (39). HS-oligosaccharides only partly saturate the heparin binding domains on the LPL molecule and, therefore do not affect further binding of LPL to cell surface HSPGs (39). All of these in vitro results were complemented by the fact that feeding animals also increases the activity of LPL as well that of heparanase-like activity in adipose tissue (39).

Movement of LPL across endothelial cells has been suggested to occur via a poorly understood process called transcytosis. Endothelial transcytosis involves endocytosis of macromolecules like LPL at the basolateral side of endothelial cells, vesicular transport across the cell, and exocytosis at the luminal surface. Much of the understanding comes from basic cellular transport processes that are applicable to various macromolecules in general. Endothelial cells lining the arterioles, capillaries and venules of glomeruli and peritubules of kidney and capillaries associated with intestinal mucosa and secretory glands are fenestrated. However, endothelial cells lining the microvessels of the heart are not fenestrated but continuous. Therefore, the transport of macromolecules across the endothelial barrier has to be either by fluid phase or transcytotic mechanisms (40). Several studies suggest that caveolae could act as ferries for macromolecules between luminal and abluminal surfaces of the endothelial cells. Caveolae are endothelial vesicles involved in the receptor-mediated endocytosis or transcytosis of macromolecules. A specific inhibition of vesicular fusion protein, NSF (N-ethylmaleimide sensitive fusion protein) by N-ethylmaleimide could prevent the macromolecular permeability, supporting a vesicular transport system across the endothelial cells (41). A combination of phosphatidylinositol-3 kinase (PI-3 Kinase) and tyrosine kinase regulated endocytosis, and SNARE-SNAP-NSF complex mediated exocytosis are indicated in this caveolar transport across endothelium (42). Additionally, involvement of actin filaments has been suggested in the caveolar transport process since cytochalasin B prevented transport of these vesicles (42). It has be speculated that binding of LPL to HSPG triggers the aggregation and distribution of HSPGs along the actin cytoskeleton. In the absence of such ligand binding, HSPGs appear distributed irregularly on the fibroblast cell surface, without any apparent co-localization with the actin cytoskeleton. Whether this organization of HSPG along the actin cytoskeleton is involved in the transcytosis of LPL from the abluminal to the luminal surface is still not known. Earlier studies in the heart demonstrated that antimitotic agents like colchicine and vinblastin inhibited the transport of LPL to the luminal surface of endothelial cells (43). Another antimitotic drug, cyclophosphamide, also had similar inhibitory effects on the secretion of LPL in rabbit hearts (44). Recently, Ewart et al. (45) demonstrated that the actin cytoskeleton is involved in the transport of LPL from within the cardiac myocytes. Because the microvascular endothelium of the heart is known to be enriched with caveolae (40), it would be interesting to apply the various above interventions to examine whether LPL translocation follows this pathway (Figure 2).

LPL IN THE HEART

In the heart, LPL gene expression and protein synthesis begins only after birth and reaches a maximum level within 3 weeks of age. The fetal heart does not express LPL (9). Synthesis, processing and translocation of LPL in the heart occurs by mechanisms similar to those of adipose tissues and has been mainly studied in experimental animals like mouse, guinea pigs, rats, and rabbits. In the adult mouse heart, LPL is synthesized and processed in cardiac myocytes (36). Similarly, in human myocardium, in situ hybridization for LPL mRNA revealed that LPL was primarily synthesized by cardiac myocytes (8). In the rat heart, cholera toxin induced LPL mRNA expression primarily in interstitial cells (46) although cardiac myocytes also exhibited a diffuse but a definite localization of LPL mRNA. Since the LPL gene has muscle specific motifs and calcium- and cAMP-responsive elements, it is likely that under normal conditions, cardiac myocytes and possibly some vascular pericytes (which comprise a portion of interstitium in the heart) could be the primary sites of LPL synthesis (8).

Distribution of immunoreactive LPL protein was observed in different compartments of myocardium. Electron microscopic studies of immunogold-labeled sections of mouse myocardium delineated that 78% of total LPL was present in the cardiac

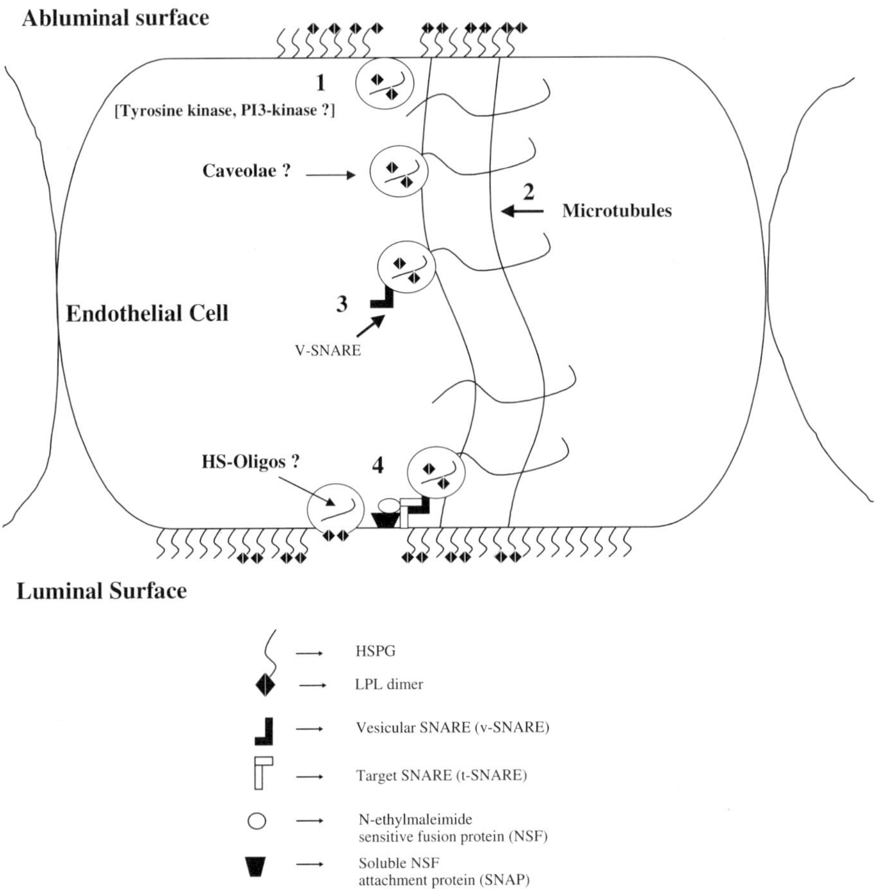

Figure 2. Scheme of probable mechanism of LPL transcytosis across endothelial cells. The transcytotic process has been depicted to involve four stages (1. Endocytosis, 2. Actin alignment, 3. Vesicular traffic along the actin cytoskeleton, and 4. Vesicle fusion and exocytosis).

myocytes, 3–6% in the interstitial space, and 18% in the capillary endothelium (36). Within the myocytes, LPL was found localized within the sarcoplasmic reticulum, Golgi complex and secretory vesicles (36). Outside the myocyte, LPL was associated with the plasma membrane and the basal surface of the capillary endothelium. LPL in the endothelium was seen inside the cells, within the vesicles and along the luminal surface of the endothelial cells (36). LPL on the luminal surface of endothelial cells were also seen associated with chylomicron particles. The functional fraction of LPL in the perfused heart was immunocytochemically localized in the vascular lumen (47). Although immunoreactivity for LPL protein was observed in endothelial cells, no mRNA expression was detected (48). Further, treatment with protein synthesis inhibitors like cycloheximide, or with transport inhibitors like colchicine reduced the LPL activity in the vascular lumen (43,49). Therefore, it was concluded that endothelial cells do not synthesize LPL and the enzyme must have been synthesized in the cardiac myocytes and translocated to the endothelial surface in the vascular lumen. Pulse-chase studies demonstrated that it takes approximately 30 minutes for the newly synthesized LPL to be translocated to the luminal surface of vascular endothelium (50).

When perfused with heparin via a Langendorff retrograde perfusion, isolated hearts release LPL. This heparin-releasable LPL was shown to occur in three phases over a 60 minute period in guinea pig hearts (49,51): 1) a rapid phase, occurring within seconds after heparin perfusion, probably from the endothelial luminal surface; 2) a shoulder of release, occurring between 2–30 minutes, probably from within and from the abluminal surface of endothelial cells; and 3) a slow steady release of LPL, probably explained by release from the site of synthesis. The rapid, heparin releasable, vascular-bound LPL fraction is also called "functional" LPL since it is involved in the hydrolysis of circulating TGRLs. It is this heparin-releasable fraction of LPL that is more sensitive to physiological (e.g. fasting and feeding, 23), and pathological (e.g. diabetes, 20) changes and this can correspondingly affect exogenous FFA supply to the heart.

LPL REGULATION

LPL synthesis and activity is regulated in a tissue specific manner during developmental stages by various physiological conditions like fasting, feeding, cold exposure, lactation etc., and by various pathological conditions like diabetes, hypertension, obesity etc. For example, LPL synthesis can be observed in the fetal liver but the adult liver does not synthesize LPL. On the contrary, heart LPL activity is very low in the fetus but reaches maximum levels within three weeks after birth (9). Several transcriptional, post-transcriptional and post-translational mechanisms have been proposed for this differential regulation of LPL.

Transcriptional regulation

The LPL gene has several cis-acting regulatory sequences in its 5′-flanking region. Regulation of LPL gene transcription involves binding of specific trans-acting factors to these cis-acting elements. Oct-1 (octamer sequence ATTTGCAT) at nucleotide −46 (relative to the transcriptional start site) is one such site which binds to trans-acting factors like OTF-1 (octamer transcription factor). Using transient transfection studies, deletion of the Oct-1 site has been shown to decrease the transcription of LPL gene. The specificity of Oct-1 and 2 protein binding to this octamer sequence is determined by the DNA sequence adjacent to the Oct-1 site (26,52). NF-Y, another protein which specifically binds to the CAAT motif at position −65, is also involved in the transcriptional regulation of LPL (52). The presence of positive (−368 to −35, increases LPL expression) and negative (−724 to −565, suppresses LPL expression) regulatory sequences in the 5′flanking region have been indicated to play a role in the tissue specific regulation of LPL (26). Similarly, LP-α/β, Ap-1 complex, and C/EBP proteins are all involved in the transcriptional regulation of LPL (53). Differences that exist in these regulatory sequences and in the expression of trans-acting factors have been postulated to play a role in tissue specific regulation of LPL in various species.

The involvement of the 3′untranslated region (3′UTR) region in the tissue specific regulation of LPL is increasingly evident from recent studies. LPL cDNA from various species including human, bovine and mouse exhibits two polyadenylation signals (corresponding to the human sequence at nucleotides 3155 and 3550) in its 3′-UTR and these sites are highly conserved in all species examined so far (54). Adipose tissue in humans expresses two LPL mRNA species (3.2 and 3.6 kb) probably due to a random choice of one of the two polyadenylation sites (54). However, skeletal and heart muscles express only the 3.6 kb mRNA form probably due to a non-random choice. In addition to humans, several other species express multiple mRNAs for LPL. However, in rat adipose and muscle tissues only the second polyadenylation site is utilized to express the 3.6 kb LPL mRNA (54). Therefore, in addition to the 5′-flanking region, the 3′UTR can be speculated to play a role in the tissue and species specific regulation of LPL expression.

Post-transcriptional regulation

Two mRNA species have so far been identified for LPL; one is 3.2 kb and the other 3.6 kb in length. When transfected in CHO cells, the longer mRNA form more efficiently translated to LPL protein that had higher specific activity than the 3.2 kb mRNA transcript (54). Steady state mRNA levels depend on message stability as well as gene transcription. Stability and translatability of mRNA determine the amount and rate of protein translation. The polyadenylation tail confers stability to mRNA. Although the exact mechanism by which the 3.6 kb mRNA translates more efficiently is not known, it is proposed that in general, changes in the secondary structure of mRNA may allow better interactions of certain trans-acting binding proteins. The 3′-UTR may also be involved in mRNA stability and in its translational efficiency (54). Hormones like insulin and epinephrine may alter the translational efficiency of mRNA by modulating mRNA-binding proteins (55).

Turnover of LPL mRNA is usually very slow under normal conditions (~40 hours). This slow turnover of mRNA means a continuous production of active LPL even when there is no physiological need. Therefore, posttranslational regulation is required to control the enzyme concentration at a level that is absolutely necessary to fulfill the physiological demand (56). The rate of LPL protein translation from its mRNA is commonly measured by ^{35}S-methionine incorporation and immunoprecipitation techniques. The increase in rate of LPL synthesis can either be dependent on or independent of mRNA levels. For example, insulin stimulated LPL synthesis in rat adipocytes is dependent on an increase in mRNA levels whereas glucose further increased LPL synthesis in these cells without altering mRNA levels (57). In another instance, the diurnal variation (both increase and decrease) in LPL mass and activity was not accompanied by corresponding changes in LPL mRNA levels indicating a posttranslational regulation (58). However, certain conditions like treatment with TNF-α, and cold/warm adaptations may markedly alter LPL mRNA production and degradation with a corresponding change in LPL mass and activity (56). LPL regulation at multiple levels such as transcriptional, pretranslational and posttranslational levels was observed in Djungarian hamsters' brown adipose tissue in response to cold adaptation. In early phases of cold adaptation posttranslational mechanisms are activated whereas, prolonged cold exposure involved posttranscriptional, pretranslational and posttranslational mechanisms (59).

Post-translational regulation

Posttranslational regulation of LPL can occur at various sites including glycosylation, turnover of LPL protein, dimerization to an active form and also through control of LPL binding sites on the endothelium. The LPL activity can also be regulated by physiological substrates such as VLDL and CHYL and breakdown products like FFA.

Glycosylation

6–7% of the mass of each molecule of LPL is contributed by carbohydrate structures. This carbohydrate is in the form of N-glycosylated sugars on the LPL protein. Core glycosylation and glucose trimming occurs in ER and further processing takes place in the Golgi complex. Inhibition of glycosylation and glucose trimming in ER by tunicamycin (prevents N-linked oligosaccharide chain transfer) and castanospermin (glucosidase I inhibitor) led to the production of inactive monomeric LPL that had low affinity for heparin. However, treatment with 1-deoxymannojirimycin (Golgi mannosidase I inhibitor) and swainsonine (inhibits Golgi processing) produced active, dimeric LPL that had high affinity for heparin. Therefore, it was concluded that glycosylation and subsequent removal of distal glucose residues was necessary but processing by the Golgi mannosidase I was not required for the production of active and dimeric LPL that had high affinity for heparin binding (60,61).

Binding sites

LPL, after secretion binds to HSPG binding sites that are present both on parenchymal and endothelial cell surfaces (62–67). Recently, the active fragment of HSPG was found to be a decasaccharide (made up of the repeating structure -[IdceA(2-SO_4)α1–4GlcNSO_4(6-SO_4)]); with a linear array of negatively charged sulfate groups. This active fragment may bind to peptide region(s) containing basic amino acid residues of LPL with high affinity (68). LPL bound to HSPGs can be displaced by a competitive ionic interaction by heparin. This release of LPL by heparin is believed to stimulate LPL secretion from the parenchymal cells. The exact mechanism by which this stimulatory effect of heparin occurs is not yet known. Binding of LPL to HSPG also stabilizes LPL activity (38). Unbound LPL present in the medium loses its activity much faster than the bound form. In vivo, LPL released into the circulation from its endothelial binding sites is subsequently taken up by the liver and degraded (69). Intravenous injection of heparin results in a release of large amount of functional LPL from all extrahepatic binding sites into the circulation. Heparin delays but does not abolish the hepatic clearance of LPL (69). In addition to heparin, LPL can also be displaced from its HSPG binding sites by physiological factors like antithrombin III, α-thrombin and its inactive derivative, DIP-α-thrombin (35). LPL that is bound to HSPGs has a higher K_m but lower V_{max} than LPL in solution. In other words, LPL in solution is more efficient as a lipolytic enzyme as compared to the endothelium-bound counterpart. This is probably due to a better accessibility of the enzyme for its substrate (e.g. VLDL, CHYL) and proposed to be an additional mechanism by which HSPG binding could regulate LPL action (70).

Glycosylphosphatidylinositol (GPI) is another binding site identified on the cell surface for LPL. GPI binding sites can be selectively cleaved by phsophatidylinositol (PI) specific phospholipase C or D (PLC or PLD). PLC is activated by insulin and therefore, incubation of 3T3-L1 adipocytes with insulin resulted in a PLC mediated release of LPL from GPI binding sites on the surface (71–73). In addition to insulin, agents like glimepiride (a sulfonylurea) also induced release of LPL anchored to GPI from rat adipocytes via activation of GPI specific phospholipase (GPI-PL). Glucose free medium completely abolished the stimulatory effect of insulin as well as glimepiride on GPI-PL and therefore on LPL release (74). This set of data indicates that increased glucose transport rather than insulin stimulates GPI-PL and release of LPL from rat adipocytes.

Other binding sites for LPL include low density lipoprotein receptor related protein (LRP), a glycoprotein (gp330), a heparin releasable protein (hrp-116), and a novel 85-kDa glycoprotein (75). Physiological importance of these non-HSPG LPL binding sites is not yet known. Similarly, another putative binding of LPL with unknown physiology has been shown to occur with α2-macroglobulin (α_2-M) in the plasma. α2-M is a broad spectrum protease inhibitor known to bind various basic proteins like nerve growth factor, basic fibroblast growth factor, cationic aspartate aminotransferase, myelin basic protein and eosinophil cationic protein. LPL, being a basic protein, also binds to α_2-M in a non-covalent manner via its heparin binding domain and thus loses its ability to bind to cell surface HSPGs. Whether this binding of LPL to α_2-M plays any physiological role is not yet known (76,77).

LPL turnover by intracellular degradation/recycling

LPL turnover by intracellular degradation is an important post-translational mechanism by which LPL activity is rapidly regulated during conditions like feeding and fasting (78). About 80% of newly synthesized LPL are degraded before being secreted. This turnover by intracellular degradation in adipocytes is a very rapid process with a $t_{1/2}$ of about 40 minutes. Degradation could occur either in a leupeptin inhibitable, lysosomal compartment or a tunicamycin inhibitable, ER compartment (23). Surface bound LPL also undergoes degradation after being internalized. Adipocytes degrade only a fraction (<28%) of total surface bound LPL and this process involves internalization of the enzyme and a subsequent degradation in lysosomal compartment (79). HSPGs mediate this process of LPL turnover by facilitating internalization of LPL by various cells including adipocytes and hepatocytes (79–81). Berryman and Bensadoun (38) demonstrated that HSPG binding sites are essential for the internalization and degradation of the enzyme by cultured CHO-K1 cells. The degree of sulfation of HSPGs can alter LPL binding. Hoogewerf et al. (80) demonstrated that a decrease in sulfation of HSPGs on the adipocytes decreased the maximum binding of LPL to the cell surface. This decreased binding of LPL to HSPGs also resulted in less degradation of the enzyme as a result of decreased internalization. Similar decreases in internalization and degradation can be achieved by releasing the surface bound LPL by heparin. Release of surface bound LPL by heparin stimulates secretion of the enzyme from within cells. In adipocytes, this secretory process diverts the newly synthesized LPL away from lysosomal compartment and thereby significantly reduces intracellular degradation. In cardiac myocytes, release of surface bound LPL does not alter the amount of intracellular degradation of LPL but in compensation, intracellular degradation of LPL in cardiac myocytes is slow (49). In addition to HSPGs, receptor-associated protein-sensitive LRP binding sites also mediate this LPL turnover process, however, it contributes less compared to proteoglycan binding sites (79).

Unlike adipocytes and cardiac myocytes, endothelial cells degrade LPL to a very small extent. Using in vitro cell cultures, endothelial cells were in fact shown to recycle the surface bound LPL in its active dimeric form (82). Involvement of HSPG binding sites is once again emphasized. The probable recycling mechanism involves internalization of HSPG-LPL complexes into an endocytotic compartment. The acidic pH in the endocytotic vesicles favors HSPG-LPL binding, thereby enabling the complex to be released back into the medium or inserted onto the cell surface. However, the following issues have yet to be clarified to substantiate the above mechanisms. Are HSPG/HS-oligosaccharides being internalized with LPL during the recycling process? If it is undegraded HSPG, then is the HSPG-LPL complex inserted back into the cell surface?

Regulation of LPL by substrates

Physiological substrates like VLDL and CHYL and lipolytic products like FFA also regulate LPL activity. Apolipoproteins present on TGRLs such as VLDL and CHYL influence their interaction with LPL. For example, binding of apolipoprotein CII (apoCII) present on the TGRL surface to LPL enhances lipolysis while, binding of apoCIII inhibits LPL activity (32). Recently, apoE, another major apolipoprotein of TGRLs, has been shown to inhibit LPL activity. LPL activity is also regulated by the substrates via a feed-back mechanism. For example, FFA released from the TGs by the lipolytic action of LPL can bind to LPL and competitively inhibit LPL activity (83). However, albumin can prevent this feed-back inhibition due to its higher affinity for FFAs (83). Another mechanism by which LPL activity can be inhibited by its substrates is by displacement of LPL from its binding sites (84). LPL bound to endothelial cells can be displaced from its binding sites by TGRLs and oleic acid. In vitro experiments demonstrate that FFA binding interferes with the LPL-heparin interaction. In addition, FFA also affects LPL binding to its activator apolipoprotein

CII (84). It is proposed that when more FFA than the tissue can utilize is released by LPL, FFA would probably bind to LPL and displace it from its binding sites, thereby regulating the enzyme activity via a negative feed-back mechanism. The above results generated by cell culture experiments were questioned due to the fact that no LPL was released when FFAs were perfused through isolated beating hearts from rats (6). Alternatively, incubation of cardiac myocytes with oleic acid resulted in a decreased LPL activity, not due to release of the enzyme from its binding sites but due to alterations in intracellular processing and secretion of the enzyme (34).

LPL REGULATION DURING FASTING, FEEDING AND DIABETES

Fasting and feeding

Fasting increases LPL activity in muscles (skeletal and cardiac) but decreases the enzyme activity in adipose tissues in different animal models such as rats, guinea pigs and hamsters. Feeding has opposite effects in these tissues (85–88). Regulation at post-transcriptional and post-translational levels has been suggested. Decrease in rat adipose LPL due to short term fasting was restored within 4 hours of refeeding. However, long term fasting (36 hr, 60 hr, and 3–5 days) took several days of refeeding before LPL levels were restored (58). It was shown that short-term fasting, similar to diurnal rhythms did not affect LPL mRNA levels (58) and was in fact due to an increase in the proportion of inactive form of LPL in adipose tissues (89). In addition, the short term fasting period was also shown to increase degradation of newly synthesized LPL and markedly decrease secretion of LPL into the medium (78). Thus, the regulation during short term fasting was at a post-translational level. Prolonged fasting (>24 hours) on the other hand, resulted in a decreased level of mRNA and thus required transcriptional regulation for the restoration of LPL activity in rat adipose tissues (58). Recent studies have further confirmed that this differential level of LPL regulation in rat adipose tissue is associated with the duration of fasting (78).

Fasting and feeding respectively increased and decreased heparin releasable fraction of heart LPL in rats. There was no change in LPL activity in soleus or extensor digitorum longus (EDL) in response to short term fasting or feeding. However, LPL activity and mRNA in skeletal muscle increased only after a 6-day fast. It was concluded that heart LPL is more sensitive to fasting/feeding than is the skeletal muscle (90,91). The increase in HR-LPL in the heart is also attributed to increased uptake of LPL from the blood (92). Although plasma LPL level was not measured in this study, uptake of exogenous ^{125}I-LPL was shown to be increased in the heart during fasting. In the mouse myocardium, immunocytochemical studies revealed that fasting induced a 5-fold increase in LPL at the luminal projections of endothelium (36). When pulsed with ^{35}S-methionine (which incorporates into newly synthesized LPL molecule) and chased with non-radioactive methionine, guinea pig hearts exhibited no difference in the rate of transport of newly synthesized [^{35}S]-LPL during fed or fasted states (49). The above studies in general support that changes in heart LPL during fasting and feeding are controlled at the posttranslational level (90–91,93).

In humans, studies were mainly done in adipose tissues and skeletal muscle. Adipose LPL decreases in humans similar to animal models during fasting, but skeletal muscle exhibits either no change or increase in LPL activity depending on the duration of fasting (53). LPL regulation in obese subjects is different in that LPL activity decreased both in adipose tissue as well as in skeletal muscle as a result of fasting. Weight reduction in obese individuals caused adipose LPL to remain elevated during fasting suggesting that the metabolic set point is primed for continued weight gain in these individuals (94,95). These alterations in LPL activity are however not accompanied by any change in mRNA or immunoreactive mass of LPL. Thus it is proposed that fasting/feeding induced changes in LPL is due to posttranslational mechanisms.

Diabetes

LPL regulation during diabetes has been well documented and is known to occur in a tissue specific manner. The following sections review tissue specific LPL regulation in adipose tissue, skeletal muscle, cardiac muscle and post-heparin plasma, during diabetes.

Adipose LPL

Adipose LPL activity has been shown to be unequivocally decreased both at the functional level and at the site of synthesis during diabetes (96). This decrease in adipose LPL was partly due to decreased immunoreactive LPL protein and steady state mRNA levels but primarily as a result of decreased catalytic activity (20). The decrease in LPL activity was reversed by insulin treatment. In vitro studies have demonstrated a direct effect of insulin on adipose LPL activity (23). Insulin increased cellular LPL activity, rate of LPL synthesis, LPL mRNA levels and HR-LPL activity on the cell surface of adipocytes and thus regulates adipose LPL activity at transcriptional, post-transcriptional, and post-translational levels. These in vitro studies are further complemented by several in vivo experiments which demonstrate that increases in plasma insulin levels (as in euglycemic, hyperinsulinemic clamps) augmented adipose LPL activity (53). In STZ-diabetic rats and non-diabetic controls, high caloric intake increased plasma insulin levels with a parallel increase in adipose LPL activity in both groups (16). This increase in LPL activity was accompanied by increases in LPL specific mRNA levels. The decreased adipose LPL in diabetic patients (both type 1 and type 2) was improved by insulin or oral hypoglycemic therapy (97). This improvement in LPL activity was due to both an increased rate of LPL synthesis and a decreased degradation of the enzyme. Since there was no change in LPL-mRNA levels due to insulin treatment, the regulation was suggested to be at a post-translational level (97).

The insulin resistance that occurs in obesity blunts the adipose LPL stimulation in response to insulin (98). This response was even more diminished in type 2 diabetics (98). Weight reduction in obesity or exercise in type 2 diabetics increased insulin sensitivity with a parallel increase in the responsiveness of adipose LPL to insulin suggesting that the stimulatory effect of insulin on adipose LPL depends on insulin sensitivity. The greater the insulin sensitivity, the better the response of adipose LPL and a threshold level of insulin sensitivity controls the enzyme response in adipose tissue (98). In this regard, it was also shown that the more severe the insulin resistance, the lower is the adipose LPL mRNA level (99). This was attributed to the inability of insulin either to stimulate transcription or to increase the intracellular LPL mRNA stability in adipose tissue in insulin resistant individuals (99). Contrary to all of the above evidence, insulin resistance and hyperinsulinemia induced by chronic high-fat feeding actually exaggerated the insulin response in adipose and muscle tissues (100). This discrepancy is probably due to differences in the severity and duration of high fat induced insulin resistance and hyperinsulinemia.

Skeletal muscle LPL

Skeletal muscle LPL activity during type 1 diabetes was found to be either decreased, not changed, or increased, depending on type of skeletal muscle and the degree and duration of diabetes studied (96). Under normal physiology of fasting/feeding cycle, insulin negatively regulates skeletal muscle LPL whereas during insulin resistance, as seen in obesity, skeletal muscle LPL is increased by insulin (98). When type 2 diabetes was present together with obesity, the severe insulin resistance that occurs did not increase the LPL activity in the skeletal muscle (98). Indeed, in type 2 diabetic patients infusion of insulin/glucose led to a blunted response on skeletal muscle LPL activity suggesting that neither plasma insulin nor glucose play an important role in the regulation of skeletal muscle LPL activity (101). Microalbuminurea, another diabetic complication, by its damaging effects on endothelial cells decreases functional LPL in type 2 diabetics (102). Albuminuria was associated with defects in HSPGs in extra-cellular matrix (ECM) and therefore type 1 diabetic patients with albuminuria were suggested to have decreased vascular LPL activity leading to hypertriglyceridemia (103). However, skeletal muscle LPL activity in diabetic patients with or without albuminuria did not differ although both groups had lower LPL activity as compared to healthy individuals. The elevated plasma TG levels were correlated to this decreased skeletal muscle LPL activity in both the diabetic groups (103).

Cardiac LPL

Cardiac LPL regulation during diabetes is mainly studied in experimental animal models. In spite of a plethora of literature on diabetes and its effect on cardiac LPL, results are inconclusive due to high variability. For example, studies on cardiac LPL regulation in alloxan/STZ-diabetes showed that both heparin-releasable, and total LPL activities (as determined in whole heart homogenate) were elevated during diabetes (104,19). Insulin treatment reversed the diabetic conditions as well as fractional and total LPL activities in the heart to normal levels. Tavangar et al. (20) demonstrated that the elevated levels of heart LPL in STZ-diabetic rats was accompanied by an increase in immunoreactive LPL protein but with decreased LPL-mRNA levels. Therefore, the elevated level of LPL activity was not due to enhanced translation of the protein but was probably due to the depressed rate of LPL turnover (degradation) in the diabetic heart. Contrary to these studies, isolated hearts from diabetic animals expressed a decreased functional LPL activity, which was reflected by a decreased lipolysis of perfused VLDL-TG (21). These alterations were normalized by in vivo as well as in vitro insulin treatments. Further, the effects of insulin could be inhibited by a protein synthesis inhibitor, cycloheximide (21). The latter set of experiments supports the idea that the decrease in functional LPL in the diabetic heart could be due to a decreased synthesis of the enzyme and that insulin can directly stimulate LPL synthesis in the heart. It is to be noted that the in vitro effects of insulin either in perfused hearts or isolated cardiac myocyte culture could not be reproduced by several subsequent studies (23,45,105–107). Nevertheless, in vivo insulin administration did stimulate LPL activity in the diabetic heart, which led to a conclusion that insulin requires a second factor to regulate cardiac LPL activity. In this regard, Ewart et al. (98,45) using cardiac myocytes from control and diabetic rats demonstrated that incubation of cells with insulin and dexamethasone (a glucocorticoid) together stimulated LPL activity. Neither insulin nor glucocorticoid by themselves had any effect on myocyte LPL. Therefore, it appears that insulin regulates heart LPL in vivo in the presence of another factor (like glucocorticoid). Liu and Severson (108) further confirmed that functional (heparin-releasable) LPL from perfused hearts as well as myocyte-associated LPL (non-functional) activities were depressed in diabetic rats. This decrease in cardiac LPL was neither accompanied by changes in steady state LPL mRNA levels and stability nor by a decrease in relative rates of LPL synthesis and turnover (degradation) (109). Also, the diabetic heart did not exhibit any changes in LPL-specific HSPG binding sites (110). The decrease in LPL activity was therefore attributed to an absolute decrease in LPL synthesis and aberrations in post-translational mechanisms resulting in accumulation of inactive enzyme (109).

Evidence supporting the idea that there is no change in heart LPL activity during diabetes has also been noted in the literature. LPL activity in the hearts of STZ-diabetic rats was not affected either by calorie intake or by the diabetic state per se (16). In summary, diabetes produced variable regulation of LPL in the heart. The disparity in the literature can be partly explained by differences in chemical agent used to induce diabetes (alloxan/STZ), dose of STZ, duration of diabetes, differences in animal models used (species and strain differences), and the techniques used to measure LPL activity (heart tissue homogenate versus isolated heart perfusion, acetone-ether extracts versus unextracted tissues, etc.) (96).

Post-heparin plasma lipolytic activity (PHPLA)

Diabetes is usually accompanied by hypertriglyceridemia in addition to elevated glucose levels. High plasma TG levels could be due either to a decreased clearance or increased secretion of TGRLs or both (111–117). The decreased clearance of TGRL from blood could partly be due to decreased LPL activity (23). PHPLA is an index of overall LPL activity contributed by various tissues like, skeletal and cardiac muscles, adipose tissues, etc. PHPLA was determined to be low in diabetic patients (118,96) and STZ-diabetic hamsters (119). Treatment of diabetes with insulin resulted in the normalization of PHPLA and plasma triglyceride levels (120). Insulin resistance and the compensatory hyperinsulinemia (often associated with type 2 diabetes) can also decrease plasma LPL activity and cause postprandial lipemia (121). Maheux et al. (1997) further demonstrated that the degree of insulin resistance was directly correlated to the degree of decrease in plasma LPL (activity and mass), and to the degree of elevations in plasma TG concentrations (99). In fact, numerous studies have shown a genetic correlation between diabetic hyperlipidemia and abnormalities in LPL activity (122,123). Specifically, HindIII restriction fragment-length polymorphism genotype of LPL is associated with insulin resistance, hypertriglyceridemia and reduced levels of HDL-cholesterol (124). Pvu II polymorphism of the LPL gene is also significantly associated with type 2 diabetes and coronary artery disease (125). Heterozygous familial lipoprotein lipase deficiency in association with hyperinsulinemia caused deleterious effects on plasma TG levels (126). A novel compound NO-1886, by elevating LPL activity without affecting the hypoinsulinemic and hyperglycemic states of diabetes, decreased plasma TG levels and increased HDL-cholesterol levels (127). This evidence at least demonstrates LPL is directly responsible for the plasma TG levels in diabetic animals. On the contrary, several reports also demonstrated an increase or no change in plasma lipase activity in diabetic patients and in experimental animal models (128,112,119). These inconsistencies could be partly due to differences in procedures to measure LPL activity, type of diabetes studied, basal insulin or TG levels in the diabetic conditions, and duration of insulin treatment and withdrawal in diabetic patients (96).

Decreased clearance of TGRLs from the circulation could also be due to factors other than defective LPL. A dissociation between LPL activity and plasma TG level was observed during diabetes (129) suggesting that factors other than LPL could contribute towards the hypertriglyceridemia. Clinical and experimental diabetes show alterations in lipoprotein structure and composition resulting in a poorer interaction with LPL and this was implicated as one of the mechanisms involved in the development of hypertriglyceridemia (130,131). Major apolipoproteins that are packaged along with the lipids in TGRLs are apoB100, B48, apoE1-5, apoA1-4 and apoC1-3 (132). Among these apolipoproteins, apoCII is a co-factor necessary for the full expression of LPL activity. ApoCIII and apoE, on the other hand, inhibit LPL activity. Changes in ratios of apoCII/apoCIII and apoCs/apoEs have been shown to alter lipolysis of TGRLs by LPL (113,131,133–134).

RECENT OBSERVATIONS

We have demonstrated that in rats made diabetic with STZ, there was an elevated peak heparin-releasable LPL activity at 2 and 12 weeks after diabetes induction. Interestingly, the higher LPL activity in diabetic rats was not secondary to an expanded cellular pool, which was dramatically, reduced (51). Next, we confirmed that: a) the increase in LPL protein originates mainly in capillary blood vessels, presumably within or at the luminal and abluminal surface of the endothelial cell, b) the intravascular heparin-releasable fraction of cardiac LPL can be acutely (hours)

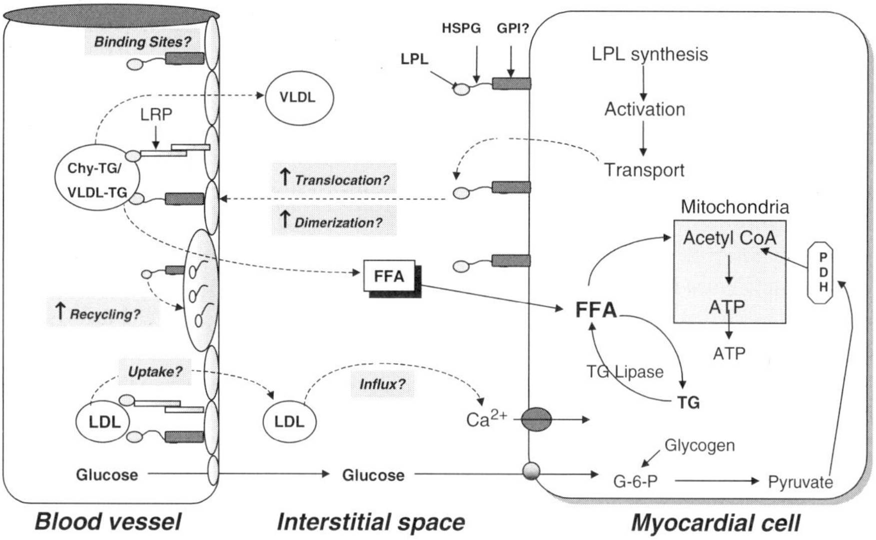

Figure 3. Schematic representation of LPL synthesis, translocation, various functions, and Its possible pathophysiological role in the diabetic heart.

regulated by short-term changes in insulin, and c) the enlarged LPL pool in the diabetic heart is functionally relevant and is capable of hydrolyzing VLDL (135,136). More recently, we present evidence that: a) hyperglycemia is an unlikely candidate for regulating cardiac LPL whose activity more closely correlates with changes in insulin levels, and b) alterations in the transport and utilization of glucose likely modulate changes in cardiac LPL activity and thereby influence free fatty acid consumption (Figure 3). Presently, the mechanism(s) by which insulin regulates LPL at the vascular endothelial cell is not known. Moreover, the role of an enhanced cardiac LPL activity in the diabetic heart is unclear.

SIGNIFICANCE

In Canada, there is an increasing prevalence of diabetes, from 2.4% in 1985 to 5% in 1989. Despite insulin therapy, diabetics in general have both a higher incidence of, and mortality from, heart disease. In addition to factors that enhance the incidence of heart disease in diabetics such as atherosclerosis, altered lipid metabolism in the heart may be a key mechanism for the pathogenesis of a specific diabetic cardiomyopathy. As changes in cardiac LPL can result in abnormal FFA supply and utilization by the heart tissue, it could potentially initiate and sustain cardiac dysfunction during diabetes. Our studies with STZ-diabetic rats indicate that even a short duration of hypoinsulinemia will result in a large increase in the functional LPL pool at the endothelial cell surface. As effective blood glucose control is always difficult in Type 1 diabetic patients, it is possible that over time, these patients are predisposed to brief periods of hypoinsulinemia/hyperglycemia. Interestingly, when compared to age- and sex-matched controls, significantly higher levels of post heparin plasma LPL have been reported in insulin-treated Type 1 patients with diabetes of 10 years or more duration (137). Hence, it is conceivable that a parallel increase in functional cardiac LPL activity in insulin-treated diabetic individuals predisposes them to premature death from cardiac disease. We aim to better understand both the role and the mechanism(s) of dysregulation of cardiac LPL activity in the overall disease process. By gaining more insight into the initial metabolic processes in the diabetic heart, we can attempt to piece together a part of the cascade of events leading to diabetic cardiomyopathy.

REFERENCES

1. Regan TJ, Weisse AB. 1992. Diabetic cardiomyopathy. J Am Coll Cardiol 19:1165–1166.
2. Rodrigues B, Xiang H, McNeill JH. 1988. Effect of L-carnitine treatment on lipid metabolism and cardiac performance in chronically diabetic rats. Diabetes 37:1358–1364.
3. Rodrigues B, Cam MC, McNeill JH. 1995. Myocardial substrate metabolism: implications for diabetic cardiomyopathy. J Mol Cell Cardiol 27:169–179.
4. van der Vusse GJ, Glatz JF, Stam HC, Reneman RS. 1992. Fatty acid homeostasis in the normoxic and ischemic heart. Physiol Rev 72:881–940.
5. Randle PJ, Hales CN, Garland PB, Newsholme EA. 1963. The glucose fatty acid cycle: its role in insulin sensitivity and the metabolic disturbances of diabetes mellitus. Lancet 1:785–789.
6. Rodrigues B, McNeill JH. 1992. The diabetic heart: metabolic causes for the development of a cardiomyopathy. Cardiovasc Res 26:913–922.
7. Eckel RH. 1989. Lipoprotein lipase. A multifunctional enzyme relevant to common metabolic diseases. N Engl J Med 320:1060–1068.
8. O'Brien KD, Ferguson M, Gordon D, Deeb SS, Chait A. 1994. Lipoprotein lipase is produced by cardiac myocytes rather than interstitial cells in human myocardium. Arterioscler Thromb 14: 1445–1451.
9. Hamosh M, Hamosh P. 1983. Lipoprotein lipase: its physiological and clinical significance. Mol Aspects Med 6:199–289.
10. Rodrigues B, Braun JE, Spooner M, Severson DL. 1992. Regulation of lipoprotein lipase activity in cardiac myocytes from control and diabetic rat hearts by plasma lipids. Can J Physiol Pharmacol 70:1271–1279.
11. Murthy VK, Bauman MD, Shipp JC. 1983. Regulation of triacylglycerol lipolysis in the perfused hearts of normal and diabetic rats. Diabetes 32:718–722.
12. Kenno KA, Severson DL. 1985. Lipolysis in isolated myocardial cells from diabetic rat hearts. Am J Physiol 249:H1024–H1030.
13. Chattopadhyay J, Thompson EW, Schmid HH. 1990. Elevated levels of nonesterified fatty acids in the myocardium of alloxan diabetic rats. Lipids 25:307–310.
14. Elkeles RS, Hambley J. 1977. The effects of fasting and streptozotocin diabetes on hepatic triglyceride lipase activity in the rat. Diabetes 26:58–60.
15. Veeraraghavan K, Murthy K, Bauman MD, Shipp J. 1983. Regulation of triacylglycerol lipolysis in the perfused hearts of normal and diabetic rats. Diabetes 32:718–722.
16. Inadera H, Tashiro J, Okubo Y, Ishikawa Y, Shirai K, Saito Y, Yoshida S. 1992. Response of lipoprotein lipase to calorie intake in streptozotocin-induced diabetic rats. Scand J Clin Lab Invest 52: 797–802.
17. Rauramaa R, Kuusela P, Hietanen E. 1980. Adipose, muscle and lung tissue lipoprotein lipase activities in young streptozotocin treated rats. Horm Metab Res 12:591–595.
18. Stam H, Schoonderwoerd K, Breeman W, Hulsmann WC. 1984. Effects of hormones, fasting and diabetes on triglyceride lipase activities in rat heart and liver. Horm Metab Res 16:293–297.
19. Nomura T, Hagino Y, Gotoh M, Iguchi A, Sakamoto N. 1984. The effects of streptozotocin diabetes on tissue specific lipase activities in the rat. Lipids 19:594–599.
20. Tavangar K, Murata Y, Pedersen ME, Goers JF, Hoffman AR, Kraemer FB. 1992. Regulation of lipoprotein lipase in the diabetic rat. J Clin Invest 90:1672–1678.

21. O'Looney P, Vander Maten M, Vahouny GV. 1983. Insulin-mediated modifications of myocardial lipoprotein lipase and lipoprotein metabolism. J Biol Chem 258:12994–13001.
22. Deshaies Y, Geloen A, Paulin A, Bukowiecki LJ. 1990. Restoration of lipoprotein lipase activity in insulin-deficient rats by insulin infusion is tissue specific. Can J Physiol Pharmacol 69:746–751.
23. Braun JE, Severson DL. 1992. Regulation of the synthesis, processing and translocation of lipoprotein lipase. Biochem J 287:337–347.
24. Rodrigues B, Severson DL. 1993. Acute diabetes does not reduce heparin-releasable lipoprotein lipase activity in perfused hearts from Wistar-Kyoto rats. Can J Physiol Pharmacol 71:657–661.
25. Liu L, Severson DL. 1995. Myocardial lipoprotein lipase activity: regulation by diabetes and fructose-induced hypertriglyceridemia. Can J Physiol Pharmacol 73:369–377.
26. Previato L, Parrott CL, Santamarina-Fojo S, Brewer HB, Jr. 1991. Transcriptional regulation of the human lipoprotein lipase gene in 3T3-L1 adipocytes. J Biol Chem 266:18958–18963.
27. Ben-Zeev O, Doolittle MH, Davis RC, Elovson J, Schotz MC. 1992. Maturation of lipoprotein lipase. Expression of full catalytic activity requires glucose trimming but not translocation to the cis-Golgi compartment. J Biol Chem 267:6219–6227.
28. Vannier C, Ailhaud G. 1989. Biosynthesis of lipoprotein lipase in cultured mouse adipocytes. II. Processing, subunit assembly, and intracellular transport. J Biol Chem 264:13206–13216.
29. Liu G, Bengtsson-Olivecrona G, Olivecrona T. 1993. Assembly of lipoprotein lipase in perfused guinea-pig hearts. Biochem J 292:277–282.
30. Scow RO, Schultz CJ, Park JW, Blanchette-Mackie EJ. 1998. Combined lipase deficiency (cld/cld) in mice affects differently post-translational processing of lipoprotein lipase, hepatic lipase and pancreatic lipase. Chem Phys Lipids 93:149–155.
31. Rothman JE, Wieland FT. 1996. Protein sorting by transport vesicles. Science 272:227–234.
32. Olivevrona T, Olivecrona GB. 1993. Lipoprotein lipase and hepatic lipase. Curr Opin Lipidol 4:187.
33. Stins MF, Maxfeild FR, Goldberg IJ. 1992. Polarized binding of lipoprotein lipase to endothelial cells: implications for its physiological actions. Arterioscler Thromb 12:1437–1446.
34. Anderson LG, Carroll R, Ewart HS, Acharya A, Severson DL. 1997. Fatty acid reduce heparin releasable LPL activity in cultured cardiomyocytes from the rat heart. Am J Physiol 273:E759–E769.
35. Shaul TC, Freidman G, Olivecrona GB, Vlodavsky I, Shavit RB. 1990. Interaction of lipoprotein lipase with sub endothelial extracellular matrix. Biochem Biophys Acta 1042:168–175.
36. Blanchette-Mackie EJ, Dwyer NK, Amende LA. 1989. Cytochemical studies of lipid metabolism: immunogold probes for lipoprotein lipase and cholesterol. Am J Anat 185:255–263.
37. Saxena U, Klein MG, Goldberg IJ. 1991. Transport of lipoprotein lipase across endothelial cells. Proc Natl Acad Sci USA 88:2254–2258.
38. Berryman DE, Bensadoun A. 1995. Heparan sulfate proteoglycans are primarily responsible for the maintenance of enzyme activity, binding, and degradation of lipoprotein lipase in Chinese hamster ovary cells. J Biol Chem 270:24525–24531.
39. Sivaram P, Paka L, Sasak A, Vanni-Reyes T, Yin B, Parthasarathy N, Wagner W, Goldberg IJ. 1997. Endothelial cell heparanase modulation of lipoprotein lipase activity. Evidence that heparan sulfate oligosaccharide is an extracellular chaperone. J Biol Chem 272:15753–15759.
40. Michel CC. 1998. Capillaries, caveolae, calcium and cyclic nucleotides: a new look at microvascular permeability. J Mol Cell Cardiol 30:2541–2546.
41. Oh P, McIntosh DP, Schnitzer JE. 1998. Dynamin at the neck of caveolae mediates their budding to form transport vesicles by GTP-driven fission from the plasma membrane of endothelium. J Cell Biol 141:101–114.
42. Niles WD, Malik AB. 1999. Endocytosis and exocytosis events regulate vesicle traffic in endothelial cells. J Membr Biol 167:85–101.
43. Chajek T, Stein O, Stein Y. 1975. Interference with the transport of heparin-releasable lipoprotein lipase in the perfused rat heart by colchicine and vinblastine. Biochim Biophys Acta 388:260–268.
44. Lespine A, Chap H, Perret B. 1997. Impaired secretion of heart lipoprotein lipase in cyclophosphamide-treated rabbit. Biochim Biophys Acta 1345:77–85.
45. Ewart HS, Severson DL. 1999. Insulin and dexamethasone stimulation of cardiac lipoprotein lipase activity involves the actin-based cytoskeleton. Biochem J 340:485–490.
46. Stein O, Stein Y, Schwartz SP, Reshef A, Chajek-Shaul T, Ben-Naim M, Friedman G, Leitersdorf E. 1991. Expression of lipoprotein lipase mRNA in rat heart is localized mainly to mesenchymal cells as studied by in situ hybridization. Arterioscler Thromb 11:857–863.
47. Pedersen ME, Schotz MC. 1980. Rapid changes in rat heart lipoprotein lipase activity after feeding carbohydrate. J Nutr 110:481–487.

48. Camps L, Reina M, Llobera M, Vilaro S, Olivecrona T. 1990. Lipoprotein lipase: cellular origin and functional distribution. Am J Physiol 258:C673–C681.
49. Liu G, Olivecrona T. 1992. Synthesis and transport of lipoprotein lipase in perfused guinea pig hearts. Am J Physiol 263:H438–H446.
50. Liu GQ, Olivecrona T. 1991. Pulse-chase study on lipoprotein lipase in perfused guinea pig heart. Am J Physiol 261:H2044–H2050.
51. Rodrigues B, Cam MC, Jian K, Lim F, Sambandam N, Shepherd G. 1997. Differential effects of streptozotocin-induced diabetes on cardiac lipoprotein lipase activity. Diabetes 46:1346–1353.
52. Currie RA, Eckel RH. 1992. Characterization of a high affinity octamer transcription factor binding site in the human lipoprotein lipase promoter. Arch Biochem Biophys 298:630–639.
53. Enerback S, Gimble J. 1993. Lipoprotein lipase gene expression: physiological regulators at the transcriptional and post-transcriptional level. Biochim Biophys Acta 1169:107–125.
54. Ranganathan G, Ong JM, Yukht A, Saghizadeh M, Simsolo RB, Pauer A, Kern PA. 1995. Tissue-specific expression of human lipoprotein lipase. Effect of the 3′-untranslated region on translation. J Biol Chem 270:7149–7155.
55. Yukht A, Davis RC, Ong JM, Ranganathan G, Kern PA. 1995. Regulation of lipoprotein lipase translation by epinephrine in 3T3-L1 cells. Importance of the 3′ untranslated region. J Clin Invest 96:2438–2444.
56. Mitchell JR, Jacobsson A, Kirchgessner TG, Schotz MC, Cannon B, Nedergaard J. 1992. Regulation of expression of the lipoprotein lipase gene in brown adipose tissue. Am J Physiol 263: E500–E506.
57. Ong JM, Kern PA. 1989. The role of glucose and glycosylation in the regulation of lipoprotein lipase synthesis and secretion in rat adipocytes. J Biol Chem 264:3177–3182.
58. Bergo M, Olivecrona G, Olivecrona T. 1996. Diurnal rhythms and effects of fasting and refeeding on rat adipose tissue lipoprotein lipase. Am J Physiol 271:E1092–E1097.
59. Klingenspor M, Ebbinghaus C, Hulshorst G, Stohr S, Spiegelhalter F, Haas K, Heldmaier G. 1996. Multiple regulatory steps are involved in the control of lipoprotein lipase activity in brown adipose tissue. J Lipid Res 37:1685–1695.
60. Masuno H, Okuda H. 1994. Role of processing of the oligosaccharide chains in the affinity of lipoprotein lipase for heparin. Biochim Biophys Acta 1212:125–128.
61. Park JW, Oh MS, Yang JY, Park BH, Rho HW, Lim SN, Jhee EC, Kim HR. 1995. Glycosylation, dimerization, and heparin affinity of lipoprotein lipase in 3T3-L1 adipocytes. Biochim Biophys Acta 1254:45–50.
62. Cheng CF, Oosta GM, Bensadoun A, Rosenberg RD. 1981. Binding of lipoprotein lipase to endothelial cells in culture. J Biol Chem 256:12893–12898.
63. Shimada K, Gill PJ, Silbert JE, Douglas WH, Fanburg BL. 1981. Involvement of cell surface heparin sulfate in the binding of lipoprotein lipase to cultured bovine endothelial cells. J Clin Invest 68:995–1002.
64. Wang-Iverson P, Brown WV. 1982. Interaction of lipoprotein lipase with cultured endothelial cells. Ann N Y Acad Sci 401:92–101.
65. Williams MP, Streeter HB, Wusteman FS, Cryer A. 1983. Heparan sulphate and the binding of lipoprotein lipase to porcine thoracic aorta endothelium. Biochim Biophys Acta 756:83–91.
66. Cisar LA, Hoogewerf AJ, Cupp M, Rapport CA, Bensadoun A. 1989. Secretion and degradation of lipoprotein lipase in cultured adipocytes. Binding of lipoprotein lipase to membrane heparan sulfate proteoglycans is necessary for degradation. J Biol Chem 264:1767–1774.
67. Chajek-Shaul T, Halimi O, Ben-Naim M, Stein O, Stein Y. 1989. Phosphatidylinositol-specific phospholipase C releases lipoprotein lipase from the heparin releasable pool in rat heart cell cultures. Biochim Biophys Acta 1014:178–183.
68. Parthasarathy N, Goldberg IJ, Sivaram P, Mulloy B, Flory DM, Wagner WD. 1994. Oligosaccharide sequences of endothelial cell surface heparan sulfate proteoglycan with affinity for lipoprotein lipase. J Biol Chem 269:22391–22396.
69. Chevreuil O, Hultin M, Ostergaard P, Olivecrona T. 1993. Depletion of lipoprotein lipase after heparin administration. Arterioscler Thromb 13:1391–1396.
70. de Man FH, de Beer F, van der Laarse A, Smelt AH, Havekes LM. 1997. Lipolysis of very low density lipoproteins by heparan sulfate proteoglycan-bound lipoprotein lipase. J Lipid Res 38: 2465–2472.
71. Eckel RH, Fujimoto WY, Brunzell JD. 1978. Insulin regulation of lipoprotein lipase in cultured 3T3-L1 cells. Biochem Biophys Res Commun 84:1069–1075.

72. Spooner PM, Chernick SS, Garrison MM, Scow RO. 1979. Insulin regulation of lipoprotein lipase activity and release in 3T3-L1 adipocytes. Separation and dependence of hormonal effects on hexose metabolism and synthesis of RNA and protein. J Biol Chem 254:10021–10029.
73. Chan BL, Lisanti MP, Rodriguez-Boulan E, Saltiel AR. 1988. Insulin-stimulated release of lipoprotein lipase by metabolism of its phosphatidylinositol anchor. Science 241:1670–1672.
74. Muller G, Dearey EA, Korndorfer A, Bandlow W. 1994. Stimulation of a glycosyl-phosphatidylinositol-specific phospholipase by insulin and the sulfonylurea, glimepiride, in rat adipocytes depends on increased glucose transport. J Cell Biol 126:1267–1276.
75. Wolle J, Ferguson E, Devall LJ, Newton RS, Saxena U. 1995. Identification of a novel 85-kDa lipoprotein lipase binding protein on human aortic endothelial cell surface. Biochem Biophys Res Commun 216:906–912.
76. Vilella E, Bengtsson-Olivecrona G, Stigbrand T, Jensen PE. 1994. Binding of lipoprotein lipase to alpha 2-macroglobulin. Biochem J 300:443–448.
77. Nielsen MS, Brejning J, Garcia R, Zhang H, Hayden MR, Vilaro S, Gliemann J. 1997. Segments in the C-terminal folding domain of lipoprotein lipase important for binding to the low density lipoprotein receptor-related protein and to heparan sulfate proteoglycans. J Biol Chem 272: 5821–5827.
78. Lee JJ, Smith PJ, Fried SK. 1998. Mechanisms of decreased lipoprotein lipase activity in adipocytes of starved rats depend on duration of starvation. J Nutr 128:940–946.
79. Obunike JC, Sivaram P, Paka L, Low MG, Goldberg IJ. 1996. Lipoprotein lipase degradation by adipocytes: receptor-associated protein (RAP)-sensitive and proteoglycan-mediated pathways. J Lipid Res 37:2439–2449.
80. Hoogewerf AJ, Cisar LA, Evans DC, Bensadoun A. 1991. Effect of chlorate on the sulfation of lipoprotein lipase and heparan sulfate proteoglycans. Sulfation of heparan sulfate proteoglycans affects lipoprotein lipase degradation. J Biol Chem 266:16564–16571.
81. Sehayek E, Olivecrona T, Bengtsson-Olivecrona G, Vlodavsky I, Levkovitz H, Avner R, Eisenberg S. 1995. Binding to heparan sulfate is a major event during catabolism of lipoprotein lipase by HepG2 and other cell cultures. Atherosclerosis 114:1–8.
82. Saxena U, Klein MG, Goldberg IJ. 1990. Metabolism of endothelial cell-bound lipoprotein lipase. Evidence for heparan sulfate proteoglycan-mediated internalization and recycling. J Biol Chem 265:12880–12886.
83. Bengtsson G, Olivecrona T. 1980. Lipoprotein lipase. Mechanism of product inhibition. Eur J Biochem 106:557–562.
84. Saxena U, Goldberg IJ. 1990. Interaction of lipoprotein lipase with glycosaminoglycans and apolipoprotein C-II: effects of free-fatty-acids. Biochim Biophys Acta 1043:161–168.
85. Robinson DS. 1960. The effect of changes in nutritional state on the lipolytic activity of rat adipose tissue. J Lipid Res 1:332–338.
86. Salaman MR, Robinson DS. 1966. Clearing-factor lipase in adipose tissue. A medium in which the enzyme activity of tissue from starved rats increases in vitro. Biochem J 99:640–647.
87. Robinson DS, Jennings MA. 1965. Release of clearing factor lipase by the perfused rat heart. J Lipid Res 6:222–229.
88. Pedersen ME, Schotz MC. 1980. Rapid changes in rat heart lipoprotein lipase activity after feeding carbohydrate. J Nutr 110:481–487.
89. Bergo M, Olivecrona G, Olivecrona T. 1996. Forms of lipoprotein lipase in rat tissues: in adipose tissue the proportion of inactive lipase increases on fasting. Biochem J 313:893–898.
90. Ong JM, Simsolo RB, Saghizadeh M, Pauer A, Kern PA. 1994. Expression of lipoprotein lipase in rat muscle: regulation by feeding and hypothyroidism. J Lipid Res 35:1542–1551.
91. Ladu MJ, Kapsas H, Palmer WK. 1991. Regulation of lipoprotein lipase in adipose and muscle tissues during fasting. Am J Physiol 260:R953 R959.
92. Olivecrona T, Bergo M, Hultin M, Olivecrona G. 1995. Nutritional regulation of lipoprotein lipase. Can J Cardiol 11 Suppl G:73G–78G.
93. Doolittle MH, Ben-Zeev O, Elovson J, Martin D, Kirchgessner TG. 1990. The response of lipoprotein lipase to feeding and fasting. Evidence for posttranslational regulation. J Biol Chem 265: 4570–4577.
94. Schwartz RS, Brunzell JD. 1981. Increase of adipose tissue lipoprotein lipase activity with weight loss. J Clin Invest 67:1425–1430.
95. Eckel RH, Yost TJ. 1987. Weight reduction increases adipose tissue lipoprotein lipase responsiveness in obese women. J Clin Invest 80:992–997.

96. O'Looney PA, Vahouny GA. 1987. Diabetes and lipoprotein lipase activity: Lipoprotein lipase, 229–246 USA: Evener Publishers.
97. Simsolo RB, Ong JM, Saffari B, Kern PA. 1992. Effect of improved diabetes control on the expression of lipoprotein lipase in human adipose tissue. J Lipid Res 33:89–95.
98. Eckel RH, Yost TJ, Jensen DR. 1995. Alterations in lipoprotein lipase in insulin resistance. Int J Obes Relat Metab Disord 19 Suppl 1:S16–S21.
99. Maheux P, Azhar S, Kern PA, Chen YD, Reuven GM. 1997. Relationship between insulin-mediated glucose disposal and regulation of plasma and adipose tissue lipoprotein lipase. Diabetologia 40:850–858.
100. Boivin A, Montplaisir I, Deshaies Y. 1994. Postprandial modulation of lipoprotein lipase in rats with insulin resistance. Am J Physiol 267:E620–E627.
101. Yost TJ, Froyd KK, Jensen DR, Eckel RH. 1995. Change in skeletal muscle lipoprotein lipase activity in response to insulin/glucose in non-insulin-dependent diabetes mellitus. Metabolism 44: 786–790.
102. Kashiwazaki K, Hirano T, Yoshino G, Kurokawa M, Tajima H, Adachi M. 1998. Decreased release of lipoprotein lipase is associated with vascular endothelial damage in NIDDM patients with microalbuminuria. Diabetes Care 21:2016–2020.
103. Hansen PM, Jensen T, Egeberg J, Lithell H, Kofoed-Enevoldsen A, Deckert T. 1997. Skeletal muscle lipoprotein-lipase activity in insulin-dependent diabetic patients with and without albuminuria. J Diabetes Complications 11:230–235.
104. Kessler J. 1963. Effect of diabetes and insulin on the activity of myocardial and adipose tissue lipoprotein lipase of rats. J Clin Invest 42:362–367.
105. Braun JE, Severson DL. 1991. Diabetes reduces heparin- and phospholipase C-releasable lipoprotein lipase from cardiomyocytes. Am J Physiol 260:E477–E485.
106. Rodrigues B, Spooner M, Severson DL. 1992. Free fatty acids do not release lipoprotein lipase from isolated cardiac myocytes or perfused hearts. Am J Physiol 262:E216–E223.
107. Ewart HS, Carroll R, Severson DL. 1997. Lipoprotein lipase activity in rat cardiomyocytes is stimulated by insulin and dexamethasone. Biochem J 327:439–442.
108. Liu L, Severson DL. 1994. Regulation of myocardial lipoprotein lipase activity by diabetes and thyroid hormones. Can J Physiol Pharmacol 72:1259–1264.
109. Carroll R, Liu L, Severson DL. 1995. Post-transcriptional mechanisms are responsible for the reduction in lipoprotein lipase activity in cardiomyocytes from diabetic rat hearts. Biochem J 310:67–72.
110. Liu L, Severson DL. 1996. Endothelial binding sites for lipoprotein lipase are not diminished in perfused hearts from diabetic rats. Can J Physiol Pharmacol 74:1204–1209.
111. Wilson DE, Zeikus R, Chan IF. 1987. Relationship of organ lipoprotein lipase activity and ketonuria to hypertriglyceridemia in starved and streptozocin-induced diabetic rats. Diabetes 36:485–490.
112. Hirano T, Mamo JC, Takeuchi H, Nagano S, Takahashi T. 1991. Correlation of insulin deficiency and hypertriglyceridemia in diabetic rats. Diabetes Res Clin Pract 12:173–180.
113. Mamo JC, Hirano T, Sainsbury A, Fitzgerald AK, Redgrave TG. 1992. Hypertriglyceridemia is exacerbated by slow lipolysis of triacylglycerol-rich lipoproteins in fed but not fasted streptozotocin diabetic rats. Biochim Biophys Acta 1128:132–138.
114. Staprans I, Pan XM, Rapp JH, Feingold KR. 1992. Chylomicron and chylomicron remnant metabolism in STZ-induced diabetic rats. Diabetes 41:325–333.
115. Duerden JM, Gibbons GF. 1993. Restoration in vitro of normal rates of very-low-density lipoprotein triacylglycerol and apoprotein B secretion in hepatocyte cultures from diabetic rats. Biochem J 294:167–171.
116. Garg A. 1994. Management of dyslipidemia in IDDM patients. Diabetes Care 17:224–234.
117. Yoshino G, Hirano T, Kazumi T. 1996. Dyslipidemia in diabetes mellitus. Diabetes Res Clin Pract 33:1–14.
118. Taskinen MR. 1987. Lipoprotein lipase in diabetes. Diabetes Metab Rev 3:551–570.
119. Ebara T, Hirano T, Mamo JC, Sakamaki R, Furukawa S, Nagano S, Takahashi T. 1994. Hyperlipidemia in streptozocin-diabetic hamsters as a model for human insulin-deficient diabetes: comparison to streptozocin-diabetic rats. Metabolism 43:299–305.
120. Bagdade JD, Porte D, Jr., Bierman EL. 1968. Acute insulin withdrawal and the regulation of plasma triglyceride removal in diabetic subjects. Diabetes 17:127–132.
121. Jeppesen J, Hollenbeck CB, Zhou MY, Coulston AM, Jones C, Chen YD, Reaven GM. 1995. Relation between insulin resistance, hyperinsulinemia, postheparin plasma lipoprotein lipase activity, and postprandial lipemia. Arterioscler Thromb Vasc Biol 15:320–324.

122. Zhang Q, Cavallero E, Hoffmann MM, Cavanna J, Kay A, Charles A, Braschi S, Marz W, Perlemuter L, Jacotot B, Galton DJ. 1997. Mutations at the lipoprotein lipase gene locus in subjects with diabetes mellitus, obesity and lipaemia. Clin Sci (Lond) 93:335–341.
123. Knudsen P, Murtomaki S, Antikainen M, Ehnholm S, Lahdenpera S, Ehnholm C, Taskinen MR. 1997. The Asn-291–>Ser and Ser-477–>Stop mutations of the lipoprotein lipase gene and their significance for lipid metabolism in patients with hypertriglyceridaemia. Eur J Clin Invest 27:928–935.
124. Ahn YI, Ferrell RE, Hamman RF, Kamboh MI. 1993. Association of lipoprotein lipase gene variation with the physiological components of the insulin-resistance syndrome in the population of the San Luis Valley, Colorado. Diabetes Care 16:1502–1506.
125. Wang XL, McCredie RM, Wilcken DE. 1996. Common DNA polymorphisms at the lipoprotein lipase gene. Association with severity of coronary artery disease and diabetes. Circulation 93: 1339–1345.
126. Julien P, Vohl MC, Gaudet D, Gagne C, Levesque G, Despres JP, Cadelis F, Brun LD, Nadeau A, Ven Murthy MR. 1997. Hyperinsulinemia and abdominal obesity affect the expression of hypertriglyceridemia in heterozygous familial lipoprotein lipase deficiency. Diabetes 46:2063–2068.
127. Tsutsumi K, Inoue Y, Shima A, Murase T. 1995. Correction of hypertriglyceridemia with low high-density lipoprotein cholesterol by the novel compound NO-1886, a lipoprotein lipase-promoting agent, in STZ-induced diabetic rats. Diabetes 44:414–417.
128. Groop PH, Elliott T, Ekstrand A, Franssila-Kallunki A, Friedman R, Viberti GC, Taskinen MR. 1996. Multiple lipoprotein abnormalities in type I diabetic patients with renal disease. Diabetes 45:974–979.
129. Chen YD, Howard J, Huang V, Kraemer FB, Reaven GM. 1980. Dissociation between plasma triglyceride concentration and tissue lipoprotein lipase deficiency in insulin-deficient rats. Diabetes 29:643–647.
130. Bar-on H, Levy E, Oschry Y, Ziv E, Shafrir E. 1984. Removal defect of very-low-density lipoproteins from diabetic rats. Biochim Biophys Acta 793:115–118.
131. O'Looney P, Irwin D, Briscoe P, Vahouny GV. 1985. Lipoprotein composition as a component in the lipoprotein clearance defect in experimental diabetes. J Biol Chem 260:428–432.
132. Breslow JL. 1989. Genetic basis of lipoprotein disorders. J Clin Invest 84:373–380.
133. Levy E, Shafrir E, Ziv E, Bar-On H. 1985. Composition, removal and metabolic fate of chylomicrons derived from diabetic rats. Biochim Biophys Acta 834:376–385.
134. Saheki S, Hitsumoto Y, Murase M, Takeuchi N, Uchida K. 1993. In vitro degradation of very low density lipoprotein from diabetic patients by lipoprotein lipase.Clin Chim Acta 217:105–114.
135. Sambandam N, Abrahani MA, St Pierre E, Al-Atar O, Cam MC, Rodrigues B. 1999. Localization of lipoprotein lipase in the diabetic heart: regulation by acute changes in insulin. Arterioscler Thromb Vasc Biol 19:1526–1534.
136. Rio ALD, Sandalio LM, Palma JM, Bueno P, Corpas FJ. 1991. Metabolism of oxygen radicals in peroxisomes and cellular implications. Free Radicals Biol. Med. 557.
137. Rutledge JC, Woo MM, Rezai AA, Curtiss LK, Goldberg IJ. 1997. Lipoprotein lipase increases lipoprotein binding to the artery wall and increases endothelial layer permeability by formation of lipolysis products. Circ Res 80:819–828.

Frontiers in Cardiovascular Health, edited by
N.S. Dhalla, A. Chockalingam,
H.I. Berkowitz & P.K. Singal
Kluwer Academic Publishers, Boston, 2003

Does Reperfusion Cause Any Injury to the Myocardium?

Petr Ostadal,[1] Irena Zdobnicka, and Naranjan S. Dhalla

Institute of Cardiovascular Sciences St. Boniface General Hospital Research Centre & Department of Physiology, Faculty of Medicine University of Manitoba, Winnipeg, Canada and [1]Department of Internal Medicine University Hospital Motol, Charles University Prague, Czech Republic

Summary. Enormous effort has been made during the past three decades to explain the pathologic events which occur upon reperfusion of the previously ischemic heart in animals. Experimental studies have described potentially harmful effects of reperfusion, a phenomenon called "reperfusion injury". It is based on the observations in different animals that some myocardial damage occurs upon reperfusion if it is not instituted within a certain time-period of the ischemic insult. Although reperfusion has been shown as the most efficient treatment strategy for acute myocardial infarction in humans, arrhythmias and myocardial depression (cardiac stunning) have been observed upon reperfusion in patients with acute myocardial infarction; these harmful effects are temporary. In fact, the hard-core evidence that reperfusion causes myocardial injury in human is lacking and this is primarily due to the fact that a host of drugs are administered before inducing reperfusion by angioplasty, thrombolytic therapy or coronary bypass surgery. The purpose of this article is to summarize the current knowledge regarding the relationship between reperfusion and reperfusion injury and their implications in clinical management. De spite abundant information concerning the reperfusion-related injury, it is not clear whether reperfusion causes further injury to the ischemia-damaged cardiomyocytes or it is the delayed effect of ischemia per se. In addition, modifications of the reperfusion conditions have not been shown to improve the long-term damage to the myocardium. Thus, some caution should be exercised in interpreting the data from animal experiments to human until long-term results on ischemia-reperfusion injury are available.

***Key words*:** reperfusion, myocardial ischemia, acute myocardial infarction, cardiac protection.

Correspondence to: Prof. Dr. N.S. Dhalla, Institute of Cardiovascular Sciences, St. Boniface General Hospital Research Centre, 351 Tache Avenue, Winnipeg, Manitoba, R2H 2A6, Canada. Tel: (204) 235-3417, Fax: (204) 233-6723, E-mail: nsdhalla@sbrc.ca.

INTRODUCTION

Restoration of blood flow to the ischemic myocardium is widely accepted as an effective approach in the clinical management of conditions associated with the ischemic heart disease. It has been repeatedly shown that early reperfusion decreases infarct size and improves prognosis of patients with acute myocardial infarction (AMI). Similarly, shorter time of cardiopulmonary by-pass improves the outcome of cardiac surgery. Introduction of reperfusion therapy into the clinical practice was, therefore, one of the milestones in the treatment strategy for AMI and in fact successful reperfusion is the life-saving intervention employed by cardiologists and cardiac surgeons all around the world. At present, reperfusion in the ischemic heart is carried out by angioplasty, thrombolytic therapy and coronary by-pass surgery. While the importance of reperfusion in the clinical management is readily apparent, the results from experimental laboratories have described harmful effects of reperfusion—a phenomenon called "reperfusion injury".

Animal studies have shown that reperfusion of the ischemic myocardium induces an injurious component counteracting the positive effect. Already in 1935 Tennant and Wigers (1) observed the reperfusion-induced fibrillation in the dog heart. Furthermore, Jennings et al. (2) described adverse structural and electrophysiologic changes in the reperfused dog heart. Hearse et al. (3) demonstrated that severe myocardial damage characterized by myofibrilar hypercontracture and sarcolemmal disruption may develop with the onset of reoxygenation of the oxygen-depleted myocardium and this phenomenon was termed "oxygen paradox". Hearse et al. (4) have also shown that the damage occurring during reperfusion was far greater than that which would happen if the ischemia would be maintained. There is an increasing body of evidence for detrimental mechanisms, which are triggered during reperfusion and cause additional damage to the cardiomyocytes already injured by ischemia. Despite abundant data describing impairment of some parameters during the period of reperfusion and despite that reperfusion injury became widely (but not generally) accepted theory, there is a lack of data showing that reperfusion is responsible for this damage. It is still not clear whether reperfusion can lethally injure the viable cells or if it just cleans the ischemia-injured area by removing the already severely damaged cells. Reperfusion-related occurrence of the injury does not provide clear-cut evidence about the cause-effect relationship between reperfusion and injury. The aim of this article is, therefore, to critically review the current knowledge concerning the reperfusion injury. It is proposed to discuss whether the reperfusion injury is caused by reperfusion per se and whether we should target our efforts to block the reperfusion-related damage to the myocardium.

DEFINITION OF REPERFUSION INJURY

The concept of reperfusion injury in the ischemic myocardium was not fully developed until 1983 when Rosenkranz and Buckberg (5) defined it as "those metabolic, functional, and structural consequences of restoring coronary arterial flow . . . that can be avoided or reversed by modification of conditions of reperfusion". Other

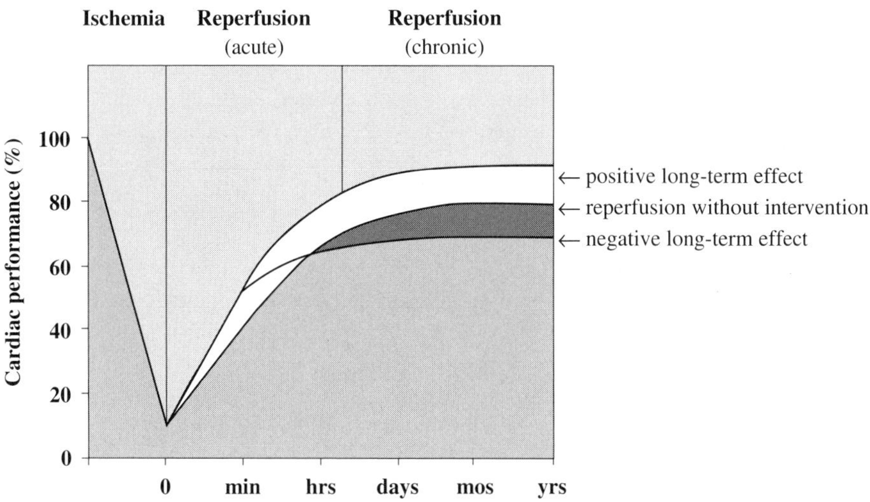

Figure 1. Schematic demonstration of the evolution of cardiac performance after ischemia and reperfusion. Even without the modification of the conditions of reperfusion cardiac performance increases during and after reperfusion. Some interventions to the conditions of reperfusion (e.g. antioxidants) cause faster recovery of cardiac performance in first minutes and hours after the onset of reperfusion (acute reperfusion). There are, however, no data available describing the long-term results (chronic reperfusion) and, therefore, it is not clear whether immediate benefit is a long-lasting effect (positive long-term effect) or it is just increased rate of recovery that is neutral or even harmful in long-term settings (negative long-term effect). Reperfusion injury = potentially harmful effect of the intervention to the conditions of reperfusion; min = minutes; hrs = hours; mos = months, yrs = years.

description of the reperfusion injury was indicated by Park and Lucchesi (6) who defined this process as "death of myocytes, alive at the time of reperfusion, as a direct result of one or more events initiated by reperfusion" as well as by Piper et al. (7) who referred to reperfusion injury as a "causal event associated with reperfusion that had not occurred during the preceding ischemic period and can be entirely attenuated by an intervention given only at the time of reperfusion". Since all major parameters of cardiac performance improve during reperfusion (8), reperfusion injury can also be defined as a difference between good trend and possible better trend (Figure 1). Not defined, however, remains the time of evaluation what is good and what is better? Most of the experimental studies have shown reperfusion injury during the short-time period of minutes and hours after the onset of reperfusion. Current evidence-based clinical medicine, built on long-time, years lasting trials, indicate that even the beneficial immediate effect can be harmful in longer-time period (Figure 1). Without the evidence of longer lasting consequences of reperfusion-induced myocardial damage, clinical medicine should not target its efforts to block these adverse acute effects of reperfusion. Moreover, without such evidence we can look at reperfusion as a healing process of previously damaged myocardial tissue by ischemia. The reperfusion involves the same mechanisms as the healing of any other tissue injury, including inflammatory response, release of oxygen free radicals and proteases. The process of healing is generally initiated by mechanisms which destroy the damaged tissue and replace it by scar. Should we suppress the healing process in the ischemic myocardium when we know from other diseases that it can produce an immediate benefit, but usually it can be harmful in long-term period? Thus, the suppression of reperfusion-related destroying mechanisms may expose the organism to the risk of life-threatening arrhythmias.

MECHANISMS OF REPERFUSION INJURY

Restoration of coronary blood flow not only provides oxygen and other substances which are essential for the survival of the ischemic myocardium, but also agents which may cause further impairment of the tissue already damaged by ischemia. At this point it is necessary to mention that these factors may not be harmful for the healthy tissue and that previous damage by ischemia is fundamental for the development of reperfusion injury (9,10). Reperfusion after a brief period of ischemia does not cause any damage and the extension of reperfusion injury positively correlates with the duration of ischemia. Potentially harmful factors could be divided into the three closely connected groups: (i) factors which are useful or even essential for normal cells but are capable of inducing further damage in already damaged cells (e.g. energy supply, pH normalization); (ii) factors which are harmful either in excess or in the cells with broken self-defense systems (e.g. free radicals, proteases); (iii) factors that are activated by ischemia-induced changes and, therefore, specifically invade damaged tissue (e.g. immune mechanisms). Besides these mechanisms (Figure 2) other important factors—microvascular injury and "no-reflow" phenomenon are related to reperfusion injury.

(i) Factors useful or essential for normal cells

Energy supply

Supply of oxygen and other essential substances lead to restoration of the intracellular energy stores. This energy is immediately used for the activation of important enzymes responsible for the ionic homeostasis of cardiomyocytes and these include sarcolemmal Na^+-K^+ ATPase, sarcolemmal Ca^{2+}-pump ATPase and sarcoplasmic reticulum Ca^{2+}-pump ATPase. If these pumps are not much damaged by ischemia, there is a sufficient capacity for cardiomyocytes to reverse the ion imbalance (7,11). On the other hand, if these mechanisms are severely injured by ischemia, there occurs an intracellular Ca^{2+}-overload and subsequent uncontrolled hypercontracture causing possibly fatal cell damage (7,11,12).

Rapid pH normalization

Ischemic cells suffer from an excess of H^+, mainly because of anaerobic metabolism and breakdown of ATP. Rapid normalization of the interstitial pH during early phase of reperfusion generates a gradient between the interstitium and cytosol and activates the mechanisms for H^+ extrusion; i.e. through Na^+-H^+ exchanger and Na^+-

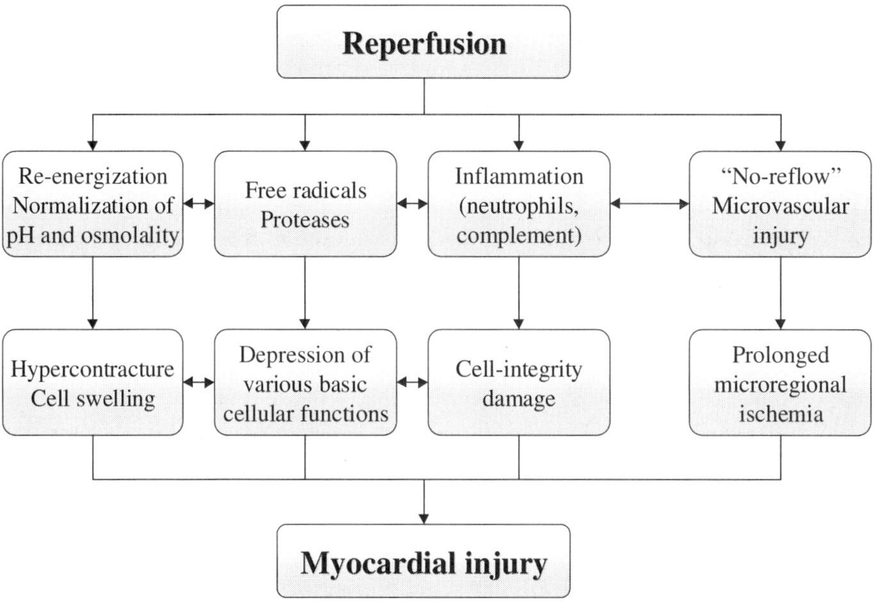

Figure 2. Schematic demonstration of pathologic mechanisms involved in the myocardial injury during reperfusion. The "reperfusion injury" is a complex interaction of (i) factors useful or even essential for normal cells but capable of inducing further damage in already damaged cells (e.g. re-energization, pH normalization); (ii) factors harmful either in excess or in the cells with broken self-defense systems (e.g. free radicals, proteases); (iii) factors that are activated by ischemia-induced changes and, therefore, specifically invade damaged tissue (e.g. mediators of inflammation). Besides these mechanisms, there occurs a microvascular injury and "no-reflow" phenomenon that in fact blocks the reperfusion and prolongs microregional ischemia.

HCO_3^- symporter. An increase in the intracellular H^+ is associated with a rise of cytosolic Na^+ and subsequent cytosolic Ca^{2+}-overload via the Na^+-Ca^{2+} exchanger. Status of ATPases responsible for the intracellular ion homeostasis is again a key factor for cell survival. In addition, decreasing the intracellular H^+ upon reperfusion diminishes the suppressive effect of acidosis on myofibrilar contraction (7,11,13).

Rapid osmolality normalization

Rapid wash out of osmotically active substances accumulated in the extracellular space during ischemia together with the occurrence of intracellular Na^+ overload leads to the generation of osmotic gradient across the sarcolemmal membrane. If the Na^+-K^+ ATPase and other enzymes involved in ion handling are damaged by ischemia and the capacity for Na^+ extrusion is not sufficient, cell swelling with all its consequences may develop (7,11). Although the question about viability of targeted cardiomyocytes remains unanswered, it is pointed out that re-energization, rapid normalization of pH and osmolality intensify the damage in already severely injured cells whereas these factors enable the recovery of less injured cells.

(ii) Factors harmful to cells with decreased self-defense systems

Oxygen free radicals

It is widely accepted that the oxygen free radicals play a major role in cellular damage during reperfusion (8,10,14–17). Oxyradicals are generated from different sources: intracellular, mainly as a side product of restored mitochondrial metabolism and extracellular, partly coming with oxygenated blood and partly from degranulation of the inflammatory cells (e.g. neutrophils and macrophages). It is important to emphasize that at the time of reperfusion, usually the cellular antioxidant-self-defense is damaged by ischemia and, therefore, such cells are very susceptible to the oxygen free radical-induced injury (18). In fact, free radicals are responsible for the depression of various cellular functions. At the sarcolemmal level, these affect different proteins, including those important for cell homeostasis as Na^+-K^+ ATPase, Ca^{2+}-pump ATPase, Na^+-Ca^+ exchanger and Na^+-H^+ exchanger; lipid peroxidation may cause defects in sarcolemma with all their consequences (8,19–21). Depression of the sarcoplasmic reticulum function due to damage of Ca^{2+}-pump ATPase, ryanodine receptor (Ca^{2+}-release channels) and Ca^{2+}-regulatory proteins may significantly decrease the ability of cardiomyocyte to restore Ca^{2+}-handling mechanisms and cell function (22–28). Mitochondrial injury is represented by lipid peroxidation and mitochondrial DNA fragmentation (29–36). Nucleus is another target for oxidative stress as DNA damage by the oxygen free radicals has been reported (36). Also contractile proteins may be depressed by oxyradicals (14).

Proteases

Activation of intracellular proteases as well as release of these enzymes from neutrophil granules have been documented during reperfusion (37,38). Proteases may damage proteins on the same level as oxygen free radicals and cause further impairment of the cardiomyocyte function (38–43). It has been well documented that oxygen free radicals and proteases are involved in the destructive processes triggered by reperfusion. On the other hand, it is reasonable to assume that the cellular defense mechanisms may already be seriously damaged to allow further destruction by these agents. Life-expectancy of such cells is not known as we do not have data showing that oxyradicals and proteases cause death of the viable cells or just accelerate destruction of the already irreversibly damaged cells.

(iii) Factors activated by ischemia-induced changes

Neutrophils

These cells represent the major component contributing to myocardial injury during reperfusion (6,44). Accumulation of neutrophils to the site of myocardial infarction was repeatedly demonstrated by histologic studies (45,46). Recruitment and activation of neutrophils in the infarcted area is subjected to the same rules as any other inflammatory process. Circulating neutrophils are attracted to the site of inflammation by chemotactic factors, which include the complement fragment C5a, interleukin-8, and transforming growth factor-α. Transendothelial migration is enabled by the expression of adhesive molecules, mainly selectin-family and CD11/CD18 from integrin family, and their interaction with activated endothelium (6,47–49). Finally, degranulation of activated neutrophils causes release of proteases, oxygen metabolites, hypochlorous acid and other cytotoxic substances and thereby enhances injury to the infarcted myocardium. Another way by which neutrophils can damage the myocardium during reperfusion is a possible participation in the "no-reflow" phenomenon by the formation of microthrombi and microvascular occlusions.

Complement system

The complement system is a major component of non-specific humoral immunity and important contributor to the inflammation occurring during reperfusion. It is a complex of more than thirty plasmatic proteins. When the activation cascade of the complement is triggered, a complicated interplay among these proteins starts, leading to release of factors responsible for amplification of the inflammatory process, chemoattraction of other immune components, and finally, the formation of membrane attack complex (MAC) capable of cell lysis induction by invading the cell membrane. Activation of this system has been reported to be implicated in reperfusion injury (50–52); however, it is pointed out that the complement is probably activated during the ischemic phase before the onset of reperfusion (53–55). Other factors have also been described to play a role in the immune response during reperfusion. Degranulation of mast cells (at least in part started already before the onset of reperfusion) causes release of important mediators such as histamine (43,47,56). Migration of monocytes as well as their maturation and production of different regulatory cytokines has also been reported (57,58) and is considered to be the contribution of monocyte/macrophage to the reperfusion injury; specific role of different cytokines has been described for this process (59,60).

Several aspects of inflammatory reaction during reperfusion should be pointed out: (i) inflammatory reaction is triggered by changes caused by ischemia, (ii) at least in marginal zone, inflammatory reaction is triggered often before the onset of reperfusion, (iii) probably most important in this context is the fact that inflammatory process is in general targeted to remove the pathologic and the damaged structures and, if necessary, replace it by scar. There are well-described immunopathologic conditions (e.g. allergy or autoimmune diseases) when excessive immune reaction may cause tissue damage; however, there is no evidence that immune reaction during reperfusion fulfils these criteria. Thus, should we block inflammation during reperfusion? It is true, for example, that immunosuppressive treatment may relieve symptoms of some acute viral infections. On the other hand, such intervention may slow down defense mechanisms with all their consequences including chronic persistence of pathogenic virus, and thereby it can be harmful in the long-term outcome.

(iv) No-reflow phenomenon and microvascular injury

This phenomenon was first reported in the heart by Krug et al. (61), who defined it as the "inability of blood to reperfuse an ischemic region, despite the removal of

Table 1. Clinical relevance of "reperfusion injury"

	Observation in humans	Clinical relevance
Reperfusion-induced arrhythmias	+	–
Reperfusion-induced stunning	+	+/–
Reperfusion-induced vascular damage	+	+
Reperfusion-induced cardiac damage	?	?

+, Published studies support this observation; –, published studies do not support this observation; +/– published studies are conflicting; ?, no data are available.

the vascular obstruction responsible for ischemia". Other mechanisms have also been reported to be involved and these include changes in structure and function of the endothelium, changes in constituents of blood, vasoconstriction, and capillary occlusion by platelets and neutrophils (44,62–64). To refer to the no-reflow phenomenon in this context may be controversial from several points. Although this event is strictly connected to the period of reperfusion, it virtually causes blockade for complete reperfusion and in fact prolongs ischemia in some regions. In contrast to the reperfusion injury, no-reflow phenomenon has clear clinical implications as the presence of no-reflow in patients with AMI is associated with worse recovery of global and regional contractility, higher incidence of arrhythmias, and development of congestive heart failure (65). Therefore it is, undoubtedly, an important target of therapeutic approaches. Collapse of microcirculation and no-reflow phenomenon have also an experimental consequence. In some experimental models (e.g. Langendorff model of the isolated heart) it may mask the genuine effect of reperfusion injury and, therefore, events that are being related to reperfusion may be caused (at least in part) by prolonged ischemia.

CLINICAL RELEVANCE OF REPERFUSION INJURY

Better understanding of the reperfusion injury from the clinical point of view was enabled by Hearse et al. (66,67), who divided the consequences of reperfusion into the four sequential events: (i) reperfusion-induced arrhythmias, (ii) myocardial stunning, (iii) lethal reperfusion-induced injury, and (iv) accelerated necrosis. This classification was later modified by Ferrari and Hearse (68), presenting the clinical relevance of the reperfusion injury in four blocks: (i) reperfusion-induced arrhythmias, (ii) reperfusion-induced stunning, (iii) reperfusion-induced vascular damage, and (iv) reperfusion-induced cardiac damage (Table 1).

(i) Reperfusion-induced arrhythmias

Reperfusion-induced arrhythmias may occur within seconds of the onset of reperfusion and are observed in different species including human (68–71). Reperfusion-related arrhythmias in the human heart are commonly seen in the open-heart surgery, cardiopulmonary bypass or after transplantation as well as after successful reperfusion in AMI. However, such arrhythmias are not an important management problem and in fact a short run of accelerated idioventricular rhythm (typical reperfusion arrhythmias in human) is an ECG marker of successful reperfusion in addition to representing the likelihood of recovery of mechanical function after thrombolysis (72).

(ii) Reperfusion-induced stunning

Myocardial stunning is defined as the mechanical dysfunction that persist after reperfusion despite the absence of irreversible damage and despite restoration of normal or near-normal coronary flow (9). It is in fact a dysfunction of the reversibly damaged myocardium that develops during ischemia and that is recovering during the period of reperfusion. Myocardial stunning may be responsible (at least in part) for the dysfunction observed in acute coronary syndrome as well as in chronic coronary artery disease (10,68,73). It is in general a well-tolerated condition (68). Recovery of contractility after AMI in majority takes place in 7–10 days (74) and if it is supposed to be treated, it usually augurs well to general treatment of heart failure. Occurrence of myocardial stunning in unstable angina and in chronic forms of ischemic heart disease is usually confused with hibernation since it is dependent on the pathologic pathways leading to cardiac dysfunction: episodes of ischemia and reperfusion on one side and fluctuating ischemia on the other side. Diagnosis of stunning in such cases is from clinical point of view an academic question; if revascularization procedure is considered, assessment of viability is indicated. The significance of possible stunning increases in the patients with critically low ejection fraction and low output syndrome, where the contractible mechanism should be stimulated. Under these circumstances, however, adequate treatment including the positive inotropic agents is a common approach irrespective of the diagnosis of stunning (68). On the other hand, if any modification of the conditions of reperfusion is proven to be efficient, these high-risk patients could definitely profit from such interventions.

(iii) Reperfusion-induced vascular damage

As described above, the presence of "no-reflow" phenomenon is associated with worse prognosis of the patients with AMI undergoing reperfusion therapy (65) and it is, therefore, a clear and important target for the development of therapeutic interventions.

(iv) Reperfusion-induced cardiac damage

It is not easy to provide a proof for the existence of lethal reperfusion injury; the majority of studies in this area are not sufficient in duration of follow up and, therefore, it is not clear whether the conditions of reperfusion influence the cardiac damage or just the rate of injury and/or recovery (66,68). Since there is a lack of evidence describing the occurrence of lethal reperfusion injury and its existence remains highly controversial even in experimental models, it is not surprising that virtually almost nothing is known about lethal reperfusion injury under clinical settings (68). Nonetheless, the real danger of reperfusion injury should not be ignored, particularly when the reperfusion of the ischemic myocardium is carried out beyond a certain time-period after the ischemic insult.

CONCLUSION

It can be concluded that despite enormous efforts to explain defects occurring during reperfusion, the clear evidence that reperfusion causes an additional injury to the ischemic myocardium, under clinical situations is still lacking. The existing literature supports the suggestion presented by Bolli (75) that the term "reperfusion injury" is actually a misnomer and that the appropriate term should be "ischemia-reperfusion injury". Although reperfusion of the acute ischemic myocardium is known to produce arrhythmias and cardiac stunning, these defects are short-lived. Since reperfusion in patients is usually carried out after administering different drugs, it is possible that the reperfusion associated defects are protected by these agents. In fact, there is no evidence to indicate that any of the reperfusion-related events fulfils the definition of reperfusion injury from the long-term point of view. Accordingly, it is suggested that (i) more data showing the long-term efficiency of different modifications of the conditions of reperfusion are required, (ii) more data about the clinical importance of reperfusion injury are needed, and (iii) careful approach to clinical experiments with respect to the identification of reperfusion injury is necessary. On the other hand, reperfusion-induced no-reflow phenomenon, which in fact blocks reperfusion and prolongs ischemia may be of great clinical importance. Since the no-reflow phenomenon is the only event related to reperfusion which has been shown to be harmful in patients with ischemic heart disease, it represents a clear target for developing therapeutic interventions.

ACKNOWLEDGEMENTS

The work described in this article was supported by a grant from the Canadian Institutes of Health Research (CIHR) Group in Experimental Cardiology. NSD holds CIHR/Pharmaceutical Research and Development Chair in Cardiovascular Research supported by Merck Frosst Canada Ltd. PO and IZ were postdoctoral fellows supported by the St. Boniface General Hospital Research Foundation.

REFERENCES

1. Tennant R, Wiggers C. 1935. The effect of coronary occlusion on myocardial contraction. Am J Physiol 112:351–361.
2. Jennings RB, Sommers HM, Smyth GA, Flack HA, Linn H. 1960. Myocardial necrosis induced by temporary occlusion of a coronary artery in the dog. Pathology 70:68–78.
3. Hearse DJ, Humphrey SM, Chain EB. 1973. Abrupt reoxygenation of the anoxic potassium-arrested perfused rat heart: a study of myocardial enzyme release. J Mol Cell Cardiol 5:395–407.
4. Hearse DJ, Humphrey SM, Bullock GR. 1978. The oxygen paradox and the calcium paradox: two facets of the same problem? J Mol Cell Cardiol 10:641–668.
5. Rosenkranz ER, Buckberg GD. 1983. Myocardial protection during surgical coronary reperfusion. J Am Coll Cardiol 1:1235–1246.
6. Park JL, Lucchesi BR. 1999. Mechanisms of myocardial reperfusion injury. Ann Thorac Surg 68:1905–1912.

7. Piper HM, Garcia-Dorado D, Ovize M. 1998. A fresh look at reperfusion injury. Cardiovasc Res 38: 291–300.
8. Dhalla NS, Golfman L, Takeda S, Takeda N, Nagano M. 1999. Evidence for the role of oxidative stress in acute ischemic heart disease: a brief review. Can J Cardiol 15:587–593.
9. Bolli R. 1990. Mechanism of myocardial "stunning". Circulation 82:723–738.
10. Bolli R, Marban E. 1999. Molecular and cellular mechanisms of myocardial stunning. Physiol Rev 79:609–634.
11. Piper HM, Garcia-Dorado D. 1999. Prime causes of rapid cardiomyocyte death during reperfusion. Ann Thorac Surg 68:1913–1919.
12. Hearse DJ, Humphrey SM, Boink AB, Ruigrok TJ. 1978. The calcium paradox: metabolic, electrophysiological, contractile and ultrastructural characteristics in four species. Eur J Cardiol 7:241–256.
13. Ladilov YV, Siegmund B, Piper HM. 1995. Protection of reoxygenated cardiomyocytes against hypercontracture by inhibition of Na^+/H^+ exchange. Am J Physiol 268:H1531–H1539.
14. Bolli R. 1998. Causative role of oxyradicals in myocardial stunning: a proven hypothesis. A brief review of the evidence demonstrating a major role of reactive oxygen species in several forms of postischemic dysfunction. Basic Res Cardiol 93:156–162.
15. Ferrari R, Ceconi C, Curello S, Cargnoni A, De Giuli F, Visioli O. 1992. Occurrence of oxidative stress during myocardial reperfusion. Mol Cell Biochem 111:61–69.
16 Ferrari R, Alfieri O, Curello S, Ceconi C, Cargnoni A, Marzollo P, Pardini A, Caradonna E, Visioli O. 1990. Occurrence of oxidative stress during reperfusion of the human heart. Circulation 81:201–211.
17. Jeroudi MO, Hartley CJ, Bolli R. 1994. Myocardial reperfusion injury: role of oxygen radicals and potential therapy with antioxidants. Am J Cardiol 73:2B–7B.
18. Dhalla NS, Elmoselhi AB, Hata T, Makino N. 2000. Status of myocardial antioxidants in ischemia-reperfusion injury. Cardiovasc Res 47:446–456.
19. Dixon IMC, Kaneko M, Hata T, Panagia V, Dhalla NS. 1990. Alterations in cardiac membrane Ca^{2+} transport during oxidative stress. Mol Cell Biochem 99:125–133.
20. Shao Q, Matsubara T, Bhatt SK, Dhalla NS. 1995. Inhibition of cardiac sarcolemma Na^+-K^+ ATPase by oxyradical generating systems. Mol Cell Biochem 147:139–144.
21. Mochizuki S, Jiang C. 1998. Na^+/Ca^{++} exchanger and myocardial ischemia/reperfusion. Jpn Heart J 39:707–714.
22. Temsah RM, Netticadan T, Chapman D, Takeda S, Mochizuki S, Dhalla NS. 1999. Alterations in sarcoplasmic reticulum function and gene expression in ischemic-reperfused rat heart. Am J Physiol 277(2 Pt 2):H584–H594.
23. Netticadan T, Temsah R, Osada M, Dhalla NS. 1999. Status of Ca^{2+}/calmodulin protein kinase phosphorylation of cardiac SR proteins in ischemia-reperfusion. Am J Physiol 277:C384–C391.
24. Lamers JMJ, Duncker DJ, Bezstarosti K, McFalls EO, Sassen LM, Verdouw PD. 1993. Increased activity of the sarcoplasmic reticular calcium pump in porcine stunned myocardium. Cardiovasc Res 27:520–524.
25. Dhalla NS, Panagia V, Singal PK, Makino N, Dixon IMC, Eyolfson DA. 1988. Alterations in heart membrane calcium transport during the development of ischemia-reperfusion injury. J Mol Cell Cardiol 20(Suppl 2):3–13.
26. Kaplan P, Hendrikx M, Mattheussen M, Mubagwa K, Flameng W. 1992. Effect of ischemia and reperfusion on sarcoplasmic reticulum calcium uptake. Circ Res 71:1123–1130.
27. Dhalla NS, Temsah R. 2001. Sarcoplasmic reticulum and cardiac oxidative stress: an emerging target for heart disease. Emerging Therapeutic Targets 5:205–217.
28. Dhalla NS, Temsah RM, Netticadan T. 2000. Role of oxidative stress in cardiovascular diseases. J Hypertens 18:655–673.
29. Ambrosio G, Zweier JL, Flaherty JT. 1991. The relationship between oxygen radical generation and impairment of myocardial energy metabolism following post-ischemic reperfusion. J Mol Cell Cardiol 23:1359–1374.
30. Lucas DT, Szweda LI. 1998. Cardiac reperfusion injury: aging, lipid peroxidation, and mitochondrial dysfunction. Proc Natl Acad Sci USA 95:510–514.
31. Griffiths EJ, Halestrap AP. 1995. Mitochondrial non-specific pores remain closed during cardiac ischaemia, but open upon reperfusion. Biochem J 307:93–98.
32. Wanagat J, Cao Z, Pathare P, Aiken JM. 2001. Mitochondrial DNA deletion mutations colocalize with segmental electron transport system abnormalities, muscle fiber atrophy, fiber splitting, and oxidative damage in sarcopenia. FASEB J 15:322–332.

33. Ozawa T, Sugiyama S, Tanaka M, Hattori K. 1991. Mitochondrial DNA mutations and disturbances of energy metabolism in myocardium. Jpn Circ J 55:1158–1164.
34. Ide T, Tsutsui H, Hayashidani S, Kang D, Suematsu N, Nakamura K, Utsumi H, Hamasaki N, Takeshita A. 2001. Mitochondrial DNA damage and dysfunction associated with oxidative stress in failing hearts after myocardial infarction. Circ Res 88:529–535.
35. Shlafer M, Kane PF, Wiggins VY, Kirsh MM. 1982. Possible role for cytotoxic oxygen metabolites in the pathogenesis of cardiac ischemic injury. Circulation 66:I85–I92.
36. Bohr VA, Dianov GL. 1999. Oxidative DNA damage processing in nuclear and mitochondrial DNA. Biochimie 81:155–160.
37. Yoshida K, Sorimachi Y, Fujiwara M, Hironaka K. 1995. Calpain is implicated in rat myocardial injury after ischemia or reperfusion. Jpn Circ J 59:40–48.
38. Cheung PY, Sawicki G, Wozniak M, Wang W, Radomski MW, Schulz R. 2000. Matrix metalloproteinase-2 contributes to ischemia-reperfusion injury in the heart. Circulation 101: 1833–1839.
39. Shibata T, Yamamoto F, Suehiro S, Kinoshita H. 1997. Effects of protease inhibitors on postischemic recovery of the heart. Cardiovasc Drugs Ther 11:547–556.
40. Yaoita H, Ogawa K, Maehara K, Maruyama Y. 1998. Attenuation of ischemia/reperfusion injury in rats by a caspase inhibitor. Circulation 97:276–281.
41. Yoshida Y, Shiga T, Imai S. 1990. Degradation of sarcoplasmic reticulum calcium-pumping ATPase in ischemic-reperfused myocardium: role of calcium-activated neutral protease. Basic Res Cardiol 85:495–507.
42. Yoshida K, Inui M, Harada K, Saido TC, Sorimachi Y, Ishihara T, Kawashima S, Sobue K. 1995. Reperfusion of rat heart after brief ischemia induces proteolysis of calspectin (nonerythroid spectrin or fodrin) by calpain. Circ Res 77:603–610.
43. Matsumura Y, Kusuoka H, Inoue M, Hori M, Kamada T. 1993. Protective effect of the protease inhibitor leupeptin against myocardial stunning. J Cardiovasc Pharmacol 22:135–142.
44. Hansen PR. 1995. Role of neutrophils in myocardial ischemia and reperfusion. Circulation 91: 1872–1885.
45. Romson JL, Hook BG, Kunkel SL, Abrams GD, Schork MA, Lucchesi BR. 1983. Reduction of the extent of ischemic myocardial injury by neutrophil depletion in the dog. Circulation 67:1016–1023.
46. Hawkins HK, Entman ML, Zhu JY, Youker KA, Berens K, Dore M, Smith CW. 1996. Acute inflammatory reaction after myocardial ischemic injury and reperfusion. Development and use of a neutrophil-specific antibody. Am J Pathol 148:1957–1969.
47. Frangogiannis NG, Youker KA, Rossen RD, Gwechenberger M, Lindsey MH, Mendoza LH, Michael LH, Ballantyne CM, Smith CW, Entman ML. 1998. Cytokines and the microcirculation in ischemia and reperfusion. J Mol Cell Cardiol 30:2567–2576.
48. Kishimoto TK, Rothlein R. 1994. Integrins, ICAMs, and selectins: role and regulation of adhesion molecules in neutrophil recruitment to inflammatory sites. Adv Pharmacol 25:117–169.
49. Simpson PJ, Todd RF, III, Fantone JC, Mickelson JK, Griffin JD, Lucchesi BR. 1988. Reduction of experimental canine myocardial reperfusion injury by a monoclonal antibody (anti-Mo1, anti-CD11b) that inhibits leukocyte adhesion. J Clin Invest 81:624–629.
50. Hill JH, Ward PA. 1969. C3 leukotactic factors produced by a tissue protease. J Exp Med 130: 505–518.
51. Yasojima K, Schwab C, McGeer EG, McGeer PL. 1998. Human heart generates complement proteins that are upregulated and activated after myocardial infarction. Circ Res 83:860–869.
52. Yasojima K, Kilgore KS, Washington RA, Lucchesi BR, McGeer PL. 1998. Complement gene expression by rabbit heart: upregulation by ischemia and reperfusion. Circ Res 82:1224–1230.
53. Pinckard RN, Olson MS, Kelley RE, DeHeer DH, Palmer JD, O'Rourke RA, Goldfein S. 1973. Antibody-independent activation of human C1 after interaction with heart subcellular membranes. J Immunol 110:1376–1382.
54. Ward PA, Zvaifler NJ. 1971. Complement-derived leukotactic factors in inflammatory synovial fluids of humans. J Clin Invest 50:606–616.
55. Rossen RD, Laughter AH, Orson FM, Flagge FP, Cashaw JL, Sumaya CV. 1985. Human peripheral blood monocytes release a 30,000 dalton factor (30 KD MF) that stimulates immunoglobulin production by activated B cells. J Immunol 135:3289–3297.
56. Linden J. 1994. Cloned adenosine A3 receptors: pharmacological properties, species differences and receptor functions. Trends Pharmacol Sci 15:298–306.
57. Birdsall HH, Green DM, Trial J, Youker KA, Burns AR, MacKay CR, LaRosa GH, Hawkins HK, Smith CW, Michael LH, Entman ML, Rossen RD. 1997. Complement C5a, TGF-beta 1, and MCP-

1, in sequence, induce migration of monocytes into ischemic canine myocardium within the first one to five hours after reperfusion. Circulation 95:684–692.
58. Kumar AG, Ballantyne CM, Michael LH, Kukielka GL, Youker KA, Lindsey ML, Hawkins HK, Birdsall HH, MacKay CR, LaRosa GJ, Rossen RD, Smith CW, Entman ML. 1997. Induction of monocyte chemoattractant protein-1 in the small veins of the ischemic and reperfused canine myocardium. Circulation 95:693–700.
59. Kukielka GL, Smith CW, LaRosa GJ, et al. 1995. Interleukin-8 gene induction in the myocardium after ischemia and reperfusion in vivo. J Clin Invest 95:89–103.
60. Kukielka GL, Smith CW, Manning AM, Youker KA, Michael LH, Entman ML. 1995. Induction of interleukin-6 synthesis in the myocardium. Potential role in postreperfusion inflammatory injury. Circulation 92:1866–1875.
61. Krug A, Du Mesnil DR, Korb G. 1996. Blood supply of the myocardium after temporary coronary occlusion. Circ Res 19:57–62.
62. Hearse DJ, Maxwell L, Saldanha C, Gavin JB. 1993. The myocardial vasculature during ischemia and reperfusion: a target for injury and protection. J Mol Cell Cardiol 25:759–800.
63. Entman ML, Smith CW. 1994. Postreperfusion inflammation: a model for reaction to injury in cardiovascular disease. Cardiovasc Res 28:1301–1311.
64. Ambrosio G, Tritto I. 1999. Reperfusion injury: experimental evidence and clinical implications. Am Heart J 138:S69–S75.
65. Ito H, Maruyama A, Iwakura K, Takiuchi S, Masuyama T, Hori M, Higashino Y, Fujii K, Minamino T. 1996. Clinical implications of the "no reflow" phenomenon. A predictor of complications and left ventricular remodeling in reperfused anterior wall myocardial infarction. Circulation 93:223–228.
66. Hearse DJ. 1990. Ischemia, reperfusion, and the determinants of tissue injury. Cardiovasc Drugs Ther 4(Suppl 4):767–776.
67. Hearse DJ, Bolli R. 1992. Reperfusion induced injury: manifestations, mechanisms, and clinical relevance. Cardiovasc Res 26:101–108.
68. Ferrari R, Hearse DJ. 1997. Reperfusion injury: Does it exist and does it have clinical relevance? J Thromb Thrombolysis 4:25–34.
69. Tanaka K, Hearse DJ. 1988. Reperfusion-induced arrhythmias in the isolated rabbit heart: characterization of the influence of the duration of regional ischemia and the extracellular potassium concentration. J Mol Cell Cardiol 20:201–211.
70. Manning AS, Hearse DJ. 1984. Reperfusion-induced arrhythmias: mechanisms and prevention. J Mol Cell Cardiol 16:497–518.
71. Goldberg S, Greenspon AJ, Urban PL, Muza B, Berger B, Walinsky P, Maroko PR. 1983. Reperfusion arrhythmia: a marker of restoration of antegrade flow during intracoronary thrombolysis for acute myocardial infarction. Am Heart J 105:26–32.
72. Hackett D, McKenna W, Davies G, Maseri A. 1990. Reperfusion arrhythmias are rare during acute myocardial infarction and thrombolysis in man. Int J Cardiol 29:205–213.
73. Bolli R. 1998. Basic and clinical aspects of myocardial stunning. Prog Cardiovasc Dis 40:477–516.
74. Ferrari R, La Canna G, Giubbini R, Milan E, Ceconi C, De Giuli F, Berra P, Alfieri O, Visioli O. 1994. Left ventricular dysfunction due to stunning and hibernation in patients. Cardiovasc Drugs Ther 8(Suppl 2):371–380.
75. Bolli R. 1992. Postischemic myocardial "stunning": pathogenesis, pathophysiology, and clinical relevance. In: Yellon DM, Jennings RB, editors. Myocardial Protection: The Pathophysiology of Reperfusion and Reperfusion Injury. New York: Raven Press, 105–149.

Frontiers in Cardiovascular Health, edited by
N.S. Dhalla, A. Chockalingam,
H.I. Berkowitz & P.K. Singal
Kluwer Academic Publishers, Boston, 2003

Fulminant Myocarditis—From Lethal Disease to Survival

Tohru Izumi, Naoyoshi Aoyama, Mototsugu Nishii,
Hitoshi Takehana, Chieko Matsuda, Ken Kohno,
Junichi Nakahata, and Takayuki Inomata

Department of Internal Medicine and Cardiology, Kitasato University School of Medicine
Sagamihara, 228-8555 Japan

Summary. Fulminant myocarditis is a representative lethal heart disease, in which patients have only been urgently rescued with the help of mechanical cardiopulmonary supports. Nevertheless, the therapeutic outcomes of fulminant myocarditis treated with PCPS has not been elucidated. Recently, a national survey was conducted to undertake these tasks by considering the current situation of patients in Japan and to propose a therapeutic guidelines for fulminant myocarditis using PCPS. Thirty (57.7%) out of 52 patients could be rescued in the survey. Important factors concerning the prognosis were the severity and improvement grade of cardiac and renal dysfunction. Based on the data, management guidelines using PCPS to improve the survival rate of fulminant myocarditis patients were published. Of the individual prognosis of patients treated with PCPS, limiting factors have not been identified even in the present survey.

Key words: Fulminant myocarditis, percutaneous cardiopulmonary support (PCPS), guideline and inflammatory cytokines.

INTRODUCTION

Just at the end of the 19th century, Dr. Fiedler gave a historic lecture of autopsied myocarditis in front of the civil hospital in Dresden, Germany (1). Since his talk, the rapidly progressing and fatal type of myocarditis had been called Fiedler's myocarditis. Recently, the disease is generally named fulminant myocarditis, and the

Correspondence: Prof. Tohru Izumi MD, FACP, Department of Internal Medicine and Cardiology, Kitasato University School of Medicine, Sagamihara, 228-8855 Japan.

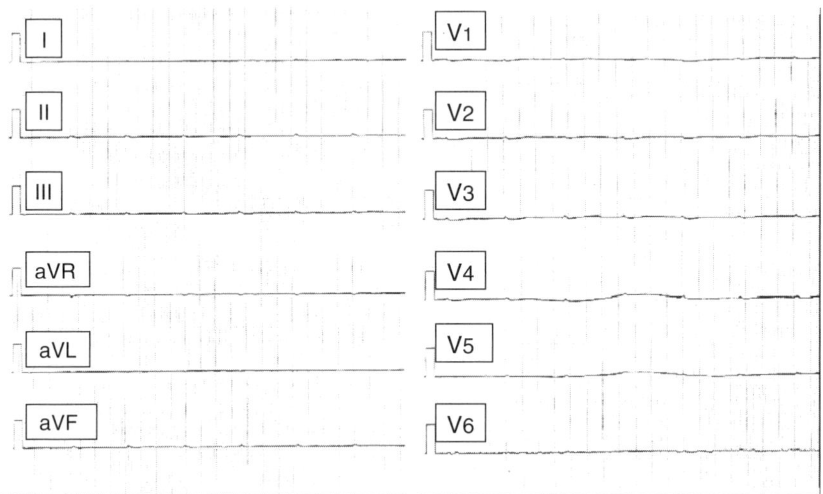

Figure 1. A representative ECG in a patient with fulminant myocarditis. The ECG documented only p waves in all 12 leads revealing ventricular asystole. Despite the fatal changes, this patient was rescued using PCPS, and he returned to normal life.

clinical entity is well known as a representative lethal heart disease. Accordingly, fulminant myocarditis is a disease, in which patients are faced with fatal cardio-pulmonary crisis caused by lethal arrhythmia and/or low output syndrome. These patients urgently require mechanical cardiopulmonary support to rescue them from cardiopulmonary crisis (2–16). Figure 1 shows a representative case of a patient with fulminant myocarditis who had an impressive ECG recorded. The ECG documented only p waves in all 12 leads, that is to say, it indicated ventricular asystole. Despite the fatal changes, this patient was rescued with PCPS, and he returned to normal social life. And another feature is documented in endomyocardial biopsies (Figure 2A). The cell infiltrates and myocardial necrosis are very serious, but this patient managed to survive too. In a case refractory to any therapies, the autopsied heart is quite different from the normal in color and form, changed into an organ similar to a clay work (Figure 2B). In the histological examination, normal myocytes have mostly disappeared (Figure 2C). For these serious patients, we are now applying mechanical cardiopulmonary support to rescue them. Conventionally, PCPS: percutaneous cardiopulmonary support is used all over the world. This circuit functions using catheter techniques. Namely the venous blood is removed from the right atrium with a catheter, and the oxygenated blood is returned into the aorta with a centrifugal pump.

Through many experiments and investigations into myocarditis, the time course of this disease is conceptually understood as shown in Figure 3. Cardiac dysfunction in the myocarditis is caused from two factors: organic changes such as myocar-

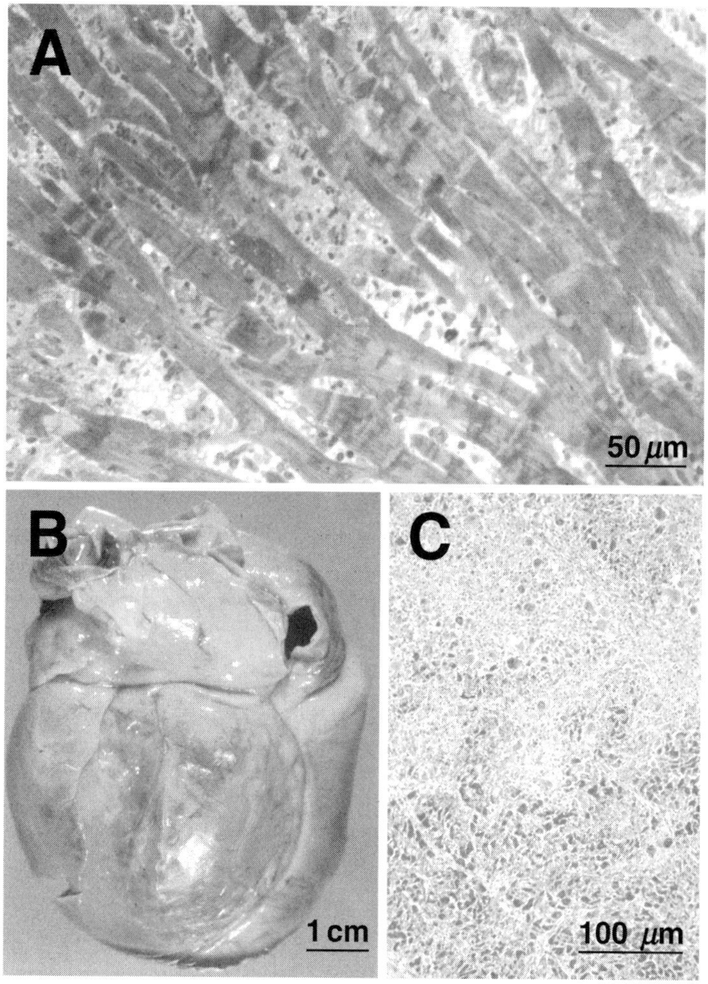

Figure 2. Histopathology of fulminant myocarditis. 2-A: Endomyocardial biopsies obtained on admission. Cell infiltrates and myocardial necrosis are dominant throughout. He also returned to normal life. 2-B: An autopsied heart refractory to any therapies. The appearance is quite different from the normal in color and form. It changes into an organ similar to clay work. 2-C: Histology in the above heart. Normal myocytes have mostly disappeared.

dial necrosis and functional disorders including cytokine inhibitions. Accordingly, practical cardiac failure seems to proceed on a curve superimposed by these two changes. Among the patients with myocarditis, serious cases may reach the fatal zone. Such cases require urgently mechanical support such as bridge therapy to survive the cardiopulmonary crisis. This understanding is the theoretical basis of PCPS use in fulminant myocarditis.

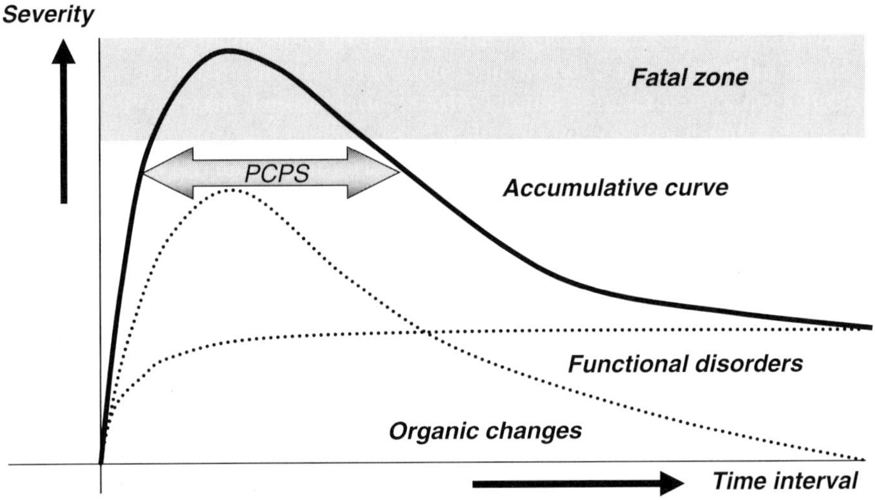

Figure 3. Time course of fulminant myocarditis. Cardiac dysfunction is caused from two factors: organic changes and functional disorders. Accordingly, practical cardiac failure is proceeding on a curve superimposed by these two changes. Fulminant cases reach up to the fatal zone. They urgently require the mechanical support as bridge therapy to survive.

JAPANESE NATIONAL SURVEY ON FULMINANT MYOCARDITIS

For three years, 1997 to 1999, a national survey on fulminant myocarditis was conducted in Japan (17). The investigators were elected from the Japanese Circulation Society. In total, fifty-two patients were enrolled in this survey from every corner of Japan. The patient age was 48 years on average. They consisted of 26 males and 26 females. Accurate diagnosis was done histologically using biopsies and autopsies. On admission, 80% of patients showed very clear consciousness. But their cardiac state was not good: 92% of them belonged to NYHA functional class IV. Consequently, PCPS use has been conducted according to a flowchart as shown in Figure 4. Namely, the indicators are divided into two scenarios: one, a life-threatening arrhythmia and the second, low output syndrome. In case of arrhythmia, cardiopulmonary resuscitation (CPR) was first undertaken. If CPR failed, PCPS was indicated. Then, in the case of low output syndrome, catecholamines (CA) and PDE-III inhibitors were maximally given, and if this was insufficient, intra-aortic balloon pumping (IABP) was added. When the additional treatment failed, PCPS was indicated.

Clinical features of these patients are as follows. Sixty-five percent of them suffered from idiopathic myocarditis, 27% the viral type, and eosinophilic myocarditis and giant cell myocarditis occupied 4%, respectively. As initial symptoms, fever was the most common, and malaise, coughing and nausea followed (Figure 5). All patients showed some ECG findings. Especially, ST-T changes were very common

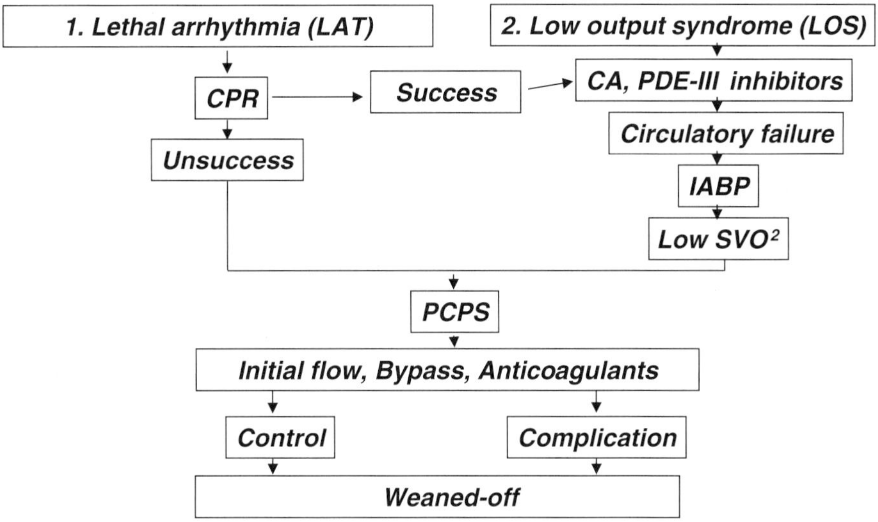

Figure 4. A flowchart of PCPS use in fulminant myocarditis. The indications are divided into two scenarios: life-threatening arrhythmia and low output syndrome. In case of arrhythmia, cardio-pulmonary resuscitation (CPR) was first undertaken. If CPR failed, PCPS was indicated. In the case of low output syndrome, catecholamines (CA) and PDE-III inhibitors were administered, and if they were not helpful, intra-aortic balloon pumping (IABP) was added. When the additional treatments failed, PCPS was indicated.

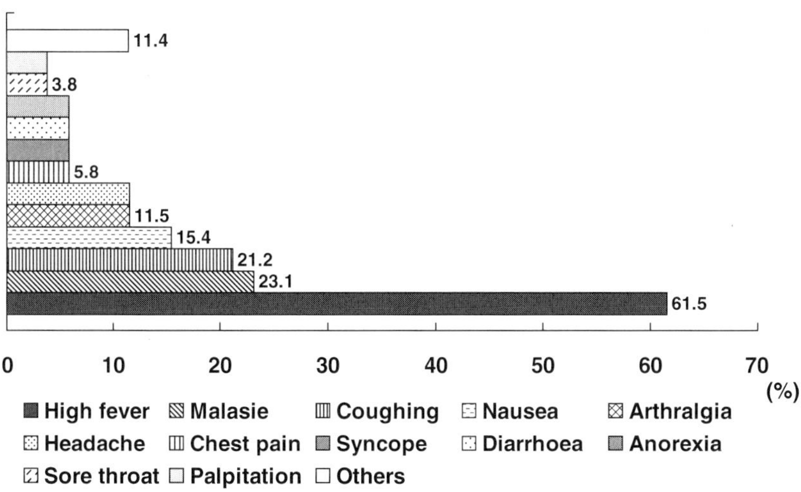

Figure 5. Initial symptoms. A high fever was very common. And malaise, coughing and nausea followed.

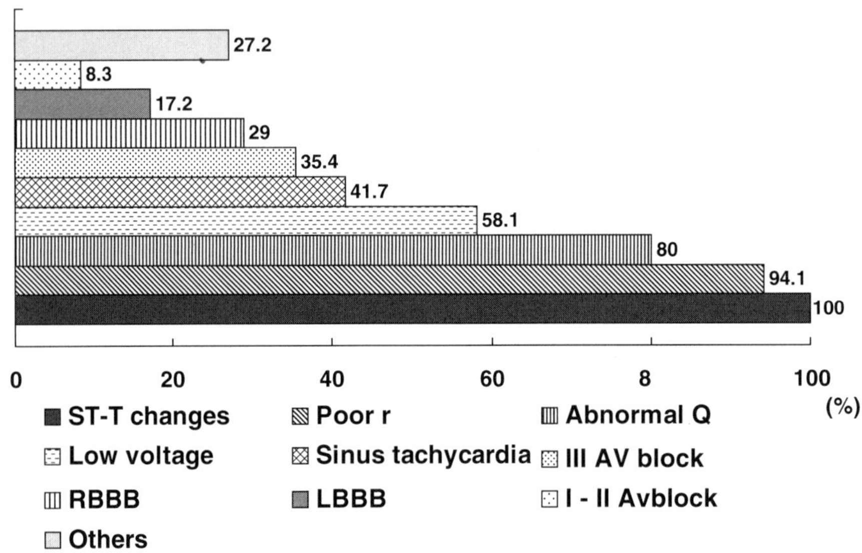

Figure 6. ECG findings. All patients showed changes. Especially, ST-T changes were very common. Poor r progression, abnormal Q and low voltage were also frequent.

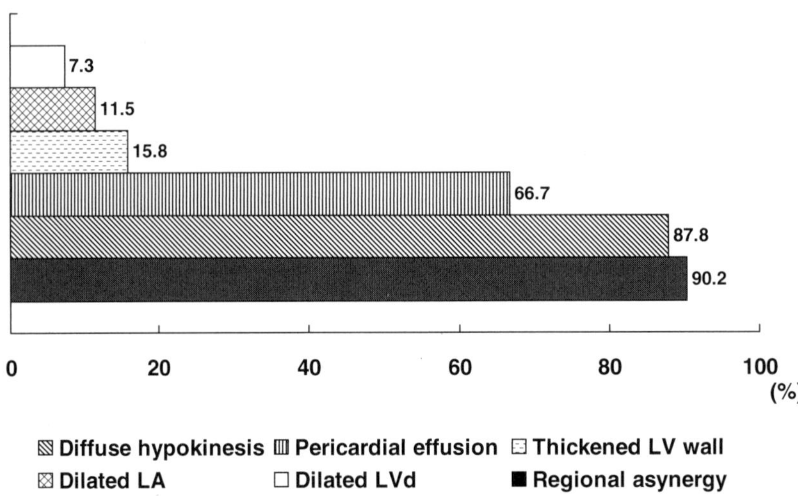

Figure 7. Echocardiogram. Diffuse hypokinesis, pericardial effusion and thickened LV wall were remarked.

in the present survey. Poor r progression in the precordial leads, occurrence of abnormal Q and low voltage appearance were also frequent (Figure 6). Many biomarkers documented the abnormalities. Elevated GOT, CRP, troponin-T (TNT), CPK and LDH were diagnostic indicators as shown in Figure 7.

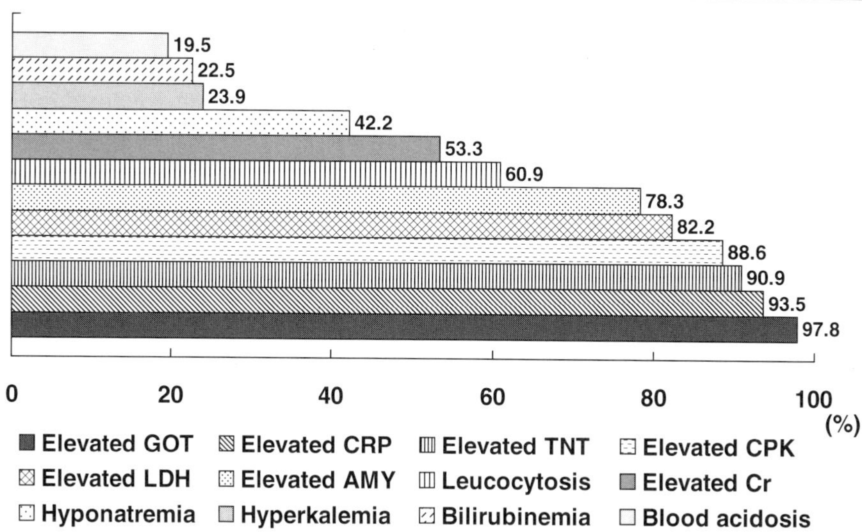

Figure 8. Biomarker abnormalities. Of these, GOT, CRP, troponin-T (TNT), CPK and LDH were diagnostic indicators.

Through this national survey, the following outline was obtained. The patient consulted the physician within 5 days (4.7 days on average) after onset. Within 0.9 day, they were referred to the cardiology department. Under the guidance of specialists, PCPS use was started either because of life-threatening arrhythmia in 24 patients or low output syndrome in 28 patients. Consequently, PCPS was continued for 7.8 days on average. By PCPS use, 30 patients could be rescued and returned to normal social life. On the other hand, unfortunately 21 patients died in the hospital, and 1 patient who suffered from an anoxic brain was accommodated in an institute. To promote the former outcome, guidelines of PCPS use for fulminant myocarditis was proposed by a Japanese investigator group based on the present survey (17). In Figure 8, the outline is introduced.

SURVIVORS AND NON-SURVIVORS

Among the data, clinical features of the survivors were investigated. The survivors were characterized by a higher heart rate, lower CPK level, less leg ischemia and multiorgan failure (MOF), lower doses of noradrenaline (NA) infusion, a lower percentage of steroid therapy, continuous hemo-diffuse filtration (CHDF) use and PCPS exchange in comparison with non-survivors. In a similar way, features of arrhythmia patients were studied. The survivor patients with lethal arrhythmia were characterized by shorter period of use, lower frequency of leg ischemia and MOF, lower levels of creatinine and NA infusion and lower percentage of gamma globulin and CHDF therapy than non-survivors. On the other hand, in survivor subgroup with low output syndrome, higher initial flow, lower incidence of leg ischemia, MOF, diffuse intravascular coagulation (DIC), acidosis and leukocytosis, lower level of

CK-MB and creatine titer were remarked in comparison with non-survivors. Next, those who could be weaned off the PCPS apparatus were studied. The survivors were especially characterized by fewer occurrences of leg ischemia and MOF, lower GOT levels and higher ejection fraction than the nonsurvivors. After PCPS therapy, patients who could complete the post stage were closely related to higher initial flow, lower frequency of leg ischemia and MOF, lower levels of creatinine and higher percentages of low voltage in ECG.

What are good parameters determining the survivor? This is a key question in the present survey. We attempted to answer also using our own experience, 10 patients. The first approach was a histological point of view focusing on cell infiltrates and myocardial necrosis in the endomyocardial biopsies. Unfortunately, histological severity did not show any significant relationships with the prognosis. Even when less severe, some patients died. Thus, biomarkers consisting of inflammatory cytokines were studied. At the present time, tumor necrotizing factor (TNF)-α, interleukin (IL)-4, IL-6, IL-8, IL-10, IL-12, soluble IL-2 receptor (sIL-2R), soluble TNF-α receptor 2 (sTNF-α R2) were evaluated. They were sampled before PCPS, at the time supported by PCPS and after being weaned-off PCPS or at the terminal stage. These biomarkers were measured according to the ELISA method and compared with two controls: normal data form the healthy individuals and disease data from patients with acute myocardial infarction who required the PCPS to rescue because of left main trunk lesions. Of these measures, several biomarkers were noticed. Presently, the serum level of IL-10 was remarked in survivors. In fulminant myocarditis, the level of IL 10 was much higher than the normal control. After the use of PCPS, the level decreased abruptly and entered into the normal range, and at the time of weaning off, the low level could be maintained. These tendencies in the survivor with fulminant myocarditis were compared with those with acute myocardial infarction (Figure 10). In those with this disease, though the level of IL-10 was much higher, noticeably the high titer did not decrease after the use of PCPS. Even at the time of weaning off, the titer did not enter into the normal range. On the other hand, in contrast with the survivors, the serum level of IL-10 was much higher in non-survivors, and even while using PCPS, the level did not normalize until the end of the protocol in survivors with acute myocardial infarction.

In experimental viral myocarditis, cytokine therapy using recombinant IL-10 is an important use to improve mortality (18). At least, in the present study, IL-10 is emerging as a helpful biomarker candidate to assess the short-time prognosis. If the titer is not very high, and then the value is very responsible to PCPS therapy, the prognosis of the patient may be fair or better. But, this tendency is quite different from that of acute myocardial infarction. The clinical usefulness will need to be reconfirmed in further studies before its pathomechanism can be discussed.

NATURAL HISTORY OF THE SURVIVORS

After discharge, the patients were followed up for approximately 3 years, 962 days on average. During the process, two patients suffered from congestive heart failure, and 1 patient had relapsed myocarditis.

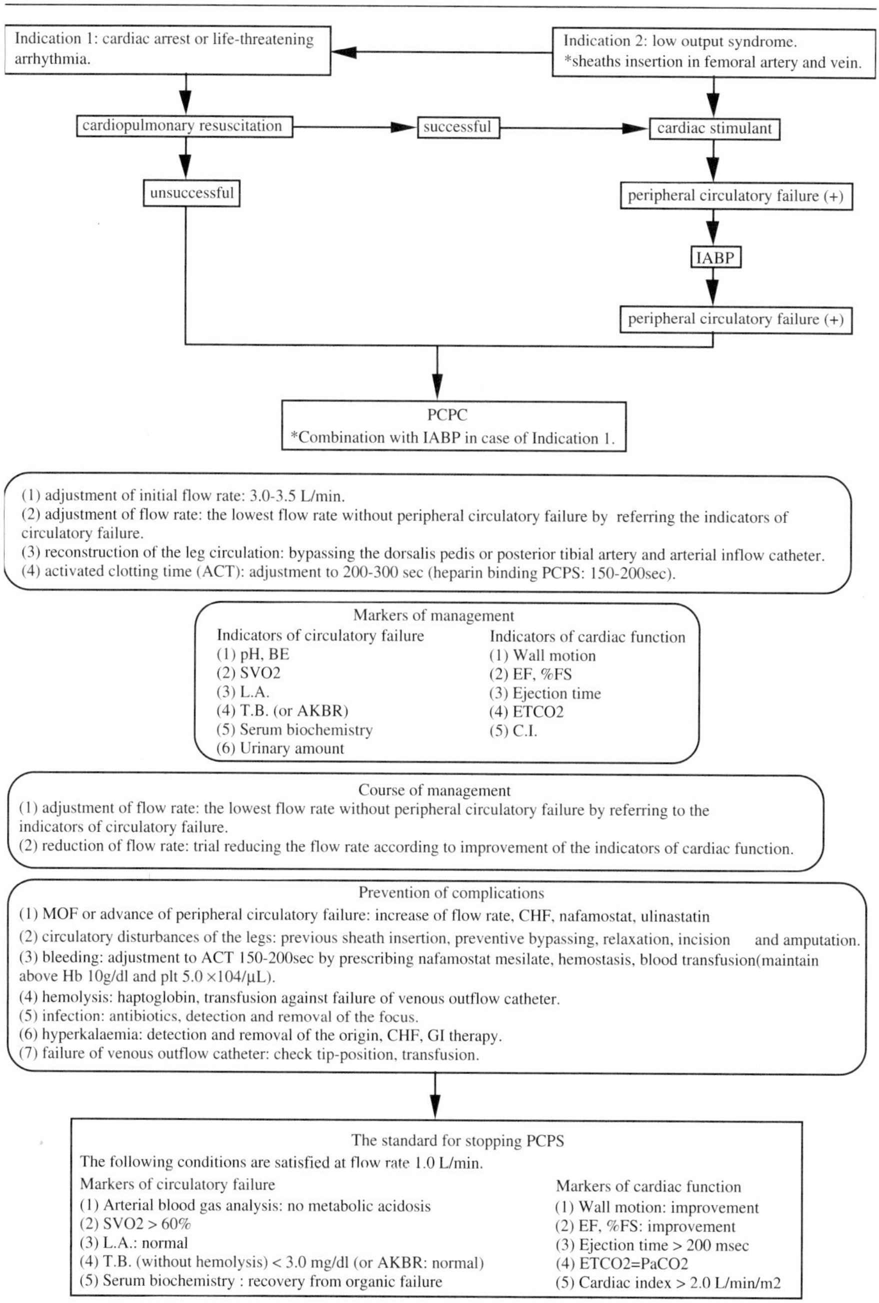

Figure 9. An outline of PCPS use for fulminant myocarditis proposed by the Japanese investigator group.

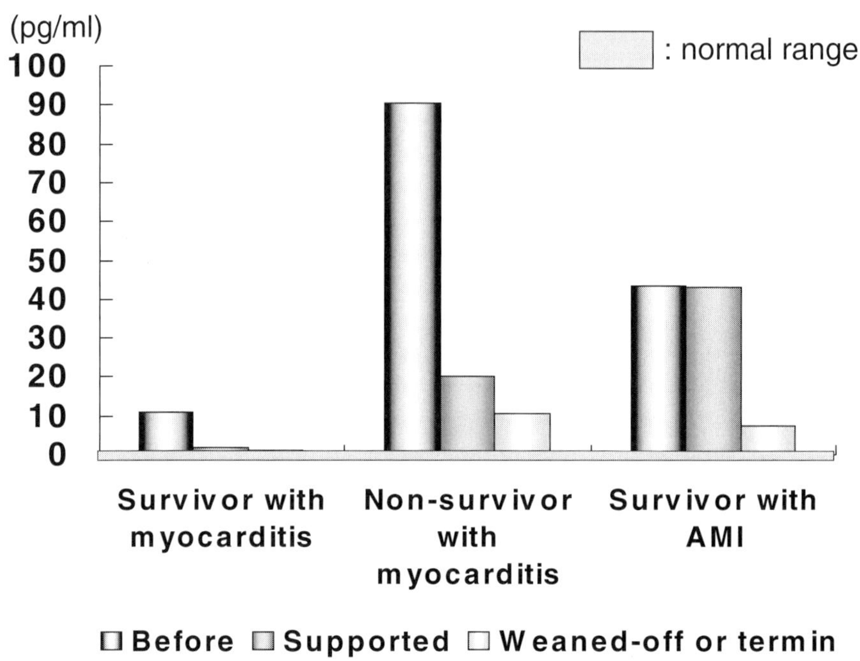

Figure 10. Serum levels of IL-10 among survivors, non-survivors and disease control. In fulminant myocarditis, the level of IL-10 was much higher than the normal control. After the use of PCPS, the level decreased abruptly and entered into the normal range, and at the time of being weaning off, the low level could be maintained. This tendency was not seen in acute myocardial infarction caused by left main trunk lesions. On the other hand, the titer of IL-10 was much higher than that in non-survivors, and even while using PCPS, the level did not normalize.

Upon discharge, the patients recovered quite well. Eighty percent of the patients belonged to NYHA I. However, three years after discharge, seventy-seven percent of the patients experienced good health, but three patients have suffered from cardiac events. From McCarthy's report (19), the fate of survivors with fulminant myocarditis is considered to be good. As we had forecast before the start of national survey, the long-term prognosis of this disease was not good. Survivors with fulminant myocarditis are still obligatory to be followed by specialists for a long period of time.

CONCLUSIONS

Through the present national survey, we could conclude the following. 1. Using PCPS, half of the patients with fulminant myocarditis could be rescued from cardiopulmonary crisis. 2. Among survivors, chronic heart failure and recurrence of myocarditis appeared. 3. Of the biomarkers assessing the efficacy of PCPS use, IL-10 might emerge as the most helpful one.

ACKNOWLEDGMENTS

This study was partly supported by a grant from the vehicles foundation of Japan (1997–1999). Also, we would like to thank Japanese investigators of fulminant myocarditis for their cooperation in achieving this national survey.

REFERENCES

1. Fiedler A. 1899. Über akute interstitielle Myokarditis. Festschrift zur Feir des 50 Jahr. Bestehens des Stadtkrankenhauses Dresden-Friedrichstadt. Dresden part 2, p. 3.
2. Starling RC, Galbraith TA, Baker PB, Howanitz EP, Murray KD, Binkley PF, Watson KM, Unverferth DV, Myerowitz PD. 1988. Successful management of acute myocarditis with biventricular assist devices and cardiac transplantation. Am J Cardiol 62:341–343.
3. Tsuboi H, Sone T, Sassa H, Itoh T, Koyama T, Takasu A, Minakuchi K. 1990. Rescue of a patient with fulminant myocarditis by percutaneous extracorporeal bypass. Jpn J Med. 29:519–522.
4. Rockman HA, Adamson RM, Dembitsky WP, Bonar JW, Jaski BE. 1991. Acute fulminant myocarditis: long-term follow-up after circulatory support with left ventricular assist device. Am Heart J 121: 922–926.
5. Grundl PD, Miller SA, del Nido PJ, Beerman LB, Fuhrman BP. 1993. Successful treatment of acute myocarditis using extracorporeal membrane oxygenation. Crit Care Med 21:302–304.
6. Morishima I, Sassa H, Sone T, Tsuboi H, Kondo J, Koyama T. 1994. A case of fulminant myocarditis rescued–by long-term percutaneous cardiopulmonary support. Jpn Circ J 58:433–438.
7. Reiss N, el-Banayosy A, Posival H, Morshuis M, Minami K, Korfer R. 1996. Management of acute fulminant myocarditis using circulatory support systems. Artif Organs 20:964–970.
8. Nagai N, Ogura R, Seki A, Kajiyama M, Masumoto H, Sasaki M. 1996. Cardiac rescue of an infant with fulminant myocarditis using extracorporeal membrane oxygenation. Jpn Circ J 60:699–702.
9. Yasu T, Murata S, Katsuki T, Fujii M, Kubo N, Ohmura N, Ino T, Saito M. 1997. Acutely severe myocarditis successfully treated by percutaneous cardiopulmonary support applied by a newly developed heparin-binding oxygenator and circuits. Jpn Circ J 61:1037–1042.
10. Kawahito K, Murata S, Yasu T, Adachi H, Ino T, Saito M, Misawa Y, Fuse K, Shimada K. 1998. Usefulness of extracorporeal membrane oxygenation for treatment of fulminant myocarditis and circulatory collapse. Am J Cardiol 82:910–911.
11. Ito M, Tanabe Y, Suzuki K, Kumakura M, Kimura K, Masani F, Aizawa Y. 1999. Left ventricular free wall rupture in acute fulminant myocarditis during long-term cardiopulmonary support. Jpn Circ J 63:397–399.
12. Kato S, Morimoto S, Hiramitsu S, Nomura M, Ito T, Hishida H. 1999. Use of percutaneous cardiopulmonary support of patients with fulminant myocarditis and cardiogenic shock for improving prognosis. Am J Cardiol 83:623–625.
13. Ueno T, Bergin P, Richardson M, et al. 2000. Bridge to recovery with a left ventricular assist device for fulminant acute myocarditis. Ann Thorac Surg 69:284–286.
14. Kohno K, Aoyama N, Shimohama T, Yoshida M, Machida Y, Fukuda N, Aizaki T, Suzuki K, Kurosawa T, Izumi T. 2000. Resuscitation from fulminant myocarditis associated with refractory ventricular fibrillation. Jpn Circ J 64:139–143.
15. Inoue Y, Kaneko H, Yoshizawa Y, Morikawa A. 2000. Rescue of a child with fulminant myocarditis using percutaneous cardiopulmonary support. Pediatr Cardiol 21:158–160.
16. Duncan BW, Bohn DJ, Atz AM, French JW, Laussen PC, Wessel DL. 2001. Mechanical circulatory support for the treatment of children with acute fulminant myocarditis. J Thorac Cardiovasc Surg 122:440–448.
17. Aoyama N, Izumi T, Hiramori K, Isobe M, Kawana M, Hiroe M, Hishida H, Kitaura Y, Imaizumi T, Japanese Investigators of Fulminant Myocarditis. 2002. Special Report from a Scientific Committee: National Survey of Fulminant Myocarditis in Japan. Therapeutic Guidelines and Long-term Prognosis of Fulminant Myocarditis Using Percutaneous Cardiopulmonary Support (PCPS). Circulation J 66:133–144.
18. Nishio R, Matsumori A, Shioi T, Ishida H, Sasayama S. 1999. Treatment of experimental viral myocarditis with Interleukin-10. Circulation 100:1102–1108.
19. McCarthy RE 3rd, Boehmer JP, Hruban RH, Hutchins GM, Kasper EK, Hare JM, Baughman KL. 2000. Long-term outcome of fulminant myocarditis as compared with acute (nonfulminant) myocarditis. N Engl J Med 342:690–695.

Frontiers in Cardiovascular Health, edited by
N.S. Dhalla, A. Chockalingam,
H.I. Berkowitz & P.K. Singal
Kluwer Academic Publishers, Boston, 2003

Homocysteine/Coronary Atherosclerosis and Cardiac Transplantation: A Case Control Study

Ramesh N. Kundur, Maureen P. Flattery, and Michael L. Hess

Medical College of Virginia Campus, Virginia Commonwealth University, Richmond, VA U.S.A.
Cardiac Transplant Group, Division of Cardiology and Cardiothoracic Surgery

Summary
Background Hyperhomocysteinemia has been implicated as an independent risk factor for atherosclerotic cardiovascular disease. Both cardiac transplantation and diabetes are associated with accelerated coronary artery disease. We therefore, designed this study to determine serum homocysteine levels in cardiac transplant recipients and patients with diabetes. We also sought to determine the relationship between hyperhomocysteinemia and renal insufficiency and its response to oral supplementation with folic acid.
Methods We measured fasting serum creatinine and homocysteine levels in 34 cardiac transplant patients, 29 patients with diabetes and 36 heart failure patients who served as controls.
Results Mean serum creatinine was significantly elevated in the heart transplant group (1.8 $\pm$ 0.5 mg/dl, $p < 0.01$) and diabetes group (1.6 $\pm$ 0.8 mg/dl, 0.02) as compared to the control group. The mean serum homocysteine level was also significantly elevated in the heart transplant group (18.1 $\pm$ 6 microM/l, $p < 0.001$) as well as diabetic group (17.1 $\pm$ 8 microM/L, $p < 0.002$) as compared to the control group (11.6 $\pm$ 5 microM/L). There was a strong correlation between the serum homocysteine level and the serum creatinine in the heart transplant group ($r = 0.5$, $p < 0.002$), diabetes group ($r = 0.8$, $p < 0.002$) as well as control group ($r = 0.8$, $p < 0.03$). However, there was a weak relationship between serum homocysteine and time since heart transplant ($r = 0.11$, $p = 0.5$). Heart transplant patients and patients in the diabetes group were treated with 1000 micrograms of oral folic acid for at least 4 weeks. There was no significant change in the homocysteine levels after the treatment.

Address all correspondences to: Michael L. Hess, MD, P.O.Box 980281, Medical College of Virginia, Richmond, VA 23298. U.S.A. Phone: 804-828-9700, Fax: 804-828-8700.
Presented in part at the XXVII World Congress of the International Society for Heart Research.

Conclusions Hyperhomocysteinemia is common among heart transplant recipients and diabetic patients. The serum homocysteine level correlates well with the degree of renal insufficiency.

***Key words*:** Homocysteine, coronary artery disease, cardiac transplantation, diabetes.

INTRODUCTION

Hyperhomocysteinemia has been implicated as an independent risk factor for atherosclerotic cardiovascular disease (1), potentially by the induction of oxygen radicals (2). These in turn could initiate endothelial injury, causing type I vascular injury and thus the initiation and propagation of the atherosclerotic process (3).

Both cardiac transplantation (4) and diabetes are associated with a rapid progression of coronary artery disease, giving rise to the term accelerated coronary artery disease. In cardiac transplant patients, it has been estimated that 50% of patients have developed coronary artery disease by five years (4).

Diabetes is well known to be associated with rapidly progressive coronary artery disease, albeit at a slower rate of progression compared to transplant vasculopathy. The mechanisms involved in the rapidly progressive coronary artery disease are unknown. We have therefore hypothesized that elevated serum homocysteine, known to be associated with atherosclerotic disease, may be present in this patient population and contribute to the pathogenesis of accelerated coronary artery disease in the heart transplant and diabetic patients.

METHODS

We enrolled 36 heart transplant recipients who presented consecutively for routine clinical follow-up. Control group consisted of 38 congestive heart failure patients with documented left ventricular ejection fraction less than 30%. Two patients were excluded in each group due to extreme values of serum creatinine. The diabetes group consisted of 29 diabetic patients with documented coronary artery disease.

We measured fasting serum total homocysteine and serum creatinine levels among patients in the heart transplant group, the control group and the diabetes group. The diagnosis of coronary artery disease was confirmed by coronary angiography performed during the previous year for clinical indications.

Results expressed as mean ± standard deviation. Linear regression analyses were used to examine the relationship between serum total homocyteine levels, serum creatinine and time since transplant. A p value <0.05 was considered statistically significant.

RESULTS

Table 1 presents the baseline clinical characteristics of the three initial groups. There were 34 heart transplant patients, 29 diabetic patients and 36 patients in the control group. The mean age and gender were not significantly different among the groups. The etiology of heart failure was not significantly different between the heart trans-

Table 1. Baseline clinical characteristics of patients in study groups

	Heart transplant group	Control group	Diabetes group
Number of patients.	34	36	29
Age (yrs.)	56.5 ± 11.3	53.6 ± 13.5	52.8 ± 13.3
Age <65 yrs.	25 (74%)	31 (87%)	22 (75%)
Age >65 yrs.	9 (26%)	5 (13%)	7 (25%)
Gender			
Male	30 (88%)	24 (66%)	11 (37%)
Female	4 (12%)	12 (34%)	18 (63%)
CHF Etiology			
Ischemic	17 (50%)	20 (50%)	N/A
Nonischemic	17 (50%)	20 (50%)	N/A
Time since transplant (yrs.)	8.2 (0.5–15 yrs.)	N/A	N/A
Diabetes Milletus	7 (22%)	6 (25%)	29 (100%)
Serum Creatinine (mg/dl)	1.8 ± 0.5	1.1 ± 0.4	1.6 ± 0.8

Continuous variables expressed as Mean ± SD.

plant group and the control group. The percentage of patients having diabetes (patients requiring therapy) was also similar among the heart transplant and the control group of patients. Average duration since heart transplant was 8.2 years with a range from 6 months to 15 years.

Serum creatinine was significantly elevated in the heart transplant group (mean 1.8 ± 0.5 mg/dl) and diabetes group (1.6 ± 0.8 mg/dl) while serum creatinine was normal in the control group (mean 1.1 ± 0.4 mg/dl).

The mean serum homocysteine level was significantly elevated among heart transplant patients (18.1 ± 7 micromol/l, normal range 5.0–15.0), diabetes group (17.1 ± 8 micromol/l) as compared to the control group (11.6 ± 5 micromol/l) (Figure 1). The serum homocysteine level compared quite well to the coronary artery disease patients reported by Schnyder et al. (5) and renal transplant patients reported by Bertoni et al. (6).

There was strong correlation between serum homocysteine level and serum creatinine in the heart transplant patients ($r = 0.5$, $p < 0.002$) (Figure 2) as well as the control group ($r = 0.8$, $p < 0.03$) (Figure 3). A strong correlation was found to exist between serum homocysteine levels and serum creatinine in the diabetes group as well ($r = 0.8$, $p < 0.002$) (Figure 4). However, there was a weak relationship between serum homocysteine and time since heart transplant ($r = 0.11$, $p = 0.5$). Heart transplant patients and patients in the diabetes group were treated with 1000 micrograms of oral folic acid for at least 4 weeks. There was no significant change in the homocysteine levels after the treatment.

In the transplant and the control group, the most significant elevation in homocysteine occurred in those patients with diabetes and concomitant renal insufficiency. Likewise, in the diabetes group, the highest elevation in homocysteine levels occurred in those patients with renal insufficiency.

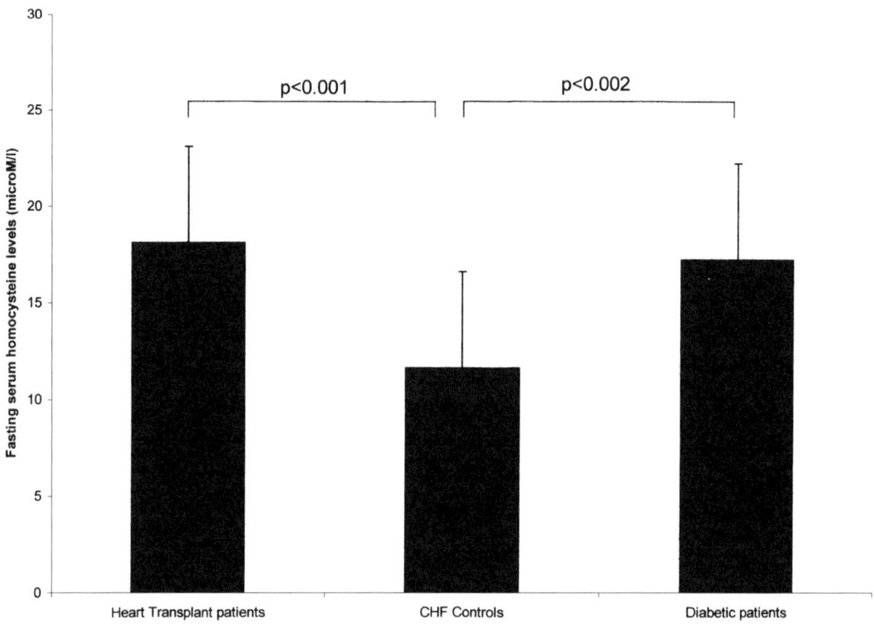

Figure 1. Elevated mean homocysteine Level in heart transplant patients (n = 34) and diabetic patients (n = 29) in comparison with CHF controls (n = 36), ($p < 0.0001$).

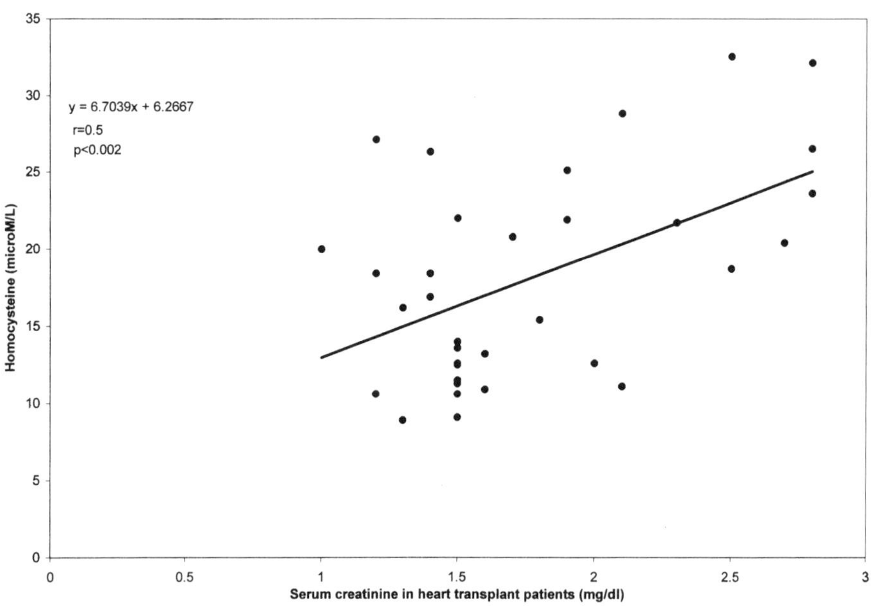

Figure 2. Linear regression plot showing a strong relationship between serum creatinine and total homocysteine levels in heart transplant patients ($r = 0.5$) ($p < 0.002$).

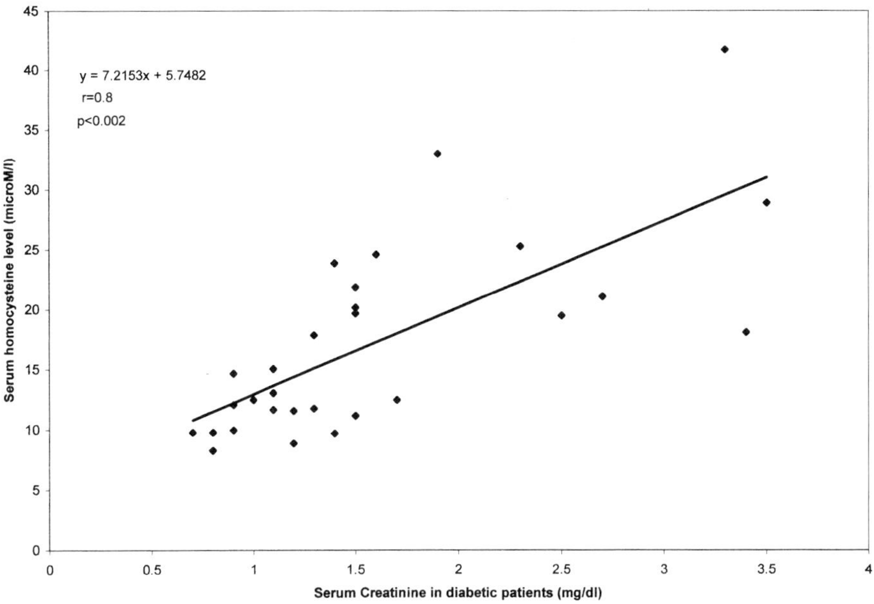

Figure 3. Linear regression plot showing a strong relationship between serum creatinine and total homocysteine levels in diabetic patients ($r = 0.8$) ($p < 0.002$).

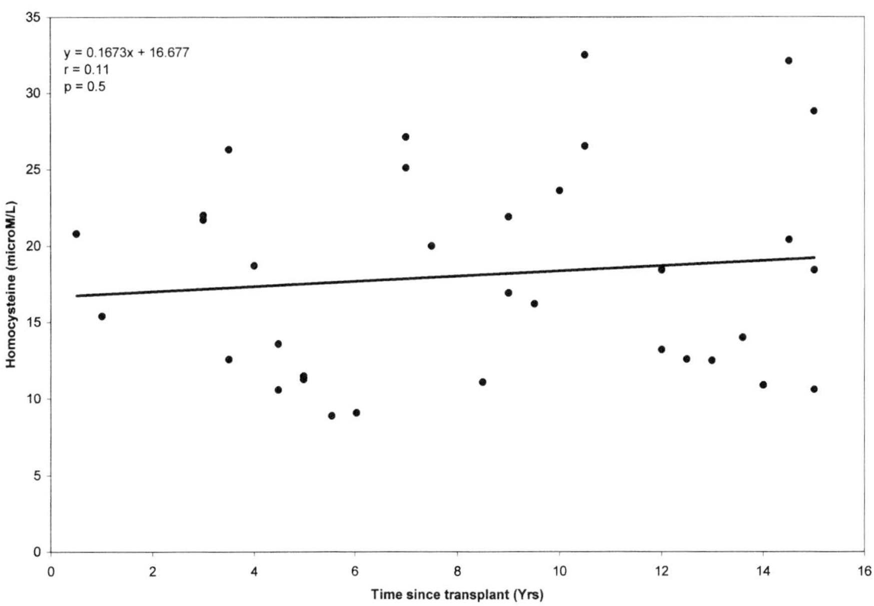

Figure 4. Linear regression plot showing a weak relationship between time since transplant (yrs) and total homocyteine levels in heart transplant patients ($r = 0.11$) ($p = 0.5$).

DISCUSSION

The principal finding of the study is that hyperhomocysteinemia is widely prevalent in heart transplant recipients. Causes of hyperhomocysteinemia could be severalfold. First, immunosuppressive agents and antimetabolites used in heart transplant patients may contribute to elevated homocysteine levels. In our study, there was a weak correlation between homocysteine level and time since transplant. Second, renal insufficiency could contribute to elevated homocysteine levels. In our study, heart transplant recipients had elevated but stable creatinine levels, suggestive of chronic renal insufficiency. There was a strong correlation between serum creatinine and serum homocysteine levels among heart transplant patients as well as diabetic patients. It is well documented that homocysteine levels are elevated in patients with renal insufficiency as well as renal transplant recipients (7). Homocysteine levels are influenced by the degree of renal impairment in patients with chronic renal failure. The cause of elevated homocysteine in renal failure may be related to altered extrarenal metabolism of homocysteine by uremic toxins rather than impaired excretion of homocysteine (8).

Another important observation made in this study is that the highest homocysteine levels were noted in patients with diabetes and concomitant renal insufficiency. This was the case in the heart transplant group as well as control group. It is well known that the onset of vascular disease or falling glomerular filtration rate may cause homocysteine levels to rise in diabetic patients (9).

Oral supplemenation with folic acid (1000 micrograms) failed to normalize homocysteine levels. Homocysteine level is modulated through a series of pyridoxal phosphate, folate and Vitamin B12 dependent pathways. Schnyder et al. (5) have demonstrated that treatment with combination of folic acid, vitamin B12 and pyridoxine significantly decreases the homocysteine level and reduces the restenosis rate after coronary angioplasty. Further study is needed to determine the impact of this combination therapy on our patient population.

REFERENCES

1. Clarke R, Daly L, Robinson K, et al. 1991. Hyperhomocysteinemia: an independent risk factor for cardiovascular disease. N Engl J Med 324:1149–1155.
2. Heinecke JW. 1999. Biochemical evidence for a link between elevated levels of homocysteine and lipid peroxidation in vivo. Curr Atherosclero Rep pp. 87–89.
3. Harker LA, Slichter SJ, Scott CR, et al. 1974. Homocysteinemia: vascular injury and arterial thrombosis. N Engl J Med 291:537–543.
4. Gallo P, Agozzino L, Angelini A, et al. 1997. Causes of late failure after heart transplantation: a ten-year survey. J Heart Lung Transplantation 16:1113–1121.
5. Schnyder G, Roffi M, Pin R, et al. 2001. Decreased rate of coronary artery restenosis after lowering of plasma homocysteine levels. N Eng J Med 345:1593–1600.
6. Bertoni E, Rosati A, Marcucci R, et al. 2001. Hyperhomocysteinemia in renal transplant patients as independent cause of endothelial damage and cardiovascular disease. Transplant Proc 33:3682–3683.
7. Sheshadri N, Robinson K. 2000. Homocysteine, B vitamins, and coronary artery disease. Med Clin North Am 84:215–237.
8. van Guldener C, Donker AJ, Jakobs C, et al. 1998. No net renal extraction of homocysteine in fasting humans. Kidney Int 54:166–169.
9. Wollesen F, Brattstrom L, Refsum H, et al. 1999. Plasma total homocysteine and cysteine in relation to glomerular filtration rate in diabetes mellitus. Kidney Int 55:1028–1035.

Frontiers in Cardiovascular Health, edited by
N.S. Dhalla, A. Chockalingam,
H.I. Berkowitz & P.K. Singal
Kluwer Academic Publishers, Boston, 2003

Drug Development Based on Functional Genomics of Overloaded Cardiomyocytes: CPT 1 vs. PPARalpha Effects of Etomoxir

Heinz Rupp, Angel Zarain-Herzberg,[1] and Bernhard Maisch

Molecular Cardiology Laboratory, Department of Internal Medicine and Cardiology Philipps University of Marburg, Marburg, Germany
[1] *Laboratorio de Biología Molecular, Departamento de Bioquímica, Facultad de Medicina, Universidad Nacional Autónoma de México, México D.F.*

***Key words*:** etomoxir, heart failure, SERCA, myosin, metabolism, PPAR, gene expression.

INTRODUCTION

Heart failure remains a fatal disease with a constantly increasing incidence. Apart from an improved therapy of acute cardiac events, a main reason is seen in the increasing age of the population that frequently is accompanied with an inadequately treated hypertension leading to a chronic pressure overload of the heart. Heart failure is the final outcome of diseases such as hypertension, coronary heart disease, myocarditis, cardiomyopathies, heart valve disorders, cardiac gene defects, diabetes and sepsis. Hypertension and cardiac hypertrophy are present in approximately 90% of patients with heart failure (1). Also after myocardial infarction, an overload occurs in the non-infarcted area leading to an adverse remodelling and thus a further functional deterioration of ventricular function. Since at present no diagnostic measures are in general use for identifying early stages of heart failure, the disease is detected often very late and after symptoms are observed. The current standard therapy is targeted at preventing the further progression of heart failure, whereby the therapy is inadequate in many patients (2). The major drug target is activation of the neuroendocrine system resulting from an impaired cardiac performance. As is the case

The review part of the present study is based on Rupp and Maisch (2002) *Herz* 27:1–8
Correspondence: Heinz Rupp, Ph.D., Molecular Cardiology Laboratory, Karl-von-Frisch-Str. 1, 35033 Marburg. Tel.: +49 6421 286 5032, Fax: +49 6421 286 8964, E-mail: Rupp@mailer.unimarburg.de.

of an acute blood loss, activation of the sympathetic nervous system, the renin angiotensin-aldosterone-system (RAAS) and the endothelin and vasopressin system occurs when cardiac function becomes impaired. Because of the complex ensuing reparation processes, a therapy which only blocks individual components of neuroendocrine activation is expected to slow progression of heart failure but not to stop it. Even if neuroendocrine activation could be prevented, only a functional state could be reached which led to neuroendocrine activation. It is, therefore, of great importance to examine unfavorable processes during the early progression of heart failure. In particular, therapeutic approaches are needed which prevent the transition from asymptomatic to symptomatic heart failure.

LEFT VENTRICULAR DYSFUNCTION AS EARLY DRUG TARGET

Pump function of the heart is often reduced during a prolonged period before symptoms of heart failure are noticed. The incidence of left ventricular dysfunction can be derived from the data of the "Strong Heart Study". A left ventricular dysfunction (ejection fraction <40%) was found in approximately 14% of all older persons (3). Screening procedures for the early identification of left ventricular dysfunction in the general population would particularly be justified if new pharmacological targets in addition to standard therapy (4) become available. The diagnostics of left ventricular dysfunction appears feasible by measuring natriuretic peptides in the serum. BNP which is formed in the loaded ventricle, is increased and rises in parallel with the functional loss of the left ventricle (5,6). Unsettled is at present whether BNP is also diagnostic for an altered gene expression of hypertrophied cardiomyocytes and whether BNP can be influenced by pharmacologic interventions interfering with a dysregulated cardiac gene expression.

PROTEIN PHENOTYPE AND SWITCH IN FUEL METABOLISM

As a consequence of cardiac hypertrophy, characteristic changes occur in gene expression of cardiomyocytes. DNA microarray studies on rats after myocardial infarction showed that the previously identified changes in myosin isozymes and Ca^{2+} pump (SERCA2) of sarcoplasmic reticulum (SR) should be considered as markers of a large group of genes expressed in an apparently coordinated manner. Also the fetal gene expression which was initially been characterized on the basis a reduced expression of alpha-myosin heavy chain (MHC) in several models of cardiac overload was observed (7). The modifications in gene expression were, however, more extensive and the concept of a fetal phenotype can account only for one aspect of the observed altered gene expression. More than 200 out of approximately 4000 genes studied were altered in the hypertrophied ischemic ventricle after myocardial infarction (7). The findings that many of the differentially expressed genes code for enzymes involved in energy metabolism might not be unexpected taking into account that they are also reduced in the fetal period (8). A repression of genes which are responsible for the oxidation of fatty acids was particularly pronounced. To this group belongs the enoyl CoA isomerase, dienoyl CoA reductase, hydroxyacyl CoA dehydrogenase, acyl CoA synthase and ketoacyl CoA thiolase (7). This coordinated repression of enzymes involved in beta-oxidation (9) indicates a reduced fatty acid utilization. Furthermore, the lipoproteinlipase and CD36, a fatty acid transporter, were repressed (7). These findings explain the observation that as a result of pressure overload, glucose utilization is increased at the expense of fatty acid utilization (10–13). The expression of genes involved in fatty acid oxidation are modulated by the transcription factor PPARalpha. Since PPARalpha was found to be reduced as a consequence of pressure overload (14), the characteristic switch in fuel metabolism has been attributed to a reduced influence of PPARalpha (15). It is intriguing that this fetal phenotype was observed also after a Coxsackie-B3 infection of the mouse (16–18). It was concluded that cardiomyocytes surviving a virus-induced damage become hypertrophied and respond with a gene expression that is characteristic of pressure overloaded hearts (18). The impaired heart function after a virus infection arises, therefore, not only from the loss of cardiomyocytes but also from an adverse molecular remodelling of cardiomyocytes.

The DNA chip data on PPARalpha regulated genes provide also a further interpretation of our studies on etomoxir which has a selective influence on the protein phenotype of hypertrophied cardiomyocytes. Etomoxir was developed as an inhibitor of the mitochondrial carnitine palmitoyltransferase-1 (CPT 1) located on the outer mitochondrial membrane. Because of the long fatty acid residue, etomoxir has also a PPARalpha agonist action (19). A CPT 1 inhibition alone would solely reduce the already diminished fatty acid oxidation of pressure overloaded hearts. Since etomoxir had a protective action on the ischemia/reperfusion injury of the kidney similarly to an established PPARalpha agonist (19), one could infer an unexplored benefit also for an overloaded heart. The question arises, therefore, whether the functional improvements due to etomoxir treatment are due to CPT 1 inhibition or some additional yet undefined influences possibly related to PPARalpha activation (20).

The further characterization of the complex effects of metabolically active drugs such as etomoxir is important, since they have been shown to increase the Ca^{2+} transport rate of SR. An inadequate SR function leads to delayed relaxation which causes not only an impaired diastolic filling of the heart but most probably also an impaired coronary perfusion. A fast relaxation is required for efficient coronary perfusion at a time when the aortic pressure is still high. Because of reduced Ca^{2+} stores of SR, also the systolic pressure development is expected to be impaired. During a chronic pressure overload, the Ca^{2+} pump activity of SR is not increased proportionally to the hypertrophy of the ventricle (21). Since the quantity of Ca^{2+} required for triggering force generation is increased proportionally to the volume of cardiomyocytes, the adverse impact of a reduced SR function raises progressively with the extent of hypertrophy. Furthermore, due to the increased diffusion distances, hypertrophied cardiomyocytes are expected to exhibit also a reduced Ca^{2+} induced Ca^{2+} release (22).

Although an unchanged SERCA2 mRNA level has been reported (23), it was found decreased in a number of studies on rabbits and rats with pressure overloaded hearts (24,25). Irrespective of the extent of a SERCA2 mRNA decrease, the fact that it is not raised in parallel with the hypertrophy is crucial for the progression of heart failure. There is also increasing evidence that a raised adrenergic activity can lead to an impaired SR Ca^{2+} transport activity (26).

CPT 1 INHIBITION AND PPARALPHA ACTIVATION BY ETOMOXIR

In a number of studies, we examined pharmacological interventions for influencing gene expression of normal and pressure-overloaded cardiomyocytes (27). Of particular interest was the question whether changes in gene expression are reflected in an altered pump function of the heart. As a marker of the fetal phenotype we used a reduced alpha-MHC expression. Contrary to previous findings, there is now clear evidence that alpha-MHC is expressed also in human ventricles and that its disappearance represents an early marker of an impaired function (28). We examined also whether a reduction in alpha-MHC proportion is accompanied by a diminished SERCA2 activity. During our recent screening studies, we focussed on etomoxir which was developed as a type II antidiabetic drug which does not have acute cardiovascular effects. Etomoxir changed neither the radio-telemeterically determined heart rate nor systolic or diastolic blood pressure of conscious rats (unpublished). Rather the action of etomoxir involves a molecular remodelling of cardiomyocytes. The time, after which half of the SR Ca^{2+} pumps is replaced is in the range of 2–3 days. An important consequnce of a short half-life observed also in proteins of the contractile machinery is that any dysregulated gene expression results in an inadequate supply of crucial proteins of the cardiomyocyte. This is probably also the cause for the microscopically observed adverse structural alterations after a prolonged pressure overload.

A chronic treatment with etomoxir increased the SR Ca^{2+} ATPase activity (29), the Ca^{2+} uptake rate (30), the number of active Ca^{2+} pumps E~P (31,32), the SERCA2 protein (31,32) and the SERCA2 mRNA abundance (25). Since etomoxir increased the SR Ca^{2+} uptake rate also in cultured neonatal cardiomyocytes (Vetter & Rupp, unpublished), a direct effect of etomoxir can be inferred. In parallel to the effect on SERCA2, the proportion of alpha-MHC or myosin V1 (2 alpha-MHC) was increased which demonstrates a coordinated expression of genes required for fast relaxation and contraction.

Although it is well accepted that etomoxir inhibits CPT 1, it remains unclear whether additional influences arising from PPARalpha activation have to be taken into account. Oxirane compounds such as methylpalmoxirate can bind and activate PPARalpha (33). In particular, the etomoxir-induced protection of renal function after ischemia has been attributed to PPARalpha activation (19). To examine putative additional influences, the CPT 1 inhibition can be bypassed by feeding etomoxir treated rats a medium-chain fatty acid diet containing nonanoate and decanoate. Medium-chain fatty acids do not require CPT 1 for their entry into mitochondria. Thus, a medium-chain fatty acid diet is expected to result in an unaltered fatty acid oxidation although CPT 1 is inhibited by etomoxir. In rats treated with etomoxir and fed a regular long-chain fatty acid containing diet, the lipid

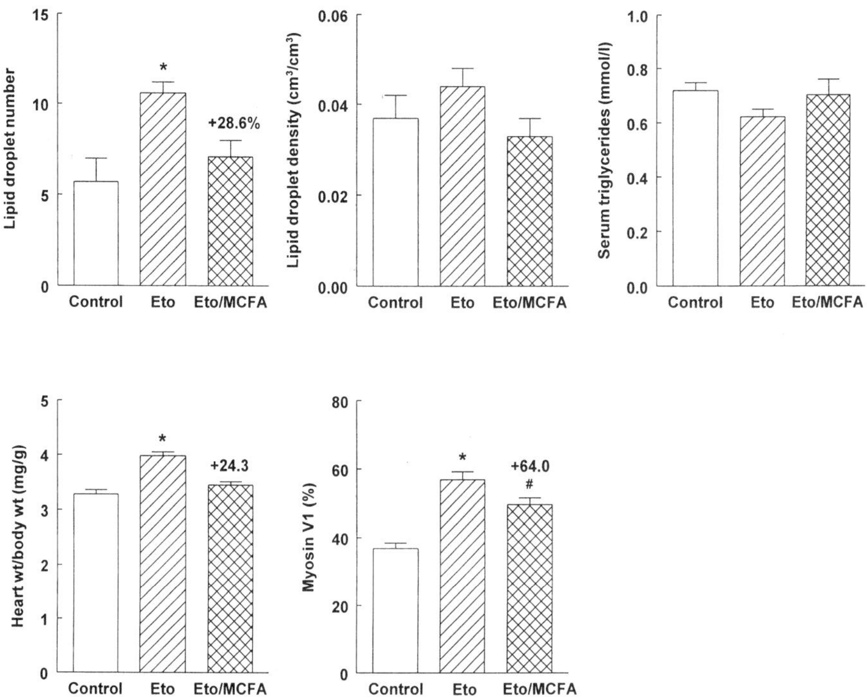

Figure 1. Comparative analysis of the effect of a medium-chain fatty acid diet on etomoxir-induced changes in left ventricular lipid droplet number and density, serum triglycerides, the heart-to-body weight ratio and myosin V1 proportion. The percentage values given on the bars of the etomoxir treated WKY rats fed a medium-chain fatty acid diet refer to the increase seen in etomoxir treated rats fed a long-chain fatty acid regular diet. Abbreviations are: Eto, etomoxir treated rats fed a long-chain fatty acid regular diet; Eto/MCFA, etomoxir treated rats fed a medium-chain fatty acid diet (50–65% C9:0, 30–40% C10:0). Data are adapted from Rupp et al. (31).

droplet number was moderately increased which was greatly prevented by exchanging the dietary long-chain fatty acids for medium-chain fatty acids (31) (Figure 1). Lipid droplet number was not significantly increased corresponding to 28.6% of the increase observed in etomoxir treated rats fed a regular diet. The lipid droplet density was increased not significantly by etomoxir which argues against an adverse lipid accumulation in the myocardium. The high dose etomoxir treatment resulted in a harmonious ventricular growth (+21% left ventricle, +17% right ventricle (31)) of the heart which, based on the observed phenotype, resembles that of swim-exercised rat hearts (34). The increase in left ventricular weight was reduced by the medium-chain fatty acid diet similarly to the lipid droplet number. Also the etomoxir-induced decrease in serum triglycerides was prevented by the medium chain fatty acid diet. By contrast, the etomoxir-induced increase in myosin V1 was prevented to a lesser extent than lipid droplet number and growth parameters suggesting that on top of CPT 1 inhibition additional influences occur. The myosin

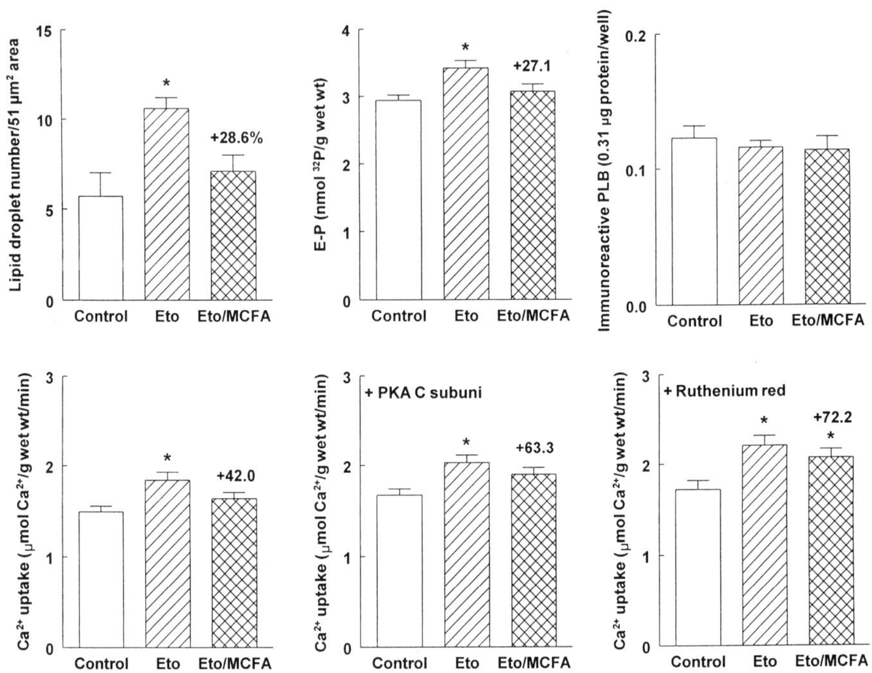

Figure 2. Comparative analysis of the effect of a medium-chain fatty acid diet on etomoxir-induced changes in left ventricular lipid droplet number, phosphorylated intermediate E~P of the SR Ca^{2+}-ATPase, immunoreactive SR phospholamban content and oxalate-supported SR Ca^{2+} uptake rate measured also in the presence of C subunit of protein kinase A or ruthenium red. The percentage values given on the bars of the etomoxir treated WKY rats fed a medium-chain fatty acid diet refer to the increase seen in etomoxir treated rats fed a long-chain fatty acid regular diet. Abbreviations are: Eto, etomoxir treated rats fed a long-chain fatty acid regular diet; Eto/MCFA, etomoxir treated rats fed a medium-chain fatty acid diet (50–65% C9:0, 30–40% C10:0). Data are adapted from Rupp et al. (31).

V1 proportion was 64% of the increase seen in etomoxir treated rats fed the regular diet.

Etomoxir increased the number of active E~P Ca^{2+} pumps of SR which was prevented to a similar extent as the lipid droplet number (Figure 2). The SR phospholamban content was not affected by etomoxir. SR Ca^{2+} uptake of ventricular homogenates was increased in etomoxir treated rats irrespective of the presence of the SR Ca^{2+} release inhibitor ruthenium red or the catalytic subunit of protein kinase A which phosphorylates phospholamban. The medium-chain fatty acid diet resulted in SR Ca^{2+} uptake rates that were in between those of etomoxir-treated and untreated rats. Since etomoxir increased SR Ca^{2+} pumps but not phospholamban, Ca^{2+} pumps can be inferred which are not inhibited by dephosphorylated phospholamban leading thereby to a higher overall SR Ca^{2+} uptake rate (35). It remains nonetheless an intriguing observation that a medium-chain fatty acid diet had a smaller effect on the SR Ca^{2+} uptake rate when compared with the SR active E~P Ca^{2+} pumps.

PUTATIVE DNA SEQUENCE CANDIDATES FOR ETOMOXIR-INDUCED CHANGES IN GENE EXPRESSION

Many studies have demonstrated that the expression of genes encoding mitochondrial fatty acid beta-oxidation enzymes is regulated at the transcriptional level in parallel with fatty acid utilization rates during cardiac development and in the hypertrophic and failing heart (36–40). CPT 1 is involved in the import of long-chain fatty acids which is a limiting regulated step in myocardial lipid beta-oxidation. It has been shown that CPT 1 gene expression is induced by long chain fatty acids in the heart by the PPARalpha transcription factor (36,37,39). PPARs belong to the steroid, thyroid, and retinoid receptor superfamily of nuclear receptors. Three members of the PPAR family have been identified, PPARalpha, PPARdelta (also called PPARbeta, FFAR or NUC1), and PPARgamma. PPARalpha is mainly expressed in the heart, skeletal muscle, liver, kidney and vascular endothelial cells (40,41). PPARalpha is involved in the control of lipoprotein metabolism, fatty acid oxidation and cellular uptake of fatty acids (41). The transcriptional activity of PPARalpha is stimulated by insulin, fibrates, phenylacetate and its analogues, and the selective agonists WY14643, JTT-501, GW2331 and PD72953 (41,42). Etomoxir is a compound that binds irreversibly to the catalytic site of CPT-1 inhibiting its activity, but also upregulates FAO enzymes (19). For the above reason and because of the chemical structure of etomoxir, it has been suggested to be a ligand for PPAR-alpha (19).

PPARs contain a central DNA-binding domain that recognizes response elements (PPREs) in the promoters of their target genes. The consensus sequence of a PPRE is 5′-TGAMCT T TGNCCT AGWTYYG-3′ (36,41,42). The core sequence is a direct repeat 5′-TGAMCT T TGNCCT-3′, where RXR binds the 5′ half site and PPAR the 3′ half site of the repeat with one nucleotide spacing between the two half sites. PPARs must form heterodimers with the 9-*cis* retinoic acid receptor (RXR) in order to be active. PPAR-RXR complexes activate transcription through a conserved PPAR carboxyl-terminal ligand binding domain (41,42).

Recent reports have demonstrated that PPARalpha is downregulated in the hypertrophied myocardium (15,43). Therefore, it has been suggested that the reduced DNA binding activity of PPARalpha may be responsible for the downregulated expression of cardiac fatty acid oxidation enzyme genes in the hypertrophied heart. In pressure overload cardiac hypertrophy, the heart shifts from a normal preference for fatty acid oxidation to an increased glucose oxidation (38,44). This response in shift of fuel utilization may initially be adaptive in the hypertrophic process. The reduced capacity to maintain lipid and energy homeostasis in the hypertrophic cardiomyocyte may, however, lead to contractile dysfunction during pathologic myocardial remodeling. The decrease in PPARalpha expression during the development of cardiac hypertrophy could contribute to the pathologic remodeling associated with contractile dysfunction of the heart. In addition, as an early response to compensate for the increased energy demand during cardiac hypertrophy, p38 activated MAPK phosphorylates PPARalpha thereby activating it. This suggests that PPARalpha is a downstream effector of p38 kinase-dependent stress-activated signaling in the cardiomyocyte (45).

It has been extensively documented that in animal models of cardiac hypertrophy and patients with heart failure, the Ca^{2+} transport by the SR as well as the mRNA expression of SERCA2 are decreased. It has been demonstrated that the decreased SERCA2 mRNA levels arise from a reduced gene transcription (46–49). It has been reported that the SERCA2 mRNA level is increased in hearts of animals treated with etomoxir (25) and in cardiomyocytes in culture (Vetter and Rupp, Zarain-Herzberg and Rupp, unpublished). The increase in SERCA2 mRNA could be regulated at the transcriptional level. As putative sequence candidates for the etomoxir-induced increase in SERCA2 expression, there are several sequences of the promoter of the SERCA2 gene which must be considered (44). Because of the possibility that etomoxir could be a PPARalpha ligand activator, this receptor is a potential candidate for the transcriptional action of etomoxir. Within 1.5 kb of the human SERCA2 regulatory region there are six regions that share homology with the PPRE consensus sequence 5′-TGAMCT T TGNCCT AGWTYYG-3′ (36). The sequence of three of these putative PPREs is highly conserved among the human, rabbit, rat and mouse SERCA2 genes (data not shown). However, it is not known if etomoxir increases the transcription of the SERCA2 gene, and if PPAR-alpha binds to those putative PPRE sequences and further experimental data are required in this respect.

Because the increased glucose utilization that results from partial CPT 1 inhibition by etomoxir, glucose metabolites such as glucose-6-phosphate and/or xylulose-5-phosphate may also increase their concentration, in turn activating intracellular signaling mechanisms that may lead to increased transcription of target genes. The glucose response sequences of the L-PK, S14 and fatty acid synthase have been well characterized (40). These regions have the consensus E-box DNA binding site (5′-CANNTG-3′) that binds the upstream stimulatory factors (USFs). USFs are basic helix-loop-helix leucine zipper (bHLHZ) transcription factors. Two USF factors named USF-1 and USF-2 have been identified. USF-1 has been shown to be expressed in the heart and may be a candidate for glucose mediated signaling (40,44). The alpha-MHC gene proximal promoter contains an E-box/USF motif (5′-CACGTG-3′) near the TATA-box. This E-box/USF motif can bind USF-1 and is necessary for high levels of basal transcription. It has been suggested that this motif may function as a glucose response element (50,51). In addition, overexpression of USF-1 increased the transcription of the cardiac alpha-MHC gene (51). The proximal SERCA2 promoter also contains a consensus E-box/USF motif (5′-CACATG-3′) just upstream from the TATA-box which can be identified as potential glucose response element (44). There are other four consensus E-box/USF sequences within the 1.5 kb SERCA2 sequence of regulatory region that may function as glucose response elements (data not shown).

Therefore, it can be suggested that the transcriptional effects of etomoxir arise from a shift in energy metabolism with increased glucose utilization and/or a PPARalpha activation (44). However, further work is required to examine the metabolites involved in the altered gene transcription. Etomoxir has also been identified as a lead compound of so-called "transcription modulators" which, via an altered gene transcription, improve the function of diseased hearts.

PARTIAL NORMALIZATION OF PRESSURE OVERLOAD-INDUCED PHENOTYPE BY ETOMOXIR

The etomoxir induced modifications in gene expression of cardiomyocytes resulted in an improved pump function of the pressure overloaded heart (52). Using a low dosage, etomoxir had a selective influence on the pressure-overloaded left ventricle of rats with banding of the ascending aorta while in sham-operated rats no significant changes were observed. Both the myocardial working capacity and the contraction and relaxation rate of the isovolumically beating heart were increased.

It was also examined whether etomoxir can improve heart function in rats with a pre-existing prolonged pressure overload which, however, does not induce pulmonary edema (53). Etomoxir treatment started 6 weeks after banding of the ascending aorta. The treatment increased the proportion of alpha-MHC and prevented the increase of the left ventricular inner volume and thus the beginning of a deleterious left ventricular dilatation. Also the maximum isovolumically developed pressure and the rate of pressure rise and decline were increased. After transforming pressure values into wall stress values, an improved myocardial function was apparent.

REDUCED PULMONARY CONGESTION AFTER ETOMOXIR TREATMENT

It was examined whether etomoxir influences the transition from compensated to decompensated cardiac hypertrophy by assessing the incidence of pulmonary edema in rats with pressure overloaded hearts (21). After a more severe constriction of the ascending aorta, a pronounced left ventricular hypertrophy (+62% to +103%) occurred which was associated with pulmonary congestion in 60–100% of rats 8, 10, 14 and 28 weeks after aortic banding. The SR Ca^{2+} uptake rate per g wet weight was reduced by 30% which was independent of phospholamban phosphorylation and inhibition of SR Ca^{2+} release. The SERCA2 protein was likewise reduced by 30%. The SR Ca^{2+} uptake rate was inversely correlated with left ventricular weight but was not influenced by the occurrence of pulmonary edema. Since the calculated SR Ca^{2+} uptake rate of the entire ventricle was not reduced, a hypertrophy proportional dilution of the SR Ca^{2+} pumps appears likely which precedes the occurrence of pulmonary edema. A treatment with etomoxir did not affect the left ventricular weight but reduced the right ventricular hypertrophy which is a consequence of pulmonary edema. In parallel, the SR Ca^{2+} uptake rate and the proportion of myosin V1 were increased. It was concluded that etomoxir represents a candidate drug for prevention of the progression of heart failure of a pressure-overloaded heart, whereby it induces an increased SR Ca^{2+} uptake rate which is nearly proportional to the hypertrophy.

IMPROVED HEART FUNCTION IN HEART FAILURE PATIENTS AFTER ETOMOXIR TREATMENT

In the first clinical etomoxir trial in patients with heart failure by Holubarsch et al., patients with impaired heart performance but without diabetes mellitus type II exhibited an improved cardiac function (54). A dose of 80 mg of etomoxir was given once daily to 10 patients suffering from heart failure (NYHA functional class II–III; mean age 55 ± 4 years; one patient with ischaemic heart disease and nine patients with dilated idiopathic cardiomyopathy; all male), in addition to standard therapy. The left ventricular ejection fraction was measured echocardiographically before and after a 3-month period of treatment. Central hemodynamics at rest and exercise (supine position bicycle) were defined by means of a pulmonary artery catheter and thermodilution. All 10 patients improved clinically; no patient had to stop taking the medication, and no patient died during the 3-month period. Maximum cardiac output during exercise increased after treatment. This increase was mainly due to an increased stroke volume (Figure 3). Resting heart rate was slightly reduced. For any given heart rate, stroke volume was significantly enhanced during exercise. The left ventricular ejection fraction increased significantly from 21.5 ± 2.6% to 27.0 ± 2.3%. Mean pulmonary pressure and pulmonary capillary wedge pressure were significantly reduced (Figure 3). Based on echocardiographic data, it was concluded that the etomoxir treatment had no influence on left ventricular muscle mass. The principal possibility of dissociating effects of CPT 1 inhibition on cardiac growth and alterations in cardiac phenotype is demonstrated also by the finding that a low dose etomoxir treatment had a specific effect in pressure overloaded hearts which was not associated with a significant left ventricular hypertrophy (52). In acute studies, etomoxir showed neither a positive inotropic effect nor vasodilatory properties (54). Thus, although the results of this small pilot study are not placebo-controlled, all patients seem to have benefitted from etomoxir treatment (54). Furthermore, no side effects were observed (54). In this respect it should be mentioned that it has been reported that etomoxir can cause lipid accumulation in the liver (55). In this study, 125 mg/kg/day (+)-etomoxir was administered for 28 days which is 8 times higher than the dose (15 mg/kg/day (+)-etomoxir for 5 weeks) used in the experiments described in Figures 1 and 2 (31). Even at this very high dose, only in two out of 6 rats a diffuse moderate panlobur steatosis was observed while in the remaining rats a minimal to mild steatosis primarily in periportal regions was described (55). A lipid accumulation might be inferred from a marked CPT 1 inhibition alone. This is, however, expected to be counteracted by the hypolipidemic action of etomoxir arising from a reduced *de novo* fatty acid synthesis most probably arising from acetyl CoA carboxylase inhibition.

This new drug approach which does not directly target neuroendocrine activation encountered great interest (56). In this respect, it should also be mentioned that POCA which preceded etomoxir has anti-arrhythmic (57) and anti-ischemic effects (58–60). Currently, the phase II "ERGO Trial" (Medigene AG) is performed to assess the therapeutic dose ot etomoxir in patients with heart failure.

PRESSURE OVERLOAD-INDUCED PHENOTYPE DOES NOT OCCUR IN FASTED RATS

For further defining metabolic signals, it was assessed whether the reduced insulin influences and associated processes occurring during intermittent fasting have any effect on the characteristics of a pressure loaded heart (61). Like a pressure over-

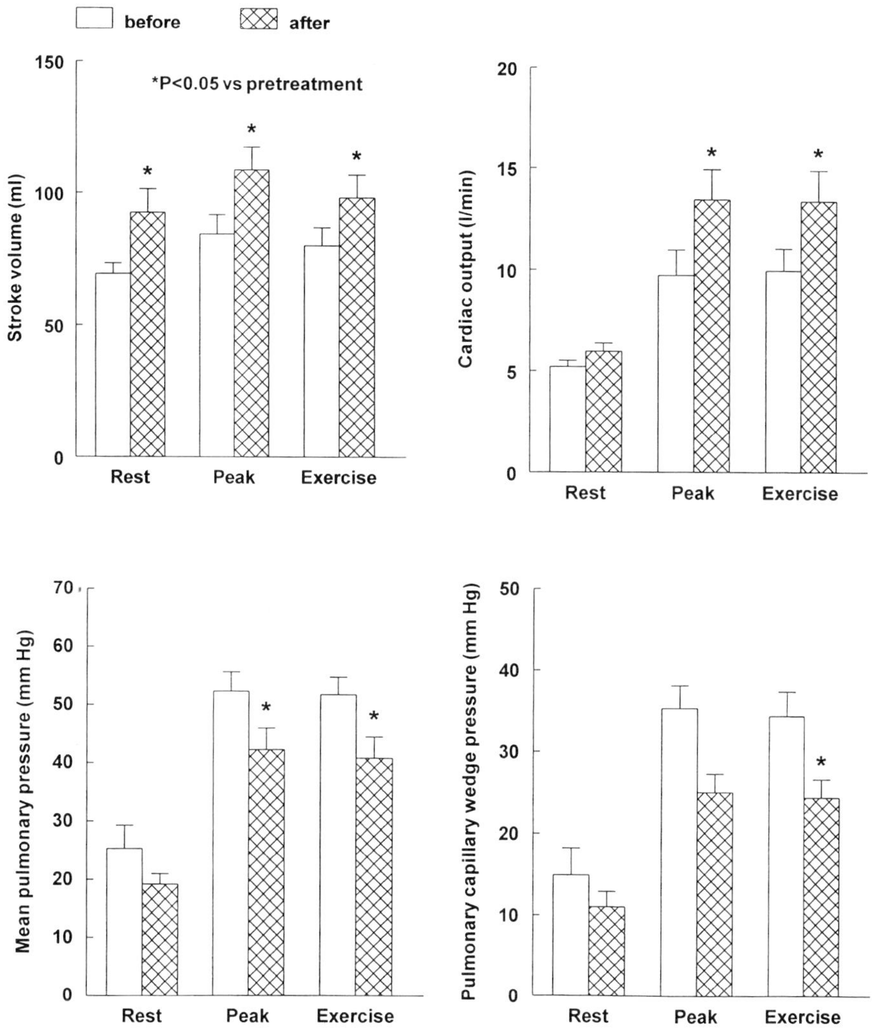

Figure 3. Hemodynamic data of patients with heart failure (NYHA class II–III) treated on top of a standard therapy with daily 80 mg etomoxir for 3 months. The significance of differences was compared with respective values before treatment. Central hemodynamics at rest and maximum exercise (supine position bicycle) were defined by means of a pulmonary artery catheter and thermodilution. Data are from Schmidt-Schweda and Holubarsch (54).

load, intermittent fasting reduced the proportion of myosin V1 and the SR Ca^{2+} stimulated ATPase activity. If both interventions were combined, the hypertrophy was not significantly changed compared with *ad libitum* fed rats. However, no additive effect was observed on myosin and SR (Figure 4). Furthermore, the administration of 0.8% sucrose in the drinking water prevented the modifications in myosin

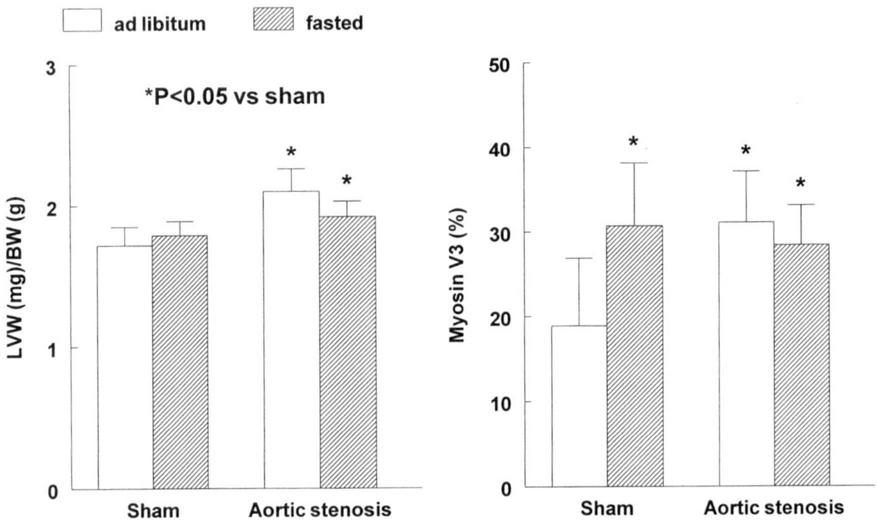

Figure 4. Caloric intake-dependent changes in the myosin V3 increase resulting from abdominal aortic stenosis. The intermittent fasting (one day feeding, one day fasting) did not affect the left ventricular hypertrophy but prevented the rise in myosin V3 proportion when compared with sham-operated intermittently fasted rats. Data are adapted from Rupp et al. (61).

and SR in rats with pressure overload, after intermittent fasting and in the group of combined interventions. The effect of sucrose appears to be mediated by incretin related signals and an enhanced insulin influence (62,63). It was concluded that intermittent fasting and a left ventricular pressure overload recruite metabolic signals which are similar in their final pathways. It can furthermore be inferred that metabolic signals are crucially involved in any dysregulated gene expression of pressure overloaded hearts.

FAILURE OF BM13.907 TO INCREASE ALPHA-MHC EXPRESSION

To examine whether the effects of etomoxir can be induced also by a compound which has been reported to increase glucose transporter translocation, rats with an abdominal aortic stenosis were treated with BM13.907 which was developed as type II antidiabetic drug (61). The treatment increased left ventricular hypertrophy but, contrary to etomoxir, reduced the proportion of alpha-MHC corresponding to an increased myosin V3 proportion (Figure 5). An inverse relationship between the increase in left ventricular weight and alpha-MHC was observed. The SR Ca^{2+} stimulated ATPase of pressure-overloaded hearts was, however, not reduced as one might infer from the reduced alpha-MHC proportion. It was concluded that an intervention which apparently leads only to an increased glucose transporter translocation amplifies the left ventricular hypertrophy arising from a pressure overload but only partially prevents the characteristic phenotype of a pressure-overloaded heart.

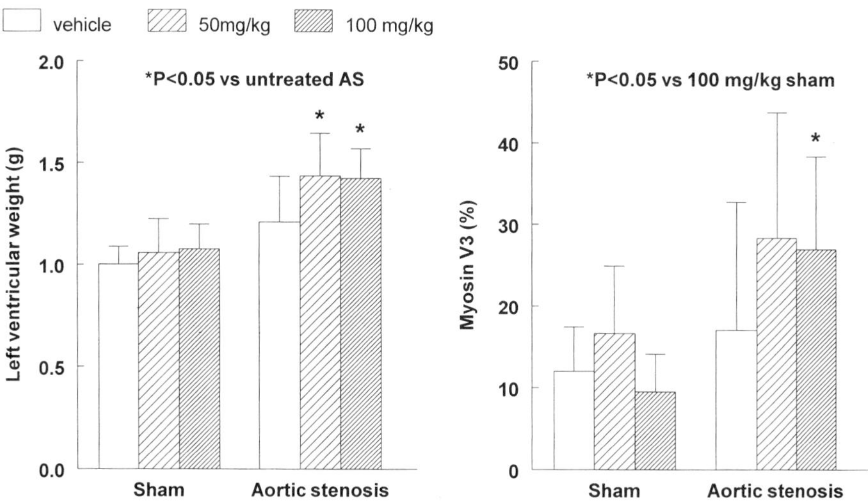

Figure 5. Effect of BM13.907 on left ventricular weight and myosin V3 proportion of rats with abdominal aortic stenosis. BM13.907 amplified the left ventricular hypertrophy but, in contrast to etomoxir, did not prevent a weight proportional rise in myosin V3 proportion which is typical of pressure-overloaded ventricles. Data are adapted from Rupp et al. (61).

NO EFFECT OF LOSARTAN ON ALPHA-MHC EXPRESSION

The question arose whether the effects of etomoxir are unique or whether they are observed also after a standard therapy for heart failure. Previous studies have shown that a beta-blockade with atenolol or alpha-blockade with terazosin could not prevent the reduced alpha-MHC expression of pressure-overloaded hearts (64). It remained unsettled whether a systemic AT_1 blockade can influence the hypertrophy and associated gene expression as a result of a fixed left ventricular afterload. Neither the concentric hypertrophy nor the reduced myocardial contractility and alpha-MHC expression were significantly influenced by the AT_1 blocker losartan (65). The expression of the fetal phenotype of pressure-overloaded hearts as exemplified by the reduced alpha-MHC expression are, therefore, not influenced by AT_1 receptors. This conclusion is supported by the findings of Yazaki et al. (66) that the left ventricular hypertrophy, fibrosis and expression of fetal genes are not altered in AT_1-knockout mice with abdominal aortic stenosis.

CAPTOPRIL SPECIFIC EFFECTS ON ALPHA-MHC EXPRESSION

It was further examined whether the ACE inhibitor quinapril changes the alpha-MHC expression and whether an ACE inhibition can retard heart failure development in rats with ascending aortic banding (67). During a 24-week observation period, quinapril reduced significantly the mortality. The characteristic reduction of the alpha-MHC expression was partially prevented only in the first few weeks. At the end of the 24-week observation period there was no difference between the quinapril and the placebo group. Irrespective of the treatment, failing hypertrophied ventricles showed an increased left ventricular volume, a further reduction in the alpha-MHC expression and a marked fibrosis as determined by an increased hydroxyproline concentration. Although the cause of the reduced mortality of the quinapril treated rats has not yet been clarified, quinapril had no influence on the expression of the fetal phenotype during a prolonged pressure overload.

It remained unsettled whether apart from ACE inhibition, other effects of ACE inhibitors have to be considered. In particular, whether raised bradykinin levels due to ACE inhibition have any effect (68). The question was also addressed whether the ACE inhibitor captopril has specific effects arising from its thiol group. In contrast to quinapril, captopril increased the proportion of alpha-MHC not only in rats with ascending aortic stenosis but also in sham-operated rats. The proportion of alpha-MHC was inversely correlated with left ventricular weight, whereby two different correlation lines for untreated and captopril treated rats were observed. A simultaneous administration of HOE 140, a bradykinin B2-receptor antagonist, had no significant effect. It was concluded that stimulation of bradykinin B2-receptors does not influence cardiac growth and MHC expression during the development of cardiac hypertrophy. Since a treatment with the ACE inhibitor lisinopril did not affect the alpha-MHC proportion (unpublished), the effects of captopril appear to be specific for a thiol-containing ACE inhibitor. It is currently not known whether captopril increased the SR Ca^{2+} uptake rate.

CONCLUSIONS

Drugs known to increase glucose oxidation of the heart increase SERCA2 and alpha-MHC expression. This favorable effect is observed in pressure overloaded hearts due to ascending aortic constriction. In contrast to other models of pressure overload such as myocardial infarction or abdominal aortic stenosis, drug interventions cannot reduce the afterload in the present model of ascending aortic constriction. Thus, an altered cardiac phenotype cannot be attributed simply to a reduced afterload as would be the case in myocardial infarction. We consider, therefore, the model of ascending aortic constriction which, depending on the severity of aortic banding, can induce pulmonary edema a prerequisite for identifying drugs which can counteract a dysregulated gene expression of the cardiomyocyte at a fixed pressure overload.

The CPT 1 inhibitor etomoxir exhibited a selective influence on contraction and relaxation parameters of pressure-overloaded hearts. The functional parameters were correlated with the proportion of alpha-MHC. Thus, the partial prevention of the fetal phenotype resulted in an improved function of the heart. Since bypassing the CPT 1 inhibition by a medium-chain fatty acid diet had a lesser effect on myosin V1 proportion than on lipid droplet number and growth parameters, it can be concluded that the action of etomoxir arises not only from CPT 1 inhibition. To what extent PPARalpha activation is involved, is currently under investigation. Since viral or inflammatory injury of the heart can also induce a fetal phenotype, metabolic modulators would be applicable also in various cardiomyopathies for increasing SERCA2 expression.

ACKNOWLEDGEMENTS

The experimental studies were supported by the German Research Foundation (Ru 245/7-1).

REFERENCES

1. Lenfant C, Roccella EJ. 1999. A call to action for more aggressive treatment of hypertension. J Hypertens Suppl 17:S3–S7.
2. Remme WJ. 1998. Towards the better treatment of heart failure. Eur Heart J 19 Suppl L:L36–L42.
3. Devereux RB, Roman MJ, Paranicas M, Lee ET, Welty TK, Fabsitz RR, Robbins D, Rhoades ER, Rodeheffer RJ, Cowan LD, Howard BV. 2001. A population-based assessment of left ventricular systolic dysfunction in middle-aged and older adults: The Strong Heart Study. Am Heart J 141:439–446.
4. Malik IS, Bhatia VK, Kooner JS. 2001. Cost effectiveness of ramipril treatment for cardiovascular risk reduction. Heart 85:539–543.
5. McDonagh TA, Robb SD, Murdoch DR, Morton JJ, Ford I, Morrison CE, Tunstall-Pedoe H, McMurray JJ, Dargie HJ. 1998. Biochemical detection of left-ventricular systolic dysfunction. Lancet 351:9–13.
6. Luchner A, Burnett JC, Jougasaki M, Hense HW, Heid IM, Muders F, Riegger GA, Schunkert H. 2000. Evaluation of brain natriuretic peptide as marker of left ventricular dysfunction and hypertrophy in the population. J Hypertens 18:1121–1128.
7. Stanton LW, Garrard LJ, Damm D, Garrick BL, Lam A, Kapoun AM, Zheng Q, Protter AA, Schreiner GF, White RT. 2000. Altered patterns of gene expression in response to myocardial infarction. Circ Res 86:939–945.
8. Kelly DP, Gordon JI, Alpers R, Strauss AW. 1989. The tissue-specific expression and developmental regulation of two nuclear genes encoding rat mitochondrial proteins. Medium chain acyl-CoA dehydrogenase and mitochondrial malate dehydrogenase. J Biol Chem 264:18921–18925.
9. Sack MN, Rader TA, Park S, Bastin J, McCune SA, Kelly DP. 1996. Fatty acid oxidation enzyme gene expression is downregulated in the failing heart. Circulation 94:2837–2842.
10. Bishop SP, Altschuld RA. 1970. Increased glycolytic metabolism in cardiac hypertrophy and congestive failure. Am J Physiol 218:153–159.
11. Taegtmeyer H, Overturf ML. 1988. Effects of moderate hypertension on cardiac function and metabolism in the rabbit. Hypertension 11:416–426.
12. Christe ME, Rodgers RL. 1994. Altered glucose and fatty acid oxidation in hearts of the spontaneously hypertensive rat. J Mol Cell Cardiol 26:1371–1375.
13. Feinendegen LE, Henrich MM, Kuikka JT, Thompson KH, Vester EG, Strauer B. 1995. Myocardial lipid turnover in dilated cardiomyopathy: a dual in vivo tracer approach. J Nucl Cardiol 2:42–52.
14. Sack MN, Disch DL, Rockman HA, Kelly DP. 1997. A role for Sp and nuclear receptor transcription factors in a cardiac hypertrophic growth program. Proc Natl Acad Sci USA 94:6438–6443.
15. Barger PM, Brandt JM, Leone TC, Weinheimer CJ, Kelly DP. 2000. Deactivation of peroxisome proliferator-activated receptor-alpha during cardiac hypertrophic growth. J Clin Invest 105:1723–1730.
16. Hamrell BB, Huber SA, Leslie KO. 1994. Reduced unloaded sarcomere shortening velocity and a shift to a slower myosin isoform in acute murine coxsackievirus myocarditis. Circ Res 75:462–472.
17. Hamrell BB, Huber SA, Leslie KO. 1995. Depressed unloaded sarcomere shortening velocity in acute murine coxsackievirus myocarditis: myocardial remodelling in the absence of necrosis or hypertrophy. Eur Heart J 16 Suppl O:31–35.
18. Taylor LA, Carthy CM, Yang D, Saad K, Wong D, Schreiner G, Stanton LW, McManus BM. 2000. Host gene regulation during coxsackievirus B3 infection in mice: assessment by microarrays. Circ Res 87:328–334.
19. Portilla D, Dai G, Peters JM, Gonzalez FJ, Crew MD, Proia AD. 2000. Etomoxir-induced PPARalpha-modulated enzymes protect during acute renal failure. Am J Physiol Renal Physiol 278:F667–F675.

20. Zarain-Herzberg A, Rupp H. 1999. Transcriptional modulators targeted at fuel metabolism of hypertrophied heart. Am J Cardiol 83:31H–37H.
21. Rupp H, Vetter R. 2000. Sarcoplasmic reticulum function and carnitine palmitoyltransferase-1 inhibition during progression of heart failure. Br J Pharmacol 131:1748–1756.
22. Wang SQ, Song LS, Lakatta EG, Cheng H. 2001. Ca2+ signalling between single L-type Ca2+ channels and ryanodine receptors in heart cells. Nature 410:592–596.
23. Yue P, Long CS, Austin R, Chang KC, Simpson PC, Massie BM. 1998. Post-infarction heart failure in the rat is associated with distinct alterations in cardiac myocyte molecular phenotype. J Mol Cell Cardiol 30:1615–1630.
24. Nagai R, Zarain-Herzberg A, Brandl CJ, Fujii J, Tada M, MacLennan DH, Alpert NR, Periasamy M. 1989. Regulation of myocardial Ca2+-ATPase and phospholamban mRNA expression in response to pressure overload and thyroid hormone. Proc Natl Acad Sci U S A 86:2966–2970.
25. Zarain-Herzberg A, Rupp H, Elimban V, Dhalla NS. 1996. Modification of sarcoplasmic reticulum gene expression in pressure overload cardiac hypertrophy by etomoxir. FASEB J 10:1303–1309.
26. Rupp H, Maisch B, Brilla CG. 1997. Schedule-induced psychological stress and molecular structures of cardiomyocytes. Am J Physiol 272:R776–R782.
27. Rupp H, Benkel M, Maisch B. 2000. Control of cardiomyocyte gene expression as drug target. Mol Cell Biochem 212:135–142.
28. Kinugawa K, Minobe WA, Wood WM, Ridgway EC, Baxter JD, Ribeiro RC, Tawadrous MF, Lowes BA, Long CS, Bristow MR. 2001. Signaling Pathways Responsible for Fetal Gene Induction in the Failing Human Heart: Evidence for Altered Thyroid Hormone Receptor Gene Expression. Circulation 103:1089–1094.
29. Rupp H, Elimban V, Dhalla NS. 1992. Modification of subcellular organelles in pressure-overloaded heart by etomoxir, a carnitine palmitoyltransferase I inhibitor. FASEB J 6:2349–2353.
30. Rupp H, Wahl R, Hansen M. 1992. Influence of diet and carnitine palmitoyltransferase I inhibition on myosin and sarcoplasmic reticulum. J Appl Physiol 72:352–360.
31. Rupp H, Schulze W, Vetter R. 1995. Dietary medium-chain triglycerides can prevent changes in myosin and SR due to CPT-1 inhibition by etomoxir. Am J Physiol 269:R630–R640.
32. Vetter R, Rupp H. 1994. CPT-1 inhibition by etomoxir has a chamber-related action on cardiac sarcoplasmic reticulum and isomyosins. Am J Physiol 267:H2091–H2099.
33. Forman BM, Chen J, Evans RM. 1997. Hypolipidemic drugs, polyunsaturated fatty acids, and eicosanoids are ligands for peroxisome proliferator-activated receptors alpha and delta. Proc Natl Acad Sci U S A 94:4312–4317.
34. Rupp H. 1989. Differential effect of physical exercise routines on ventricular myosin and peripheral catecholamine stores in normotensive and spontaneously hypertensive rats. Circ Res 65: 370–377.
35. Vetter R, Kott M, Rupp H. 1995. Differential influences of carnitine palmitoyltransferase-1 inhibition and hyperthyroidism on cardiac growth and sarcoplasmic reticulum phosphorylation. Eur Heart J 16 Suppl C:15–19.
36. Mascaro C, Acosta E, Ortiz JA, Marrero PF, Hegardt FG, Haro D. 1998. Control of human muscle-type carnitine palmitoyltransferase I gene transcription by peroxisome proliferator-activated receptor. J Biol Chem 273:8560–8563.
37. Brandt JM, Djouadi F, Kelly DP. 1998. Fatty acids activate transcription of the muscle carnitine palmitoyltransferase I gene in cardiac myocytes via the peroxisome proliferator-activated receptor alpha. J Biol Chem 273:23786–23792.
38. Barger PM, Kelly DP. 2000. PPAR signaling in the control of cardiac energy metabolism. Trends Cardiovasc Med 10:238–245.
39. van der Lee KA, Vork MM, De Vries JE, Willemsen PH, Glatz JF, Reneman RS, van der Vusse GJ, van Bilsen M. 2000. Long-chain fatty acid-induced changes in gene expression in neonatal cardiac myocytes. J Lipid Res 41:41–47.
40. van Bilsen M, van der Vusse GJ, Reneman RS. 1998. Transcriptional regulation of metabolic processes: implications for cardiac metabolism. Pflugers Arch 437:2–14.
41. Bishop-Bailey D. 2000. Peroxisome proliferator-activated receptors in the cardiovascular system. Br J Pharmacol 129:823–834.
42. Djouadi F, Brandt JM, Weinheimer CJ, Leone TC, Gonzalez FJ, Kelly DP. 1999. The role of the peroxisome proliferator-activated receptor alpha (PPAR alpha) in the control of cardiac lipid metabolism. Prostaglandins Leukot Essent Fatty Acids 60:339–343.

43. Kanda H, Nohara R, Hasegawa K, Kishimoto C, Sasayama S. 2002. A nuclear complex containing PPARalpha/RXRalpha is markedly downregulated in the hypertrophied rat left ventricular myocardium with normal systolic function. Heart Vessels 2000;15(4):191–196 15:191–196.
44. Zarain-Herzberg A, Rupp H. 2002. Therapeutic potential of CPT I inhibitors: cardiac gene transcription as a target. Expert Opin Investig Drugs 11:345–356.
45. Barger PM, Browning AC, Garner AN, Kelly DP. 2001. p38 mitogen-activated protein kinase activates peroxisome proliferator-activated receptor alpha: a potential role in the cardiac metabolic stress response. J Biol Chem 276:44495–44501.
46. Qi M, Shannon TR, Euler DE, Bers DM, Samarel AM. 1997. Downregulation of sarcoplasmic reticulum Ca(2+)-ATPase during progression of left ventricular hypertrophy. Am J Physiol 272:H2416–H2424.
47. Ribadeau Dumas A, Wisnewsky C, Boheler KR, Ter Keurs H, Fiszman MY, Schwartz K. 1997. The sarco(endo)plasmic reticulum Ca(2+)-ATPase gene is regulated at the transcriptional level during compensated left ventricular hypertrophy in the rat. C R Acad Sci III 320:963–969.
48. Takizawa T, Arai M, Yoguchi A, Tomaru K, Kurabayashi M, Nagai R. 1999. Transcription of the SERCA2 gene is decreased in pressure-overloaded hearts: A study using in vivo direct gene transfer into living myocardium. J Mol Cell Cardiol 31:2167–2174.
49. Aoyagi T, Yonekura K, Eto Y, Matsumoto A, Yokoyama I, Sugiura S, Momomura S, Hirata Y, Baker DL, Periasamy M. 1999. The sarcoplasmic reticulum Ca2+-ATPase (SERCA2) gene promoter activity is decreased in response to severe left ventricular pressure-overload hypertrophy in rat hearts. J Mol Cell Cardiol 31:919–926.
50. Ojamaa K, Samarel AM, Klein I. 1995. Identification of a contractile-responsive element in the cardiac alpha-myosin heavy chain gene. J Biol Chem 270:31276–31281.
51. Xiao Q, Ojamaa K. 1998. Regulation of cardiac alpha-myosin heavy chain gene transcription by a contractile-responsive E-box binding protein. J Mol Cell Cardiol 30:87–95.
52. Turcani M, Rupp H. 1997. Etomoxir improves left ventricular performance of pressure-overloaded rat heart. Circulation 96:3681–3686.
53. Turcani M, Rupp H. 1999. Modification of left ventricular hypertrophy by chronic etomoxir treatment. Br J Pharmacol 126:501–507.
54. Schmidt-Schweda S, Holubarsch C. 2000. First clinical trial with etomoxir in patients with chronic congestive heart failure. Clin Sci (Colch) 99:27–35.
55. Steiner S, Wahl D, Mangold BL, Robison R, Raymackers J, Meheus L, Anderson NL, Cordier A. 1996. Induction of the adipose differentiation-related protein in liver of etomoxir-treated rats. Biochem Biophys Res Commun 218:777–782.
56. Bristow M. 2000. Etomoxir: a new approach to treatment of chronic heart failure. Lancet 356: 1621–1622.
57. Corr PB, Creer MH, Yamada KA, Saffitz JE, Sobel BE. 1989. Prophylaxis of early ventricular fibrillation by inhibition of acylcarnitine accumulation. J Clin Invest 83:927–936.
58. Lopaschuk GD, Wall SR, Olley PM, Davies NJ. 1988. Etomoxir, a carnitine palmitoyltransferase I inhibitor, protects hearts from fatty acid-induced ischemic injury independent of changes in long chain acylcarnitine. Circ Res 63:1036–1043.
59. Lopaschuk GD, McNeil GF, McVeigh JJ. 1989. Glucose oxidation is stimulated in reperfused ischemic hearts with the carnitine palmitoyltransferase 1 inhibitor, Etomoxir. Mol Cell Biochem 88:175–179.
60. Lopaschuk GD, Spafford M. 1989. Response of isolated working hearts to fatty acids and carnitine palmitoyltransferase I inhibition during reduction of coronary flow in acutely and chronically diabetic rats. Circ Res 65:378–387.
61. Rupp H, Elimban V, Dhalla NS. 1998. Differential influence of fasting and BM13.907 treatment on growth and phenotype of pressure overloaded rat heart. Mol Cell Biochem 188:209–215.
62. Fukase N, Takahashi H, Manaka H, Igarashi M, Yamatani K, Daimon M, Sugiyama K, Tominaga M, Sasaki H. 1992. Differences in glucagon-like peptide-1 and GIP responses following sucrose ingestion. Diabetes Res Clin Pract 15:187–195.
63. Rupp H, Maisch B. 1999. Radiotelemetric characterization of overweight-associated rises in blood pressure and heart rate. Am J Physiol 277:H1540–H1545.
64. Jacob R, Brandle M, Dierberger B, Rupp H. 1991. Functional consequences of cardiac hypertrophy and dilatation. Basic Res Cardiol 86 Suppl 1:113–130.
65. Turcani M, Rupp H. 1998. Development of pressure overload induced cardiac hypertrophy is unaffected by long-term treatment with losartan. Mol Cell Biochem 188:225–233.

66. Harada K, Komuro I, Shiojima I, Hayashi D, Kudoh S, Mizuno T, Kijima K, Matsubara H, Sugaya T, Murakami K, Yazaki Y. 1998. Pressure overload induces cardiac hypertrophy in angiotensin II type 1A receptor knockout mice. Circulation 97:1952–1959.
67. Turcani M, Rupp H. 2000. Heart failure development in rats with ascending aortic constriction and angiotensin-converting enzyme inhibition. Br J Pharmacol 130:1671–1677.
68. Turcani M, Rupp H. 2000. Bradykinin (B2) independent effect of captopril on the development of pressure overload cardiac hypertrophy. Mol Cell Biochem 212:219–225.

Frontiers in Cardiovascular Health, edited by
N.S. Dhalla, A. Chockalingam,
H.I. Berkowitz & P.K. Singal
Kluwer Academic Publishers, Boston, 2003

Mutational Profiles and Molecular Etiologies of Hypertrophic Cardiomyopathy and Dilated Cardiomyopathy in Asian Populations

Akinori Kimura,[1] Manatsu Ito-Satoh,[1] Takeharu Hayashi,[1] Megumi Takahashi,[1] Takuro Arimura,[1] Michio Yasunami,[1] Su Yeoun Lee,[2] Tae Hong Hwang,[2] Won-Ha Lee,[2] and Jeong-Euy Park[2]

[1] *Department of Molecular Pathogenesis, Medical Research Institute, Tokyo Medical and Dental University, Tokyo 101-0062, Japan*
[2] *Cardiology Division, Cardiovascular Institute, Samsung Seoul Hospital, Sungkyunkwan University School of Medicine, Seoul 135-230, Korea*

Summary. Idiopathic cardiomyopathy (ICM) had been defined as the cardiac disease of unknown etiology. There are two major clinical phenotypes of ICM; hypertrophic cardiomyopathy (HCM) and dilated cardiomyopathy (DCM). During the last decade, a considerable progress has been made for identifying gene mutations as the causes of HCM and DCM. We have searched for mutations in the known disease genes for ICM in Japanese and Korean patients with HCM or DCM, and identified a considerable number of disease-related mutations in a portion of HCM patients and a few DCM patients. In addition, our recent candidate gene approach has revealed that mutations in the titin gene cause both HCM and DCM, and functional analyses of the titin mutations have suggested that the HCM-related and DCM-related mutations would lead to stiff sarcomere and loose sarcomere, respectively. The notion that HCM is a disease of stiff sarcomere can also be supported by that most of the HCM-related mutations in the genes for sarcomeric proteins increase the calcium sensitivity of muscle contraction, i.e. cardiac muscles are contracted under relatively low calcium concentration. In other words, HCM-related sarcomere mutations may lead to relatively stiff sarcomere under physiological condition. On the other hand, most of the DCM-related mutations in Z-disc elements would manifest with loose sarcomere, which may lead to relatively

Corresponding Author: Akinori Kimura, M.D. Ph.D., Department of Molecular Pathogenesis, Medical Research Institute, Tokyo Medical and Dental University, 2-3-10, Kandasurugadai, Chiyoda-ku, Tokyo 101-0062, Japan. Tel: +81-3-5280-8056, Fax: +81-3-5280-8055, E-mail: akitis@mri.tmd.ac.jp.

inefficient transmission of power through the Z-disc, then, DCM at least in part can be considered as a disease of loose sarcomere. In this concept, cardiac hypertrophy in HCM can also be considered as compensatory response against the excess overload, and the decompensation could be occurred later, while DCM can be considered as to be with less compensatory hypertrophy and earlier decompensation than HCM.

Key words: idiopathic cardiomyopathy, gene mutation, sarcomere, hypertrophic cardiomyopathy, dilated cardiomyopathy.

INTRODUCTION

Idiopathic cardiomyopathy (ICM) is a heterogeneous disease defined as a cardiac disease of unknown etiology. There are two major clinical phenotypes of ICM; hypertrophic cardiomyopathy (HCM) and dilated cardiomyopathy (DCM). HCM is characterized by left ventricular hypertrophy and diastolic dysfunction or reduced compliance of ventricles, accompanied by disarrays of myocytes and of myofibrils. On the other hand, DCM is characterized by ventricular dilatation and systolic dysfunction, and is often accompanied by myocyte hypertrophy and interstitial fibrosis. It is well known that a part of HCM patients would develop DCM-like phenotype in their later clinical courses; such condition is considered as burnout phase of HCM and called as dilated HCM. The classification of ICM is based on the clinical findings and not on the etiology, then the pathogenesis of this heterogeneous disease had been difficult to be understood.

Recent studies on molecular genetics have now revealed, by linkage studies in multiplex families and by candidate gene approaches, that gene mutations can be the direct causes of HCM and DCM (1). Family history of the disease can be found in about half of HCM patients and in about 20–35% of cases. So far, many different disease genes, in which mutation could be found in the ICM patients, were reported (1). This means that mutations in any of these genes cause ICM phenotypes, and such information about the genetic etiology of HCM or DCM has enabled us to speculate about the pathogenesis of this heterogeneous cardiac disease.

We have investigated for gene mutations in Japanese and Korean patients with HCM or DCM, and identified many disease-related mutations in the known disease genes. These mutations are in part correlated with severity of clinical manifestations and survival prognosis. In addition, we could identity a novel disease gene for both HCM and DCM, That is the titin gene. We found several different titin mutations in the HCM patients and DCM patients. Because one of the HCM-related mutations and the other DCM-related mutation were located at the actinin binding domain of titin in close to each other, we performed functional studies to demonstrate how the mutations affect the affinity of titin to actinin, by using yearst-2-hybrid assays. In addition, another DCM-related titin mutation found in telethonin binding domain was also tested for the functional change. These functional studies demonstrated a fundamental difference between the HCM-related and DCM-related mutations (2,3).

Here, we summarize our current data for mutational profiles of HCM and DCM in Asian populations. From the recent findings in our laboratory as well as those in the literatures, we now propose that HCM is the disease of stiff sarcomere, while DCM is the disease of loose sarcomere.

MUTATIONS FOUND IN THE PATIENTS WITH HCM

More than half of HCM patients have family history of HCM or sudden unexpected cardiac death consistent with autosomal dominant inheritance, suggesting that a single gene mutations is the cause of HCM in each patient or multiplex family. In 1990, the first HCM-linked mutation in the gene for cardiac beta-myosin heavy chain (*MYH7*) was found in a large multiplex family of HCM (4). Since then, *MHY7* has been extensively investigated for the mutations in HCM and is now well recognized as the major disease gene for HCM (1). However, *MYH7* mutations can not be identified in all of the HCM families, nor did they show the linkage of HCM to *MYH7* locus, revealing the locus heterogeneity of HCM and suggesting the presence of other disease genes (1).

The linkage studies in the HCM families non-linked to MYH7 as well as candidate gene analyses were taken to identify the other disease genes. By these approaches, mutations in the cardiac troponin T gene (*TNNT2*), alpha-tropomyosin gene (*TPM1*) and cardiac myosin binding protein-C gene (*MYBPC3*), have been shown to cause HCM (5–7). On the other hand, candidate gene approaches have revealed several other disease genes, i.e. mutations in genes for ventricular myosin essential light chain (*MYL3*), ventricular myosin regulatory light chain (*MYL2*), cardiac troponin I (*TNNI3*), cardiac alpha-actin (*CACT*), and titin (*TTN*) also cause HCM (2,8–10).

It has recently revealed that mutations in the gamma subunit of AMP-activated protein kinase gene (*PRKAG2*) are associated with cardiac hypertrophy resembling to HCM (11). This is the disease gene for the previously reported 7q3-linked HCM (12), but recent biochemical analyses have demonstrated that *PRKAG2* mutations cause glycogen storage disease of cardiac muscle and not HCM (13). Moreover, two other possible disease genes have recently been reported; one is the myosin-light chain kinase gene (*MYLK2*) (14) and the other is the alpha myosin heavy chain gene (*MYH6*) (15). Therefore, more than 10 different genes are so far listed-up as the disease genes for HCM.

We have searched for mutations in these disease genes, except for *PRKAG2*, *MYLK2* and *MYH6*, in a large panel of HCM patients collected form Japan and Korea; 184 proband cases of familial HCM and 110 sporadic cases. As listed in Table 1, disease-related mutations were identified in 47% of familial cases and in 14% of sporadic cases. It may be noted here that we have used SSCP method for screening the mutations, then there is a possibility that not all of mutations could be identified because the efficacy of SSCP in defecting a point mutation is about 90%. Nevertheless, we found 61 different disease-related mutations in 122 probands of HCM (Table 2). Some mutations are commonly found in several different families, but most of the mutations were specific to each proband or family, so-called private mutations.

Table 1. Frequency of disease-related mutations in the known disease genes in Oriental HCM

Gene symbol	coding protein	% mut. in familial cases (n = 184)	% mut. in sporadic cases (n = 110)
MYH7	b-myosin heavy chain	17.9	1.8
TNNT2	troponin T	10.9	2.7
TPM1	tropomyosin	0.5	0.0
MYBPC3	myosin binding protein	12.5	4.5
MYL3	essential light chain	1.1	1.8
MYL2	regulatory light chain	1.1	0.0
TNNI3	troponin I	2.7	2.7
CACT	cardiac actin	0.0	0.0
TTN#1	titin	0.5	0.9
PRKAG2	AMP-act PK	nt#2	nt
MYLK2	MLC kinase	nt	nt
MYH6	a-myosin heavy chain	nt	nt

#1; only the Z-disc region and N2-B region had been tested for mutational screening (3).
#2; not tested.

Table 2. Clinical phenotypes of hypertrophic cardiomyopathy gene mutations

Gene death	no. of mutation	no. of family	IVST (mm)	dilated HCM	sudden
MHY7 variable	28	55	21 ± 7	variable	
TNNT2 variable	8	20	16 ± 5	frequent	
TPM1	1	1	13 ± 2	not found	rare
MYBPC3	14	32	19 ± 7	rare	rare
MYL3	1	3	12 ± 2	rare	rare
MYL2	1	2	15 ± 6	variable	rare
TNNI3	6	7	15 ± 2	not found	rare
TTN found	2	2	16 ± 2	not found	not

IVST: interventricular septal thickness.

The clinical manifestations of HCM could be variable depending on which gene is mutated (locus difference) and where the mutations is in the disease gene (allelic difference). Table 2 shows the locus differences, demonstrating that cardiac hypertrophy was more evident in the patients with mutations in *MYH7* or *MYBPC3*. In contract, relatively mild hypertrophy was noted for the other cases including those with *TNNT2* mutations. On the other hand, the transmission to dilated HCM was relatively frequent in the *TNNT2* cases but can also be found in *MYH7* and *MYL2* cases, while the sudden deaths were mostly found in *MYH7* or *TNNT2* cases. These clinical features were similar to those reported in Caucasian patients (16–18).

The allelic differences were also found, as an example is the cumulative survival curve of individuals having *MYH7* mutations (Figure 1). Several *MYH7* mutations were associated with poor survival prognosis, while some other mutations were not. The differences in the survival prognosis could not be explained by the nature of mutations, e.g., presence of charge alterations as speculated by Watkins et al. (16).

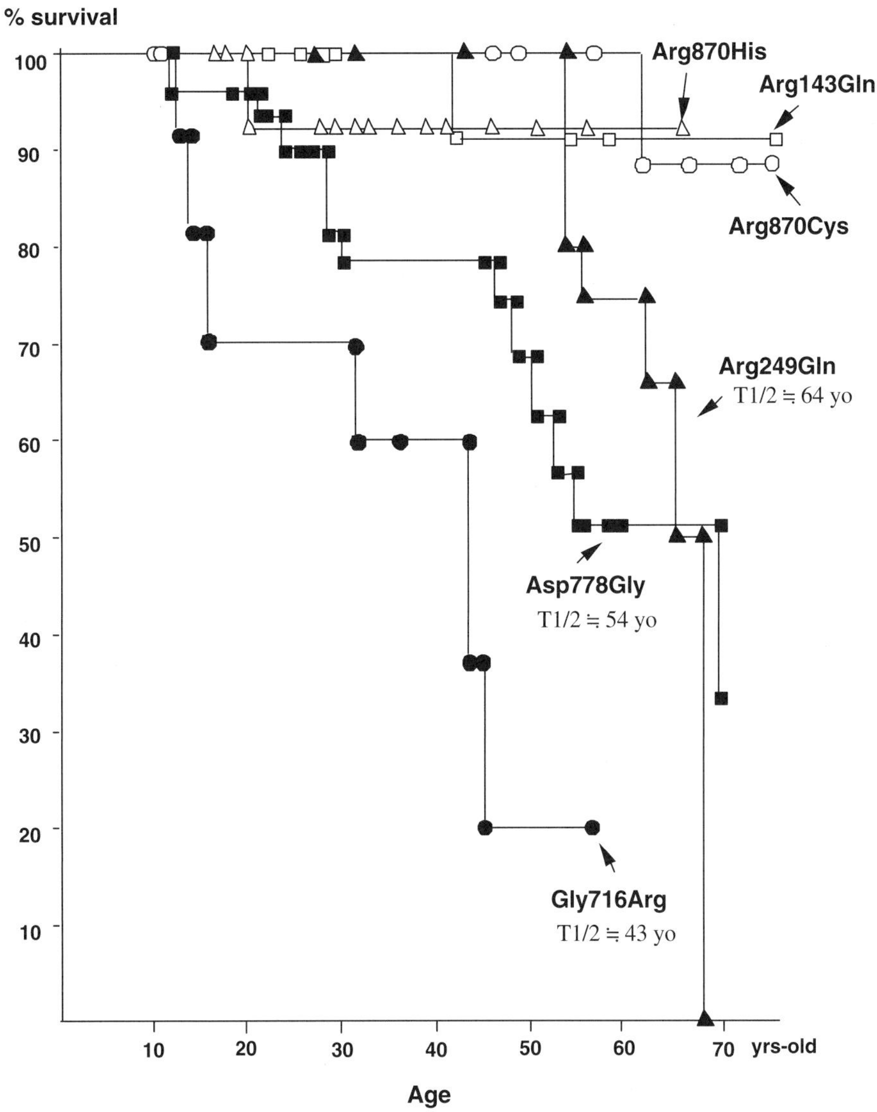

Figure 1. Cumulative survival curve of individuals having *MYH7* mutations. The cumulative curves were drawn according to the clinical history and family history of patients' relatives from 2 families with Arg870Cys, 4 families with Arg870His, 2 families with Arg143Gln, 4 families with Asp778Gly, 1 family with Arg249Gln, and 1 family with Gly716Arg.

Rather it appears that the mutations associated with poor prognosis were found in or around the functionally most important domains of myosin heavy chain, such as the ATP-binding domain, actin-interacting domain, and light-chain interacting domains (19).

Table 3. Frequency of disease-related mutations in the known disease genes in Oriental DCM

Gene symbol	coding protein	% mut. familial cases (n = 32)	% mut. sporadic cases (n = 100)
CACT	cardiac actin	0.0	0.0
DES	desmin	3.1	0.0
DMD	dystrophin	0.0	3.0
LMNA	lamin A/C	0.0	nt#1
SAGD	delta-sarcoglycan	0.0	nt
MYH7	b-myosin heavy chain	0.0	nt
TNNT2	troponin T	0.0	nt
TPM1	tropomyosin	0.0	nt
VCL	vinculin	0.0	0.0

#1; not tested.

MUTATIONS FOUND IN THE PATIENTS WITH DCM

It is also known about 20–35% of DCM cases can be considered as monogenic diseases, and autosomal dominant transmission is most often observed in familial DCM, although X-linked recessive or autosomal recessive inheritance was found in some families (20). As were the cases with HCM families, linkage studies and/or candidate gene analyses have been taken to decipher the disease genes for DCM families. It is now revealed that mutations in *LMNA* (lamin A/C), *DES* (desmin), *SAGD* (delta-sarcoglycan), and *VCL* (metavinculin) cause autosomal dominant DCM (21–24). In addition, mutations in *CACT*, *TNNT2*, *MYH7*, and *TMP1* have also been shown to cause DCM (25–27), although the mutations in these genes are different from those identified in HCM (1). However, it remains unknown why and how the mutations in the same gene could cause different clinical phenotypes, HCM or DCM. On the other hand, autosomal recessive DCM and similar phenotypes, mainly found in childhood, are caused by mutations in CPTase II, plakoglobin, or desmoplakin (28–30). X-linked DCM is caused by mutations in *DMD* (dystrophin) or *G4.5* (tafazzin) (31,32). It should be noted here that the *G4.5* mutations were reported only in childhood.

We have had searched for mutations in 9 different disease genes for DCM (Table 3), because mutations in those genes were reported in adult DCM. As shown in Table 3, our systematic analyses in 32 proband patients of familial DCM and 100 sporadic DCM patients have shown that mutations in these known DCM genes are rarely found in the Asian patients, both in the familial and sporadic cases. In our analyses, *DMD* mutations were found in the sporadic patients. They developed DCM at the ages of 30's and none of them showed skeletal muscle disease phenotypes, as reported for X-linked DCM caused by the *DMD* mutation (31). On the other hand, a *DES* mutation was found in a familial DCM patient. Although a *DES* mutation was reported to manifest with restrictive phenotype (22), our case showed typical DCM phenotypes and not restrictive phenotype (data will be described elsewhere). These analyses have demonstrated the disease heterogeneity of DCM in Asian populations and suggested that there should be other disease genes for DCM.

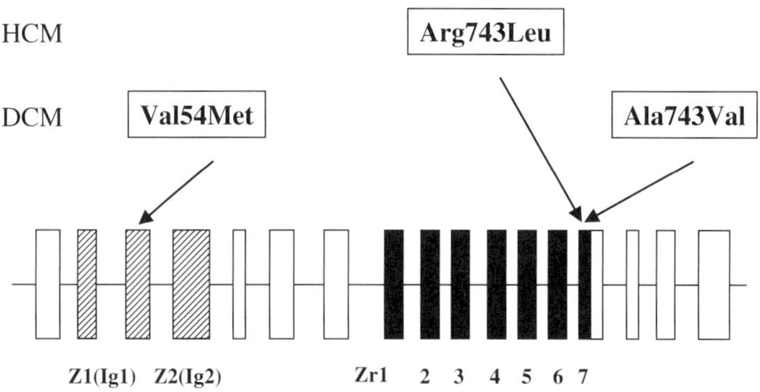

Figure 2. ***Schematic representation of titin mutations in the Z-disc region.*** The exon/intron organization of the Z-disc region is indicated. Numbers indicated amino acid positions in the cardiac titin isoforms. Mutations found in HCM or DCM patients are indicated. Exons are represented by filled boxes.

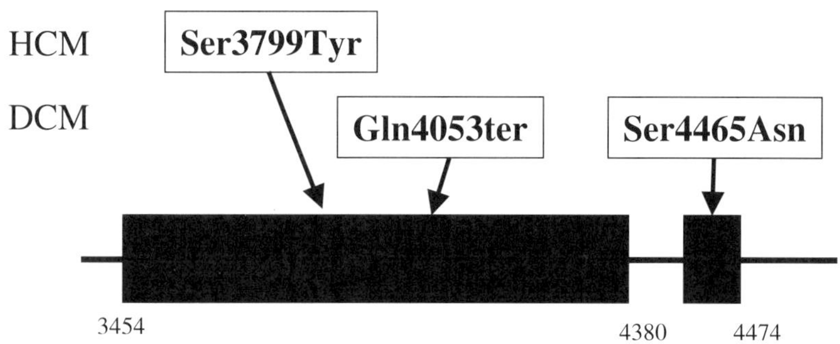

Figure 3. ***Schematic representation of titin mutations in the N2-B region.*** The exon/intron organization of the N2-B region is indicated. Numbers indicated amino acid positions in the cardiac titin isoforms. Mutations found in HCM or DCM patients are indicated. Exons are represented by filled boxes.

IDENTIFICATION OF TITIN MUTATIONS IN BOTH HCMAND DCM

Because we have previously reported an HCM-related titin mutation in the Z-disc region (2), and because several HCM genes could also be the DCM gene (1), we searched for mutations in the titin gene (*TTN*) in the Asian patients with DCM (3). Our analysis of *TTN* for the Z-disc region and N2-B region revealed two Z-disc region mutations in familial DCM cases (Figure 2) and the other two N2-B region mutations in sporadic DCM cases (Figure 3). Although the previously identified titin mutation in the Z-disc region was found in a sporadic HCM case (2), another N2-B region mutation (Ser3799Tyr, Figure 3) was found in a sibling case of familial HCM. These analyses have revealed that mutations in *TTN* could be found in a few cases of HCM and DCM, even when only about 10% of the entire gene region was investigated, suggesting that *TTN* might be a major disease gene for ICM, especially for DCM (3).

FUNCTIONAL ALTERATIONS CAUSED BY TITIN MUTATIONSIN THE Z-DISC REGION

At the same time as we have reported the titin mutations in DCM (3), Gerull et al. also reported two other titin mutations linked to DCM in two large multiplex families (33). It is then confirmed that the titin mutation can cause DCM in humans. One of the DCM mutations we identified in the N2-B region was a termination mutation (Figure 3). It is worth noting that a termination mutation in the N2-B region of titin was recently reported to cause a cardiac contraction defect in zebrafish (34). It also is interesting to note that an insertion mutation in the N2-A region of titin was also recently found in the *mdm* mouse that is characterized by skeletal myopathy (35). These observations suggested that a mutations in the heart-specific N2-B region causes cardiac phenotype, while a mutation in the non-heart-specific N2-A region may also express skeletal muscle phenotype.

Because a DCM-related titin mutation (Ala743Val) was found very near to the HCM-related mutation (Arg740Leu) (Figure 2), it was a good model to investigate why and how the mutations in the same gene could cause different clinical phenotypes. We then performed an yeast-two-hybrid (Y2H) assay to examine the functional changes caused by these mutations in interacting with actinin, because both mutations were located in the actinin-binding domain of titin (36). The DCM-related mutation decreased the affinity to actinin, in clear contract to that the HCM-related mutation increased the affinity (Figure 4). These observations have indicated that the mutations in the same gene exert the opposite functional alterations in HCM and DCM. A similar finding was also reported for *TNNT2* mutations in HCM or DCM. The HCM-related mutations increased calcium sensitivity of ATPase activity (37) or muscle contraction (38), whereas the DCM-related mutation decreased the calcium sensitivity of contraction (38). The other DCM-related mutation (Val54Met) observed in a familial DCM case (Figure 2) was located in the telethonin-binding domain (39), prompting us to investigate the functional alternation in binding to telethonin caused by the mutation, by using the Y2H assay. It was revealed that the DCM-related mutation decreased the affinity to telethonin (Figure 4).

Based on these findings along with that most of the HCM-related sarcomere mutations cause increased calcium sensitivity of muscle contraction (1), i.e., muscles are lender to be in contraction under relatively low calcium concentration at the diastolic phase, HCM may be considered as the disease of stiff sarcomere. In contrast, the titin and telethonin mutations described here in DCM decreased the affinity of telethonin-titin-actinin complex. The functional change reported for DCM-related *TNNT2* mutation was a decreased calcium sensitivity of muscle contraction, an opposite change to the HCM-related mutation (38). These observations along with the findings of dystrophin gene defects in X-linked-DCM and dys-

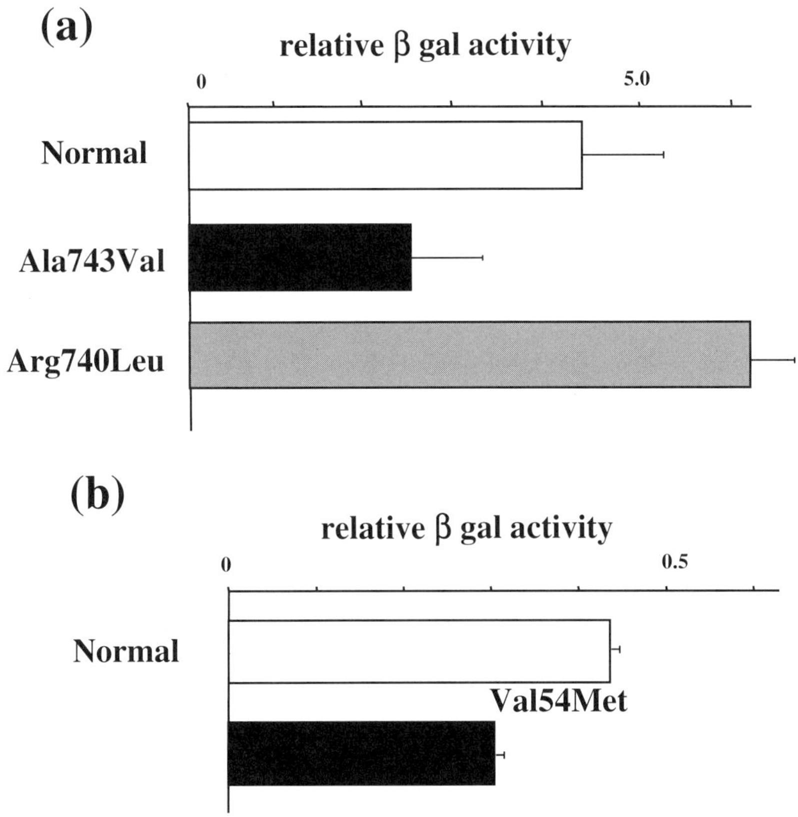

Figure 4. ***Functional analysis of titin mutations found in the Z-disc region.*** (a) Results of Y2H assays between actinin and titin with or without mutation. The DCM-related mutation (Ala743Val) reduced and the HCM-related mutation (Arg740Leu) increased the affinity to actinin. (b) Y2H assays showed that the Val54Met mutation of titin reduced the affinity to telethonin.

trophin cleavage by enterovirus in myocarditis (40) suggest that DCM at least in part can be a disease of loose sarcomere, as is speculated for the muscle LIM protein deficient mice (41).

ACKNOWLEDGEMENTS

This work was supported by Grant-in-Aids from the Ministry of Education, Culture, Sports, Science and Technology, Japan, a research grant from the Ministry of Health, Labour and Welfare, Japan, a grant for the joint research project from Japan Society for the Promotion of Science and Korean Science and Engineering Foundation, and a research grant from Heiwa-Nakajima Foundation.

REFERENCES

1. Seidman JG, Seidman C. 2001. The genetic basis for cardiomyopathy: from mutation identification to mechanistic paradigms. Cell 104:557–567.
2. Satoh M, Satoh M, Takahashi M, Sakamoto T, Hiroe M, Marumo F, Kimura A. 1999. Structural analysis of the titin gene in hypertrophic cardiomyopathy: identification of a novel disease gene. Biochem Biophys Res Commun 262:411–417.
3. Itoh-Satoh M, Hayashi T, Nishi H, Koga Y, Arimura T, Ueda K, Hohta S, Nouchi T, Takahashi M, Hiroe M, Marumo F, Imaizumi T, Yasunami M, Kimura A. 2002. Titin mutations as the molecular basis for dilated cardiomyopathy. Biochem Biophys Res Commun 291:385–393.
4. Geisterfer-Lowrance AA, Kass S, Tanigawa G, Vosberg HP, McKenna W, Seidman CE, Seidman JG. 1990. A molecular basis for familial hypertrophic cardiomyopathy: a beta-cardiac myosin heavy chain gene missense mutation. Cell 62:999–1006.
5. Thierfelder L, Watkins H, MacRae C, Lamas R, McKenna W, Vosberg HP, Seidman JG, Seidman CE. 1994. Alpha-tropomyosin and cardiac troponin T mutations cause familial hypertrophic cardiomyopathy. Cell 77:701–712.
6. Watkins H, Conner D, Thierfelder L, Jarcho JA, MacRae C, McKenna WJ, Maron BJ, Seidman JG, Seidman CE. 1995. Mutations in the cardiac myosin binding protein-C gene on chromosome 11 cause familial hypertrophic cardiomyopathy. Nature Genet 11:434–437.
7. Bonne G, Carrier L, Bercovici J, et al. 1995. Cardiac myosin binding protein-C gene splice acceptor site mutation is associated with hypertrophic cardiomyopathy. Nature Genet 11:438–440.
8. Poetter K, Jiang H, Hassanzadeh S, Master SR, Chang A, Dalakas MC, Rayment I, Sellers JR, Fananapazir L, Epstein ND. 1996. Mutations in either essential or regulatory light chain of myosins are associated with a rare myopathy in human heart and skeletal muscle. Nature Genet 13:63–69.
9. Kimura A, Harada H, Park JE, Nishi H, Satoh M, Takahashi M, Hiroi S, Sasaoka T, Ohbuchi N, Nakamura T, Koyanagi T, Hwang TH, Choo JA, Chung KS, Hasegawa A, Nagai R, Okazaki O, Nakamura H, Matsuzaki M, Sakamoto T, Toshima H, Koga Y, Imaizumi T, Sasazuki T. 1997. Mutations in the cardiac troponin I gene associated with hypertrophic cardiomyopathy. Nature Genet 16: 379–382.
10. Mogensen J, Klausen IC, Pedersen AK, Egeblad H, Bross P, Kruse TA, Gregersen N, Hansen PS, Baandrup U, Borglum AD. 1999. Alpha-cardiac actin is a novel disease gene in familial hypertrophic cardiomyopathy. J Clin Invest 103:R39–R43.
11. Blair E, Redwood C, Ashrafian H, Oliveira M, Broxholme J, Kerr B, Salmon A, Ostman-Smith I, Watkins H. 2001. Mutations in the gamma 2 subunit of AMP-activated protein kinase cause familial hypertrophic cardiomyopathy: evidence for the central role of energy compromise in disease pathogenesis. Hum Mol Genet 10:1215–1220.
12. MacRae CA, Ghaisas N, Kass S, et al. 1995. Familial hypertrophic cardiomyopathy with Wolff-Parkinson-White syndrome maps to a locus on chromosome 7q3. J Clin Invest 96:1216–1220.
13. Arad M, Benson DW, Perez-Atayde AR, McKenna WJ, Sparks EA, Kanter RJ, McGarry K, Seidman JG, Seidman CE. 2002. Constitutively active AMP kinase mutations cause glycogen storage disease mimicking hypertrophic cardiomyopathy. J Clin Invest 109:357–362.
14. Davis JS, Hassanzadeh S, Winitsky S, Lin H, Satorius C, Vemuri R, Aletras AH, Wen H, Epstein ND. 2001. The overall pattern of cardiac contraction depends on a spatial gradient of myosin regulatory light chain phosphorylation. Cell 107:631–641.
15. Niimura H, Patton KK, McKenna WJ, Soults J, Maron BJ, Seidman JG, Seidman CE. 2002. Sarcomere protein gene mutations in hypertrophic cardiomyopathy of the elderly. Circulation 105:446–451.
16. Watkins H, Rosenzweig A, Hwang DS, Levi T, McKenna W, Seidman CE, Seidman JG. Characteristics and prognostic implicaions of myosin missense mutations in familial hypertrophic cardiomyopathy. N Engl J Med 326:1108–1114.
17. Watkins H, McKenna WJ, Thierfelder L, et al. 1995. Mutations in the genes for cardiac troponin T and alpha-tropomyosin in hypertrophic cardiomyopathy. N Engl J Med 332:1058–1064.
18. Niimura H, Bachinski LL, Sangwatanaroj S, Watkins H, Chudley AE, McKenna W, Kristinsson A, Roberts R, Sole M, Maron BJ, Seidman JG, Seidman CE. 1998. Mutations in the gene for cardiac myosin-binding protein C and late-onset familial hypertrophic cardiomyopathy. N Engl J Med 338:1248–1257.
19. Rayment I, Rypniewski WR, Schmidt-Base K, Smith R, Tomchick DR, Benning MM, Winkelmann DA, Wesenberg G, Holden HM. 1993. Three-dimensional structure of myosin subfragment-1: a molecular motor. Science 261:50–58.

20. Mestroni L, Rocco C, Gregori D, Sinagra G, Di Lenarda A, Miocic S, Vatta M, Pinamonti B, Muntoni F, Caforio AL, McKenna WJ, Falaschi A, Giacca M, Camerini. 1999. Familial dilated cardiomyopathy: evidence for genetic heterogeneity. J Am Coll Cardiol 34:181–190.
21. Fatkin D, MacRae C, Sasaki T, Wolff MR, Porcu M, Frenneaux M, Atherton J, Vidaillet HJ Jr, Spudich S, De Girolami U, Seidman JG, Seidman C, Muntoni F, Muehle G, Johnson W, McDonough B. 1999. Missense mutations in the rod domain of the lamin A/C gene as the causes of dilated cardiomyopathy and conduction-system disease. N Engl J Med 341:1715–1724.
22. Li D, Tapscoft T, Gonzalez O, Burch PE, Quinones MA, Zoghbi WA, Hill R, Bachinski LL, Mann DL, Roberts R. 1999. Desmin mutation responsible for idiopathic dilated cardiomyopathy. Circulation 100:461–464.
23. Tsubata S, Bowles KR, Vatta M, Zintz C, Titus J, Muhonen L, Bowles NE, Towbin JA. 2000. Mutations in the human delta-sarcoglycan gene in familial and sporadic dilated cardiomyopathy. J Clin Invest 106:655–662.
24. Olson TM, Illenberger S, Kishimoto NY, Huttelmaier S, Keating MT, Jockusch BM. 2002. Metavinculin mutations alter actin interaction in dilated cardiomyopathy. Circulation 105:431–437.
25. Olson TM, Michels VV, Thibodeau SN, Tai YS, Keating MT. 1998. Actin mutations in dilated cardiomyopathy, a heritable form of heart failure. Science 280:750–752.
26. Kamisago M, Sharma SD, DePalma SR, Solomon S, Sharma P, McDonough B, Smoot L, Mullen MP, Woolf PK, Wigle ED, Seidman JG, Seidman CE. 2000. Mutations in sarcomere protein genes as a cause of dilated cardiomyopathy. N Engl J Med 343:1688–1696.
27. Olson TM, Kishimoto NY, Whitby FG, Michels VV. 2001. Mutations that alter the surface charge of alpha-tropomyosin are associated with dilated cardiomyopathy. J Mol Cell Cardiol 33:723–732.
28. Taroni F, Verderio E, Fiorucci S, Cavadini P, Finocchiaro G, Uziel G, Lamantea E, Gellera C, DiDonato S. Molecular characterization of inherited carnitine palmitoyltransferase II deficiency. Proc Natl Acad Sci USA 89:8429–8433.
29. Norgett EE, Hatsell SJ, Carvajal-Huerta L, Cabezas JC, Common J, Purkis PE, Whittock N, Leigh IM, Stevens HP, Kelsell DP. 2000. Recessive mutation in desmoplakin disrupts desmoplakin-intermediate filament interactions and causes dilated cardiomyopathy, woolly hair and keratoderma. Hum Mol Genet 9:2761–2766.
30. McKoy G, Protonotarios N, Crosby A, Tsatsopoulou A, Anastasakis A, Coonar A, Norman M, Baboonian C, Jeffery S, McKenna WJ. 2000. Identification of a deletion in plakoglobin in arrhythmogenic right ventricular cardiomyopathy with palmoplantar keratoderma and woolly hair (Naxos disease). Lancet 355:2119–2124.
31. Towbin JA, Hejtmancik JF, Brink P, Gelb B, Zhu XM, Chamberlain JS, McCabe ER, Swift M. 1993. X-linked dilated cardiomyopathy. Molecular evidence of linkage to the Duchenne muscular dystrophy (dystrophin) gene at the Xp21 locus. Circulation 87:1854–1865.
32. Bione S, D'Adamo P, Maestrini E, Gedeon AK, Bolhuis PA, Toniolo D. 1996. A novel X-linked gene, G4.5, is responsible for Barth syndrome. Nature Genet 12:385–389.
33. Gerull B, Gramlich M, Atherton J, McNabb M, Trombitas K, Sasse-Klaassen S, Seidman JG, Seidman C, Granzier H, Labeit S, Frenneaux M, Thierfelder L. 2002. Mutations of TTN, encoding the giant muscle filament titin, cause familial dilated cardiomyopathy. Nature Genet 30:201–204.
34. Xu X, Meiler SE, Zhong TP, Mohideen M, Crossley DA, Burggren WW, Fishman MC. 2002. Cardiomyopathy in zebrafish due to mutation in alternatively spliced exon of titin. Nature Genet 30:205–209.
35. Garvey SM, Rajan C, Lerner AP, Frankel WN, Cox GA. 2002. The muscular dystrophy with myositis (mdm) mouse mutation disrupts a skeletal muscle-specific domain of titin. Genomics 79:146–149.
36. Gregorio CC, Trombitas K, Centner T, Kolmerer B, Stier G, Kunke K, Suzuki K, Obermayr F, Herrmann B, Granzier H, Sorimachi H, Labeit S. 1998. The NH2 terminus of titin spans the Z-disc: interaction with a novel 19-kD ligand (T-cap) is required for sarcomere integrity. J Cell Biol 143:1013–1027.
37. Yanaga F, Morimoto S, Ohtsuki I. 1999. Ca2+ sensitization and potentiation of the maximum level of myofibrillar ATPase activity caused by mutations of troponin T found in familial hypertrophic cardiomyopathy. J Biol Chem 274:8806–8812.
38. Morimoto S, Lu QW, Harada K, Takahashi-Yanaga F, Minakami R, Ohta M, Sasaguri T, Ohtsuki I. 2002. Ca (2+)-desensitizing effect of a deletion mutation delta K210 in cardiac troponin T that causes familial dilated cardiomyopathy. Proc Natl Acad Sci USA 99:913–918.

39. Mues A, van der Ven PF, Young P, Furst DO, Gautel M. 1998. Two immunoglobulin-like domains of the Z-disc portion of titin interact in a conformation-dependent way with titin. FEBS Lett 428: 111–114.
40. Badorff C, Lee GH, Lamphear BJ, Martone ME, Campbell KP, Rhoads RE, Knowlton KU. 1999. Enteroviral protease 2A cleaves dystrophin: evidence of cytoskeletal disruption in an acquired cardiomyopathy. Nature Med 5:320–326, 1999.
41. Arber S, Hunter JJ, Ross J Jr, Hongo M, Sansig G, Borg J, Perriard JC, Chien KR, Caroni P. 1997. MLP-deficient mice exhibit a disruption of cardiac cytoarchitectural organization, dilated cardiomyopathy, and heart failure. Cell 88:393–403.

II. Nutrition, Metabolism and Cardiovascular Health

Frontiers in Cardiovascular Health, edited by
N.S. Dhalla, A. Chockalingam,
H.I. Berkowitz & P.K. Singal
Kluwer Academic Publishers, Boston, 2003

Flavanol-Rich Foods and Cardiovascular Health

Carl L. Keen,[1,2]* Roberta R. Holt,[1] Fernando Carrasquedo,[1] M. Eric Gershwin,[2] Tin K. Mao,[2] and Harold H. Schmitz[3]

Departments of Nutrition[1], and Internal Medicine[2], University of California, Davis, One Shields Avenue, Davis, California, 95616, USA; Analytical and Applied Sciences, Mars Incorporated[3], 800 High Street, Hackettstown, New Jersey, USA

Summary. Fruit and vegetables provide fiber, antioxidants, micronutrients, and phytochemicals that separately or in combination, influence vascular health. Flavonoids are the largest, and most widely distributed class of phytochemicals. Several epidemiology studies have observed an inverse association between flavonoid intake and risk of cardiovascular mortality. Flavonoids can be subdivided into six different classes. One class, the flavanols, is commonly found in foods such as grapes, red wine, tea and cocoa. Recent studies have looked at the potential of these foods to influence vascular health in a positive fashion. In this paper, we discuss evidence for the hypothesis that the consumption of flavanol-rich foods can reduce the risk for CVD through a multiplicity of mechanisms, including changes in: antioxidant defense mechanisms, vascular reactivity, cytokine production, and platelet function.

Key words: Flavanols, red wine, cocoa, tea, cardiovascular health.

INTRODUCTION

In their dietary guidelines, the American Heart Association strongly endorse the consumption of five or more servings of a variety of fruits and vegetables per day to reduce the risk of cardiovascular disease (CVD) (1). This recommendation is based on numerous epidemiology studies that have associated fruit and vegetable intake with reduced risks of heart disease, stroke and hypertension (1). Fruit and vegetables provide fiber, antioxidants, micronutrients, and phytochemicals that separately or in combination, influence vascular health. Flavonoids are the largest, and most widely distributed class of phytochemicals. Recently, flavonoids garnered the attention of scientists, after several epidemiology studies observed an inverse association

This work is supported in part by grants from the National Institute of Health (DK-35747) and Mars Incorporated.
Address correspondence to: Carl L Keen, Department of Nutrition, University of California, Davis, One Shields Avenue, Davis, CA 95616-8669. Tel: 530-752-6331, Fax: 530-752-8966, Email: clkeen@ucdavis.edu.

between flavonoid intake and risk of cardiovascular mortality. Flavonoids can be subdivided into six different classes. One class, the flavanols, is commonly found in foods such as grapes, red wine, tea and cocoa. Recent studies have looked at the potential of these foods to influence vascular health in a positive fashion. The common structure of all classes of flavonoids consists of two aromatic rings linked by on oxygen heterocycle (2). This structure provides flavonoids with a redox chemistry that allows flavonoids to not only act as free radical scavengers, but it also allows for their possible interaction with numerous enzyme systems, receptors, and intracellular signaling cascades. In this paper, we discuss evidence for the hypothesis that the consumption of flavanol-rich foods can reduce the risk for CVD through a multiplicity of mechanisms, including changes in: oxidant defense mechanisms, vascular reactivity, cytokine production, and platelet function.

EFFECTS ON ANTIOXIDANT STATUS

Inflammation is now considered to be a key player in the development and progression of CVD, and it is thought to have a critical role in the initiation and progression of disease, such as, hypertension and diabetes, that can compromise vascular health (3,4). Inflammation produces large amounts of localized free radicals that can modify nearby cell membranes, proteins and lipoproteins, eventually resulting in cellular damage that progresses to disease. The oxidant defense system limits the damage caused by an oxidant insult through the concerted use of numerous enzymes, small molecular weight antioxidants and vitamins (5). Because of their redox chemistry, dietary flavanols can also provide further protection.

Several different assays are used to determine the antioxidant potential of foods. A summary of the antioxidant effects of the flavanols can be found in Table 1. Bearden et al., used the ORAC assay to compare the antioxidant activity of cocoa powder, green tea, blueberry, garlic, and strawberry. The greatest amount of antioxidant activity was observed with cocoa powder followed by green tea (1000 and 800 ORAC units, respectively), whereas the other foods tested typically provided antioxidant activities less then 100 ORAC units (6). Interestingly, similar types of flavonoids can be found in both tea and cocoa. Green tea provides the flavanols (+)-catechin (catechin), (−)-epicatechin (epicatechin), (−)-epigallocatechin-3-gallate (EGCG), (−)-epigallocatechin (EGC), and (−)-epicatechin-3-gallate (ECG), while the fermentation process used in black tea production results in the polymerization of the tea flavanols to theaflavins and thearubigin (7). Similar to tea, cocoa contains the flavan-3-ols, catechin and epicatechin, and the oligomers of these monomeric units known as the procyanidins. To date, oligomers up to the decamer have been isolated, and identified in cocoa (8). Interestingly, as is discussed later in this paper the bioactivities of the oligomers can be markedly different.

Like cocoa, red wine also contains flavanols and procyanidins, in addition to other flavonoid classes, such as flavonols and flavanone. The "French Paradox" refers to the observation by Renaud and De Lorgeril that segments of the French population have a low incidence of CVD, despite being characterized with diets that are rich in fat (9). Frankel and colleagues first suggested that it might be the phenolic

Table 1. Antioxidant protection of flavanols

Model System	Flavanol or Food (with reference)
Antioxidant Capacity	
ORAC, in vitro	Cocoa (6), Green Tea (6), Procyanidins (93)
TEAC, in vitro	Blueberries (94), Blackberries (94), Red Wine (95)
TRAP, in vitro	Red Wine (18,96), Tea, Mate (96), Chocolate and Chocolate Liquor (93)
Plasma ORAC, FRAP, TEAC	Strawberries (97), Red Wine (97)
Plasma TRAP	Dealcoholized Red Wine (98), Chocolate (15)
Plasma ORAC (chronic feeding study)	Cocoa (16)
Plasma FRAP	Black and Green Tea (19)
Lipid and Lipoprotein	
Copper Induced LDL or liposome oxidation, in vitro	Red Wine (99,100), Dealcholized Red Wine (10), Catechin (11), Epicatechin (11,21), Procyanidins (6,11–13), Epicatechin gallate, Epigallocatechin gallate, Theaflavins (21)
Peroxyl-Radical Induced LDL or liposome oxidation, in vitro	Red Wine (18), Green Tea (18), Black Tea (18,101), Procyanidins (12)
Cell-mediated LDL oxidation, in vitro	Epicatechin, Epigallocatechin, Epicatechin gallate, Epigallocatechin gallate, Theaflavins (21), Procyanidins (13)
TBARS, in vitro	Red Wine (100), Epicatechin, Epigallocatechin, Epicatechin gallate, Epigallocatechin gallate (21), Procyanidins (12)
Copper Induced LDL oxidation, ex vivo	Red Wine (27,29,31), Dealcoholized Red Wine (28), Black Tea (20,21), Green Tea (22), Procyanidins (42), Cocoa (16,17), Grape Juice (26)
Peroxyl-Radical Induced LDL oxidation, ex vivo	Cocoa (17)
TBARS, ex vivo	Red Wine (27), Dealcholized Red Wine (27), Chocolate (15)
Protein	
Peroxynitrite scavenging of liver homogenates	Epicatechin, Catechin, Red Wine (102)
RBC Hemolysis	Grape Seeds (103), Procyanidins (14), Cocoa extract (14)
Protein oxidation	Green tea extract (104,105), Epigallocatechin gallate (105,106)
DNA	
①8-OH2′dG	Theaflavins (107), Epigallocatechin gallate (108)
Comet Assay	Theaflavins (107), Epigallocatechin gallate (109)

substances present in red wine that may contribute to this "French Paradox", since the phenols present in red wine had the ability to inhibit copper catalyzed LDL-oxidation (10). Teissedre et al. expanded on these findings, observing that the flavanols appear to have a greater ability to inhibit LDL-oxidation relative to the flavonols found in wine. In addition, they showed that only certain procyanidin dimers and trimers have similar antioxidant ability as the monomers, suggesting that differences in binding characteristics, and therefore biological activity, may exist with the procyanidins (11). Lotito et al., tested this concept by measuring the protective effects of cocoa procyanidins on liposome oxidation. Their investigation found that the antioxidant capacity of the procyanidins was influenced by oligomer chain length. They also observed that the degree of protection provided by the different oligomers was influenced by the type of oxidation system used. When 2,2′-azo-bis (2-amidinopropane) dihydrochloride (AAPH) was used as the radical initiator (produces radicals in the aqueous phase), the highest amount of protection was observed with the lower number of monomeric units (e.g. dimers, trimers, monomers). In contrast, with 2,2′-azobis (2,4-dimethylvaleronitrile) (AMVN) initiation (produces radicals in the lipid phase) the higher chained oligomers provided the greatest amount of protection (12). Subsequent to the above work, Pearson et al. reported that the higher cocoa oligomers provided better protection against copper-catalyzed LDL oxidation at 1 uM than did monomers, suggestive of a chelating effect, however, all monomers and procyanidins provided near complete inhibition at a concentration of 5 uM, suggestive that mechanisms other than chelation may also be involved (13). When another oxidation system was used (human endothelial cell mediated oxidation), the monomers and dimers provided the strongest protection (13). While the precise mechanisms underlying the antioxidant effects of flavonoids have yet to be identified, the above studies suggest that a varied combination of flavonoids and procyanidins in the diet may represent the best way to combat the diverse array of oxidative insults that are in the environment.

The above promising in vitro data has been shown to translate in part to in vivo models. Plasma antioxidant capacity was observed to increase as soon as 30 minutes after rats were given 100 mg of a cocoa extract, and remained elevated four hours later (14). In the same study, the cocoa extract was observed to protect against red blood cell hemolysis (14). Wang et al., observed a dose dependent increase in plasma antioxidant capacity, and a dose related reduction in 2-thiobarbituric acid reactive substances (TBARS), when increasing amounts of a flavanol-rich chocolate were given to healthy adult human subjects (15) (Figure 1). Likewise, longer-term feeding studies with a flavanol-rich cocoa has been reported to be associated with an increase total plasma antioxidant capacity (16), and reductions in the susceptibility of LDL to ex vivo oxidation (16,17). Importantly, in the above chronic studies there were no differences observed between the control- and cocoa-fed groups in total cholesterol, triglycerides, and LDL and HDL levels. Similar to cocoa, tea consumption has been reported to result in increases in plasma antioxidant capacity (18,19), however, the results for tea are mixed with respect to ex vivo LDL oxidation. The results for LDL oxidation appear to be dependent on the amounts of tea given, and study design. An acute dose of green tea and black tea (1.37 and 1.44 g of total polyphenols, respec-

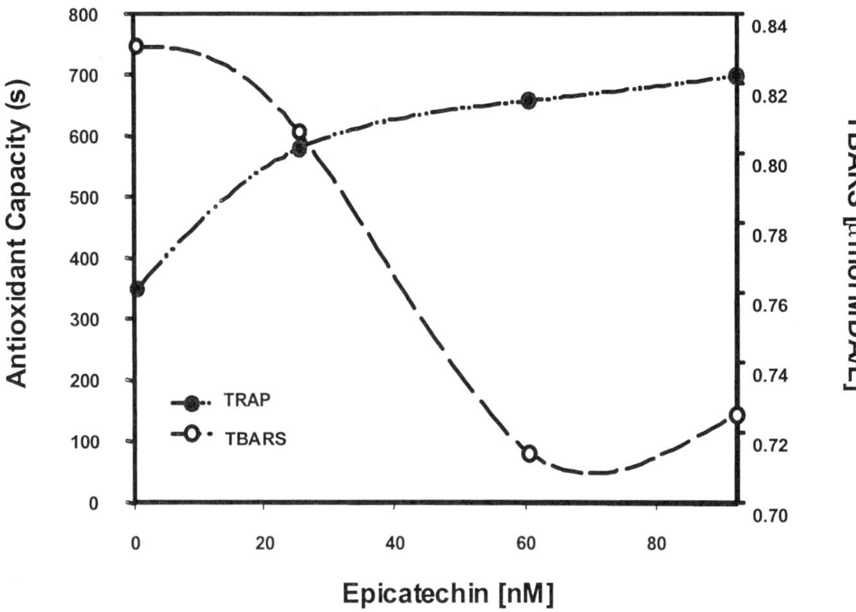

Figure 1. Plasma TBARS values are, and antioxidant capacity is, and epicatechin levels 6h after flavanol-rich chocolate consumption. Plasma TBARS values expressed as malondialdehyde equivalents (μmol/L). Plasma antioxidant capacity expressed as changes in lag time(s) before chemiluminescence is observed. A weak positive correlation ($r = 0.37$, $P < 0.03$) was observed between 6h plasma antioxidant capacity and 6h epicatechin levels after a total flavanol and procyanidin load of 558mg. A weak positive correlation ($r = 0.34$, $P < 0.03$) was observed between 6h plasma TBARS levels and 6h epicatechin levels after consuming 105g of flavanol-rich chocolate (15).

tively) provided a slight protective effect with black tea, but not with green tea (20). Ishikawa et al., observed a decrease in the susceptibility of copper-induced LDL to oxidation after subjects were given approximately 5 cups/day (750mL; 376mg total flavanols) of black tea for 4 weeks (21), and similar results were observed when subjects were given a green tea extract (300mg twice daily) for one week (22). In contrast, Van Het Hof et al., observed no significant changes in LDL oxidation after subjects consumed 8 cups (0.5g of tea solids/cup) of green or black tea for 3 days (23). In addition, no effect of tea consumption was observed on other markers of lipid oxidation, including plasma TBARS concentrations (22), and plasma F_2-isoprostanes (24,25).

While purple grape juice has shown the ability to reduce LDL oxidation in patients with CVD (26), studies observing the in vivo effects of red wine consumption on LDL oxidation are complicated by the alcohol content of the wine, in that the alcohol can potentially act as an prooxidant. The acute ingestion of dealcoholized red wine has been reported to result in a reduction in the susceptibility of LDL to oxidation after an acute ingestion (18). Similar effects have been reported following the chronic consumption of alcohol for two (27), or five weeks (28).

When alcohol is retained in the red wine, some investigators have seen positive acute and chronic effects (27,29), while others have seen no change (30), or even a shortening in lag times, compared to controls (31). These observed differences point to the need to have a thorough food analysis of the test product for proper interpretation of final results. The study by van Golde used a Spanish Valdepeñas wine with no stated alcoholic content, although they used a alcohol control of 12%, that represented the average of the wines used. In addition, the concentration of the polyphenol content of the wines used in this study was not reported (31). The acute study by Natella et al., used a Rubesco D.O.C. wine with a 12% alcohol content, and a measured total polyphenol content providing a total dose of 1280 mg (29), while the short term study by Cacceta et al., used a Cabernet Shiraz of 13% alcoholic content and an approximate polyphenol dose of 600 mg (30). Finally, the chronic study by Nigdikar et al., used a French Cabernet of 10% alcohol and a daily polyphenol dose of 600 mg (27). Although total polyphenol content as measured by the Folin assay gives a good approximation, an even better measurement would be the analysis of known key wine components using HPLC or GC-MS. Only Caccetta et al., and Nigdikar et al., provided this type of analysis, with the former study focusing on phenolic compounds only (30), and the later study providing analysis for eight different flavonoids, plus total procyanidins, anthocyanidins, and phenolic acids (27). This type of analysis is important, given that marked differences are observed between cultivars and regions for the flavanols epicatechin and catechin (32), and the polyphenol resveratrol (33). These flavonoids have been reported to have important biological effects in vitro, and as will be discussed in the following section, found in plasma after the consumption of certain flavanol-rich foods.

FLAVANOL BIOAVAILABILITY

Flavanols are distinct from other flavonoid classes, because they do not appear as glycosides, instead, they are present in foods in the aglycone form, or as oligomers, or can be esterified with gallic acid (34,35). In the circulation, the flavanols predominately exist in conjugated forms. From rat studies, using both in situ and isolated intestinal preparations, it has been established that the flavanols are first absorbed into the epithelial cell layer, then glucuronidated by urindine-5′-diphosphate glucuronosyltransferase (UGT) in the intestinal mucosa (35–37). It is also evident that the flavanols can be methylated by catechol-o-methyltransferases (COMT) present in the small intestine, but to a lesser extent then glucuronidation (35,37). In the liver, further conjugation can take place by COMT, as well as sulfation by phenolsulfotransferase (PST) (35,36). Eventually, the conjugated flavanols are excreted into the bile or urine.

Feeding studies have confirmed the presence of the conjugates in the plasma and urine of human subjects. Typically after a single dose, the flavanols rapidly reach peak levels in the plasma within 1–2 hours after consumption, and are predominately non-methylated conjugates (5,38,39). However, which non-methylated conjugate is detected in the greatest amount appears to be dependent on the type of flavanol present. Lee and coworkers (40) reported that after subjects consumed a total of 235 mg of flavanol EGCG (88 mg), EGC (82 mg), ECG (33 mg) and epicatechin (32 mg) in green tea, only EGC, EGCG, and epicatechin were detected in the plasma. Interestingly, EGCG and epicatechin were predominately sulfate conjugates, whereas, EGC was mostly glucuronidated. This appears to be in agreement with the observations of Baba et al. (39), who reported that epicatechin in cocoa was sulfated in a greater amount then glucuronide. However, the greatest conjugate in the plasma after cocoa consumption was a combination of both sulfide and glucuronide conjugation (39), which was not measured in the Lee et al. study (40). Similar conjugation patterns are observed with catechin after red wine consumption. One hour after consuming a glass of red wine containing 35 mg of catechin, the predominant conjugates are the nonmethylated conjugates, with glucuronide plus sulfide detected in the greatest amount (~60%) followed by sulfate (~20%) and glucuronide (~10%) conjugation (38). Similar to plasma, the flavanols are predominately non-methylated conjugates, however, they are mainly excreted in the sulfated form (39,40).

Studies have shown dose-response increases in plasma non-methylated epicatechin. Richelle et al., observed that the consumption of 40 g and 80 g of chocolate produced a plasma epicatechin concentration of 383 nmol/L and 700 nmol/L, respectively (41). Similar results were shown after subjects consumed chocolate containing 46 mg, 92 mg, and 138 mg of epicatechin, producing a plasma epicatechin level of 133 nmol/L, 258 nmol/L and 355 nmol/L, respectively (15). Larger doses of epicatechin can produce plasma non-methlyated epicatechin concentrations in the micromolar range as soon as 1 hour after cocoa consumption (39,42,43). It is important to note that the flavanols are rapidly removed from the plasma, so that by 24 hours post consumption they are non-detectable (39). Only EGC has been observed in the plasma after an overnight fast, and only after consuming either multiple doses of tea (every two hours, 3 doses total) (44), and after a two daily cups of tea for one week (22).

There is evidence that certain flavanols are better absorbed than others. Lee et al. (40) reported that while EGC and EGCG were present in similar concentration in a green tea drink, plasma EGC was greater in concentration, by approximately 2 fold, then EGCG. In the same study, epicatechin and ECG, were also present in the tea at the same concentration, but only epicatechin could be detected in the plasma (40). Similar results have been reported for cocoa. After human subjects consumed a cocoa beverage containing epicatechin and catechin in a 1 : 1 ratio, peak plasma catechin levels were <10% of the peak epicatechin concentration (42,43) (Figure 2). Since cocoa contains a high amount of procyanidins, it is possible that epicatechin may be formed as a breakdown product which could contribute to the above observation. Given that epicatechin and catechin can have different biological activities, further research is clearly warranted on this subject, as well as, the possibility that the two flavanols differ in their absorption or metabolism.

Although a number of papers have looked at the bioavailability of the monomeric flavanols, there is limited information concerning the metabolism of the procyani-

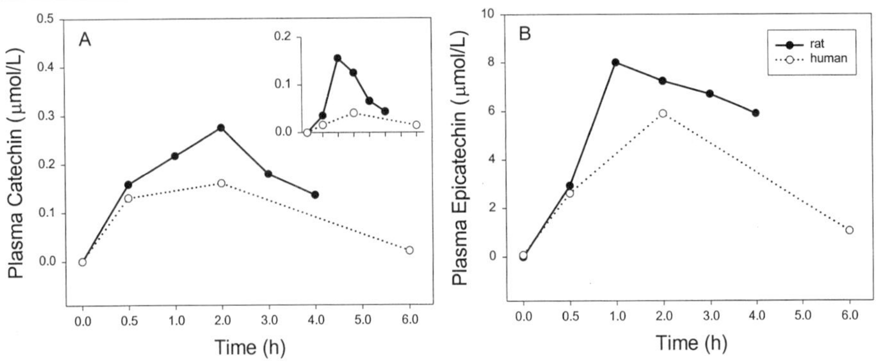

Figure 2. Mean plasma catechin (A) and plasma epicatechin (B) levels in both rat and human. The human subjects (n = 5) were given an approximate dose of cocoa monomers and dimers of 4 mg/kg (body weight = $kg^{3/4}$). The rats (n = 5–6) were given 100 mg of a cocoa extract, with an estimated (rat weight = $kg^{3/4}$) monomer and dimer dose of 29 mg/kg. Inset: rat and human dimer B2 plasma concentrations μmol/L (14,43).

dins, theaflavins, and thearubigins. Some studies have used radiolabelled techniques to indicate that extracts containing procyanidins are bioavailable (45,46). However, these techniques do not answer the question of whether the procyanidins are depolymerized, or remain intact before absorption. Recent studies have shown the vulnerability of cocoa procyanidins to the acidic and alkaline conditions or the stomach and intestine (47,48). Two types or procyanidin dimers are present in cocoa, dimer B2 and dimer B5. Zhu et al., observed that although the dimers are more stable then the other oligomers, they can degrade to epicatechin, and experience intraflavan bond conversion (e.g., dimer B2 convert to dimer B5) in the acidic conditions of the stomach. In addition, dimer B5 is more susceptible to conversion and degradation then dimer B2 (48). Complementing the above study, using a dimers fraction (containing dimer B2 and B5), Spencer et al., perfused a 50 uM dimers solution for 90 minutes through isolated rat small intestine. Small amounts (<1%) of the procyanidin dimers B2 and B5 were observed to pass through the rat enterocytes, with 95.8% of the total passing flavanols being unconjugated epicatechin (49). Consistent with these in vitro findings, dimer B2 was detected in relatively modest concentrations in the plasma relative to the flavanol monomers, after human subjects were given a cocoa dose containing relatively large amounts of monomers and dimers (42,43), and in rats given an extract of cocoa (14). In the latter study, small amounts of dimer B5 were also detected (14). Similarly, the theaflavins in green tea can be detected in minute amounts in the plasma after human subjects consumed large amounts of this compound (700 mg, equivalent to 30 cups of tea) (50).

EFFECTS ON ENDOTHELIAL FUNCTION

The vascular endothelium regulates hemostasis, by maintaining vasomotor tone, and through its influence on platelet function and leukocyte adherence. Under normal physiological conditions several mediators are released from the endothelium, such as, endothelin, prostacylin (PGI_2), nitric oxide (NO), and adenosine (51). Shear stress, ischemia and reperfusion, inflammation, and disease states, such as, atherosclerosis, diabetes and hypertension can disrupt the endothelium. As a result, the endothelium can no longer produce its regulatory mediators, and therefore can no longer regulate vascular tone, and an overall prothrombotic state ensues.

Because of their ability to act as antioxidants, it is possible that flavanols can in part improve endothelial function through the reduction of oxidative damage. However, other mechanisms may also be involved. For example, several investigators have reported that the flavanols can stimulate endothelium-dependent relaxation by increasing nitric oxide production. A fraction containing flavanols and procyanidins isolated from red wine, was observed to produce significant endothelium-dependent relaxation in rat aortic rings (52). Epicatechin also produced endothelium-dependent relaxation that was abolished with the use of the NO inhibitor, N^G-Nitro-L-arginine methyl ester (L-NAME) (53). The cocoa procyanidins also produced endothelium-dependent relaxation, and in addition, it has been reported that they increase the activity of endothelial nitric oxide synthase activity (NOS), as measured by the citrulline assay (54).

Advances in non-invasive ultrasound techniques have allowed investigators to look at endothelium function, in vivo, in human subjects. This technique known as flow mediated dialation (FMD), has been shown to be influenced by nitric oxide (55) released under shear stress conditions. Using this technique, black tea was given to patients with coronary artery disease (CAD), and FMD was measured after 2 hours of tea or water consumption (450 mL) or after four weeks (450 mL, twice daily) in a crossover design. Both acute and chronic tea consumption significantly improved endothelium function in these subjects compared to baseline levels, and compared to when the subjects were given just water as a control (56). Endothelium function was also improved after CAD patients consumed purple grape juice for 14 days, despite confounding factors such as subject use of antioxidant vitamins and lipid-lowering medications (26).

EFFECTS ON CYTOKINE PRODUCTION

It is generally accepted that inflammation plays a significant role in the initiation and promotion of various cardiovascular disorders that are mediated, in part, by cytokines (57–59). Human atherosclerotic plaques express a cytokine profile dominated by the proinflammatory type, which includes interferon (IFN)-γ, interleukin (IL)-1α and β, tumor necrosis factor (TNF)-α, and IL-6 (58). Long term exposure of proinflammatory cytokines can be functionally and structurally detrimental to the myocardium, and (57–59) therefore elevated levels of these soluble mediators of inflammation are associated with a poor prognosis in heart failure (60,61). Therapeutic avenues to attenuate or counteract pronounced levels of proinflammatory cytokines include the use of specific (i.e., TNF-binding protein) or global (IL-10) cytokine antagonists (59). However, emerging evidence suggests that certain flavanols from cocoa may have the ability to reduce the production of certain proinflamma-

Table 2. Cytokine modulation by cocoa flavanols

Cytokine	Flavanol(s)	Effect	Level of Detection	PBMC	Reference
IL-2	Pentamer Hexamer Heptamer	inhibition	mRNA	PHA-stimulated	(62, 63)
IL-1β	Monomer Dimer Trimer Tetramer	inhibition	protein/mRNA	PHA-stimulated	(63, 69)
IL-4	Pentamer Hexamer Heptamer Octamer Nonamer Decamer	stimulation	protein	resting	(63, 70)
	Monomer	stimulation	protein	PHA-stimulated	(63, 70)
TGF-β	All (monomer-decamer)	stimulation (low producers) inhibition (high producers)	protein protein	resting resting	(64) (64)
IL-5	Monomer Dimer Trimer Tetramer Pentamer	stimulation	protein	PHA-stimulated	(78)

tory cytokines, while they can stimulate the production of select antiinflammatory cytokines such as tumor growth factor (TGF)-β and IL-4. The modulatory effects of the cocoa flavanols can be found in Table 2.

Distinct fractions of cocoa flavanols and procyanidins have been shown to effectively suppress the production of cytokines (IL-1β and IL-2) that promotes inflammation (62–64). Interleukin (IL)-2 is involved with the regulation of T-cell activation, and is important for the initiation of the immune response. However, chronic exposure to aberrantly high levels of IL-1β is considered a major contributor to endothelial dysfunction (65). Currently, it is thought that IL-1β can initiate a cascade of events that lead to the production of proatherogenic C-reactive protein (66), which is generally accepted as a sensitive indicator for predicting CVD (67). Compounding the above problem, foam cell formation is in part mediated by IL-1 (4,68). Given the above, it is reasonable to suggest that reductions in IL-1β production could attenuate the progression of atherosclerosis. Mao and colleagues recently reported that the in vitro culture of PHA-stimulated peripheral blood mononuclear cells (PBMCs) with pentameric through decameric cocoa procyanidins dramatically inhibited the IL-2 mRNA transcript expression (62,63). However, under similar experimental parameters, the flavanols and smaller procyanidins (monomer through tetramer) appeared more efficacious at suppressing IL-1β protein secretion (63,69).

Cocoa flavanols can also modulate the levels of antiinflammatory cytokines (IL-4 and TGF-β). The larger procyanidins (pentamer through decamer) were shown to enhance IL-4 protein levels from resting PBMCs (63,70). However, in PHA-stimulated PBMCs only monomer augmented IL-4 secretion (63,70). Interestingly, the effects of the cocoa flavanols and procyanidins on the production of TGF-β are dependent on the amount of baseline production from resting PBMCs. Individuals with low baseline levels of TGF-β were stimulated by the individual fractions to enhance TGF-β levels, whereas TGF-β secretion from high baseline subjects was inhibited by the cocoa procyanidins and flavanols (64).

TGF-β is a multifunctional protein that may be involved in a variety of physiological processes (71,72). In particular, it has been receiving attention as a mediator of cardiovascular protection by actively maintaining the normal physiological phenotype of endothelial cells and smooth muscle cells in the arterial vessel wall (73). However, excess production TGF-β can cause extracellular matrix accumulation that is unfavorable in the injured vessel wall, consequently leading to cardiac fibrosis (74). Therefore, the above results suggest cocoa can promote cardiovascular homeostasis by modulating the levels of TGF-β.

Accumulating epidemiological evidence has implicated that periodontal disease is associated with the development of CVD (75,76). Chronic infections, such as periodontitis, induce inflammatory immune responses which may contribute to coronary atherogenesis (77). In periodontal diseases, a humoral response involving IgA is considered protective in pathogenesis (78). Furthermore, the cytokine responsible for the growth and differentiation of B lymphocytes into IgA-producing plasma cells is IL-5 (79). Recently, it has been shown that the smaller cocoa flavanols and procyanidins (monomer through pentamer) can augment mitogen-induced secretion of IL-5 (80).

EFFECTS ON PLATELET ACTIVATION

Given the prominent role of platelets in the development and manifestation of acute myocardial infarction, stroke and venous thromboembolism, several antiplatelet strategies have recently been developed to prevent secondary events. Antiplatelet therapies involving aspirin, clopidogrel, low molecular weight heparins, and glycoprotein IIb/IIIa inhibitorss have been shown to be effective against thrombi formation (81). However, except for the case of aspirin, these antiplatelet therapies are employed as ways to prevent secondary, but not primary thromboembolic events. Several studies suggest that besides providing antioxidant vitamins, certain fruits and vegetables may provide protection against thrombosis due to their flavanol content (Table 3). For example, ex vivo platelet aggregation was reduced after subjects consumed approximately 450 mL of purple grape juice for either one, or two, weeks (82,83). Cocoa was able to reduce ADP/collagen and epinephrine/collagen platelet-related primary hemostasis, within hours after subjects consumed either high (897 mg) or moderate amounts of cocoa flavanols (220 mg) (84–86). It is important to note that similar positive effects were not observed with black tea (56,87); whether or not the differential effects of these beverages on platelet function are due to differences in tea flavanol composition, compared to that of cocoa and grape juice, merits further study.

Table 3. Effects of food flavanols on platelet function

Red Wine	
↓	cyclic flow reduction, in vivo (110)
↓	ADP- and thrombin-induced aggregation, in vitro (111)
↓	Platelet thromboxane B2 production (111)
Dealcoholized Red Wine	
↓	Epinephrine-induced P-selectin expression, in vitro (112)
Grape Juice	
↓	cyclic flow reduction, in vivo (110,113)
↓	ADP- and thrombin-induced aggregation, in vitro (111)
↓	Collagen-induced platelet aggregation, ex vivo (83,113)
↓	ADP-induced aggregation, ex vivo (82)
↓	Platelet-derived superoxide release (82)
↓	Platelet PKC-dependent protein phosphorylation (82)
↑	Platelet-derived NO release (82)
Cocoa	
↓	ADP- and epinephrine-induced GPIIb/IIIa expression (84,112)
↓	Epinephrine-induced GPIIb/IIIa expression (86)
↓	ADP-induced P-Selectin expression (84, 112)
↓	Microparticle formation (84)
↓	ADP-collagen-induced primary hemostasis (85,86)
↓	Epinephrine-collagen-induced primary hemostasis (84,85)
Black Tea	
↓	Soluble P-Selectin levels (87)

At present, the mechanism by which flavanols exert their anti-aggregatory effect remain unknown. In the circulation, platelet quiescence is maintained, in part, with nitric oxide and prostacylin produced from the intact endothelium (88). Platelet aggregation occurs when agonists, such as, ADP, collagen and thrombin, initiates receptor-mediated release of secretory granules, conformational changes in platelet cytoskeleton, and glycoprotein IIa/IIIb (GP IIa/IIIb) binding to fibrinogen, allowing for platelet to platelet interaction (89). The anti-aggregatory effects observed with cocoa were shown to be due, in part, to a reduction in the ADP and epinephrine induced expression of the activated conformation of the GPIIa/IIIb surface protein (84,86). In addition, cocoa was able to reduce GPIIa/IIIb expression to a similar, but lesser extent as low-dose aspirin (81 mg) (86). However, GP IIa/IIIb is an end step to platelet aggregation, therefore the question remains do flavanols inhibit the initiating steps of platelet aggregation or just simply prevents fibrinogen receptor (GP IIa/IIIb) binding?

Several mechanistic possibilities exist, including the possibility that the flavanols are working through an antioxidant mechanism. For example, superoxide anion is known to enhance platelet aggregation, and can bind to nitric oxide to form peroxynitrite (86). Interestingly, Freedman et al. observed that purple grape juice consumption reduced platelet superoxide anion release, with a corresponding increase in platelet nitric oxide production, and a reduction in platelet aggregation (82). In addition, catechin has been shown to reduce platelet aggregation and hydrogen

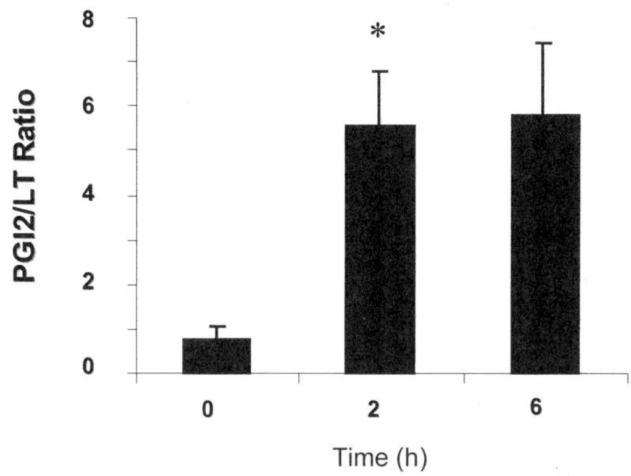

Figure 3. The ratio of plasma prostacylin (6-keto-prostaglandin-$F_{1\alpha}$) to leukotriene at baseline (0 hour) and 2 and 6 hours after consuming 25 g of semi-sweet chocolate chips in 18 healthy adult subjects.
*Significantly different from baseline, $P < 0.05$ (Repeated measure ANOVA and Tukey's all-pairwise comparison test) (85).

peroxide production, in vitro (90). These studies suggest that the flavanols may exert their antioxidant effects through their well described antioxidant activities, however, it is possible that flavanols may act through other non-antioxidant mechanisms. Purple grape juice has been reported to reduce platelet protein kinase C activity (82). Importantly, cocoa flavanols and procyanidins have been reported to inhibit human platelet 12-lipoxygenase (91). An inhibition of 12-lipoxygenase, could in part explain the observations of Schramm et al. (92) and Holt et al. (85) that the ratio of plasma prostacyclin to leukotriene increases in human subjects following the consumption of flavanol-rich chocolate (85,92) (Figure 3).

CONCLUSIONS

During the last several years, a body of data has been accumulated that supports the concept that flavanols have an ability to behave as antioxidants, as well as an ability to influence cytokine levels, vascular tone and platelet function. Collectively, work in this area is providing strong support for the hypothesis that the consumption of flavanol-rich foods may be associated with a reduced risk for vascular disease. While in vitro studies provide information on the action of the aglycones, further research is needed to define the actions of the biologically present conjugate forms. In addition, work is needed to better define which flavanol, or combination of flavanols, are providing the observed biological effects. Given the complex nature of cardiovascular disease, it is important to consider the fact that a multiplicity of factors are probably contributing to the positive health effect of these important nutrients. The flavanols provide a great diversity of biological action that deserves further attention in focused clinical studies on cardiovascular disease prevention.

REFERENCES

1. Krauss RM, Eckel RH, Howard B, Appel LJ, Daniels SR, Deckelbaum RJ, Erdman Jr. JW, Kris-Etherton P, Goldberg IJ, Kotchen TA, Lichtenstein AH, Mitch WE, Mullis R, Robinson K, Wylie-Rosett J, St Jeor S, Suttie J, Tribble DL, Bazzarre TL. 2000. AHA dietary guidelines Revision 2000. A statement for healthcare professionals from the nutrition committee of the American Heart Association. Circulation 102:2284–2299.
2. Bravo L. 1998. Polyphenols: Chemistry, dietary sources, metabolism and nutritional significance. Nutr Rev 56:317–333.
3. Libby P. 2000. Changing concepts of atherogenesis. J Int Med 247:349–358.
4. Ross R. 1999. Atherosclerosis-an inflammatory disease. N Engl J Med 340:115–126.
5. Rein D, Lotito S, Holt RR, Keen CL, Schmitz HH, Fraga CG. 2000. Epicatechin in human plasma: in vivo determination and effect of chocolate consumption on plasma oxidation status. J Nutr 130:2109S-2114S.
6. Bearden MM, Pearson DA, Rein D, Chevaux KA, Carpenter DR, Keen CL, Schmitz HH. 2000. Potential cardiovascular health benefits of procyanidins present in chocolate and cocoa. In: Caffeinated Beverages: Health Benefits, Physiological Effects, and Chemistry. Ed. Parliment TH, Ho C-T, Schieberle P, 177–186. Washington DC: American Chemical Society.
7. Kris-Etherton P, Keen CL. 2002. Evidence that the antioxidant flavonoids in tea and cocoa are beneficial for cardiovascular health. Curr Opin Lipidol 13:41–49.
8. Hammerstone JF, Lazarus SA, Mitchell AE, Rucker R, Schmitz HH. 1999. Identification of procyanidins in cocoa (Theobroma cacao) and chocolate using high-performance liquid chromatography/mass spectrometry. J Ag Food Chem 47:490–496.
9. Renaud S, De Lorgeril M. 1992. Wine, alcohol, platelets, and the French paradox for coronary heart disease. Lancet 339:1523–1526.
10. Frankel E, Kanner J, German J, Parks E, Kinsella J. 1993. Inhibition of oxidation of human low-density lipoprotein by phenolic substances in red wine. Lancet 341:454–457.
11. Teissedre PL, Frankel EN, Waterhouse AL, Peleg H, German JB. 1996. Inhibition of in vitro human LDL oxidation by phenolic antioxidants from grapes and wines. J Sci Food Agric 70:55–61.
12. Lotito SB, Actis-Goretta L, Renart L, Caligiuri M, Rein D, Schmitz HH, Steinberg FM, Keen CL, Fraga CG. 2000. Influence of oligomer chain length on the antioxidant activity of procyanidins. Biochem Biophys Res Commun 276:945–951.
13. Pearson DA, Schmitz HH, Lazarus SA, Keen CL. 2001. Inhibition of in vitro low-density lipoprotein oxidation by oligomeric procyanidins present in chocolate and cocoas. In: Methods in Enzymology. Ed. Packer L, 350–360. New York: Academic Press.
14. Zhu QY, Holt RR, Lazarus SA, Orozco T, Keen CL. 2002. Inhibitory effects of cocoa flavanols and procyanidin oligomers on free radical-induced erythrocyte hemolysis. Exp Biol Med 227:321–329.
15. Wang JF, Schramm DD, Holt RR, Ensunsa JL, Fraga CG, Schmitz HH, Keen CL. 2000. A dose-response effect from chocolate consumption on plasma epicatechin and oxidative damage. J Nutr 130:2115S–2119S.
16. Wan Y, Vinson JA, Etherton TD, Proch J, Lazarus SA, Kris-Etherton P. 2001. Effects of cocoa powder and dark chocolate on LDL oxidative susceptibility and prostaglandin concentrations in humans. Am J Clin Nutr 74:596–602.
17. Osakabe N, Baba S, Yasuda A, Iwamoto T, Kamiyama M, Takizawa T, Itakura H, Kondo K. 2001. Daily cocoa intake reduces the susceptibility of low-density lipoprotein to oxidation as demonstrated in healthy human volunteers. Free Rad Res 34:93–99.
18. Serafini M, Laranjinha JA, Almeida LM, Maiani G. 2000. Inhibition of human LDL lipid peroxidation by phenol-rich beverages and their impact on plasma total antioxidant capacity in humans. J Nutr Biochem 11:585–590.
19. Leenan R, Roodenburg A, Tijburg L, Wiseman S. 2000. A single dose of tea with or without milk increases plasma antioxidant activity in humans. Eur J Clin Nutr 54:87–92.
20. Hodgson JM, Puddey IB, Croft KD, Burke V, Mori TA, Abu-Amsha Caccetta R. 2000. Acute effects of ingestion of black and green tea on lipoprotein oxidation. Am J Clin Nutr 71:1103–1107.
21. Ishikawa T, Suzukawa M, Ito T, Yoshida H, Ayaori M, Nishiwaki M, Yonemura A, Hara Y, Nakamura H. 1997. Effect of tea flavonoid supplementation on the susceptibility of low-density lipoprotein to oxidative modification. Am J Clin Nutr 66:261–266.

22. Miura Y, Chiba T, Miura S, Tomita I, Umegaki K, Ikeda M, Tomita T. 2000. Green tea polyphenols (flavan 3-ols) prevent oxidative modification of low density lipoproteins: An ex vivo study in humans. J Nutr Biochem 11:216–222.
23. Van Het Hof KH, Wiseman SA, Yang CS, Tijburg LB. 1999. Plasma and lipoprotein levels of tea catechins following repeated tea consumption. Proc Soc Exp Biol Med 220:203–209.
24. O'Reilly JD, Mallet AI, McAnlis GT, Young IS, Halliwell B, Sanders TA, Wiseman H. 2001. Consumption of flavonoids in onions and black tea: lack of effect on F2-isoprostanes and autoantibodies to oxidized LDL in healthy humans. Am J Clin Nutr 73:1040–1044.
25. Hodgson JM, Croft KD, Mori TA, Burke V, Beilin LJ, Puddey IB. 2002. Regular ingestion of tea does not inhibit in vivo lipid peroxidation in humans. J Nutr 132:55–58.
26. Stein JH, Keevil JG, Wiebe DA, Aeschlimann S, Folts J. 1999. Purple grape juice improves endothelial function and reduces the susceptibility of LDL cholesterol to oxidation in patients with coronary artery disease. Circulation 100:1050–1055.
27. Nigdikar SV, Williams NR, Griffin BA, Howard AN. 1998. Consumption of red wine polyphenols reduces the susceptibility of low-density lipoproteins to oxidation in vivo. Am J Clin Nutr 68: 258–265.
28. Chopra M, Fitzsimons PE, Strain JJ, Thurnham DI, Howard AN. 2000. Nonalcoholic red wine extract and quercetin inhibit LDL oxidation without affecting plasma antioxidant vitamin and carotenoid concentrations. Clin Chem 46:1162–1170.
29. Natella F, Ghiselli A, Guidi A, Ursini F, Scaccini C. 2001. Red wine mitigates the postprandial increase of LDL susceptibility to oxidation. Free Radic Biol Med 30:1036–1044.
30. Caccetta RA-A, Croft KD, Beilin LJ, Puddey IB. 2000. Ingestion of red wine significantly increases plasma phenolic acid concentrations but does not acutely affect ex vivo lipoprotein oxidizability. Am J Clin Nutr 71:67–74.
31. van Golde PH, Sloots LM, Vermeulen WP, Wielders JP, Hart HC, Bouma BN, van de Wiel A. 1999. The role of alcohol in the anti low density lipoprotein oxidation activity of red wine. Atherosclerosis 147:365–370.
32. Goldberg DM, Karumanchiri A, Tsang E, Soleas GJ. 1998. Catechin and epicatechin concentrations of red wines: Region and cultivar-related differences. Am J Enol Vit 49:23–34.
33. Goldberg DM, Ng E, Yan J, Karumanchiri A, Soleas GJ, Diamandis E. 1996. Regional differences in resveratrol isomer concentration of wines from various cultivars. J Wine Res 7:13–24.
34. Hollman PC. 2001. Evidence for health benefits of plant phenols: local or systemic effects? J Sci Food Agric 81:842–852.
35. Donovan JL, Crespy V, Manach C, Morand C, Besson C, Scalbert A, Remesy C. 2001. Catechin is metabolized by both the small intestine and liver of rats. J Nutr 131:1753–1757.
36. Piskula MK, Terao J. 1998. Accumulation of (-)-epicatechin metabolites in rat plasma after oral administration and distribution of conjugation enzymes in rat yissues. J Nutr 128:1172–1178.
37. Kuhnle G, Spencer JP, Schroeter H, Shenoy B, Debnam E, Srai SK, Rice-Evans C, Hahn U. 2000. Epicatechin and catechin are o-methylated and glucuronidated in the small intestine. Biochem Biophys Res Commun 277:507–512.
38. Donovan JL, Bell JR, Kasim-Karakas S, German JB, Walzem RL, Hansen RJ, Waterhouse AL. 1999. Catechin is present as metabolites in human plasma after consumption of red wine. J Nutr 129:1662–1668.
39. Baba S, Osakabe N, Yasuda A, Natsume M, Takizawa T, Nakamura T, Terao J. 2000. Bioavailability of (-)-epicatechin upon intake of chocolate and cocoa in human volunteers. Free Rad Res 33: 635–641.
40. Lee M-J, Wang Z-Y, Li H, Chen L, Sun Y, Gobbo S, Balentine D, Yang CS. 1995. Analysis of plasma and urinary tea polyphenols in human subjects. Cancer, Epid, Biomark Prev 4:393–399.
41. Richelle M, Tavazzi I, Enslen M, Offord E. 1999. Plasma kinetics in man of epicatechin from black chocolate. Eur J Clin Nutr 53:22–26.
42. Steinberg FM, Holt RR, Schmitz HH, Keen CL. 2002. Cocoa procyanidin chain length does not determine ability to protect LDL from oxidation when monomer units are controlled. J Nutr Biochem 13:645–652.
43. Holt RR, Lazarus SA, Sullards M, Zhu QY, Schramm DD, Hammerstone JF, Fraga CG, Schmitz HH, Keen CL. 2002. Procyanidin dimer B2 (epicatechin-(4b-8)-epicatechin) in human plasma after the consumption of a flavanol-rich cocoa. Am J Clin Nutr 76:798–804.
44. Warden BA, Smith LS, Beecher GR, Balentine D, Clevidence BA. 2001. Catechins are bioavailable in men and women drinking black tea throughout the day. J Nutr 131:1731–1737.

45. Laparra J, Michaud J, Masquelier J. 1977. Etude pharmacocinetique des oligomeres flavanoliques. Plant Med Phytother 11:133–142.
46. Jimenez-Ramsey L, Rogler J, Housley T, Butler L, Elikin R. 1994. Absorption and distribution of ^{14}C-labeled condensed tannins and related sorghum phenolics in chickens. J Agric Food Chem 42:963–967.
47. Spencer JP, Chaudry F, Pannala AS, Srai S, Debnam E, Rice-Evans C. 2000. Decomposition of cocoa procyanidins in the gastric milieu. Biochem Biophys Res Commun 272:236–241.
48. Zhu QY, Holt RR, Lazarus SA, Ensunsa JL, Hammerstone J, Schmitz HH, Keen CL. 2002. Stability of the flavan-3-ols epicatechin and catechin and related dimeric procyanidins derived from cocoa. J Agric Food Chem 50:1700–1705.
49. Spencer JP, Schroeter H, Shenoy B, Srai SK, Debnam E, Rice-Evans C. 2001. Epicatechin is the primary bioavailable form of the procyanidin dimers B2 and B5 after transfer across the small intestine. Biochem Biophys Res Commun 285:588–593.
50. Mulder TP, van Platerink CJ, Wijnand SP, van Amelsvoort JM. 2001. Analysis of theaflavins in biological fluids using liquid chromatography-electrospray mass spectrometry. J Chromatog B 760:271–279.
51. Becker B, Heindl B, Kupatt C, Zahler S. 2000. Endothelial function and hemostasis. Z Kardiol 89:160–167.
52. Andriambeloson E, Magnier C, Haan-Archipoff G, Lobstein A, Anton R, Beretz A, Stoclet JC, Andriantsitohaina R. 1998. Natural dietary polyphenolic compounds cause endothelium-dependent vasorelaxation in rat thoracic aorta. J Nutr 128:2324–2333.
53. Huang Y, Chan NW, Lau CW, Yao XQ, Chan FL, Chen ZY. 1999. Involvement of endothelium/nitric oxide in vasorelaxation induced by purified green tea (-)-epicatechin. Biochim Biophys Acta 1427:322–328.
54. Karim M, McCormick K, Kappagoda CT. 2000. Effects of cocoa procyanidins on endothelium-dependent relaxation. J Nutr 130:2105S–2108S.
55. Joannides R, Haefeli WE, Linder L, Richard V, Bakkali EH, Thuillex C, Luscher TF. 1995. Nitric oxide is responsible for flow-dependent dilatation of human peripheral conduit arteries in vivo. Circulation 1995:1314–1319.
56. Duffy S, Vita J, Holbrook M, Swerdloff P, Keaney Jr JF. 2001. Effect of acute and chronic tea consumption on platelet aggregation in patients with coronary artery disease. Arterioscler Thromb Vasc Biol 21:1084–1089.
57. Kaplan RC, Frishman WH. 2001. Systemic inflammation as a cardiovascular disease risk factor and as a potential target for drug therapy. Heart Dis 3:326–332.
58. Pockley AG. 2002. Heat shock proteins, inflammation, and cardiovascular disease. Circulation 105:1012–1017.
59. Selzman CH, Miller SA, Harken AH. 2001. Therapeutic implications of inflammation in atherosclerotic cardiovascular disease. Ann Thorac Surg 71:2066–2074.
60. Torre-Amione G, Kapadia S, Benedict C, Oral H, Young JB, Mann DL. 1996. Proinflammatory cytokine levels in patients with depressed left ventricular ejection fraction: a report from the Studies of Left Ventricular Dysfunction (SOLVD). J Am Coll Cardiol 27:1201–1206.
61. Sharma R, Coats AJ, Anker SD. 2000. The role of inflammatory mediators in chronic heart failure: cytokines, nitric oxide, and endothelin-1. Int J Cardiol 72:175–186.
62. Mao TK, Powell J, Van De Water J, Keen CL, Schmitz HH, Gershwin ME. 1999. The influence of cocoa procyanidins on the transcription of interleukin-2 in peripheral blood mononuclear cells. Int J Immunotherapy 15:23–29.
63. Mao TK, Van De Water J, Keen CL, Schmitz HH, Gershwin ME. 2000. Cocoa procyanidins and human cytokine transcription and secretion. J Nutr 130:2093S–2099S.
64. Mao TK, Van De Water J, Keen CL, Schmitz HH, Gershwin ME. 2003. Cocoa flavanols and proryanidis related oligomers promote TGF-beta1 homeostasis in peripheral blood mononuclear cells. Exp Biolmed (Maywood) 228:93–99.
65. Holm T, Aukrust P, Andreassen AK, Ueland T, Brosstad F, Froland SS, Simonsen S, Gullestad L. 2000. Peripheral endothelial dysfunction in heart transplant recipients: possible role of proinflammatory cytokines. Clin Transplant 14:218–225.
66. SoRelle R. 2002. Tea for all? Circulation 105:E9109–E9110.
67. Blake GJ, Ridker PM. 2001. High sensitivity C-reactive protein for predicting cardiovascular disease: an inflammatory hypothesis. Eur Heart J 22:349–352.
68. Dinarello CA, Wolff SM. 1993. The role of interleukin-1 in disease. N Engl J Med 328:106–113.

69. Mao TK, Powell J, Van De Water J, Keen CL, Schmitz HH, Hammerstone JF, Gershwin ME. 2000. The effect of cocoa procyanidins on the transcription and secretion of interleukin 1 beta in peripheral blood mononuclear cells. Life Sciences 66:1377–1386.
70. Mao TK, Powell J, Van De Water J, Keen CL, Schmitz HH, Gershwin ME. 2000. Effect of cocoa procyanidins on the secretion of interleukin-4 in peripheral blood mononuclear cells. J Med Food 3:107–114.
71. MacLellan WR, Brand T, Schneider MD. 1993. Transforming growth factor-beta in cardiac ontogeny and adaptation. Circ Res 73:783–791.
72. Border WA, Noble NA. 1994. Transforming growth factor beta in tissue fibrosis. N Engl J Med 331:1286–1292.
73. Grainger DJ, Metcalfe JC. 1997. Transforming growth factor-beta and cardiovascular protection. In: The endothelium in clinical practice. Ed. Rubanyi GM, Dzau VJ, 203–243. New York: Marcel Dekker Inc.
74. Lijnen PJ, Petrov VV, Fagard RH. 2000. Induction of cardiac fibrosis by transforming growth factor-beta(1). Mol Genet Metab 71:418–435.
75. Beck JD, Slade G, Offenbacher S. 2000. Oral disease, cardiovascular disease and systemic inflammation. Periodontol 23:110–120.
76. Joshipura K, Ritchie C, Douglass C. 2000. Strength of evidence linking oral conditions and systemic disease. Compend Contin Educ Dent Suppl 21:12–23.
77. De Nardin E. 2001. The role of inflammatory and immunological mediators in periodontitis and cardiovascular disease. Ann Periodontol 6:30–40.
78. Kinane DF, Lappin DF, Koulouri O, Buckley A. 1999. Humoral immune responses in periodontal disease may have mucosal and systemic immune features. Clin Exp Immunol 115:534–541.
79. Salvi S, Holgate ST. 1999. Could the airway epithelium play an important role in mucosal immunoglobulin A production? Clin Exp Allergy 29:1597–1605.
80. Mao TK, Van De Water J, Keen CL, Schmitz HH, Gershwin ME. 2002. Effect of cocoa flavanols and their related oligomers on the secretion of interleukin-5 in peripheral blood mononuclear cells. J Med Foods 5:17–22.
81. Rauch U, Osende JI, Fuster V, Badimon JJ, Fayad Z, Chesebro JH. 2001. Thrombus formation on atherosclerotic plaques: Pathogenesis and clinical consequences. Ann Intern Med 134:224–238.
82. Freedman JE, Parker III C, Li L, Perlman JA, Frei B, Ivanov V, Deak LR, Iafrati MD, Folts J. 2001. Select flavonoids and whole juice from purple grapes inhibit platelet function and enhance nitric oxide release. Circulation 103:2792–2798.
83. Keevil JG, Osman HE, Reed JD, Folts JD. 2000. Grape juice, but not orange juice or grapefruit juice, inhibits human platelet aggregation. J Nutr 130:53–56.
84. Rein D, Paglieroni TG, Wun T, Pearson DA, Schmitz HH, Gosselin R, Keen CL. 2000. Cocoa inhibits platelet activation and function. Am J Clin Nutr 72:30–35.
85. Holt RR, Schramm DD, Keen CL, Lazarus SA, Schmitz HH. 2002. Flavonoid-rich chocolate and platelet function. JAMA 287:2212–2213.
86. Pearson D, Paglieroni T, Rein D, Wun T, Schramm DD, Wang JF, Holt RR, Gosselin R, Schmitz HH, Keen CL. 2002. The effects of flavanol-rich cocoa and aspirin on ex vivo platelet function. Thromb Res 106:191–197.
87. Hodgson J, Puddey IB, Mori T, Burke V, Baker R, Beilin L. 2001. Effects of regular ingestion of black tea on haemostasis and cell adhesion molecules in humans. Eur J Clin Nutr 55:881–886.
88. Vanhoutte P-M, Boulanger C-M, Mombouli J-V. 1995. Endothelium-derived relaxing factors and converting enzyme inhibition. Am J Cardio 76:3E–12E.
89. Colman RW, Clowes AW, George JN, Hirsch J, Marder VJ. 2001. Overview of Hemostasis. In: Hemostasis and thrombosis: basic principles and clinical practice. Ed. Colman RW, Hirsh J, Marder VJ, Clowes AW, George JN, 3–16. New York: Lippincott Williams & Wilkins.
90. Pignatelli PP, Fabio M, Celestini A, Lenti L, Chiselli A, Gazzsaniga PP, Violi F. 2000. The flavonoids quercetin and catechin synergistically inhibit platelet function by antagonizing the intracellular production of hydrogen peroxide. Am J Clin Nutr 72:1150–1155.
91. Schewe T, Sadik C, Klotz L-O, Yoshimoto T, Kuhn H, Sies H. 2001. Polyphenols of cocoa: Inhibition of mammalian 15-lipoxygenase. Biol Chem 382:1687–1696.
92. Schramm DD, Wang JF, Holt RR, Ensunsa JL, Gonsalves JL, Lazarus SL, Schmitz HH, German JB, Keen CL. 2001. Chocolate procyanidins decrease the leukotriene-prostacyclin ratio in humans and human aortic endothelial cells. Am J Clin Nutr 73:36–40.

93. Adamson GE, Lazarus SA, Mitchell AE, Prior RL, Cao G, Jacobs PH, Kremers BG, Hammerstone JF, Rucker RB, Ritter KA, Schmitz HH. 1999. HPLC method for the quantification of procyanidins in cocoa and chocolate samples and correlation to total antioxidant capacity. J Agric Food Chem 47:4184–4188.
94. Sellappan S, Akoh CC, Krewer G. 2002. Phenolic compounds and antioxidant capacity of Georgia-grown blueberries and blackberries. J Agric Food Chem 50:2432–2438.
95. Laundrault N, Poucheret P, Ravel P, Gasc F, Cros G, Teissedre PL. 2001. Antioxidant capacities and phenolics levels of French wines from different varieties and vintages. J Agric Food Chem 49: 3341–3348.
96. Actis-Goretta L, Mackenzie GG, Oteiza PI, Fraga CG. 2002. Comparative study on the antioxidant capacity of wines and other plant-derived beverages. Ann NY Acad Sci 957:279–283.
97. Cao G, Russell R, Lischner N, Prior R. 1998. Serum antioxidant capacity is increased by consumption of strawberries, spinach, red wine or vitamin C in elderly women. J Nutr 128:2383–2390.
98. Serafini M, Maiani G, Ferro-Luzzi A. 1998. Alcohol-free red wine enhances plasma antioxidant capacity in humans. J Nutr 128:1003–1007.
99. Ivanov V, Carr A, Frei B. 2001. Red wine antioxidants bind to human lipoproteins and protect them from metal ion-dependent and -independent oxidation. J Agric Food Chem 49:4442–4449.
100. Miyagi Y, Miwa K, Inoue H. 1997. Inhibition of human low-density lipoprotein oxidation by flavonoids in red wine and grape juice. Am J Cardio 80:1627–1631.
101. Cherubini A, Beal MF, Frei B. 1999. Black tea increases the resistance of human plasma to lipid peroxidation in vitro, but not ex vivo. Free Radic Biol Med 27:381–387.
102. Alvarez S, Zaobornyj T, Actis-Goretta L, Fraga CG, Boveris A. 2002. Polyphenols and red wine as peroxynitrite scavengers. Ann NY Acad Sci 957:271–273.
103. Carini M, Aldini G, Bombardelli E, Morazzoni P, Facino RM. 2000. UVB-induced hemolysis of rat erythrocytes: protective effect of procyanidins from grape seeds. Life Sciences 67:1799–1814.
104. Nakagawa T, Yokozawa T, Terasawa K, Shu S, Juneja LR. 2002. Protective activity of green tea against free radical- and glucose-mediated protein damage. J Agric Food Chem 50:2418–2422.
105. Hu M, Skibsted LH. 2002. Kinetics of reduction of ferrylmyoglobin by (-)-epigallocatechin gallate and green tea extract. J Agric Food Chem 50:2998–3003.
106. Nagasawa T, Hayashi H, Fujimaki N, Nishizawa N, Kitts D. 2000. Induction of oxidatively modified proteins in skeletal muscle by electrical stimulation and its suppression by dietary supplementation of (-)-epigallocatechin gallate. Biosci Biotechnol Biochem 64:1004–1010.
107. Feng Q, Torii Y, Uchida K, Nakamura Y, Hara Y, Osawa T. 2002. Black tea polyphenols, theaflavins, prevent cellular DNA damage by inhibiting oxidative stress and suppressing cytochrome P450 1A1 in cell cultures. J Agric Food Chem 50:212–220.
108. Fiala E, Sodum R, Bhattacharya M, Li H. 1996. (-)-Epigallocatechin gallate, a polyphenolic tea antioxidant, inhibits peroxynitrie-mediated formation of 8-oxodeoxyguanosine and 3-nitrotyrosine. Experientia 15:922–926.
109. Johnson MK, Loo G. 2000. Effects of epigallocatechin gallate and quercetin on oxidative damage to cellular DNA. Mut Res 459:211–218.
110. Demrow HS, Slane PR, Folts JD. 1995. Administration of wine and grape juice inhibits in vivo platelet activity and thrombosis in stenosed canine coronary arteries. Circulation 91:1182–1188.
111. Pace-Asciak C, Rounova O, Hahn S, Diamandis E, Goldberg D. 1996. Wines and grape juices as modulators of platelet aggregation in healthy human subjects. Clin Chim Acta 15:163–182.
112. Rein D, Paglieroni TG, Pearson DA, Wun T, Schmitz HH, Gosselin R, Keen CL. 2000. Cocoa and wine polyphenols modulate platelet activation and function. J Nutr 130:2120S–2126S.
113. Osman HE, Maalej N, Shanmuganayagam D, Folts J. 1998. Grape juice but not orange or grapefruit juice inhibits platelet activity in dogs and monkeys. J Nutr 128:2307–2312.

Frontiers in Cardiovascular Health, edited by
N.S. Dhalla, A. Chockalingam,
H.I. Berkowitz & P.K. Singal
Kluwer Academic Publishers, Boston, 2003

Benefits of Dietary Fiber for Cardiovascular Disease and Diabetes

Qiming Shao and Pamela M. Keagy

Processed Foods Research,
Western Region Research Center,
USDA, 800 Buchanan St.
Albany, CA USA 94710

Summary. Cardiovascular disease (CVD) and diabetes are chronic diseases distributed worldwide. Both of them share of some common risk factors and have some common pathophysiological changes. CVD and diabetes are a huge burden on the health care system of every government and its population. Therefore, the early prevention and treatment of diabetes, insulin resistance and CVD has a significant role for public health and the health care system. Dietary fiber has received recognition for reducing the risk of developing both CVD and diabetes. The implication is that dietary fiber may have therapeutic benefits in prediabetic metabolic conditions and in preventing the cardiovascular complications. The effect of dietary fiber on the common risk factors and possibly relative gene expression may reduce the morbidity of these diseases. However, the amount of total dietary fiber consumed and the chemical and physiological properties of different fiber sources will determine the effectiveness in prevention or treatment of CVD, insulin resistance or type 2 diabetes.

***Key words*:** Dietary fiber, cardiovascular disease, diabetes.

INTRODUCTION

Cardiovascular disease (CVD) is the most common problem confronting those with type 2 diabetes mellitus. Diabetes, a known independent risk factor for CVD, is associated with a high incidence of CVD and with high short-and long-term mortality. Diabetes increases the risk of all clinical manifestations of CVD, including

Address for Correspondence: Qiming Shao, M.D., Ph.D, Processed Foods Research, Office: 510-559-5704, Fax: 510-559-5777, E-mail: qshao@pw.usda.gov.

hypertension, dyslipidemia, abnormalities, cardiac, function and homeostatis. If diabetic patients have heart disease, the mortalities are dramatically increased. In diabetic patients, 60% of related conditions are attributed to cardiovascular complications and CVD is responsible for more than 60% of mortalities (1). Although many approaches have been pursued along with numerous medications, no medication or method can completely prevent or cure CVD or later stage diabetes. The cost of treatment is a tremendous burden to every government and its people. Therefore, it is important to seek adequate prevention or treatment of both CVD and diabetes. Most importantly, the occurrence of coexisting risk factors should be treated intensively through lifestyle modification.

There is no question that lifestyle can greatly influence the incidence of CVD and diabetes (2). Clinical and epidemiological data has demonstrated that nutritional factors play an important role in the prevention and therapeutic treatment of CVD (3) and diabetes (2). The nutritional approach to CVD and diabetes is an important adjunct to traditional pharmaceutical intervention in decreasing the morbidity and mortality of both diseases as well as minimizing the economic and social costs associated with these diseases. Dietary fiber, an important component of the diet, may have a valuable effect related to both CVD and diabetes. This review will focus on the relationship of dietary fiber with CVD and diabetes, two of the leading causes of mortality and morbidity in developed countries.

OVERVIEW OF CARDIOVASCULAR DISEASE, DIABETES AND INSULIN RESISTANCE

Cardiovascular disease is the leading cause of death in developed nations and is rapidly increasing in prevalence in developing countries. In the United States, more than 3 million people have congestive heart failure (CHF) and more than 500,000 new cases are presented yearly. Approximately 30–40% of patients with CHF are hospitalized every year. The mortality rates from cardiovascular disease exceed 1 million annually in the United States and the 5-year mortality after diagnosis was reported to be about 60% in men and 45% in women. Cardiovascular diseases account for the largest disease-related health cost, with an estimated total cost exceeding $120 billion per annum (4). Diabetes is also a significant public health problem, which affects approximately 16 million Americans (5), of which 83% have non-insulin dependent type 2 diabetes or mature onset diabetes. Epidemiological studies performed over the past 40 years have shown that the prevalence of diagnosed diabetes has increased dramatically worldwide (6). Within the United States, the diabetes rate increased 30% from 1990–1998 (7). Besides increasing the risk of cardiovascular disease (8), diabetes leads to other complications including blindness, end-stage renal disease, and lower limb amputations. The economic burden of diabetes in the world is enormous. The cost of diabetes management is over $98 billion in the USA alone (9).

Insulin resistance is a metabolic disorder that is increasing worldwide. Insulin resistance can be linked to the etiology of diabetes, obesity, hypertension, dyslipidemia, cardiovascular disease and other abnormalities (10,11). Insulin resistance occurs when much higher levels of insulin than normal are required to maintain plasma glucose homeostasis (12). To maintain normal blood glucose, the pancreas secretes additional insulin. In some cases (about 1/3 of the people with insulin resistance), when the body cells resist or do not respond to high levels of insulin, glucose builds up in the blood, resulting in high blood glucose or type 2 diabetes. Since insulin resistance usually develops long before these diseases appear, identifying, preventing and reducing insulin resistance has great prevention value. In addition, better prevention and treatment of diabetes and insulin resistance may result in reduced coronary heart disease. Therefore, reduction of insulin resistance should be an equally important part of the management of type 2 diabetes and cardiovascular disease.

THE RELATIONSHIP BETWEEN CARDIOVASCULAR DISEASE AND DIABETES

Cardiovascular disease and diabetes have a reciprocal cause and effect relationship. They are each other's frequent and costly complication with associated poor outcomes (13). Cardiovascular disease (CVD) is the major cause of the morbidity and mortality associated with diabetes. Among those with diabetes, the relative risk of CVD was doubled in men and tripled in women compared to those without diabetes (1,14,15). Women with diabetes lose their CVD advantage relative to men (16). The risks of death from all causes and fatal CHD were dramatically increased. One 20 year follow up survey indicated that age-adjusted relative risks of overall mortality were higher in women with a history of diabetes and no CHD at baseline (17). The seven year incidence of myocardial infarction is approximately 5 fold and the re-infarction rate was doubled in patients with diabetes compared to those without diabetes (18).

COMMON DISORDERS OF CORONARY HEART DISEASE AND DIABETES

Striking parallels exist in risk factors between coronary artery diseases and type 2 diabetes mellitus. Some common disorders in CHD and diabetes include: dyslipidemia, obesity, hyperinsulinemia and bile acid metabolism abnormalities.

CHOLESTEROL, LIPOPROTEINS AND DYSLIPIDEMIA

Cholesterol is an extremely important biological molecule that serves as a precursor for the synthesis of steroid hormones and bile acids. Cholesterol is synthesized in the liver and intestine apart from dietary cholesterol. Acetyl-CoA synthetase, hydroxymethylglutaryl-CoA (HMG-CoA) synthetase and HMG-CoA reductase play an important role in regulating cholesterol synthesis. Cholesterol is transported by lipoproteins. Based on the physical properties of density and electrophoretic mobility, the lipoprotein is classed to four types: Chylomicrons and very low density lipoprotein (VLDL), which are triglyceride–rich lipoproteins, low density lipoprotein (LDL) and high density lipoprotein (HDL). LDLs carry cholesterol from the liver, where it is made, to the cells, where it is used; HDLs may carry excess cholesterol back to the liver for breakdown and excretion. LDL-bound cholesterol is primarily responsible for deposits in arteries that can lead to coronary heart disease, angina pectoris, myocardial infarction, or stroke. On the other hand, HDL does not form such deposits and may actually retard or reduce the buildup of cholesterol plaque.

DYSLIPIDEMIA

Dyslipidemia plays a major role among the many factors that are involved in the pathogenesis of arteriosclerosis in diabetes and cardiovascular disease. Mixed hyperlipidemia is commonly seen and involves: 1) increased serum triglycerides; 2) increased very low density (VLDL) triglycerides and VLDL cholesterol; 3) increased low density lipoprotein (LDL) cholesterol; 4) reduced high density lipoprotein (HDL) cholesterol and; 5) elevated levels of apolipoprotein (19). About 20% of patients with type 2 diabetes have hypertriglyceridemia or low HDL-cholesterol levels (20). Risk of coronary heart disease decreases with reduced LDL levels: LDL > 130 mg% is associated with higher risk, LDL between 100–130 mg% indicates borderline risk and LDL < 100 mg% indicates lower risk (21). Increased hepatic VLDL production and impaired catabolism of triglyceride-rich particles contribute to hyper-triglyceridemia (22). Elevated triglyceride and low HDL levels greatly increase the risk of CVD and diabetes. Subsequent formation of small dense LDL particles leads to increased atherogenicity, since small dense LDL particles remain in the circulation longer and are susceptible to oxidation. Oxidized LDL particles are taken up by macrophages in the vessel wall. LDL cholesterol lowering therapy can decrease angiographic progression of coronary heart disease and decrease clinical events (23). A prospective study showed that dyslipidemia presented in 89% of diabetic patients and LDL had a positive relation to CVD incidence.

HDL-cholesterol level is of particular significance in patients with type 2 diabetes (24). Every 1-mg/dL decrease in HDL-cholesterol is associated with a 2% decreased risk of coronary artery disease in men and 3% decreased risk in women. Conversely, low HDL-cholesterol has also been found linked to increased risk of ischemic stroke, the degree of carotid arteriosclerosis and increased arteriosclerosis progression (25). In most cases, diabetic dyslipidemia is preceded by hyperinsulinemia resulting from insulin resistance.

OBESITY

Obesity, despite becoming a recognized epidemic in the United States and many countries around the world cannot be necessarily defined, measured, and treated in a simplified fashion. Obesity has been shown to increase the risk or be associated with numerous conditions from cardiovascular disease and type II diabetes. Body mass index (BMI) is one of the methods to calculate if the body is obesity or not. The higher BMI, the stronger risk factor for the development of type 2 diabetes and CVD. Commonly defined adults obesity is now as a body mass index (BMI) >30 kg/m^2 and is closely linked to non-insulin-dependent diabetes mellitus (NIDDM) or type 2 diabetes (26). Obesity, especially intraabdominal adiposity, is associated with increased free fatty acid plasma concentrations, which exert a major negative effect on insulin sensitivity at both muscular and hepatic sites (27). Both obesity and type 2 diabetes are major causes of morbidity and mortality from atherogenic microvascular disease, and they are independent risk factors for coronary heart disease. The major complications of obesity come under the heading of the metabolic syndrome, which includes dyslipidemia, hypertension, insulin resistance and an increase in plasma glucose. The clinical consequences of the metabolic syndrome are coronary heart disease, type 2 diabetes and its complications, fatty liver, cholesterol gallstones, and possibly some forms of cancer (28). Since obesity is a major risk factor for CVD, the increasing prevalence and degree of obesity in all developed countries has the potential to significantly offset the current efforts to decrease the CVD burden in our population. Additionally, the risk of type 2 diabetes mellitus tends to increase sharply with an increase of the obesity (29). Conversely, weight loss can improve diabetic glycaemic control and insulin resistance (30). Research is currently in progress to better understand the molecular mechanisms that could explain the relationship between environmental and genetic factors that lead from obesity to arteriosclerosis and cardiovascular events (31).

HYPERINSULINEMIA

Hyperinsulinemia is an endocrine disorder characterized by a high insulin level and a failure of blood sugar control mechanisms. It occurs as tissues become less responsive to insulin actions that lower blood glucose levels. Progressively greater concentrations of insulin are required to maintain normal blood glucose levels, until normal levels can no longer be maintained. The ability of hyperinsulinemia to maintain glucose tolerance is a mixed blessing. Insulin resistance and compensatory hyperinsulinemia are associated with a variety of abnormalities, including varying degrees of glucose intolerance, dyslipidemia and high blood pressure. These abnormalities are major risk factors for CVD, as confirmed by several researchers (32–34).

BILE METABOLISM, BILE ACID METABOLISM DISORDERS AND GALLSTONES

Bile is a complex fluid containing water, electrolytes and a battery of organic molecules including bile acids, cholesterol, phospholipid and bilirubin. It is carried from the liver through bile ducts to the gallbladder, where it is stored for secretion into the small intestine. Bile is critical for the digestion and absorption of fats and fat-soluble vitamins in the small intestine. Bile acids are either excreted (only a small percentage) or reabsorbed by the gut and returned to the liver (enterohepatic circulation). Significant physiological functions of bile acids include: emulsification of dietary triglycerides, the elimination of excess cholesterol, and dissolution of cholesterol in bile to prevent cholesterol precipitation in the gallbladder and gallstone formation. The major quantitative pathway maintaining cholesterol homeostasis is controlled by hepatic parenchymal cells, which express cholesterol-7alpha-hydroxylase (CYP7A1) thereby regulating the conversion of cholesterol into bile acids.

Diabetes, gallstones and dyslipidaemia are widespread and metabolically related. Alterations in lipid metabolism are seen in plasma, liver and bile in both CVD and diabetes which can result in the formation of gallstones (35). A link between insulin and cholesterol gallstone disease has often been suspected but never demonstrated. When compared 173 individuals with prevalent gallstones to 284 controls, Scragg et al. (36) showed that an increased risk of gallstones was associated with increased plasma insulin values independent of plasma triglyceride values. An Italian population case study reported that insulin was associated with gallstones in individuals without a clinical diagnosis of diabetes and serum glucose <7 mmol/l (37). A more direct study showed that one week of daily long acting insulin injections doubled the cholesterol gallstone incidence in hamsters fed a lithogenic diet (38). Although diabetes is important to the formation of the gallstones, Pacchioni et al. (39) reported that obesity, which often accompanied type 2 diabetes, was a stronger risk factor for gallstones than type 2 diabetes.

DIETARY FIBER

There is no single accepted definition of dietary fiber. Dietary fiber is a term used to describe a variety of plant substances that are resistant to digestion by mammalian enzymes. One of the suggested definitions is: "dietary fiber consists of the remnants of edible plant cells, polysaccharides, lignin, and associated substances resistant to digestion by the alimentary enzymes of humans and animals (40–42). Dietary fiber components can be characterized by their behavior in aqueous solutions as soluble or insoluble. Soluble dietary fiber, which is soluble in water, includes components of noncellulosic polysaccharides such as pectins gums, mucilages, algal polysaccharides, and some hemicelluloses. Insoluble dietary fiber, which is insoluble in water, consists mainly of cell wall components including cellulose, hemicelluloses, and lignin (43). Dietary fiber can also be classified as fermentable or nonfermentable, which is related to the degree of the fermentation by anaerobic bacteria in the large intestine. Soluble fiber is more fermentable than insoluble fiber. Between 1972 and 1976, the role of the dietary fiber was expanded to be used in health-related hypotheses, which is that a high intake of fiber-containing foods is directly related to or associated with a low incidence of many diseases. Dietary fiber is available in the human diet through a wide variety of food sources, such as vegetable, fruits, whole grains, nuts, legumes as well as grains such as oat and wheat bran (42). Components of dietary fiber vary with the source of the fiber. The relationship between dietary fiber and chronic disease has led to an increased interest in the effect of high fiber foods on risk factors. Although the recommended dietary fiber intake is about 20–35 g/day/person, the actual fiber intake in the population is much lower, only 10–15 g/day/person (44).

DIETARY FIBER AND CARDIOVASCULAR DISEASE

The relationship of dietary fiber and cardiovascular diseases was explored in the early 60s when Keys et al. (45) reported that blood cholesterol was reduced by about 5% in healthy adult men when consuming 15g/day of pectin. In 1972, Trowell (46) supported this hypothesis by showing that a high fiber diet is protective for hyperlipidemia and ischemic heart disease. Kromhout et al. (47) confirmed that an increase in dietary fiber can significantly reduce the mortality of coronary heart disease in a 10-year follow up study. Today, the association of dietary fiber with reduced CVD is well accepted. Several epidemiological and experimental studies have shown a protective effect of dietary fiber on coronary artery disease (48–50). Among these, the prospective 10 year nurses health study of 68782 US women indicated that higher fiber intake, particularly from cereal sources, reduces the risk of CHD (48). A 12 year investigation showed that the ischemic heart disease mortality was reduced 25% after a 6 gm increment in daily fiber intake independent of other dietary variables, including calories, fat, cholesterol, protein, carbohydrate, alcohol, calcium, and potassium (50). The sources of dietary fiber providing protection from CVD include whole grains (51–54), guar, glucomannans, pectins, oat betaglucan, psyllium (55), nuts (56), fruits as well as vegetables (57). Although the association between dietary fiber and coronary heart disease is mainly due to the effect of nutrition on serum lipids and lipoproteins (58,59), the influence of dietary fiber on insulin resistance could be another major mechanism for the prevention and treatment of the CVD (60).

DIETARY FIBER EFFECTS ON DIABETES AND INSULIN RESISTANCE

There is no question of that increasing consumption of dietary fiber shows promise in the management of type 2 diabetes (61,62). Since the 1970s, a great deal of interest has been focused on the effect of dietary fiber on glucose and fat metabolism. Jenkins et al. (63) observed that 36 g of wheat fibre, pectin, or guar gum fed to healthy volunteers for 2 weeks significantly lowered the mean serum lipids. In the succeeding study, they tested the glucose tolerance in patients with or without the addition of guar, pectin, gum tragacanth, and methylcellulose (equal to 15 g fiber). The results illustrated that the blood glucose and serum insulin concentrations were reduced. In addition, the peak rises of the blood glucose are associated with the viscosity of the fiber (64). Sufficient beta-glucan in a meal flattened the postprandial glycemic and insulinemic excursions and favorably influenced the plasma lipid levels in patients with type 2 diabetes (65). The effect of dietary fiber on insulin resistance has also been reported. Our own study showed that psyllium, reduced the insulin resistance (measured by hyperinsulinemic euglycemic clamp) caused by high fat diets in rats and prevented much of the increase in fasting plasma insulin level (66). Song and colleagues (67) showed that psyllium increases insulin sensitivity by increasing in skeletal muscle GLUT-4 content. The dietary fiber from konjac-mannan ameliorates glycemic control, blood lipid profile, and systolic blood pressure in high-risk diabetic individuals, possibly improving the effectiveness of conventional treatment in type 2 diabetes (68). A controversial study reported that three-month treatment with 15 grams of guar gum had no effect on metabolic control and insulin sensitivity in patients with type 1 diabetes (69).

DIETARY FIBER EFFECTS ON THE RISK FACTORS OF CVD AND DIABETES

Since hypercholesterolemia, dyslipidemia, abnormalities of bile composition and hyperinsulinemia are risk factors of both cardiovascular disease and diabetes; the modulation of these factors with dietary fiber will contribute to the prevention and treatment these chronic diseases (70).

CHOLESTEROL AND LIPOPROTEINS

One of the most recognized physiological effects of soluble dietary fiber is to lower cholesterol, which was observed in several epidemiological and clinical trials. The role of dietary fiber in the modulation of blood lipid concentrations was initially explored in the 1960s (45). The serum cholesterol level was reduced by administration of guar gum for 2 weeks in hyperlipidemia patients (71). A meta-analysis indicates that viscous fiber significantly reduced total blood cholesterol concentrations without influencing the HDL and triglyceride levels (72). Serial studies conduct by Kahlon and colleagues (73–76) demonstrated that rice bran, oat bran and barley fractions all significantly lowered cholesterol in hamsters fed with 0.3–0.5% of cholesterol and 8–10% of fat. To date, it is well established that certain sources of dietary fiber independent of the fat or carbohydrate content of the diet, can lower serum cholesterol concentrations. In a study of 278 subjects, diets containing fiber from Konjac-mannan were given for two 3-week treatment periods separated by a 2-week washout, decreases in serum cholesterol, total/HDL ratio, LDL/HDL ratio, and LDL were observed (68). The soluble dietary fiber, guar gum, has proved an ability to lower the plasma cholesterol and change the lipoprotein profile. Rats fed guar gum diets significantly lower levels of blood serum cholesterol, triacylglycerols, and an increase in HDL-cholesterol with a substantial elevation of the HDL/LDL cholesterol ratio (77). Consuming a large amount of rye bread notably reduced serum total and LDL cholesterol concentrations in men (78).

DIETARY FIBER EFFECTS ON BILE ACID METABOLISMS AND GALLSTONES

Among the dietary fibers that affect bile acid metabolism, the most investigated source is a soluble dietary fiber from psyllium husks. Psyllium increases bile acid excretion, increases bile acid synthesis and reduces bile acid absorption. The effect of psyllium on cholesterol-7-alpha-hydroxylase (CYP7A1) was investigated because CYP7A1 regulates the pathway through which cholesterol is converted into bile acids (79). 5% dietary psyllium increased the activity of cholesterol 7alpha-hydroxylase. Apart from the above, psyllium also lowered serum cholesterol concentration by increasing the excretion of fecal bile acids and total steroids, and up-regulation of bile acid biosynthesis. A similar experiment proved that psyllium also significantly lowered liver cholesterol (80). Moreover, psyllium increases CYP7A1 and Hydroxymethylglutaryl Reductase (HMGR) mRNA levels, in addition to decreasing serum cholesterol (81,82). The fecal bile acid and total steroid excretion as well as total intestinal bile acids were significantly greater in rats fed psyllium-containing diets compared to 0% psyllium-fed rats (80,82). Other dietary fibers such as oat beta-glucan and pectin also have an effect on bile acid excretion (83,84).

In addition to the hypocholesterolemic effects, dietary fiber has a protective role in reducing cholesterol gallstone formation (85), which is related to its effect on bile and, most importantly, on bile acid metabolism as well as several limit enzymes. Psyllium, a soluble dietary fiber, significantly prevented the gallstone formation in high cholesterol fed hamsters (86). There was a 100% formation of gallstones in hamsters fed 15% butterfat and 5% corn oil. The gallstone formation was reduced from 100% to 0% if 8% psyllium or hydroxyproplymethylcellulose was added to this high fat diet. Ground barley, contributing 8% beta glucan to the diet, reduced gallstone formation to 50% in the same high fat diet (87). In addition to prevent the gallstone formation in hamsters, psyllium also prevented the cholesterol gallstone formation in dogs fed with a high cholesterol diet (88).

DIETARY FIBER AND OBESITY

Dietary fiber may influence obesity in many ways. One effect of dietary fiber on obesity may be to aid in control of energy intake and thereby reduce the risk for development of obesity. Obese individuals may exhibit a greater reduction of energy intake and body weight loss on high fiber diets. Dietary fiber, especially soluble fiber, may act through energy dilution or enhance satiation to reduce energy intake (89). A 10 year multicenter population-based cohort study showed that dietary fiber intake had linear associations with body weight, waist-to-hip ratio fasting insulin and 2-hour postglucose insulin adjusted for body mass index. They concluded that fiber consumption predicted insulin levels, weight gain, and other CVD risk factors more strongly than did total or saturated fat consumption (90). In a recent review, Howarth and Saltzman (91) summarized that consumption of an additional 14 g/day fiber for >2 days is associated with a 10% decrease in energy intake and body weight loss of 1.9 kg over 3 months. Although soluble dietary fiber is a potentially important factor contributing to the stable energy balance and obesity prevention, the influence of dietary fiber on energy regulation remains controversial. The clinical metabolic investigations have given conflicting results on the effects of soluble fiber on energy regulation. A meta-analysis indicated a non-significant difference in patients receiving guar gum compared with patients receiving placebo and this data suggests that guar gum is not efficacious for reducing body weight (92). The conflicting results may be caused by the different dietary fiber components used in the studies and lack of adequate controls to restrict subjects' consumption of other dietary components that may have affected energy regulation.

DIETARY FIBER AND RELATIVE GENE EXPRESSION

Research on the effect of nutrients on gene expression has been advanced with the use of molecular and cellular techniques. As more genes are discovered that may affect diabetes, CVD and insulin resistance (93), the chance that dietary fiber can affect these genes also increases. Dietary fiber may act directly to influence these genes, or indirectly influence gene regulation or act through specialized insulin signaling pathways pathways (94–96). Fukashima et al. (97) demonstrated that rats fed mushroom fiber or beet fiber for 4 weeks had significantly lower hepatic LDL receptor mRNA concentrations compared to rats given cellulose. The succeeding study showed different sources of mushroom fibers (maitake (Grifola frondosa) fiber (MAF), shiitake (Lentinus edodes) fiber, enokitake (Flammulina velutipes) fiber) considerably lowered serum cholesterol and hepatic low-density lipoprotein (LDL) receptor mRNA when fed to rats for 4 weeks (98). Feeding 30% of dietary fiber significantly increased the levels of glucose-stimulated circulating HGH and upregulated levels of mouse intestinal proglucagon gene expression in the jejunum, ileum, and colon (99). In order to determine the mechanism by which soluble fiber consistently lowers plasma total and LDL-cholesterol, Horton JD et al. (100) observed the effect of dietary psyllium on hepatic 7 alpha-hydroxylase, 3-hydroxy-3-methylglutaryl coenzyme A (HMG CoA) reductase and LDL receptor expression in the hamster. After feeding 7.5% dietary psyllium to hamsters, the hepatic 7 alpha-hydroxylase activity and mRNA were increased by 3–4-fold compared with the animals fed with same amount of cellulose. Although dietary psyllium did not increase hepatic LDL receptor expression in animals fed the cholesterol-free, very-low-fat diet, it did increase (or at least restore) receptor expression that had been downregulated by dietary cholesterol and triglyceride. Similar results was reported by Buhman KK et al. (82) also confirmed that that psyllium can affect the hepatic cholesterol 7alpha-hydroxylase (CYP7A) mRNA, 3-hydroxy-3-methylglutaryl CoA reductase (HMGR) mRNA, ileal apical sodium-dependent bile acid transporter (ASBT) mRNA and this affect is in a dose-dependent manner. Rhubarb-fibre feeding accelerated the fecal bile-acid loss and diminished the gall-bladder bile-acid pool in both the normal and the cholesterol-fed mice. The increase in the bile-acid excretion was positively correlated with an increased activity as well as mRNA abundance of cholesterol 7 alpha-hydroxylase (101). Another study showed that fed rats with 15% beet fiber for 14 days, ileal apolipoprotein A-I and A-IV mRNA levels were significantly lower than in animals that had been fed no fiber (102).

THE AMOUNT AND THE TYPE OF FIBER ARE IMPORTANT

The beneficial effect of soluble dietary fiber also depends on the amount of fiber consumed and fiber type. Within limits, diets high in dietary fiber have greater effects on the risk factors than diets containing moderate amounts of dietary fiber (103). The relative risk associated with fiber intake was reported in a 230,006 person-year prospective study. A higher intake of dietary fiber was associated with a lower risk of CVD and MI (49). Similarly, after age-adjustment, the relative risk for major CHD events was lower in women with the highest quintile of total dietary fiber intake (median, 22.9 g/d) compared with women in the lowest quintile (median, 11.5 g/d). Viscosity of the dietary fiber is also important. Viscous water-soluble fiber appears to have a greater potential to reduce postprandial blood glucose, insulin, and serum lipid levels than insoluble fiber. Jenkins et al. (82) noticed that treatment in diabetic with either guar or pectin, (equivalent to 12 g fibre), the greatest flattening of the glucose response was seen with guar, but this effect was abolished when hydrolysed non-viscous guar was used (104). Tappy et al. (105) gave type 2 diabetic patients breakfast cereals with 4.0, 6.0, and 8.4 g beta-glucan, the observed that plasma glucose peaks after the breakfast cereal were 67%, 42%, and

38%, of the control respectively which has an inverse linear relationship between dose of beta-glucan and plasma glucose peak or area under the glucose curve. Similar to the effect on CVD, the impact of soluble dietary fiber on diabetes is associated with the concentration or amount of fiber. In addition, fed moderate levels of soluble fiber and insoluble fiber (25 g fiber/day) or higher levels of soluble and insoluble fiber (50 g fiber/day, which contains 50% of soluble fiber) for 6 weeks to type 2 diabetes patients with. The patients in the high fiber group had significantly lower fasting plasma and urinary glucose levels as well as lower total cholesterol, triglyceride and VLDL cholesterol levels (65).

Cereal foods with low glycaemic index such as pasta and oats are beneficial for people with diabetes and might lower plasma lipids. Human experiments have clearly shown that oat fibre tends to lower plasma total and LDL cholesterol but that wheat fibre does not (106). In summary, the possible health benefits of dietary fiber in reducing the risk of CVD, insulin resistance and diabetes have been reported. However, the present consumption of dietary fiber (10–15 g/day) is less than that recommended (20–35 g/day) for expected health benefits. In addition, the underlying mechanisms of the beneficial effects of dietary fiber on CVD, insulin resistance and diabetes are far from clear. Therefore, there is a continuing need and opportunity for further research and education in the area.

REFERENCES

1. Howard BV, Magee MF. 2000. Diabetes and cardiovascular disease. Current Atherosclerosis Reports 2:476–481.
2. Tuomilehto J, Lindstrom J, Eriksson JG, Valle TT, Hamalainen H, Ilanne-Parikka P, Keinanen-Kiukaanniemi S, Laakso M, Louheranta A, Rastas M, Salminen V, Uusitupa M. 2001. Prevention of type 2 diabetes mellitus by changes in lifestyle among subjects with impaired glucose tolerance. N Engl J Med 344:1343–1350.
3. Pearson TA, Osorio D, Bronw K. 2000. Nutritional intervention in cardiovascular disease: new challenges and opportunities. Curr Atherosler Rep 2:515–520.
4. Anderson JW, Hanna TJ, Peng X, Kryscio RJ. 2000. Whole grain foods and heart disease risk. J Am Coll Nutr (Suppl 3):291S–299S.
5. NIH-NIDDK. 2000. Diabetes statistics. 15.
6. Harris MI. Diabetes in America: 1998. Epidemiology and scope of the problem. Diabetes Care (Suppl 3):C11–C14.
7. Mokdad AH, Ford ES, bowman BA, Nelson DE, Engelgau MM, Vinicor F, Marks JS. 2000. Diabetes trends in the US:1990–1998. Diabetes Care: 23:1278–1283.
8. Goldberg RB. 2000. Hyperlipidemia and cardiovascular risk factors in patients with type 2 diabetes. Am J Manag Care (Suppl 13):S682–S691.
9. American Diabetes Association. 1998. Economic consequences of diabetes mellitus in the US in1997. Diabetes Care 21:296–309.
10. Molle DE, Flier JS. 1991. Insulin resistance: mechanisms, syndromes, and implications. N Engl J Med 325:938–948.
11. O'Doherty R, Steein D, Foley J. 1997. Insulin resistance. Diabetologia 40:B10–B15.
12. Reaven GM. 1993. Role of insulin resistance in the pathophysiology of non-insulin dependent diabetes mellitus. Diabet/metab Rev 9(Suppl 1):5S–12S.
13. Harris SB, Zinman B, Hanley A, Gittelsohn J, Hegele R, Connelly PW, Shah B, Hux JE. 2002. The impact of diabetes on cardiovascular risk factors and outcomes in a native Canadian population. Diabetes Res Xclin Pract 55:165–173.
14. Stamler J, Vaccaro O, Neaton JD, Wentworth D. 1993. Diabetes, other risk factors, and 12-year cardiovascular mortality for men screened in the multiple risk factor intervention trial. Diabetes Care 16:434–444.

15. Schernthaner G. 1996. Cardiovascular mortality and morbidity in type-2 diabetes mellitus. Diabetes Res Clin Pract 31(Suppl):S3–S13.
16. Leibson C. 1999. Loss of the female advantage with cardiovascular disease for woman with diabetes. Lupus 8:351–355.
17. Hu FB, Stampfer MJ, Solomon CG, Liu S, Willett WC, Speizer FE, Nathan DM, Manson JE. 2001. Arch Intern Med 161:1717–1723.
18. Haffner SM, Lehto S, Ronnemaa T, Pyorala K, Laakso M. 1998. Mortality from coronary heart disease in subject with type 2 diabetes and in nondiabetic subjects with and without prior myocardial infarction. N Engl L Med 339:229–234.
19. Erkelens DW. 2001. Insulin resistance syndrome and type 2 diabetes mellitus. Am J Cardiol 88: 38J–42J.
20. Laakso M. 1997. Dyslipidemia, morbidity, and mortality in non-insulin-dependent diabetes mellitus. Lipoproteins and coronary heart disease in non-insulin-dependent diabetes mellitus. J Diabetes Complications 11:137–141.
21. Udawat H, Goyal RK, Maheshwari S. 2001. Coronary risk and dyslipidemia in type 2 diabetic patients. J Assoc Physicians India 49:970–973.
22. Austin MA. 1998. Plasma triglyceride as a risk factor for cardiovascular disease. Can J Cardiol (Suppl B):14B–17B.
23. Bittner V. 2001. Treatment of dyslipidemia in pre- and postmenopausal women with and without known atherosclerotic cardiovascular disease. Curr Cardiol Rep 3:401–407.
24. Franceschini G. 2001. Epidemiologic evidence for high-density lipoprotein cholesterol as a risk factor for coronary artery disease. Am J Cardiol 88:9N–13N.
25. Maron DJ. 2000. The epidemiology of low levels of high-density lipoprotein cholesterol in patients with and without coronary artery disease. Am J Cardiol 86:11L–14L.
26. Serrano Rios M. 1998. Relationship between obesity and the increased risk of major complications in non-insulin-dependent diabetes mellitus. Eur J Clin Invest (Suppl l2):14–17.
27. Scheen AJ. 2000. From obesity to diabetes: why, when and who? Acta Clin Belg 55:9–15.
28. Grundy SM. 2000. Metabolic complications of obesity. Endocrine 13:155–165.
29. Bloomgarden ZT. 2000. Obesity and diabetes. Diabetes Care 23:1584–1590.
30. Leong KS, Wilding JP. 1999. Obesity and diabetes. Baillieres Best Pract Res Clin Endocrinol Metab 13:221–237.
31. Abate N. 2000. Obesity and cardiovascular disease. Pathogenetic role of the metabolic syndrome and therapeutic implications. J Diabetes Complications 14:154–174.
32. Meigs JB, Mittleman MA, Nathan DM, Tofler GH, Singer DE, Murphy-Sheehy PM, Lipinska I, D'Agostino RB, Wilson PW. 2000. Hyperinsulinemia, Hyperglycemia, and Impaired Hemostasis: The Framingham Offspring Study JAMA 283:221–228.
33. Lakka HM, Lakka TA, Tuomilehto J, Sivenius J, Salonen JT. 2000. Hyperinsulinemia and the risk of cardiovascular death and acute coronary and cerebrovascular events in men: the Kuopio Ischaemic Heart Disease Risk Factor Study. Arch Intern Med 160:1160–1168.
34. Arrants J. 1994. Hyperinsulinemia and cardiovascular risk. Heart Lung 23:118–122.
35. Zhao JC, Xiao LJ, Zhu H, Shu Y, Cheng NS. 1998. Changes of lipid metabolism in plasma, liver and bile during cholesterol gallstone formation in rabbit model. World J Gastroenterol 4:337–339.
36. Scragg RK, Calvert GD, Oliver JR. 1984. Plasma lipids and insulin in gall stone disease: a case-control study. Br Med J 289:521–525.
37. Misciagna G, Guerra V, Di Leo A, Correale M, Trevisan M. 2000. Insulin and gallstones: a population case control study in southern Italy. Gut 47:144–147.
38. Dubrac S, Parquet M, Blouquit Y, Gripois D, Blouquit MF, Souidi M, Lutton C. 2001. Insulin injections enhance cholesterol gallstone incidence by changing the biliary cholesterol saturation index and apo A-I concentration in hamsters fed a lithogenic diet. J Hepatol 35:550–557.
39. Pacchioni M, Nicoletti C, Caminiti M, Calori G, Curci V, Camisasca R, Pontiroli AE. 2000. Association of obesity and type II diabetes mellitus as a risk factor for gallstones. Dig Dis Sci 45:2002–2006.
40. Eastwood MA, Pass more R. 1983. Dietary fiber. Lancet 2:202–206.
41. Prosky L. 2000. What is dietary fiber? J AOAC Interna 83:985–987.
42. Dreher ML. 2001. Dietary fiber overview. In: Handbook of dietary fiber. Ed Cho SS and Dreher ML. 1–16. New York Marcel Dekker, Inc.
43. McKee LH, Latner TA. 2000. Underutilized sources of dietary fiber: a review. Plant Foods for Human Nutrition 55:285–304.

44. Pilch SM. 1987. Physiological effects and health consequences of dietary fiber. pp. 149–157. Life Sciences Research office, Bethesda MD.
45. Keys A, Grande F, Anderson JT. 1961. Fiber and pectin in the diet and serum cholesterol concentrations in man. Proc Soc Exp Biol Med 106:555–558.
46. Trowell H. 1972. Ischemic heart disease and dietary fiber. Am J Clin Nutr 25:926–932.
47. Kromhout D, Bosschieter E, de Lezenne Coulander C. 1982. Dietary fiber and 10-year mortality from coronary heart disease, cancer and all causes: the Zutphen study. Lancet 2:518–522.
48. Wolk A, Manson JE, Stampfer MJ, Colditz GA, Hu FB, Speizer FE, Hennekens CH, Willett WC. 1999. Long-term intake of dietary fiber and decreased risk of coronary heart disease among women. JAMA 281:1998–2004.
49. Liu S, Buring JE, Sesso HD, Rimm EB, Willett WC, Manson JE. 2002. A prospective study of dietary fiber intake and risk of cardiovascular disease among women. J Am Coll Cardiol 39:49–56.
50. Khaw KT, Barrett-Connor E. 1987. Dietary fiber and reduced ischemic heart disease mortality rates in men and women: a 12-year prospective study. Am J Epidemiol 126:1093–1102.
51. Slavin JL, Jacobs D, Marquart L, Wiemer K. 2001. The role of whole grains in disease prevention. J Am Diet Assoc 101:780–785.
52. Liu S, Stampfer MJ, Hu FB, Giovannucci E, Rimm E, Manson JE, Hennekens CH, Willett WC. 1999. Whole-grain consumption and risk of coronary heart disease: results from the Nurses' Health Study. Am J Clin Nutr 70:412–419.
53. Jacobs DR, Pereira MA, Meyer KA, Kushi LH. 2000. Fiber from whole grains, but not refined grains, is inversely associated with all-cause mortality in older women: the Iowa women's health study. J Am Coll Nutr 19(Suppl 3):326S–330S.
54. Jenkins DJ, Kendall CW, Vuksan V, Augustin LS, Mehling C, Parker T, Vidgen E, Lee B, Faulkner D, Seyler H, Josse R, Leiter LA, Connelly PW, Fulgoni V 3rd. 1999. Effect of wheat bran on serum lipids: influence of particle size and wheat protein. J Am Coll Nutr 18:159–165.
55. Jenkins DJ, Kendall CW, Axelsen M, Augustin LS, Vuksan V. 2000. Viscous and nonviscous fibers, nonabsorbable and low glycaemic index carbohydrates, blood lipids and coronary heart disease. Curr Opin Lipidol 11:49–56.
56. Kris-Etherton PM, Zhao G, Binkoski AE, Coval SM, Etherton TD. 2001. The effect of nuts on coronary heart disease risk. Nutr Rev 4:103–111.
57. Jenkins DJ, Kendall CW, Popovich DG, Vidgen E, Mehling CC, Vuksan V, Ransom TP, Rao AV, Rosenberg-Zand R, Tariq N, Corey P, Jones PJ, Raeini M, Story JA, Furumoto EJ, Illingworth DR, Pappu AS, Connelly PW. 2001. Effect of a very-high-fiber vegetable, fruit, and nut diet on serum lipids and colonic function. Metabolism 50:494–503.
58. Pyorala K, Pedersen TR, Kjekshus J, Faergeman O, Olsson AG, Thoreirsson G. 1997. Cholesterol lowering with simvastatin improves prognosis of diabetic patients with coronary heart disease. Diabetes Care 20:614–620.
59. Sacks FM, Pfeffer Am, Moye LA, Rouleau JL, Rutherford JD, Cole TG, Brown L, Warnica JW, Arnold JMO, Wun C-C, Davis BR, Braunwald E. 1996. The effect of pravastatin on coronary events after myocardial infarction in patients with average cholesterol levels. N Engl J Med 335:1001–1009.
60. Savaiano DA, Story JA. 2000. Cardiovascular disease and fiber: is insulin resistance the missing link? Nutr Rev 58:356–358.
61. KarlstrÖm B, Vessby B, Asp NG, Boberg M, Gustafsson IB, Lithell, Werner I. 1984. Effects of an increased content of cereal fiber in the diet of type II (non-insulin-dependent) diabetic patients. Diabetologia 26:272–277.
62. Chandalia M, Garyg A, Lutjohann D, von Bergmann K, Grundy SM, Brinkley LJ. 2000. Beneficial effects of high dietary fiber intake in patients with type 2 diabetes mellitus. N Engl J Med 342:1392–1398.
63. Jenkins DJ, Newton C, Leeds AR, Cummings JH. 1975. Effect of pectin, guar gum, and wheat fibre on serum-cholesterol. Lancet 1:1116–1117.
64. Jenkins DJ, Wolever TM, Leeds AR, Gassull MA, Haisman P, Dilawari J, Goff DV, Metz GL, Alberti KG. 1978. Dietary fibres, fibre analogues, and glucose tolerance: importance of viscosity. Br Med J 6124:1392–1394.
65. Bourdon I, Yokoyama W, Davis P, Hudson C, Backus R, Richter D, Knuckles B, Schneeman BO. 1999. Postprandial lipid, glucose, insulin, and cholecystokinin responses in men fed barley pasta enriched with beta-glucan. Am J Clin Nutr 69:55–63.
66. Shao Q, Keagy PM, Yokoyama W, Kahlon T, Hudson C. 2002. Psyllium, a viscous soluble dietary decreases insulin resistance in rats. FASEB J A630–A631.

67. Song YJ, Sawamura M, Ikeda K, Igawa S, Yamori Y. 2000. Soluble dietary fibre improves insulin sensitivity by increasing muscle GLUT-4 content in stroke-prone spontaneously hypertensive rats. Clin Exp Pharmacol Physiol 27:41–45.
68. Vuksan V, Sievenpiper JL, Owen R, Swilley JA, Spadafora P, Jenkins DJ, Vidgen E, Brighenti F, Josse RG, Leiter LA, Xu Z, Novokmet R. 2000. Beneficial effects of viscous dietary fiber from konjac-mannan in subjects with the insulin resistance syndrome: results of a controlled metabolic trial. Diabetes Care 23:9–14.
69. Bruttomesso D, Biolo G, Inchiostro S, Fongher C, Briani G, Duner E, Marescotti MC, Iori E, Tiengo A, Tessari P. 1991. No effects of high-fiber diets on metabolic control and insulin-sensitivity in type 1 diabetic subjects. Diabetes Res Clin Pract 13:15–21.
70. Garber AJ. 2000. Attenuating cardiovascular risk factors in patients with type 2 diabetes. Am Fam Physician 62:2633–2642.
71. Jenkins DJ, Leeds AR, Slavin B, Mann J, Jepson EM. 1979. Dietary fiber and blood lipids: reduction of serum cholesterol in type II hyperlipidemia by guar gum. Am J Clin Nutr 32:16–18.
72. Bromn L, Rosner B, Willett WW, Sacks FM. 1999. Chlesterol-lowering effects of dietary fiber: a meta-analysis. Am J Clin Nutr 69:30–42.
73. Kahlon TS, Saunders RM, Chow FI, Betschart AA. 1990. Influence of rice Bran, Oat Bran, and wheat bran on cholesterol and triglycerides in hamsters. Cereal Chemistry 67:439–443.
74. Kahlon TS, Chow FI, Sayre RN, Betschart AA. 1992. Chlesterol lowering in hamsters fed rice bran at various levels, defatted rice bran and rice bran oil. J Nutr 122:513–519.
75. Kahlon TS, Saunders RM, Sayre RN, Chow FI, Chiu MM, Betschart AA. 1992. Chlesterol-lowering affects rice bran and rice bran oil fractions in hypercholesterolemia hamsters Cereal Chemistry 69:485–489.
76. Kahlon TS, Chow FI, Knuckles BE, Chiu MM. 1993. Chlesterol-lowering effects in hamsters of ß-glucan-enriched barley fraction, dehulled whole barley, rice bran and oat bran and their combinations. Cereal Chemistry 70:435–440.
77. Frias AC, Sgarbieri VC. 1998. Guar gum effects on food intake, blood serum lipids and glucose levels of Wistar rats. Plant Foods Hum Nutr 53:15–28.
78. Leinonen KS, Poutanen KS, Mykkanen HM. 2000. Rye bread decreases serum total and LDL cholesterol in men with moderately elevated serum cholesterol. J Nutr 130:164–170.
79. Trautwein EA, Rieckhoff D, Kunath-Rau A, Erbersdobler HF. 1998. Psyllium, not pectin or guar gum, alters lipoprotein and biliary bile acid composition and fecal sterol excretion in the hamster. Lipids 33:573–582.
80. Buhman KK, Furumoto EJ, Donkin SS, Story JA. 1998. Dietary psyllium increases fecal bile acid excretion, total steroid excretion and bile acid biosynthesis in rats. J Nutr 128:1199–1203.
81. Matheson HB, Colon IS, Story JA. 1995. Cholesterol 7 alpha-hydroxylase activity is increased by dietary modification with psyllium hydrocolloid, pectin, cholesterol and cholestyramine in rats. J Nutr 125:454–458.
82. Buhman KK, Furumoto EJ, Donkin SS, Story JA. 2000. Dietary psyllium increases expression of ileal apical sodium-dependent bile acid transporter mRNA coordinately with dose-responsive changes in bile acid metabolism in rats. J Nutr 130:2137–2142.
83. Lia A, Hallmans G, Sandberg AS, Sundberg B, Aman P, Andersson. 1995. Oat beta-glucan increases bile acid excretion and a fiber-rich barley fraction increases cholesterol excretion in ileostomy subjects. Am J Clin Nutr 62:1245–1251.
84. Garcia-Diez F, Garcia-Mediavilla V, Bayon JE, Gonzalez-Gallego J. 1996. Pectin feeding influences fecal bile acid excretion, hepatic bile acid and cholesterol synthesis and serum cholesterol in rats. J Nutr 126:1766–1771.
85. Thornton JR, Emmett PM, Heaton KW. 1983. Diet and gallstones: effects of refined and unrefined carbohydrate diets on bile cholesterol saturation and bile acid metabolism. Gut 24:2–6.
86. Zhang JX, Lundin E, Hallmans G, Bergman F, Westerlund E, Petterson. 1992. Dietary effects of barley fiber, wheat bran and rye bran on bile composition and gallstone formation in hamsters. APMIS 100:553–557.
87. Shao Q, Keagy PM, Knuckle B, Chiu M, Kahlon T, Yokoyama W, Hudson C. 2002. Dietary fiber reduced insulin resistance induced by a high fiber diet in hamsters. Cereal Chemistry (in Press).
88. Schwesinger WH, Kurtin WE, Page CP, Stewart RM, Johnson R. 1999. Soluble dietary fiber protects against cholesterol gallstone formation. Am J Surg 177:307–310.
89. Pasman WJ, Saris WH, Wauters MA, Westerterp-Plantenga MS. 1997. Effect of one week of fibre supplementation on hunger and satiety ratings and energy intake. Appetite 29:77–87.
90. Ludwig DS, Pereira MA, Kroenke CH, Hilner JE, Van Horn L, Slattery ML, Jacobs DR Jr. 1999.

Dietary fiber, weight gain, and cardiovascular disease risk factors in young adults. JAMA 282: 1539–1546.
91. Howarth NC, Saltzman E, Roberts SB. 2001. Dietary fiber and weight regulation. Nutr Rev 59:129–139.
92. Pittler MH, Ernst E. 2001. Guar gum for body weight reduction: meta-analysis of randomized trials. Am J Med 110:724–730.
93. Moller DE, Bjorrek C, Vidal-Pulg A. 1996. Candidate genes for insulin resistance. Diabetes Care 19:396–400.
94. Briggs S, Spiller GA. 1998. Dietary fiber, glucose tolerance, and diabetes related new therapy emerges. Food Product Development 12:81–82.
95. Cousins RJ. 1999. Nutritional regulation of gene expression. Am J Med 106:20S–23S.
96. Toleeler M. 1993. Diet and diabetes. Diabetes/Metabolism Rev. 9:93–108.
97. Fukushima M, Nakano M, Morii Y, Ohashi T, Fujiwara Y, Sonoyama K. 2000. Hepatic LDL receptor mRNA in rats is increased by dietary mushroom (agaticus bisporus) fiber and sugar beet fiber. J Nutr 130:2151–2156.
98. Fukushima M, Ohashi T, Fujiwara Y, Sonoyama K, Nakano M. 2001. Cholesterol-lowering effects of maitake (Grifola frondosa) fiber, shiitake (Lentinus edodes) fiber, and enokitake (Flammulina velutipes) fiber in rats. Exp Biol Med 226:758–765.
99. Nian M, Gu J, Irwin DM, Drucker DJ. 2002. Human glucagon gene promoter sequences regulating tissue-specific versus nutrient-regulated gene expression. Am J Physiol Regul Integr Comp Physiol 282:R173–R183.
100. Horton JD, Cuthbert, Spady DK. 1994. Regulation of hepatic 7α-hydroxylase expression by dietary psyllium in the hamster. L Clin Invest 93:2084–2092.
101. Goel V, Cheema SK, Agellon LB, Ooraikul B, Basu TK. 1999. Dietary rhubarb (Rheum rhaponticum) stalk fibre stimulates cholesterol 7 alpha-hydroxylase gene expression and bile acid excretion in cholesterol-fed C57BL/6J mice. Br J Nutr 81:65–71.
102. Sonoyama K, Nishikawa H, Kiriyama S, Niki R. 1995. Apolipoprotein mRNA in liver and intestine of rats is affected by dietary beet fiber or cholestyramine. J Nutr 125:13–19.
103. McIntosh M, Miller CA. 2001. Diets containing food rich in soluble and insoluble fiber improves glycemic control and reduces hyperlipidemia among patients with type 2 diabetes mellitus. Nutr Rev 59:52–55.
104. Wursch P, Pi-Sunyer FX. 1997. The role of viscous soluble fiber in the metabolic control of diabetes. A review with special emphasis on cereals rich in beta-glucan. Diabetes Care 20:1774–1780.
105. Tappy L, Gugolz E, Wursch P. 1996. Effects of breakfast cereals containing various amounts of ß-glucan fibers on plasma glucose and insulin responses in NIDDM subjects. Diabetes Care 19:831–834.
106. Truswell AS. 2002. Cereal grains and coronary heart disease. Eur J Clin Nutr 56:1–14.

Frontiers in Cardiovascular Health, edited by
N.S. Dhalla, A. Chockalingam,
H.I. Berkowitz & P.K. Singal
Kluwer Academic Publishers, Boston, 2003

Nutrition and the Brain-Heart Connection

Ram B. Singh,[1] Kumar Kartikey,[2] Mahmood Moshiri,[3] Narankar S. Neki,[4] Udai P. Singh,[5] Adarsh Kumar,[6] Daniel Pella,[7] and Shanti S. Rastogi[8]

Medical Hospital and Research Centre, Moradabad, Subharti Medical College, Meerut(UP)[1,2,5,8]; *Cardiovascular Centre, Tehran, Iran*[3]; *Government Medical College, Amritsar*[4,6]; *Safaric University, Kosice, Slovakia*[7]

Summary. The various mechanisms that may explain the association between brain-heart connection and nutrition, leading to abnormal heart rate variability (HRV) and blood pressure variability (BPV) resulting into increased morbidity and mortality due to cardiovascular diseases (CVD), are reviewed. Medline search til December, 2001 and articles published in various national and international journals were reviewed. Experts working in the field were also consulted. There is compelling evidence that saturated and total fat and sedentary behaviour can enhance sympathetic activity and increase the secretion of catecholamine and serotonin, whereas omega-3 fatty acid supplementation may enhance parasympathetic activity and increase the secretion of acetylecholine in the hippocampus. While increased sympathetic activity has adverse effects on HRV and BPV, increased parasympathetic activity has beneficial effects and can directly inhibit sympathetic tone. A large body of evidence is available demonstrating that abnormal HRV measured over a 24 hour period, or for 7 days, provides information on the risk of subsequent death in subjects with and without heart disease. There is a need to study 7-day record by Holter cardiac monitoring to further elucidate the role of HRV in the pathogenesis of CVD. Meditation, beta blockers, ACE inhibitors, n-3 fatty acids, trimetazidine and oestrogen may have a beneficial influence on HRV. However, no definite and specific therapy is currently available to improve the prognosis for patients with abnormal HRV and blood pressure variability (BPV). Low HRV has been most commonly associated with a risk of arrhythmias and arrhythmic death, unstable angina, myocardial infarction, progression of heart failure and atherosclerosis. There is a need to develop a consensus on the measure of HRV for clinical purposes and whether 7-day record is necessary and practical. New analysis methods based on nonlinear dynamics may be more useful in risk stratification. More precise insight into the patho-physiological link between HRV and nutri-

Corresponding Author: Dr. R.B. Singh, MD, Professor of Medicine, Subharti Medical College, Civil Lines, Moradabad-10(UP) 244001, India. E-mail: icn@mickyonline.com.

tion may be applied to clinical practice and used to direct therapy for prevention of disease risk.

Key words: heart rate variability, circadian rhythm, sudden death, heart failure.

INTRODUCTION

A molecular biological clock, situated in the brain's suprachiasmatic nucleus, appears to control the rhythm for everyday life. It is under the strong influence of daily light and darkness, and under weak influence of plasma melatonin levels secreted by the pineal gland. A clinical event occurs when our autonomic system is not able to control the adverse effects of the sympathetic nervous system (1–3). Triggering of suprachiasmatic nucleus due to nutrients and other environmental factors may activate sensors, receptors and hormones (pineal gland, pituitary functions and adrenal secretions) resulting into adverse effects on circadian variations, heart rate variability (HRV) and blood pressure variability (BPV) (1–5). There is evidence that saturated and total fat intake may enhance sympathetic activity with an increase in catecholamine, cortisol, serotonin and oxidative stress, whereas treatment with omega-3 fatty acids can inhibit sympathetic activity by enhancing parasympathetic activity and increased secretion of acetylecholine in the hippocampus (1). Depression, type A behaviour and stress may be associated with a deficiency of antioxidant vitamins E and C, beta-carotine, zinc, and magnesium as well as a rise in oxidative damage, resulting into a greater risk of heart disease (1–3). The role of a time-adjusted drug intake, especially in the early morning, was also known to ancient Indian physicians (5–8). In Ayurveda, drinking large amounts of water in the early morning is advised and appears to be an attempt to increase vagal tone due to gastric distention (6–8). In one industrial population, Pell and D'Alonzo (9) were the first to discuss the existence of a peak in the morning hours, in a study of acute myocardial infarction (AMI). The subsequent reports from other countries and the extensive data by WHO in the report of myocardial infarction Community Registers (10–12) from 19 European centers, clearly demonstrated a peak incidence of the onset of chest pain due to AMI from 8:01 to 11:00 a.m. with a ratio of approximately 2:1. In one study from India (5), in 605 patients of AMI, those who had Q wave infarction (n = 174) showed that 39% had the onset between 6.00 a.m. to 12.00 noon. In a more recent study among 202 patients of AMI, the incidence of onset of chest pain was highest in the second quarter of the day (41.0%), mainly between 4:00 a.m. to 8:00 a.m. which was followed by fourth quarter, usually after large meals (28.2%). Emotion, the second trigger (43.5%) was more common in patients with the onset of chest pain in the second quarter of the day (51.8%). Cold weather was a predisposing factor in 29.2% and hot temperature (>40 degree C) was common in 24.7% of the patients. Blood pressure was also lower in the night and morning while it increased in the daytime. Various triggers responsible for circadian rhythms and cardiovascular events have been described by us (1–3).

In one recent study (10), a total of 65 patients of angina pectoris, free from other diseases and drug free, were Holter monitored for 24 hours. A total of 30 patients were also monitored on isosorbide-5 mononitrate (IS-5-MN) and on metaprolol, respectively. A total of matched healthy subjects served as controls. Spectral components of HRV were analysed hourly, with special reference to the rapid changes of autonomic tone during the night and early morning hours. During the night/morning hours, healthy controls demonstrated faster high frequency maximum velocity and higher high frequency gradient than angina patients. Metoprolol and IS-5-MN increased the high frequency gradient and metoprolol tended to increase the maximum velocity. Metoprolol substantially decreased the low frequency/high frequency gradient, velocity and maximum velocity. It is clear that rapid vagal withdrawal seemed to be a sign of a healthy autonomic nervous system in the control group with healthy subjects. However, it was significantly lower in angina patients. While both drugs tended to normalize vagal withdrawal, metoprolol slowed down the rapid increase in sympathetic predominance in the morning in angina patients.

VARIATIONS IN CIRCADIAN RHYTHM AND BRAIN-HEART INTERACTION

HRV refers to the regulation of sinoatrial node, which is the natural pacemaker of the heart by the sympathetic and parasympathetic branches of the autonomic nervous system. It is possible that beat-to-beat fluctuations in the cardiac rhythm provide us with an indirect measure of heart health as defined by the degree of balance in sympathetic and vagus nerve activity. BPV and HRV may be quantified by around-the-clock serial measurement of blood pressure and heart rate as well as Holter electrocardiographic monitoring in the ward or clinic; these may be analysed by computer-implemented curve-fitting to assess the about 24 hour (circadian) variation among other rhythmic and chaotic components of the time structure (chronome) (2). As mentioned earlier, circadian, circannual, circaseptan (about 7 days) and other variations in the incidence of adverse, notably vascular events such as acute myocardial infarction (AMI), ischemia, sudden cardiac death and strokes have been noted in many studies (9–36). A casual blood pressure measurement or a casual electrocardiogram, accompanied by another check-up in 2 years may be misleading. An over-swinging of the blood pressure along the 24 hour scale or HRV may then be missed. This excessive circadian amplitude called circadian hyper-amplitude-tension (CHAT) (2) constitutes a new disease risk syndrome warranting screening, diagnosis and treatment. With or without the chronome adjusted mean value (MESOR), the circadian double amplitude, a measure of the extent of predictable change within a day, is also a predictor of vascular disease risk. An excessive amplitude was associated with an elevated left ventricular mass index in a retrospective chronometaanalysis of data from 424 patients (2,23) and with an increase in morbid events in a prospective 6 year follow-up study on 297 patients (24), as well as results obtained on the laboratory model of the stroke-prone spontaneously hypertensive rats (25). CHAT may be associated with a 720% increased risk of stroke (2,22). It seems that single measurement of blood pressure, or a single electrocardiogram should be replaced by an around-the-clock profile for a week or longer. In a recent study (33) in 86 adults, blood pressure records were obtained at 3 hour intervals for

7 days in each subject. The prevalence of MESOR hypertension was 12.0% and one known hypertensive had CHAT. These variations in blood pressures are risk factors for stroke and cardiac events.

There is clinical evidence that patients with decreased HRV die earlier than those with normal variability. It is possible that an understanding of mechanisms linking abnormal HRV to increased mortality might lead to specific therapeutic strategies which may reduce the risk of death for high risk patients. Recent studies indicate that low HRV is a predictor of arrhythmic cardiac death, myocardial infarction, rapid progression of atherosclerosis and death from heart failure (29–32). There are circadian rhythms for plasma levels of catecholamines, renin, angiotensin, aldosterone and serotonin (30–36). HRV appears to be quite important because it provides a trigger and other environmental factors (37–58). HRV also provides a window to study the hearts ability to respond to normal regulatory impulses which may influence its rhythm. Therefore, a primary focus of clinical work, as well as studies, is in finding out or modifying the balance in regulatory impulses from the vagus nerve and the sympathetic nervous system. Many studies are trying to find out the role of chemoreceptors, thermoreceptors, and the renin-angiotensin system (34–36).

NUTRITIONAL FACTORS AND BRAIN HEART CONNECTION

The brain-heart interaction through HRV as well as BPV appears to be under the influence of age, health status, lifestyle and nutritional factors (37–44). Christensen and co-workers (37) were the first to investigate the effect of dietary supplementation with n-3 fatty acids on HRV. Dietary n-3 fatty acids, in a randomized controlled trial in 81 patients with postmyocardial infarction, significantly increased HRV compared with controls indicating that an increased vagal cardiac tone may be beneficial in these patients. In a further study (38), these investigators reported that without dietary supplementation with n-3 fatty acids, there was a positive correlation between HRV and the content of n-3 fatty acids (docosahaexaenoic acid, DHA) in platelets in postmyocardial infarction patients with left ventricular dysfunction. This study also showed a negative correlation between the ratio of arachidonic acid /DHA and SDNN which is in line with earlier results, showing that this ratio is high in the heart muscle of men who die of SCD compared with controls (39). The increment in HRV seemed to be due to the intake of 1 fish meal per week with an increase in SDNN from 103 ms to 122 ms. Singh and co-workers in one randomized, controlled intervention trial (40), among 118 (fish oil group) and 122 (control group) patients with acute myocardial infarction, showed that treatment with fish oil was associated with significant reduction in cardiac events in the intervention group compared to control group (30 vs. 56, $P < 0.02$) after a follow-up of 1 year. While the majority of cardiac events were reported in the second (35.7 vs. 16.0%, $P < 0.01$) and fourth (28.5 vs. 16%, $P < 0.05$) quarters of the day compared to first (16.0%) and third (19.6%) quarter of the day, in control group, no such association was observed in fish oil group. The findings suggest that fish oil administration may have modulated circadian rhythm of cardiac events. Similar trends were reported in a randomized trial with coenzyme Q10 and placebo (n =

73 vs. 71) during a follow up of 4 weeks (41). The exact mechanism by which n-3 fatty acids increase HRV is not known but in vitro studies suggest that these fatty acids have beneficial effects on cardiac myocytes and neurones, similar to calcium blockers (42). There is strong evidence that n-3 fatty acids may inhibit sympathetic nervous activity and increase vagal tone which enhances the secretion of acetylecholine, resulting into increased HRV (43). However, all n-3 fatty acids do not provide the protection against adverse effects of autonomic dysfunction (43). In a recent intervention trial (44), treatment with alpha-linolenic acid which is a short chain n-3 fatty acids, showed no benefit in patients with low HRV. In a more recent study by Christensen et al. (45), each of the 291 patients that were referred for coronary angiography had completed a food questionnaire regarding fish and wine intake. The n-3 fatty acid composition of granulocyte membranes and of adipose tissue was measured and 24 hour HRV was analysed. Fish intake was positively associated with the level of n-3 fatty acids in adipose tissue. Significant positive correlation were found between HRV indices and the levels of n-3 fatty acids in granulocytes. Wine intake was also positively correlated with HRV, but this correlation was no longer significant after controlling for the cellular level of n-3 fatty acids. The positive association between n-3 fatty acids and HRV in patients with CAD indicates that n-3 fatty acids have a protective effect against HRV and possibly sudden cardiac death. It has been demonstrated that n-3 fatty acids incorporate in the phospholipids of the cell membrane and stabilize the excitatory neurones, cardiomyocyte and arterial smooth muscle as well as endothelial cells (43).

It is likely that adverse effects of elevated fatty acids, hyperglycemia, insulin resistance, obesity, pollution and exercise on HRV and BPV are modulated by interactions of multiple nutritional factors in providing the benefit. Some of these factors can independently have adverse effects on variability and other factors, such as exercise training, breathing exercises, meditation and drug therapy may be beneficial (29,44–58).

The effects of physical activity, exercise training, and breathing patterns have been studied in a number of studies (46–50). The heart beats about 100,000 times each day in human adults and changes in the cardiac frequency are of diagnostic importance among other features of circulation. Exercise training as part of a comprehensive cardiac rehabilitation program has been shown to improve morbidity and mortality rates in patients after myocardial infarction. It is possible that benefits of cardiac rehabilitation may be achieved through an altered cardiovascular autonomic tone. Exercise training has beneficial effect on autonomic tone whereas Duru and co-workers (47) reported no marked benefit of physical training on HRV. In this recent study, 25 men with an acute myocardial infarction and a low ejection fraction were randomly assigned to enter or not to enter a training program in a regional rehabilitation centre. HRV was evaluated before and after 1 and 2 months of training, and at 12 months. Resting heart rate was significantly decreased and the percentage of R-R intervals differing >50 ms from the proceeding one was also increased significantly after the training. The standard deviation of R-R intervals tended to increase but frequency domain indexes remained unchanged.

HRV is often recorded without measuring respiration; slow breaths might artificially increase low frequency power in RR interval and falsely mimic sympathetic activation (48,49). In 12 healthy volunteers, Benardi et al. (48) evaluated the effect of free talking and reading, silently and aloud, on respiration, RR and blood pressure. They also compared spontaneous breathing to controlled breathing and mental arithmetic, silent or aloud. The power in the so-called low and high frequency bands in RR and blood pressure was obtained from autoregressive power spectrum analysis. Compared with spontaneous breathing, reading silently increased the speed of breathing and decreased mean RR and RR variability and increased BP. Reading aloud, free talking and mental arithmetic aloud shifted the respiratory frequency into the low frequency band, thus increasing low frequency % and decreasing high frequency % to a similar degree in both RR and respiration with decrease in mean RR but with minor differences in crude RR variability. It is clear that simple mental and verbal activities markedly affect HRV through changes in respiratory frequency.

Age, sedentary habits, coronary artery disease, hypertension, diabetes, obesity, insulin resistance, pollution, hyperlipidemia, and hyperglycemia are risk factors of decreased HRV, and most of these factors are under influence of diet and lifestyle (54–58). We know that increased plasma fatty acids can stimulate sympathetic nervous system in animals. A recent study (54), in healthy subjects (20 intervention and 10 controls) were randomly assigned to receive an infusion of lipid emulsion or saline in the two groups respectively. Lipid emulsion infusion was associated with a rise in plasma epinephrine and norepinephrine concentrations in the experimental group compared to controls. The increase in plasma fatty acids was associated with a significant decline in RR interval and in total power. Analysis of different components of HRV showed that lipid emulsion infusion stimulated low frequency components at the second hour and at the third hour. Therefore, the low frequency/high frequency ratio was significantly stimulated at the second and the third hour. Such results persisted, although attenuated, when the study was repeated in association with propranolol infusion. It is possible that hyperlipidemia may stimulate cardiac autonomic nervous system activity resulting into a decrease in HRV (54).

The Framingham Heart Study was designed to examine the association of HRV with blood glucose levels in a population-based sample (55) because previous studies had demonstrated a reduced HRV among diabetics. Holter electrocardiography was done in 1919 subjects and HRV variables included the SD of normal RR intervals (SDNN), high frequency (HF, 0.15 to 0.40 Hz) and low frequency (LF, 0.04 to 0.15 Hz) power, and LF/HF ratio were inversely related to plasma glucose levels. SDNN and LF and HF powers were reduced in diabetes and in subjects with impaired fasting glucose levels (55). Short-term increases in particle air pollution have been associated with increases in daily cardiovascular mortality and morbidity in studies from cities throughout the industrialized world (58). We understand that in response to particle exposure, heart rate or rhythm abnormalities without hypoxia or respiratory distress may be present, indicating that particle air pollution may influence cardiovascular function. In one study (58), among 21 Boston residents, the association between ambient pollution levels and cardiovascular function through HRV were studied. The protocol involved 25 minutes per week of continuous Holter electrocardiographic monitoring. The findings showed that particle and ozone exposure may decrease vagal tone, resulting in reduced HRV (58).

ARRHYTHMIAS AND BRAIN-HEART INTERACTION

An acute precipitating trigger, present in the brain's suprachiasmatic nucleus and a chronic electrical instability of the myocardium, appear to be important in the pathogenesis of sudden cardiac death (SCD). Although sudden death has been commonly attributed to arrhythmias, recent data based on stored electrocardiograms (ECGs) of patients with implantable cardioverter defibrillators indicate that more than half of the deaths defined as sudden were not arrhythmic (59). The incidence of both non-sudden and sudden death among patients surviving AMI has declined significantly during the past two decades (59). Low HRV may be a better marker for increased risk of arrhythmic events than any other non-invasive measure. Prospective follow-up studies (60) indicate that low HRV is an independent predictor of SCD. Despite the general acceptance that low HRV is a marker of increased risk of arrhythmic death, there are many problems associated with the interpretation of the results that are used to support this hypothesis. Since all sudden deaths are not arrhythmic and the exact incidence of such deaths is low, even a large multicentre curve may not be able to give a definite answer regarding the value of HRV as a predictor of sudden arrhythmic death. In most of the randomized, controlled trials with n-3 fatty acids rich agents, there was a beneficial effect on SCD.

It seems that HRV is lower in patients with arrhythmias than in controls. However, significant overlapping in the measures of HRV was noted between the two groups and there may be some problems in careful matching of the patients with respect to all possible variables which can influence HRV. Ambulatory recordings suggest that HRV is altered before the spontaneous onset of ventricular tachyarrhythmia events indicating that low HRV may predispose to the onset of arrhythmias, or at least mark the presence of a transient trigger. Unfortunately, such studies are based on a small number of selected patients in which Holter ECG has been recorded for only 24 to 48 hours. Therefore, it would be important to further record Holter ECG for 7 days to be more definite regarding the role of HRV in the pathogenesis of arrhythmias. Animal experiments (61) have convincingly shown that abnormal autonomic regulation predisposes to life-threatening rhythm disturbances. Acute coronary occlusion in experimental models has been used to demonstrate the role of autonomic nervous system in the genesis of arrhythmias (61–62). The responses of autonomic nervous system to coronary occlusion have been found to predict ischaemia-induced ventricular fibrillation. During subsequent coronary occlusion in dogs without prior myocardial necrosis, the baseline reflex autonomic function, expressed as baroreflex sensitivity, has been shown to predict ventricular fibrillation, whereas baseline tonic autonomic function expressed as HRV does not (61).

Acute coronary artery occlusion during balloon angioplasty may cause variable and unpredictable alterations in HRV in humans (63). Although baseline HRV has no influence on ischemia-induced complex ventricular premature activity, the response of the HRV to acute coronary occlusion may be a predisposing factor. However, a 7-day record would be necessary to make final decision. In conclusion, these observations support the view that the responses of the autonomic nervous system to acute hemodynamic changes or ischemia may be more important in the genesis of life-threatening arrhythmias than the baseline autonomic regulation expressed as HRV. Available studies up to present time present no proof that patients with abnormal HRV have a greater risk of the life threatening ectopic activity (64,65). It is possible that low HRV measured as standard deviation of normal interval (SDNN) in conjunction with decreased ejection fraction has a low accuracy *for* prevention of SCD. However, heart rate dynamics, at the onset of ventricular tachyarrhythmias as retrieved from implantable cardioverter-defibrillators in patients with CAD may have better accuracy. Randomized, controlled intervention studies in the patients with abnormal HRV would be necessary to confirm the hypothesis of an association between low HRV and vulnerability to arrhythmic death (65).

CARDIOVASCULAR EVENTS AND BRAIN-HEART INTERACTION

Early detection of cardiac autonomic neuropathy permits individual risk stratification. HRV and baroreflex sensitivity are suggested to be superior to classic autonomic testing in that they detect neuropathy earlier with greater reliability. The Low SDNN has been demonstrated to be a predictor of death in the elderly. Data in younger subgroups indicate that low HRV indicates the occurrence of adverse cardiac events. One prospective study in Tokyo examined 297 patients for blood pressure variability who were followed up every 6 months, for 6 years for adverse vascular events (24,66). The incidence of ischaemic stroke and nephropathy was much higher in patients with an excessive swinging. All these studies, which included random samples of subjects from the general population, have shown that abnormal HRV and BPV predict various vascular events such as angina pectoris, myocardial infarction, and stroke mortality. More studies would be necessary to confirm that abnormal BPV is not only a marker of stroke but also predict cardiac events.

Several noninvasive methods have prognostic information regarding mortality and new coronary events after AMI. The practical for clinical decision making in the immediate post MI period is however less evident after thrombolysis. In a recent study (67) by Jensen-Urstad et al., a total of 100 patients who received thrombolysis after AMI, were studied by a 24 hour Holter recording with ST-analysis and analysis of HRV after a week of hospitalization. Mortality, nonfatal infarction, and the need for revascularization were followed for 12 months. A total of 6 patients died, 7 had nonfatal reinfarction and 23 were revascularized. Inability to perform an exercise test and an ejection fraction <40% were the only parameters separating those who died and the survivors. No method, including HRV, could predict a non-fatal infarction. A positive symptom limited exercise test, ST-depression on Holter ECG and reversibility on myocardial perfusion scintigraphy predicted the need for revascularization. It is not clear how many patients died due to SCD or due to arrhythmias. It is clear that analysis of HRV provides adequate information regarding prognosis, which is as good as a stress test and echocardiography, without any additional benefit.

BRAIN HEART INTERACTION AND PROGRESSION OF HEART FAILURE

The syndrome of congestive heart failure (CHF) entails complex autonomic and hormonal responses. Profound abnormalities in autonomic function, characterized by sympathetic overactivity and parasympathetic withdrawal, exert direct deleterious effects on the heart and contribute to progressive circulatory failure. In a recent study (68), by Burger and Aronson, in 64 patients with decompensated CHF, time and frequency domaine HRV indices were obtained from 24 hour Holter recording. Neurohormonal activation was assessed by measuring plasma renin activity, aldosterone and norepinephrine levels. In the time domaine, norepinephrine correlated negatively with average NN interval, SDNN and SDANN. In the frequency domaine, norepinephrine was negatively associated with total power and ultra low power. No correlation was found between indices indicative of parasympathetic modulation, except for a borderline correlation with the high frequency power. It is clear that reduced HRV may be associated with increased norepinephrine levels in patients with severe CHF.

Left ventricular hypertrophy and heart failure are a common mechanism of death among patients surviving a large AMI. Earlier studies did not give consideration that low HRV may be a prognostic marker of death from progressive heart failure. Reduced HRV and elevated heart rate reflect the degree of neurohumoral activation caused by impaired cardiac pump function. Therefore, they may influence left ventricular remodeling and the progression of heart failure. One large study revealed that low SDNN predicts deaths due to progressive heart failure but not the sudden death in patients with congestive heart failure (68). HRV has been shown to be decreased in patients with heart failure (68). In one study among 424 patients, each subject provided an echocardiogram in addition to a 24 hour ambulatory blood pressure profile (23). The left ventricular mass index was significantly elevated in subjects with CHAT compared to other subjects.

In chronic CHF, attenuated heart rate response to exercise, a manifestation of chronotropic incompetence contributes to limiting exercise capacity. A recent study (69), by Roche and co-workers, was conducted in 21 patients of CHF to evaluate the respective role of chronic attenuation of cardiac vagal tone associated with depressed baroreflex sensitivity or affected cardiac sympathetic responsiveness in CHF patients with chronotropic incompetence. All patients performed a symptom limited exercise test with measurement of gas exchange and chronotropic incompetence was noted in 14 patients. Although, there was no significant difference in baroreflex sensitivity, low frequency power of HRV in normalized units and SDNN were significantly lower in chronotropic incompetence patients. It is possible that basal depressed cardiac sympathetic tone contribute more closely than depressed baroreflex sensitivity to the impaired heart rate response to exercise. In healthy men, atrial natriuretic peptide infusion attenuates reflex increases in muscle sympathetic nerve activity and reduces low frequency components of HRV spectral power. Sympathoinhibitory actions have been documented in CHF, but the effects on the variability of muscle sympathetic nerve activity and HRV have not been described.

Increased tissue and systemic elaboration of cytokines have an important role in the pathogenesis of CHF through diverse mechanisms. Since cytokines are known to act at the neuronal levels in both the peripheral and central nervous system, there is a need to find out whether increased cytokines concentrations are associated with autonomic dysfunction that characterizes heart failure. In a further study by Aronson et al. (70), in 64 patients with decompensated CHF, autonomic function was assessed using time and frequency domaine HRV measures obtained from 24 hour Holter recordings. Plasma levels of norepinephrine, tumor necrosis factor-alpha and interleukin-6 were measured in all the patients. While TNF-alpha showed no correlation, interleukin-6 was inversely correlated with the time domaine parameters of SDNN and SDANN and with frequency domaine parameters of total power and ultra low frequency power. However, no correlation was observed between interleukin-6 and parasympathetic modulation. It is possible that the ability of long-term HRV parameters to better reflect activation of diverse hormonal systems may explain their greater prognostic power for risk stratification in patients with CHF.

BRAIN-HEART INTERACTION AND PROGESSION OF ATHEROSCLEROSIS

There is recent evidence in humans that decreased HR V and elevated 24 hour heart rate predict the progression of coronary atherosclerosis as assessed in serial quantitative coronory angiograms.

Rapid heart rate has been reported to predispose to the rapid progression of atherosclerosis in several animal models (71–73). It seems that adverse effects on hemodynamic factors due to low HRV and increased heart rate may be responsible for greater risk of atheroma development. Progression of coronary lesions has been shown to occur from the effects of heart rate on blood flow dynamics in the arterial wall (71–73). The influence of low HRV and elevated heart rate on the progression of atherosclerosis may well explain the finding that reduced SDNN is the predictor of late mortality better than early mortality in AMI patients treated with thrombolytic therapy. Sudden arrhythmic death occurs most often in the early phase after acute cardiovascular events and the progression of atherosclerosis. The occurrence of new coronary events is more likely the mechanisms of death which later follow (74). Type II diabetes and cardiac transplant recipients also have low HRV and greater heart rate which are associated with rapid progression of coronary artery disease.

NUTRITIONAL AND OTHER MECHANISMS OF BRAIN-HEART INTERATION

It is possible that neurohumoral activation and altered sympathovagal interaction, due to changes in the fatty acid, as well as phospholipid content of cell membranes of neurones and cardiac cells are the most common mechanisms of abnormal HRV of patients with heart disease. Suprachiasmatic nucleus, present in the brain is under strong influence of daylight and darkness and plasma melatonin levels secreted by the pineal gland. It may also be under influence of fatty acids, aminoacids and glucose. These nutrients are the chemical substances that are necessary to life processes such as metabolism, reproduction, motility and sensation. The nutrients found in food cannot be detected unless they interact specifically with appropriate components such as ligand binding proteins that may be linked to processes for their uptake or utilization. Glucose provides both energy to pancreatic beta cells and generates a signal that promotes insulin secretion. The functions may also be separate as in the use of glutamic acid for neuronal protein synthesis or for neurotransmission. Total and saturated fatty acids enhance sympathetic activity and catecholamines secretion and n-3 fatty acids increase the vagal activity and acetylecholine secretion. The melatonin secretion increases with darkness at night, which is beneficial to neurohumoral system, resulting into increased vagal tone and greater secretion of acetylcholine. However, daylight is associated with increased plasma concentration of cortisol and higher sympathetic activity resulting into cardiovascular dysfunction. Therefore, eating a heavy breakfast in the morning in conjunction with stress of the day and daylight may have multifold adverse effects on the brain-heart dysfunction resulting into greater cardiac events in the second quarter of the day. It seems that abnormal HRV may predict various causes of death as neurohumoral and sympathetic activation which contribute to arrhythmogenesis, cardiac events, stroke, progression of heart failure and atherogenesis. The biochemical factors responsible for these events may be greater levels of plasma cortisol, growth hormones, catecholamines, serotonin, angiotensin, renin, aldosterone which have a higher plasma concentration in the second quarter of the day when there is maximum sympathetic activity. The concentrations of protective factors such as, bradykinin, tissue plasminogen activator plasminogen activator inhibitor, magnesium, potassium, vitamin E and C and melatonin are lower in daytime (34–36). These disturbances in the biochemical factors may be associated with increased platelet aggregation, viscosity, hematocrit and hemoglobin as well as in greater heart rate, blood pressure, coronary artery tone, stroke volume and cardiac output and vascular resistance. It is possible that interaction of these biochemical factors with pathophysiological responses may result into sudden arrhythmic death, myocardial infarction, varient angina, transient myocardial ischaemia, progression of heart failure and heart failure death, as well as stroke and stroke death. Progression of atherosclerosis, as well as rupture of atheroma and thrombosis may also result due to these biochemical cardiovascular dysfunctions.

METHODOLOGY FOR MEASUREMENT OF HEART RATE VARIABILITY

There is no consensus about the best available index of HRV for clinical use. The Task Force of the North American Society of Pacing and Electrophysiology and the European Society of Cardiology have unified and standardized the methodology of HRV (75). Noisy data, artifacts, trends and ectopic beats are the major practical problems encountered in HRV measurements. A single HRV index would be an ideal method for clinical work that could be calculated reliably on the basis of a simple, widely available analytical method (75–81).

One of the commonly used prognostic HRV index is the SDNN analysed over a 24 hour period (59). The geometric triangular analysis method, developed by Malik et al. (76), perform as well as the traditional time domain analysis methods for risk stratification and do not suffer from the bias of human editing, but they are not widely available in commercial analysis systems. Poincare plot analysis of R-R intervals allows visual and quantitative analysis of instantaneous and continuous R-R interval variability and also provide more powerful prognostic information on patients with heart failure and on arrhythmic risk than the traditional time domaine methods (59). Spectral analyses of HRV allows assessment of frequency specific fluctuations in heart rate behaviour and provides prognostic information beyond the time-domain measures. The spectral methods are invalidated for wide clinical application by their numerous technical problems than in statistical or geometrical methods. Although all the statistical, geometrical and spectral measures of HRV differ in their manner of computation and analysis, these methods are fundamentally based on moment statistics and describe the magnitude of HRV. The average 24 hour heart rate also correlated relatively well with all the traditional measures of HRV (74). The prognostic information provided by the average 24 hour heart rate is almost as powerful as that obtained from a measurement of time domain HRV.

Several studies indicate that nonlinear dynamics may be involved in the genesis of HRV (77–79). But the clinical applicability of the methods based on nonlinear dynamics has not been tested in large scale studies until recently. Analysis of l/f characteristics (the inverse power-law slope) has provided prognostic information beyond the traditional HRV measures in two populations (59).

However, data on the patients with depressed left ventricular function indicate that fractal analysis of HRV produces more authentic prognostic information than the traditional nonspectral and spectral measures (63). Altered fractal properties of R-R intervals have also needed to compare the prognostic value and clinical utility of the various traditional and new HRV measures before the ideal index can be introduced for clinical intervention purposes (79–81).

In one study (81), Storck et al. studied the impact of ectopics on HRV analysis and the ability of filter algorithm to correct this. Power spectral analysis of synthetic data with an increasing proportion of ectopic beats and 24 hour Holter recordings from 98 healthy subjects and 93 post myocardial infarction patients was done with and without digital filtering and interpolation of error in the data stream. The analysis of HRV was seriously hampered by less than 1% of ectopic beats. A filter algorithm based on detection and linear interpolation of ectopic beats and other noise in the data stream, corrected effectively for the extravariability related to non-normal beats. The software could automatically process over 124 hour files in one batch. HRV analysis should include filtering for ectopic beats even with a small number of such beats. It is possible to make a fast analysis automatically in huge clinical series, which makes it possible to use the method both clinically and in epidemiological studies.

NUTRITIONAL AND OTHER FACTORS IN THE MANAGEMENT OF BRAIN-HEART FUNCTION

There is no definite management of circadian rhythms, HRV and BPV. However, one study by Watanabe and coworkers showed that meditation may have a beneficial effect on BPV (29). Exercise training, breathing exercises, trimetazidine, beta-blockers, ACE-inhibitors, n-3 fatty acids, oestrogens, ubiquinone, spironolactone have been observed to have beneficial effect on HRV and BHV (37–43). Experimental evidence suggests that aldosterone may have detrimental effects on the autonomic nervous system, especially during the morning hours. It is possible that spironolatone therapy given in addition to angiotensin converting enzyme inhibition may improve survival in CHF. In a recent study (82) by Yee et al., 28 patients with NYHA class II and III heart failure received 50 mg spirolactone daily and placebo for 4 weeks each, in a double-blind crossover fashion. After each treatment phase, a full circadian assessment was undertaken of its autonomic effects. Spironolactone significantly reduced all indices of QT dispersion. The reductions in Qtcmax, QTd and QTcd were greatest at 6 a.m. In addition, spironolactone had favourable autonomic effects which were limited to morning including heart rate reduction and improvement in HRV. Betablockers in CHF act by improving autonomic dysfunction however, patients with profound neurohumoral abnormalities derive better survival benefit. In one study (83) by Aronson and Burger, time and frequency domain HRV indices were obtained from 24 hour Holter recordings and compared to assess the role of betablockade in 199 patients with decompensated heart failure. All HRV indices were markedly suppressed but were substantially higher in patients who were on betablockers. Time domain measures parasympathetic cardiac activity, the percentage of RR intervals with >50 ms variation and the squire root of mean squired differences of successive R-R intervals were higher in betablocker group. Spectral analysis revealed that the total power and ultra low frequency power were significantly higher in patients on betablockers (82% vs 59%). The high frequency power, a spectral index of parasympathetic modulation, was 41% higher in the betablocker group. Norepinephrine and interleukin-6 levels were substantially lower in patients on betablockers (28% and 61% respectively), although these differences were not significant. It is clear that betablockers improve the impaired cardiac autonomic regulation during high sympathetic stress of decompensated CHF which plays an important role in the protection of myocardium and prevention of arrhythmias during transient increases in sympathetic activity. In a further study (84) by Lin et al., sequential 24-hour Holter recordings were obtained at baseline and 1 and 3 months after addition of atenolol therapy for advanced congestive heart failure in 10 patients. The slope and intercept of the regression line of power-law behaviour, the short and intermediate term of detrended flucturated analysis, the approximate entropy and the standard frequency spectra of the 24 hour were compared sequentially, as well as with those in 12 age-matched normal controls. The results showed that the slope and the intercept of the regression line of power law behaviour and the short term detrended fluctuated analysis; the approximate entropy increased after 3 months of atenolol treatment. The evolution of the slope or intercept of the regression line of the HRV power spectrum did not correlate with the echocardiographic or clinical cardiac function or with frequency spectral components of the HRV. It is possible that betablocker therapy upregulated the fractal behaviour control of the HRV in patients with advanced congestive heart failure.

In acute MI, HRV is depressed due to increased sympathetic activity and/or decreased parasympathetic tone resulting into electrophysiological changes such as increased ventricular late potentials in the cardiovascular system. In one recent study (85) by Ulgen and co-workers, the effect of trimetazidine (20 mg thrice daily) was studied in 64 patients suffering from first Q, wave infarction. In 64 patients, 31 received trimetazidine plus other drugs while the remaining 33 patients were studied as controls. After treatment, HRV parameters reflecting parasympathetic activity were significantly higher in the trimetazidine group, whereas the low frequency component indicating sympathetic activity was similar in both groups. In addition, low frequency/high frequency ratio showing sympatho-vagal balance was significantly decreased in the trimetazidine group. It is clear that there is a beneficial role for betablockers, trimetazidine, spironolactone, n-3 fatty acids and meditation in the management of HRV. However, large randomized and controlled intervention trials would be necessary to confirm the beneficial effect of these agents on HRV.

REFERENCES

1. Singh RB, Weydahl K, Otsuka K, Watanabe S, Yano H, Mori H, Ichimaru Yo, Mitsutake G. 2001. Can nutrition influence heart rate and blood pressure variability. Biomedicine and Pharmacother J 55:7–18.
2. Halberg F, Cornelissen G, Halberg J, Fink H, Chen CH, Otsuka K, Watanabe Y, Kumagai Y, Syutkina EV, Kawasaki T, Uezono K, Zaho Z, Schewartzkoft O. 1998. Circadian hyper-Amplitude-Tension, CHAT: a disease risk syndrome of anti aging medicine. JAAM 1:239–259.
3. Singh RB, Pella D, Neki NS, Mestutake G, Niaz MA, Rastogi SS. 2003. Mechanism of acute myocardial infarction study. Bio Med Pharmacother J 56 (in press).
4. Vaidya AB, Bhatt MA. 1999. Chronobiology of ischaemic heart disease events: relevance of ancient insights in human lifestyle. J Asso Phys India 47:629–630.
5. Mehta SR, Das S, Karloopia SD, Mathur P, Dham SK, Raghunathan D. 1998. The circadian pattern of ischaemic heart disease in Indian population. J Asso Phys India 46:767–777.
6. Charaka Samhita (Charka, 600 BC). 1981. Translated by Sharma PV, Chaukhambha Orientalia, Varanasi, Delhi.
7. Sushruta Samhita (Sushruta, 600 BC). 1989. Translated by Bhisagratna Chaukhambha Sanskrit Series Office, Varanasi Vol 1–3.
8. Atharveda Samhita (3000–5000 BC). 1984. William Dwight Whitney, Ed. Charles Pockwell, Lanman, Harvard Oriental Series, Motilal Banarsidass, Delhi.
9. Pell S, D, Allonzo CA. 1963. Acute myocardial infarction in a large industrial population. JAMA 185:831–838.
10. Wennerblom B, LKurje L, Karsson T, Tygesen H, Vahisalo R, Hjamarson A. 2001. Circadian variation of heart rate variability and the rate of autonomic change in the morning hours in healthy subjects and angina patients. Int J Cardiol 79:61–69.
11. Churisna SK, Ganelina IE. 1975. On the distribution of incidence of acute myocardial within a 24-hour period. Kardiologia 15:115–118.
12. WHO International Study Group. 1976. Myocardial infarction community register. In: Public Health in Europe, Copenhagen, Regional office for Europe, 5:1–232.

13. Christ M, Seyffart K, Wehling M. 1999. Attenuation of heart rate variability in postmenopausal women on progestin containing hormone replacement therapy. Lancet 353:1939–1940.
14. La Rovere MT, Bigger Jr, Marcus FL. 1998. Baroreflex sensitivity and heart-rate variability in prediction of total cardiac mortality after myocardial infarction. Lancet 351:478–484.
15. Bigger JT Jr, Fleish JL, Steinman RC, Rolnitzsky LM, Kleiger RE, Rottman JN. 1992. Frequency domain measures of heart period variability and mortality after myocardial infarction. Circulation 85:164–171.
16. Rosano GM, Patrizi R, Leonardo F, Ponkowski P, Collins P, Sarrel PM, Chierchia SL. 1996. Effect of oestrogen replacement therapy in heart rate variability and heart rate in healthy postmenopausal women. Am J Cardiol 80:815–817.
17. Thombson DR, Blandord RL, Sutton TW, Merchant PR. 1985. Time onset of chest pain in acute myocardial infarction. Int J Cardiol 7:139–146.
18. Willich SN, Goldberg JG, Maclure M, Petrriello I, Muller JE. 1992. Increased onset of sudden cardiac death in the first 3 hours after awakening. Am J Cardiol 70:65–68.
19. Becker RC, Corrao JM. 1989. Circadian variations in cardiovascular disease. Clev Clin J Med 56:676–680.
20. Braunwald E. 1998. Unstable angina: an etiologic approach to management. Circulation 98: 2219–2222.
21. Muller JE, Befler GH, Stone PH. 1989. Circadian variation and triggers of onset of acute cardiovascular disease. Circulation 4:733–740.
22. Otsuka K (ed). 1998. Chronome and Janus-Medicine. Heart Rate Variability (HRV) and BP variability (BPV) from a view point of chronobiology and ecology. Medical Review, Tokyo, p. 213.
23. Chen CH, Ting CT, Lin SJ, Itsu TL, Chuo P, Kuo HS, Wang SP, Yin FCP, Chang MS. 1995. Relation between diurnal variation of blood pressure and left ventricular mass in a Chinese population. Am J Cardiol 75:1239–1243.
24. Otsuka K, Cornelissen G, Halberg F, Oehlert G. 1997. Excessive circadian amplitude increases risk of ischaemic stroke and nephropathy. J Med Eng Tech 21:23–30.
25. Kumagai Y, Shiga T, Sunaga K, Conelissen G, Ebihara A, Halberg F. 1992. Usefulness of circadian amplitude of blood pressure in predicting hypertensive cardiac involvement. Chronobiologia 19: 43–58.
26. Feign VL, Nititin Yu P, Vinogrodova TE. 1997. Solar and geomagnetic activities: are there associations with stroke occurrence. Cerebro Vas Dis 7:345–348.
27. Otsuka K, Cornelissen G, Halberg F. 1997. Age, gender and fractal scaling in heart rate variability. Clin Sci 93:299–308.
28. Otsuka K, Cornelissen G, Halberg F. 1997. Circadian rhythmic scaling of heart rate variability in health and coronary artery disease. Clin Cardiol 20:631–638.
29. Watanabe Y, Conelissen G, Halberg F, Saito Y, Fukuda K, Otsuka K, Kikuchi T. 1996. Chronobiometric assessment of autogenic training effects upon blood pressure and heart rate. Perceptual and Motor Skill 83:1395–1410.
30. Tamura K, Kohna I, Saito Y, Wakasugi K, Achiwa S, Imanishi Y, Cugini P, Halberg F. 1991. Antihypertensive individualized therapeutic strategy. Diffesa Sociale 6:109–124.
31. Manfredini R, Gallerani M, Portaluppi F, Salmi R, Fesim C. 1997. Chronobiological patterns of onset of acute cerebrovascular disease. Thromb Res 88:451–463.
32. Cohen MC, Rohtla KM, Lavery CE, Muller IE, Mittleman MA. 1997. Metaanalysis of the morning excess of acute myocardial infarction and sudden cardiac death. Amer J Cardiol 79: 1512–1516.
33. Singh RB, Niaz MA, Kartikey K, Cornelissen G, Halberg F, Otsuka K, Schwartzkoft O. 2001. Prevalence and determinants of blood pressure variability in a population of North India. Biomedicine and Pharmacother, (Abstract) 55: p. 24.
34. Kukreja RS, Datta BN, Chakravarti RN. 1981. Catechoamine-induced aggravation of aortic and coronary atherosclerosis in monkeys. Atherosclerosis 40:291–298.
35. Cugini P, Letizia C, Searvo D. 1988. The circadian rhythmicity of serum angiotensin converting enzyme: its phasic relation with circadian cycle of plasma renin and aldosterone. Chronobiologia 15:229–232.
36. Veglio F, Pitrandice R, Ossola M, Vignani A, Angili A. 1997. Circadian rhythm of the angiotensin coverting enzyme activity in serum of healthy adult subjects. Chronobiologia 14:21–25.
37. Christensen IH, Gustenhoff P, Komp E, Aaroe I, Tofgt E, Moller I, Rasmusenn K, Dyerberg I, Schmidt

EB. 1996. Effect of fish oil on heart rate variability in survivors of myocardial infarction. Br Med I 312:677–678.
38. Christensen IH, Komp E, Aaroe I, Toft E, Moller I, Rasmusen K, Dyerberg I, Schmidt EB. 1997. Fish consumption, n-3 fatty acids in cell membranes, and heart rate variability in survivors of myocardial infarction with left ventricular dysfunction. Am I Cardiol 79:1670–1672.
39. Gudbjarnason S. 1989. Dynamics of n-3 fatty acids in phospholipids of heart muscle. I Intern Med 225(Suppl):117–128.
40. Singh RB, Niaz MA, Sharma IP, Kumar R, Rastogi V, Moshiri M. 1997. Randomized, double blind, placebo controlled trial of fish oil and mustard oil in patients with suspected acute myocardial infarction. The Indian experiment of infarct survival. Cardiovasc Drug Ther 11:485–491.
41. Singh RB, Wander GS, Rastogi A, Shukla PK, Mittal A, Sharma IP, Mehrotra SK, Kapoor R, Chopra RK. 1998. Randomized, double blind, placebo controlled trial of coenzyme Q10 in patients with acute myocardial infarction. Cardiovasc Drug Ther 12:347–353.
42. Pepe S, Bogdonor K, Hallaq H, Spurgeon H, Leaf A, Lakatta E. 1994. Omega-3 polyunsaturated fatty acids modulates dihydropyridine effects on L-type Ca-channels, cytosolic Ca and contraction in adult rat cardiac myocytes. Proc Natl Acad Sci USA 91:8832–8836.
43. Chin JPF. 1994. Marine oils and cardiovascular reactivity. Prostaglandins Leukot Essent Fatty Acids 50:211–222.
44. Christensen JH, Christensen MS, Toft E, Dyerberg J, Schmidt EB. 2001. Alpha-linolenic acid and heart rate variability. Nutr Metab Cardiovasc Dis 10:57–61.
45. Christensen JH, Skou HA, Fog L, Hansen V, Vesterlund T, Dyerberg J, Toft E, Schmidty EF. 2001. Marine n-3 fatty acids, wine intake, and heart rate variability in patients referred for coronary angiograph. Circulation 103:623–635.
46. Perini R, Milesi S, Fisher NM, Pendergast DR, Veicsteinas A. 2000. Heart rate variability during dynamic exercise in elderly males and females. Eur J Appl Physiol 82:8–15.
47. Duru F, Chandinas R, Dziekan G, Goebbels U, Myers J, Dubach P. 2000. Effect of exercise training on heart rate variability in patients with new onset left ventricular dysfunction after myocardial infarction. Am Heart J 140:157–161.
48. Bernardi L, Wdowczyk-Szule J, Vaenti C, Castoldi S, Passino C, Spadacini G, Sleight P. 2000. Effects of controlled breathing, mental activity and mental stress with or without verbalization on heart rate variability. J Am Coll Cardiol 35:1462–1469.
49. Garcia-Conzalez MA, Vazquez' Seisdedos C, Pallas-Areny R. 2000. Variations in breathing patterns increase low frequency contents in HRV spectra. Physiol Meas 21:417–423.
50. Mortara A, La Rovere MT, Pinna GD, Maestri R, Capomolla S, Cobelli F. 2000. Non selective beta-adrenergic blocking agent, carvedilol, improves arterial baroflex gain and heart rate variability in patients with stable chronic heart failure. J Am Coll Cardiol 36:1612–1618.
51. Kruger C, Landerer V, Zugck C, Ehmke H, Kubler W, Haass M. 2000. The bradycardic agent zatebrandine enhances baroreflex sensitivity and heart rate variability in rats early after myocardial infarction. Cardiovasc Res 45:900–912.
52. Weydahl A, Conelissen G, Halberg F, Siegelova J, Kumagai Y, Otsuka K. 1998. Chronobiologic optimization of exercise physiology and practice guided by heart rate variability. Scripta Medica (BRNO), 71:215–230.
53. Korkmaz ME, Muderrisoglu H, Ulucam, Ozin B. 2000. Effects of spironolactone on heart rate variability and left ventricular systolic function in severe ischemic heart failure. Am J Cardiol 86: 649–653.
54. Paolisso G, Manzella D, Rizzo MR, Ragno E, Barbieri M, Varricchio G, Varricchio M. 2000. Elevated plasma fatty acid concentrations stimulate the cardiac autonomic nervous system in healthy subjects. Am J Clin Nutr 72:723–730.
55. Singh JP, Larson MG, O'Donnell CJ, Wilson PF, Tsuji H, Lloyd-Jones DM, Levy D. 2000. Association of hyperglycemia with reduced heart rate variability (The Framingham Heart Study). Am J Cardiol 86:309–311.
56. Lanza GA, Giordano A, Pristipino C, Calcagni ML, Meduri G, Trani C, Franceschini R, Crea F, Troncone L. 2000. Relationship between myocardial 1231-metaiodobenzyl-guanidine scientigraphic uptake and heart rate variability in patients with syndrome X. Ital Heart J 1:221–225.
57. Paolisso G, Manzella D, Montano N, Gambradella A, Varricho M. Plasma leptin concentrations and cardiac autonomic nervous system in healthy subjects with different body weights. J Clin Endocrinol Metab 85:1810–1814.
58. Gold DR, Litonjua A, Schwartz J, Lovett E, Larson A, Nearing B, Allen G, Verrier M, Cherry R, Verrier R. 2000. Ambient pollution and heart rate variability. Circulation 101:1267–1273.

59. Kleiger RE, Miller JP, Bigger JT Jr, Moss AJ for the Multicentre Post Infarction Research Group. 1987. Decreased heart rate variability and its association with increased mortality after acute myocardial infarction. Am J Cardiol 59:256–262.
60. Bigger JT Jr, Fleiss JL, Rolnitzky LM, Steinman RC. 1993. Frequency domain measures of heart period variability to assess risk of late myocardial infarction. J Am Coll Cardiol 21:296–304.
61. Schwartz Pl, La Rovere MT, Vanoli E. 1992. Autonomic nervous system and sudden cardiac death: experimental basis and clinical observations for post-myocardial infarction risk stratification. Circulation 85(Suppl 1):77–91.
62. Schwartz Pl, Billman GE, Stone HL. 1984. Autonomic mechanisms in ventricular fibriliation induced by myocardial ischemia during exercise in dogs with a healed myocardial infarction. An experimental preparation for sudden cardiac death. Circulation 69:780–790.
63. Bonnemeier H, Hartmann F, Wiegant UK, Irmer C, Kurz T, Tolg R, Katus HA, Richardt G. 2000. Heart rate variability in patients with acute myocardial infarction undergoing primary coronary angioplasty. Am J Cardiol 85:815–820.
64. Lucreziotti S, Gavazzi A, Scolsi L, Inserra C, Klersy C, Campana C, Ghio S, Vanoli E, Tavazzi L. 2000. Five-minute recording of heart rate variability in severe chronic heart failure: correlates with right ventricular function and prognostic implications. Am Heart J 139:1088–1095.
65. Stein PK, Domitrovich PP, Kleiger RE, Schechtman KB, Rottman JN. 2000. Clinical and demographic determinants of heart rate variability in patients post myocardial infarction: insights from the cardiac arrhythmia suppression trial (CAST). Clin Cardiol 23:187–194.
66. Otsuka K, Conelissen G, Halberg F. 1996. Predictive value of blood pressure dipping and swinging with regard to vascular disease risk. Clin Drug Investag 11:20–31.
67. Jensen-Urstadf M, Samad BA, Jensen-Ursted K, Hulting J, Ruiz H, Bouvier F, Hojer J. 2001. Risk assessment in patients with acute myocardial infarction. J Intern Med 249:527–537.
68. Burger AJ, Aronson D. 2001. Activity of neurohormonal system and its relationship to autonomic abnormalities in decompensated heart failure. J Card Fail 7:122–128.
69. Roch F, Pichot V, Da Costa A, Isaaz K, Costes F, Dall Acqua T, Duverney D. 2001. Chronotopic incompetence response to exercise in congestive heart failure, relationship with cardiac autonomic status. Clin Physiol 21:335–342.
70. Aronson D, Mittleman MA, Burger AJ. 2001. Interleukin-6 levels are inversely correlated with heart rate variability in patients with decompensated heart failure. J Cardiovasc Electrophysiol 12:301–302.
71. Beere PA, Glagov S, Zarins CK. 1984. Retarding effect of lowered heart rate on coronary atherosclerosis. Science 226:180–182.
72. Kaplan JR, Manuck SB, Clarkson TB. 1987. The influence of heart rate on coronary atherosclerosis. J Cardiovasc Pharm 10(Suppl 2):S100–S102.
73. Caro CG, Fitz-Gerald JM, Schroter RC. 1969. Arterial wall shear and distribution of early atheroma in man. Nature 223:1159–1161.
74. Myerburg RJ, Kessler KM, Castellanos A. 1992. Sudden cardiac death. Structure, function, and time-dependence of risk. Circulation 85(Suppl 1):2–20.
75. Task Force of the European Society of Cardiology and the North American Society of Pacing and Electrophysiology. 1996. Heart rate variability, Standards of measurement, physiological interpretation and clinical use. Circulation 93:1043–1065.
76. Malik M, Hantkova K, Camm AJ. 1995. Practicality of postinfarction risk assessment based on time-domain measurement of heart rate variability. In: Heart Rate Variability. Ed. Malik M, Camm AJ, 393–406. Armonk, NY: Futura.
77. Goldberger AL. 1996. Non linear dynamics for clinicians; chaos theory, fractals and complexity at the bedside. Lancet 347:1312–1314.
78. Goldberger AL, West BJ. 1987. Fractals in physiology and medicine. Yale J Biol Med 60:421–435.
79. Camm AJ, Karam R, Pratt CM. 1998. The azimilide post-infarct survival evaluation (ALIVE) trial. Am J Cardiol 81:35–39.
80. Nisam S, Mower M. 1998. ICD trials; an extraordinary means of determining patients risk? PACE 21:1341–1346.
81. Storck N, Ericson M, Lindblad L, Jensen-Urstad M. 2001. Automatic computerized analysis of heart rate variability with digital filtering of ectopic beats. Clin Physiol 21:15–24.
82. Yee KM, Pringle SD, Struthers A. 2001. Circadian variation in the effects of aldosterone blockade on heart rate variability and QT dispersion in congestive heart failure. J Am Coll Cardiol 37: 1800–1807.
83. Aronson D, Burger AJ. 2001. Effect of beta blockade on autonomic modulation of heart rate and neurohormonal profile in decompensated heart failure. Ann Noninvasive Electrocardiol 6:98–106.

84. Lin LY, Lin JL, Du CC, Lai LP, Tseng Yz, Huang SK. 2001. Reversal of deteriorated fractal behaviour of heart rate variability by beta-blocker therapy in patients with advanced congestive heart failure. Cardiovasc Electrophysiol 12:33–35.
85. Ulgen MS, Akdemir O, Toprak N. 2001. The effects of trimetazidine on heart rate variability and signal-averaged electrocardiography in the early period of acute myocardial infarction. Int J Cardiol 77:255–262.

Frontiers in Cardiovascular Health, edited by
N.S. Dhalla, A. Chockalingam,
H.I. Berkowitz & P.K. Singal
Kluwer Academic Publishers, Boston, 2003

Vitamin D and Atherosclerosis: A Noteworthy Link

Chandrasekharan Cheranellore Kartha and S. Rajasree

Division of Cellular and Molecular Cardiology
Sree Chitra Tirunal Institute for Medical Sciences & Technology
Trivandrum—695011, India

Summary. A number of studies indicate a possible relationship of vitamin D with atherosclerotic diseases. Jim Moon, Bandy and Davison in 1992 observed that the epidemic of ischemic heart disease in North America paralleled the increased use of vitamin D and decreased availability of dietary magnesium. Linden had earlier found a direct correlation of dietary intake of the vitamin with susceptibility for myocardial infarction and suspected that the known hypercholestrolemic effect of the vitamin may be the mechanism. Animal experiments suggest vitamin D to be arteriotoxic. Massive doses of vitamin D induce atherosclerotic lesions in a number of animal species. Lesions similar to those in humans are found when animals are fed hypercholestrolemic diet, given large doses of vitamin D and exposed to nicotine.

The major source of vitamin D in adults is vitamin D synthesized in the skin through exposure to the sun. In tropical environment there is a possibility of high level of solar exposure and enhanced serum levels of vitamin D in the population. We explored the relation between serum level of 25-hydroxy vitamin D_3 and ischemic heart disease in a case-control study involving 143 patients with either angiographic evidence of coronary artery disease or patients with acute myocardial infarction and 70 controls, all men in the age group of 45–65 years. Serum levels of 25-hydroxy vitamin D_3, calcium, inorganic phosphate, cholesterol, low-density lipoprotein and triglycerides were elevated in a higher proportion of patients, compared to controls. Serum level of 25-OH-D_3 above 222.5 nmol/L (89 ng/ml) was observed in 59.4% of cases compared to 22.1% in controls ($p < 0.001$). Elevated serum 25 hydroxy vitamin D_3 levels (≥222.5 nmol/L, ≥89 ng/ml) are associated with a 3.18 fold (95% confidence interval of Odds Ratio: 1.31–7.73) increased rate of ischemic heart disease.

Address for Correspondence: Professor CC Kartha, MD, Professor & Head, Division of Cellular and Molecular Cardiology, Sree Chitra Tirunal Institute for Medical Sciences & Technology, Trivandrum—695011, India. Telephone: 91 471 2524608, Fax: 91 471 2446433, E-mail: cckartha@sctimst.ker.nic.in.

Considering the causal relation among calcium, vitamin D and arteriotoxicity, further investigations are warranted to probe whether the elevated serum levels of 25OH-vitamin D_3 observed in patients with ischemic heart disease in a tropical environment has any pathogenic significance.

Key words: Atherosclerosis, Cardiovascular Disease, Vitamin D, Tropical environment.

INTRODUCTION

A common feature of atherosclerosis is calcification of the arterial wall. For two centuries, coronary arterial calcification was considered to be the very essence of coronary sclerosis. Rudolf Virchow noted that vascular calcification was similar to bone formation and described atherosclerotic coronary lesion as an ossification and not mere calcification.

Arterial calcification and its role in atherogenesis were neglected in later years when it was realized that cholesterol and lipoproteins are more important in atherogenesis. With the development of angiographic techniques, arterial calcification was more easily recognized but was considered a manifestation of the later stages of the degenerative process of atherosclerosis. Atherosclerotic calcification is commonly regarded as a passive process of adsorption or precipitation, merely a secondary effect of advanced atherosclerotic degenerative process.

Atherosclerotic calcification begins as early as the second decade of life immediately after the formation of the fatty streak. Calcific deposits are however, found more frequently and in greater amounts in elderly individuals and in more complex lesions.

One of the most curious aspects of arterial calcification is its intimate association with atherosclerosis. The reason for this connection is completely unknown. High-resolution imaging studies using digital subtraction cinefluoroscopy (DSC), and ultrafast computed tomography (1–4) have revealed that calcification appears in atherosclerotic lesions much earlier than what was previously believed. Contrary to the earlier view that arterial calcification signifies dying cells, Doherty and Detrano hypothesized that arterial calcification is an organized, regulated process with cellular and molecular mechanisms similar to organized formation of bone (5). The mineral in atherosclerotic calcification is hydroxyapatite, the same mineral as in bone.

The molecular basis for arterial calcification has been extensively investigated (6). The role of mineralization in the pathogenesis and fate of the coronary plaque is unknown. The suspicion that calcium is involved in the atherogenic process is long standing, and has been reinforced by the finding in recent years that calcium antagonists and chelating agents can impede the process of atherogenesis in experimental animals (7). In man there is some evidence that calcium antagonists retard the progress of atherosclerosis.

VITAMIN D AND ARTERIAL CALCIFICATION

An important regulator of bone calcification and potentially of atherosclerotic calcification is the hormone $1,25(OH)_2D_3$, the most active form of vitamin D. Vitamin

D is formed from the precursor 7-dehydrocholesterol through ultraviolet activation in the skin and it is speculated that perhaps oxidized form of cholesterol may mimic some of the molecular actions of vitamin D. It is also known that vitamin D ingested in the diet is carried in the circulation bound to lipoproteins. Thus, entry of lipoproteins into the artery wall may also facilitate entry and accumulation of the promineralization factor vitamin D in the arterial wall.

Calcitriol, $1,25(OH)_2D_3$, the most active metabolite of vitamin D, because of its lipid solubility and low molecular weight, passes readily through the cell membrane into the interior of the cell, where there are specific receptors to which it attaches. The receptor–sterol complexes then migrate into the nucleus of the cell, interacts with DNA, and then alter the transcriptional activity of the gene (8).

In the classical target tissue, $1,25(OH)_2D_3$ receptor binding and nuclear association results in transcription of new mRNA species (9–12). The induced proteins usually include one or more calcium binding proteins (13–15).

Receptors have been identified for $1,25(OH)_2D_3$ in a wide variety of tissues including the arterial wall (16). J. Merke and colleagues documented the presence of specific vitamin D receptor (VDR) in cultured bovine aortic endothelial cells (17). Their data reveal that endothelial cells are a target site for both $1,25(OH)_2D_3$ production and receptor mediated actions. Authors comment that endothelial cells have the molecular machinery to react to $1,25(OH)_2D_3$. Because injury to the endothelial lining is a key facet of the current theory on the pathogenesis of atherosclerosis, a negative or positive influence of $1,25(OH)_2D_3$ in the re-endothelialization process could be of great significance in determining formation of atherosclerotic plaques.

POSSIBLE ROLE OF VITAMIN D TOXICITY IN THE PATHOGENESIS OF CARDIOVASCULAR DISEASES

Several lines of evidences point to a possible relationship between vitamin D toxicity and cardiovascular diseases. Jim Moon, Bandy and Davison in 1992 drew attention to the epidemic of ischemic heart disease (IHD) in North America, which directly paralleled with the increased use of vitamin D (18).

In 1917 the curative effect of cod liver oil in rickets was documented. Six years later, the import of fish liver oil in the United States of America (USA) rose from 500,000 gallons to 2.5 million gallons. Next year onwards the use of UV-irradiated milk was introduced in the USA. During the years 1948 to 1972 the manufacture of vitamin D rose from 35 lb to 14,000 lb. During the latter part of this period, vitamin D_2 was added to baked foods, breakfast cereals, milk, poultry products, baby foods and non-alcoholic beverages. Vitamin D tablets containing 200 IU were commonly sold in drug stores at that time. Along with the excessive delivery of vitamin D, there was also a continually declining intake of magnesium thanks to the use of magnesium deficient artificial fertilizers and many processing procedures that decreased magnesium content in foods. Moon, Bandy and Davison argue that the epidemic of IHD in North America is related to the increased use of vitamin D. Interestingly, from 1970 onwards, that is, ten years after Food Drug Act considered legislation to limit the amounts of vitamin D delivered to the USA, death rate from IHD in the USA began to decline.

Epidemiological studies have found correlation of moderately high vitamin D intake with the pathogenesis of cardiovascular disease. V. Linden examined in Tromso, Norway the data of patients with myocardial infarction and found a correlation between moderately high intake of vitamin D with increased incidence of myocardial infarction, renal calcinosis and urolithiasis (19). He concluded that, where intake of natural foods rich in vitamin D is common, there is increased incidence of hypercholesterolemia and susceptibility to sudden death from IHD. Linden emphasized the involvement of vitamin D in coronary disease and suspected that the known hypercholesterolemic effect of vitamin D might be the mechanism.

Hywel Davies in a provocative article focused on the early events in atherosclerosis that occur in coronary arteries of transplanted hearts (20). Coronary arterial intima, following injury undergoes a sequence of changes before the appearance of lipids. The first stage is intimal hyperplasia and disruption of the internal elastic laminae. Then the medial smooth muscle cells migrate in to the intima. Lipid incursion occurs later. The lesion seen in transplant arteriopathy is indistinguishable morphologically from that which is found in classical atherosclerosis. The early intimal and medial changes may be immune mediated in the arteries of transplanted hearts. Davies argues that a search for the cause of atherosclerotic diseases should focus on the pre-lipid stages. The lipids are possibly complicating rather than causative factors. According to Davies mitogens such as vitamin D may also catalyze the aberration of the normal mechanisms controlling cellular proliferation (20).

There are also several studies, which contradict the view that vitamin D is a causative factor for atherosclerotic heart disease. Schmidt et al. (1977) observed in their study that there is no difference between serum 25-OH-D_3 levels in patients with myocardial infarction (MI) and the levels in controls (21). Scragg and co-workers found an inverse association between plasma 25-hydroxyvitamin D_3 and myocardial infarction in a community based case-control study (22). While K.E. Watson et al. reported an inverse correlation of $1{,}25(OH)_2D_3$ with the extent of vascular calcification in patients with coronary artery disease, Y. Arad et al. did not find any correlation between serum levels of calcium, $1{,}25(OH)_2D_3$ or parathyroid hormone (PTH) to coronary calcification or to the extent of coronary stenosis (23,24).

EXPERIMENTAL EVIDENCES FOR ARTERIOTOXICITY OF VITAMIN D

Arteriotoxicity of vitamin D has been known for many years. There are experimental data that indicate a causative role for vitamin D in atherosclerosis. Several studies have been conducted in animals by oral feeding or intravenous injection of vitamin D metabolites and observing the pathological changes in the cardiovascular system. W. Donath and De Langen showed that vitamin D significantly alters the formation of atheroma in rabbits (25). High doses of vitamin D changes the concentration of both cholesterol and total lipids in blood and induces hyperphosphatemia, factors which favor the formation of atheroma.

Investigations in rats by Eisenstein and Groff indicate effects similar to those observed in rabbits (26). Massive doses produce a marked increase in serum calcium and seromucoid levels. There is increased calcareous deposition in the heart, kidneys and blood vessels together with accumulation of polysaccharides at those sites. M.G. Hass et al. induced medial calcification with secondary mesenchymal reactions in aortas of rabbits by feeding or injection of high doses of vitamin D for 4 weeks (27). Extensive atherosclerotic lesions were seen by Bajwa, Morrison and Ershoff (1971) in the aorta and coronary artery in rats on vitamin D supplemented diet after 6 weeks (28). Lesions were mostly in the media and consisted of degeneration, calcification, plaque formation, metachromatosis and lysis and fragmentation of the elastic lamina. Some of the surviving animals had subintimal mesenchymal cell proliferation in the vessels. T. Toda, Leszczynski and Kummerow used swine and rabbits to study the possible role of vitamin D_3 in the initiation and development of atherosclerosis (29). In swine, sequential aortic changes were examined with the aid of electron microscope. Fibromuscular intimal thickening was seen in the ascending and thoracic aorta of the swine fed 62,500 IU vitamin D_3/Kg of diet for three months. Three months after vitamin D_3 withdrawal, atherosclerotic lesions were found. In rabbits, pronounced aortic smooth muscle cell necrosis developed after forced feeding 10,000 IU of vitamin D_3 daily. Serum analysis indicated that blood calcium did not differ from that of animals fed corn oil alone, but the level of serum 25-OH-D_3, measured by high pressure liquid chromatography (HPLC) was 30 times more than that in the control animals. These data suggest that cholecalciferol (the oxidized sterol with vitamin D_3 activity) affects the integrity of the arterial wall.

M.R. Hughes et al. have suggested that in vitamin D toxicity, target tissues are responding to high plasma concentration of 25-OH-D_3 (30). When concentration is high, 25-OH-D_3 can bind to VDR and mimic the actions of 1,25$(OH)_2D_3$. M.J. Beckman and co-workers demonstrated that VDR up regulation occurs in vitamin D excess (31). VDR up regulation may play a significant role in the pathogenesis of hypervitaminosis D by enhancing target cell responsiveness. E. Koh et al. have shown the presence of 1,25$(OH)_2D_3$ receptor in rat coronary artery smooth muscle cells and also dose dependent enhancement of proliferation and change in shape of the smooth muscle cells when exposed to 1,25$(OH)_2D_3$ (16). I. Tsutomu and Hiroyuki found that 1,25$(OH)_2D_3$ stimulates calcium uptake in vascular smooth muscle cells (32). The effect is dose dependent at physiological concentrations and is specific for the sterol.

In experiments in rabbits Rajasree and colleagues observed that calcific lesions in aortas are also associated with significant up regulation of 1,25$(OH)_2D_3$ receptors in aortic media as well as enhanced uptake of ^{45}Ca in medial smooth muscle cells (33). Calcium levels in aorta correlate with the tissue levels of vitamin D receptor (VDR) and ^{45}Ca uptake by smooth muscle cells, which demonstrate that greater tissue VDR concentration, is associated with increased tissue responsiveness. These findings support the hypothesis that in hypervitaminosis D, the toxic effect of elevated 25-OH-D_3 is mediated by up regulation of VDR in aortic media resulting in enhanced VDR/hormone binding and consequent increased uptake of calcium by medial smooth muscle cells. Increased tissue responsiveness because of accumulation of $1,25(OH)_2D_3$ cannot however be ruled out given the earlier observation that an excess concentration of 25-OH-D_3 does competitively inhibit degradation of $1,25(OH)_2D_3$, thus increasing the level of the active metabolite in the tissues (31).

RELEVANCE OF VITAMIN D TOXICITY IN A TROPICAL ENVIRONMENT

It is accepted that the major source of vitamin D is skin exposed to the UV β rays contained in sunlight. Given the global differences in UV radiations and in dietary sources of vitamin D, disparities in vitamin D status can be expected among populations of different regions of the world. One undeniable feature of the equatorial region is that there is much sunlight and the intensity of UV radiation is high and continuous. Exposure of skin for 5–8 hours spread over 11 weeks can raise vitamin D levels in serum from 10 ng/ml to 100 ng/ml (34). Repeated total body exposures causing mild erythema raise plasma 25-OH-D_3 concentration as much as long-term ingestion of 10,000 IU of vitamin D per day does (35).

There are also other possible sources of vitamin D in the tropics. Vitamin D status of cow's milk depends on exposure to sun. In winter the vitamin D levels in cow's milk are reported to be 4 IU/ quarts where as in summer it is 40 IU/quarts. Plants too are good sources of vitamin D. *Cestrum diurnum* and *Solanum malacoxylon* have calcinogenic properties (36). Vitamin D activity in *Cestrum diurnum* naturalized at Hyderabad in Central India was found to be 3 times higher than the activity reported from the West (37). Planktons in tropical environment (collected from Hussain Sagar Lake, Hyderabad) are rich in vitamin D and vitamin D levels are high when compared to western data (38). Fish liver also contains high concentration of vitamin D. The levels differ according to geographical climate.

On these bases we felt that the population of Kerala state in southern India would be ideal to investigate the relationship between vitamin D and ischemic heart disease. Kerala is situated in the coastal belt near the equator (approximate latitude 8°N, longitude 74°E). There is abundant sunshine throughout the year, with high level of ultraviolet radiation. Despite skin pigmentation, the likelihood of substantial cutaneous synthesis of vitamin D is high. The average consumption of fish and sterol-containing tubers (e.g.: cassava) is high in this region and this too might result in a higher vitamin D status. We explored the relation between serum level of 25-hydroxyvitamin D_3 and ischemic heart disease in a case-control study involving 143 patients with either angiographic evidence of coronary artery disease or patients with acute myocardial infarction and 70 controls, all men in the age group of 45–65 years (39). Fasting blood samples were collected, serum separated and serum levels of 25-hydroxyvitamin D_3 was measured by protein binding radioligand assay. Serum levels of cholesterol, triglyceride, calcium, magnesium and inorganic phosphate were also determined. Prevalence of diabetes, hypertension and smoking history was noted. Statistical comparisons of variables between cases and controls were done using Chi-squared tests. Multivariate logistic regression analysis was done to examine the association of ischemic heart disease with serum levels of 25-hydroxyvitamin D_3 controlling for selected variables. Serum levels of 25-hydroxyvitamin D_3, calcium, inorganic phosphate, cholesterol, low density lipoprotein and triglycerides were elevated in a higher proportion of patients, compared to controls. Serum levels of 25-OH-D_3 above 222.5 nmol/L (89 ng/ml) were observed in 59.4% of cases compared to 22.1% in controls ($p < 0.001$). Elevated serum 25-hydroxyvitamin D_3 levels (≥222.5 nmol/L, ≥89 ng/ml) are associated with a 3.18 fold (95% confidence interval of Odds Ratio; 1.31–7.73) increased rate of ischemic heart disease (39).

Results of our study suggest that vitamin D may play a role as one of the risk factors for ischemic heart disease in patients in a tropical environment. Vitamin D is not an essential dietary component for the vast majority of people in the tropics and relatively small excess may be toxic in the long term. An average sized adult probably needs 100 or 200 units of vitamin D_3 per day from all sources including sunshine. M.F. Holick has pointed out that brief casual exposure of the face, arms and hands to sunlight is equivalent to ingesting 200 IU of vitamin D and repeated solar exposure causing mild erythema raises plasma 25 hydroxyvitamin D_3 concentrations as much as does the long term ingestion of 10,000 IU of vitamin D_3 per day (35). W.F. Loomis calculated that mere exposure of the skin of the cheeks of fair, thin-skinned children provides about 400 units daily, a conclusion confirmed by Holick et al. (40,41).

Serum 25 hydroxyvitamin D_3 levels are enhanced after short-term ultraviolet exposure either from natural sunlight (42) or artificial ultraviolet irradiation (43). Increased plasma levels of 25 hydroxyvitamin D_3 have been reported in two individuals exposed to tropical sunlight, during a vacation of one week (44). In another study, the average circulating levels of 25 hydroxyvitamin D_3 were found to rise in lifeguards after a minimum of four weeks of prolonged exposure to sunlight (45).

Skin pigment melanin is believed to act as a protective barrier against sunlight and UV exposure. Observations, in Blacks and Asian subjects following repeated exposure to UV radiation suggest that pigmentation has no significant effect on cutaneous synthesis of vitamin D (46). Clemens and co-workers found that skin melanin limits the role of skin vitamin D formation, but serum vitamin D_3 levels, could be raised in individuals with dark skin by increasing the amount of simulated solar radiation (47). The melanogenic response may be insufficient to inhibit cutaneous synthesis of vitamin D in persons who have continuous and prolonged or repeated solar exposure as in tropical regions.

Ultraviolet light, however strong and prolonged, cannot make people toxic to vitamin D, which may be true in adapted, indigenous populations, though not necessarily perhaps in people with very fair skin. If this is true, then the relevant factor has to be oral consumption of D_2 from plants, tubers etc. or $1,25(OH)_2D_3$ from plants as seen in enzootic calcinosis. Since the oral route bypasses the natural control mechanisms, on top of an already elevated blood level of $25(OH)_2D_3$ from sunshine the oral contribution could push the levels up to toxic ones (48,49). These factors would possibly explain the difference between our findings and those of Scragg et al. in a community in New Zealand (50).

Given the contradictory observations in two populations with dissimilar patterns of solar exposure and dietary practice, further research is needed before conclusions can be made about the relation between 25 hydroxyvitamin D_3 and ischemic heart disease. Our findings have possible pathogenic significance in the context of observations by L.B. Liu et al., that pathological lesions similar to human atherosclerosis were found in arteries of rhesus monkeys fed a hypercholesterolemic diet, given vitamin D_3 and exposed to nicotine (51). Given the causal relation among calcium, vitamin D and arteriotoxicity, further investigations are warranted to probe whether the elevated serum levels of 25 hydroxyvitamin D_3 observed in patients with ischemic heart disease in a tropical environment, has any pathogenic significance.

REFERENCES

1. Agatston AS, Janowitz WR, Hildner FJ, Lusmer WR, Viamonta M, Detrano R. 1990. Quantification of coronary artery calcium using ultrafast computed tomography. J Am Coll Cardiol 15:827–832.
2. Tanenbaun SR, Kondor GT, Vaselik KE. 1989. Detection of calcific deposits in coronary arteries by ultrafast computed tomography and correlation with angiography. Am J Cardiol 63:870–872.
3. Breen JF, Sheedy DF, Schwartz RS, Stanson AW, Kaufmann RB, Moll PP, Rumberger JA. 1992. Coronary artery calcification detected with ultrafast CT as an indication of coronary artery disease. Radiology 185:435–439.
4. Stary HE. 1990. The sequence of cell and matrix changes in atherosclerotic lesions of coronary arteries in the first forty years of life. Eur Heart J (Suppl E):3–19.
5. Doherty TM, Detrano RC. 1994. Coronary arterial calcification as an active process, a new perspective on an old problem. Calcif Tissue Int 54:224–230.
6. Jono S, Nishizawa Y, Shioi A, Morii H. 1998. 1,25 dihydroxyvitamin D3 increases in vitro vascular calcification by modulating secretion of endogenous parathyroid hormone-related peptide. Circulation 98:1302–1306.
7. Fleckenstein GG, Thimm F, Frey M, Czirfusz A. 1994. Role of calcium in atherosclerosis—Experimental evaluation of anti arteriosclerosis potencies of calcium antagonists. Basic Research in Cardiology (Suppl I) 89:145–159.
8. Alberts B, Bray D, Lewis J, Raff M, Roberts K, Watson JD. 1994. Steroids and the cell. In: Molecular Biology of the Cell. 729–30. New York, Garland Publishing Inc.
9. Emtage JS, Lawson DEM, Kodicek E. 1973. Vitamin D induced synthesis of mRNA for calcium binding protein. Nature 246:100–101.
10. Hausler MR, Mc Cain T. 1977. Basic and clinical concepts related to vitamin D metabolism and action. N Eng J Med 297:974–983 and 1041–1050.
11. Walters MR, Hunziker W, Norman AW. 1980. Unoccupied 1,25 dihydroxy vitamin D_3 receptors: Nuclear cytosol ratio depends on ionic strength. J Biol Chem 255:6799–6805.
12. Franceschi RT, Simpson RV, Deluca HF. 1981. Binding protein for vitamin D metabolites. Serum carriers and intracellular receptors. Arch Biochem Biophys 210:1–13.
13. Wasserman RH, Taylor AW. 1960. Vitamin D_3 induced calcium binding protein in chick intestinal mucosa. Science 152:791–793.
14. Siebert P, Hunziker W, Norman AW. 1982. Cell free translation analysis of the vitamin D dependent calcium binding protein mRNA activity present in total RNA and polysomal extracts from chick intestine. Arch Biochem Biophys 219:286–296.
15. Norman AW, Roth J, Orch L. 1982. The vitamin D endocrine system. Steroid metabolism, Hormone receptors and Biological Response. Endocr Rev 3:331–336.
16. Koh E, Morimoto S, Fukuo K, Itoh K, Hironaka T, Shiraishi T, Onishi T, Kumara Y. 1988. 1,25 dihydroxy vitamin D_3 binds specifically to rat vascular smooth muscle cells and stimulates their proliferation in vitro. Life Sciences 42:215–223.
17. Merke J, Milde P, Lewicka S, Hugel U, Klaus G, Mangelsdorf DJ, Haussler MR, Rauterberg EW, Ritz E. 1989. Identification and regulation of 1,25 dihydroxy vitamin D_3 receptor activity and biosynthesis of 1,25 dihydroxy vitamin D_3. Studies in cultured bovine aortic endothelial cells and human dermal capillaries. J Clin Invest 83:1903–1915.
18. Moon J, Bandy B, Davison AJ. 1992. Hypothesis: Etiology of atherosclerosis and osteoporosis: Are imbalances in the calciferol endocrine system implicated? J Am Coll Nutr 11:567–583.
19. Linden V. 1974. Vitamin D and myocardial infarction. Br Med J 3:647–658.

20. Davies H. 1989. Coronary heart disease. The significance of coronary pathology in infancy and the role of mitogens such as vitamin D. Med Hypothesis 30:179–185.
21. Schmidt GH, Goosen J, Lindle F, Seidal D. 1977. Serum 25 hydroxy cholecalciferol in myocardial infarction. Atherosclerosis 26:55–58.
22. Scragg R, Jackson R, Holdaway IM, Lim T, Beaglehole R. 1990. Myocardial infarction is inversely associated with 25-dihydroxy Vitamin D_3 levels. A community based study. Int J Epidemiol 19:59–63.
23. Watson KE, Abrolat ML, Malone LN, Hoeg MM, Doherty T, Detrano R, Demer L. 1997. Active serum vitamin D levels are inversely correlated with coronary calcification. Circulation 96:1755–1760.
24. Arad Y, Spadaro LA, Roth M, Scordo J, Goodman K, Sherman S, Lerner G, Newstein D. 1998. Serum concentration of calcium, 1,25-vitamin D and parathyroid hormone are not correlated with coronary calcifications. An electron beam computed tomography study. Coronary Artery Disease 9:513–518.
25. Donath W, De Langen C. 1956. Vitamin D sclerosis of the arteries and the danger of different forms of arterioclerosis. Acta Med Scand 156:317–325.
26. Eisenstein R, Groff W. 1957. Experimental hypervitaminosis D: Hypercalcemia, hypermucoproteinemia and metastatic calcification. Proc Soc Exp Biol Med 94:441–444.
27. Hass MG, Trueheart RE, Taylor BC, Stump M. 1958. An experimental histological study of hypervitaminosis D. Am J Pathol 34:395–431.
28. Bajwa GS, Morrison LM, Ershoff BH. 1971. Induction of aortic and coronary athero-arteriosclerosis in rats fed a hypervitaminosis D, cholesterol-containing diet. Proc Soc Exp Biol Med 138:975–982.
29. Toda T, Leszczynski DE, Kummerow FA. 1983. The role of 25-OH-vitamin D_3 in the induction of atherosclerosis in swine and rabbit by hypervitaminosis D. Acta Pathol Jpn 33:37–44.
30. Hughes MR, Baylink DJ, Jones PG, Haussler MR. 1976. Radioligand receptor assay for 25 hydroxyvitamin D_2/D_3 and 1,25 dihydroxyvitamin D_2/D_3. Applications to hypervitaminosis D. J Clin Invest 58:61–70.
31. Beckman MJ, Horst RH, Reinhardt TA, Beitz DC. 1990. Upregulation of the intestinal 1,25 dihydroxyvitamin D_3 receptor during hypervitaminosis D. A comparison between vitamin D_2 and vitamin D_3. Biochem Biophys Res Comm 169:910–915.
32. Tsutomu I, Hiroyuki K. 1988. 1,25 dihydroxyvitamin D3 stimulates $^{45}Ca^{2+}$ uptake by cultured vascular smooth muscle derived from rat aorta. Biochem Biophys Res Commun 152:1388–1394.
33. Rajasree S, Umashankar PR, Lal AV, Sankara Sarma, Kartha CC. 2002. 1,25-dihydroxyvitamin D_3 receptor is upregulated in aortic smooth muscle cells during hypervitaminosis D. Life sciences 70:1777–1788.
34. Davie M, Lawson DEM. 1980. Assessment of plasma 25-hydroxyvitamin D_3 response to ultraviolet irradiation over a controlled area in young and elderly subjects. Clin Sci 58:235–242.
35. Holick MF. 1992. Vitamin D-Solar rays, The Milky Way, or both? New Eng J Med 326:1213–1214.
36. Boland RL. 1986. Plant as a source of vitamin D3 metabolites. Nutr Rev 44:1–8.
37. Prema TP, Raghuramulu N. 1993. Vitamin D-like activity in Cestrum diurnum grown in Hyderabad, India. J Sci Food Agric 62:21–27.
38. Sunitha RD, Raghuramalu N. 1994. Provitamins D and vitamin D in plankton. (Abstract) 9th Workshop on vitamin D. 226.
39. Rajasree S, Rajpal K, Kartha CC, Sarma PS, Raman Kutty V, Iyer CSP, Girija G. 2001. Serum 25-hydroxyvitamin D_3 levels are elevated in South Indian patients with heart disease. Eur J Epidemiol 17:567–571.
40. Loomis WF. 1967. Skin pigment regulation of vitamin D biosynthesis in man. Science 57:501–506.
41. Holick MF, Mac Laughlin JA, Doppeet SH. 1981. Regulation of cutaneous previtamin D_3 photosynthesis in man: Skin pigment is not an essential regulator. Science 211:590–592.
42. Sedrani SH, Elidrissy T, El Arabi KM. 1983. Sunlight and vitamin D status in normal Saudi subjects. Am J Clin Nutr 38:129–132.
43. Matsuoka LY, Wortsman J, Hollis BW. 1990. Sun tanning and cutaneous synthesis of vitamin D_3. J Lab Clin Med 116:87–90.
44. Shepard R, Horst RL, De Luca H. 1979. Determination of vitamin D and its metabolites in plasma from normal and anephric man. Biochem J 182:55–69.
45. Haddad JG, Chyu KJ. 1971. Competitive protein binding radio assay for 25-hydroxycholecalciferol. J Clin Endocrinol 33:992–995.

46. Stamp TCB. 1975. Factors in human vitamin D nutrition and in the production and cure of classical rickets. Proc Nutr Soc 34:119–130.
47. Clemens TL, Henderson SL, Adams JS, Holick MF. 1982. Increased skin pigment reduces the capacity of skin to synthesize vitamin D_3. Lancet 1:74–76.
48. Stamp TCB, Haddad TG, Twigg CA. 1977. Comparison of oral 25-hydroxycholecalciferol, vitamin D and ultraviolet light as determinants of circulating 25-hydroxyvitamin D. Lancet 1:1341–1343.
49. Kummerow FA. 1979. Nutrition, imbalance and angiotoxins as dietary risk factors in coronary heart disease. Am J Nutr 32:58–83.
50. Scragg R, Holdaway I, Jackson R, Lim T. 1992. Plasma 25-hydroxyvitamin D_3 and its relation to physical activity and other heart disease risk factors in the general population. Ann Epidemiol 2:697–703.
51. Liu LB, Taylor CB, Peng SK, Mikkelson B. 1979. Experimental arteriosclerosis in Rhesus monkeys induced by multiple risk factors: cholesterol, vitamin D and nicotine. Arterial wall 5:25–32.

Frontiers in Cardiovascular Health, edited by
N.S. Dhalla, A. Chockalingam,
H.I. Berkowitz & P.K. Singal
Kluwer Academic Publishers, Boston, 2003

Congestive Heart Failure as Metabolic Disease

Josef Moravec

Laboratoire d'Energétique et de Cardiologie cellulaire
INSERM

Summary. The aim of the present paper is to recall some of our previous data which bring an evidence that hearts of rats with 3-mo-old aorto-caval fistula are metabolically restricted. Due to a 40 per cent depletion of tissue L-carnitine, related to impaired carrier-mediated carnitine transport, they are unable to utilize correctly both carbohydrates and long-chain fatty acids during in vitro per fusicus. This results in substrate limitation of their oxidative phosphorylation reflected by decreased VO_{2max}. At the same time, when supplied with 10 mM glucose, insulin and 1.2 mM palmitate, volume-overloaded hearts seem to operate at significantly higher $\Delta G'_{ATP}$ at each workload studied. The limitation of oxidative phosphorylation disappears when octanoate instead of palmitate is used for the in vitro perfusions. This short-chain fatty acid bypasses mitochondrial carnitine acyltransferases and, thus, improves mitochondrial NADH availability. This, per se, improves the kinetics of oxidative phosphorylation and left ventricular performance of volume-overloaded hearts. The long-term administration of propionyl-L-carnitine which restores tissue levels of L-carnitine has similar effects. In this latter case, we observe an acceleration of palmitate oxidation and an improved coupling between glycolysis and glucose oxidation. This recovery of both fatty acid and carbohydrate utilization improves mitochondrial NADH availability and, thus, increases VO_{2max} of volume-overloaded hearts. At the same time, cytololic phosphorylation potential and ADP_f become regulatory again. The restitution of energy transfer from metabolic substrates to cytosolic adenine nucleotides is thus associated with an acceleration of ATP turnover and with a significant improvement of left ventricular function. Our data suggest that the pathogenesis of congestive heart failure may involve a metabolic component, i.e. the simultaneous inhibition of long-chain fatty acid and glucose oxidation, which results in the kinetic failure of oxidative phosphorylation. It follows that appropriate pharmacological interventions that

Address for Correspondance: Dr. Josef Moravec, 13, rue Ernest Fabrègue 69009 Lyon-St. Rambert France. phone/fax: +33-450-81-0804, E-mail: moravec@wanadoo.fr improve mitochondrial NADH availability and, thus, the kinetics of oxidative phosphorylation may be used to delay the transition from cardiac hypertrophy to congestive heart failure. Prospective molecular mechanisms which may explain the recovery of contractile function in substrate-repleted mechanically-overloaded hearts are briefly discussed.

Key words: Cardiac hypertrophy, Congestive heart failure, Fatty acid oxidation rate, Glucose oxidation rate, Glycolysis rate, Kinetics of oxidative phosphorylation, L-carnitine.

INTRODUCTION

The adaptation of the heart to long-lasting mechanical overload proceeds via load-induced activation of protein kinase C and the subsequent upregulation of genes encoding for different protooncogenes (1,2). These early alterations are believed to trigger the initiation of compensatory cardiac hypertrophy and contribute to the appropriate remodelling of intracellular organelles (shift of myosin heavy chains from V_1 to V_3 isoforms, expression of skeletal α-actin, etc . . .). At the same time, the re-expression of genes encoding for different fetal proteins, including atrial and brain natriuretic factors (ANF, BNF) regularly occurs in ventricular cardiomyocytes exposed to mechanical overload (1–3). While MHC transition from fast (V_1) to slow (V_3) isoforms is believed to improve the efficiency of cardiac contractions (4), the elevated circulating ANF levels may, in turn, maintain natriuresis and blood pressure in a range permitting to moderate the outcome of surgically-induced overload to the heart. As concerns the principal metabolic changes encountered in mechanically-overloaded hearts, they have been told to serve the same finality as the above described upregulation of so-called fetal program (5). This may be, particularly, the case of downregulation of the subset of genes encoding for enzymes involved in control of long-chain fatty acid oxidation that occurs early after the onset of mechanical overload (6). Accompanying decreased rates of long-chain fatty acid oxidation (7,8), an acceleration of glucose utilization has been predicted by Taegtmeyer and Overturff (5). In analogy with control hearts, where an inhibition of fatty acid oxidation was shown to decrease intramitochondrial acetyl-CoA/CoA and $NAD^+/NADH$ ratios, a stimulation of pyruvate dehydrogenase complex could be expected (9). The end result would be an improved coupling between glycolysis and glucose oxidation resulting in decreased H^+ production from glycolytically generated ATP. While the reduction of fatty acid contribution to ATP production may decrease oxygen wasting, the suppression of intracellular accumulation of protons can further improve cardiac efficiency decreasing H^+/Na^+ and Na^+/Ca^{2+} exchanges (10). All of these metabolic adaptations, if they occur in hypertrophied hearts, could be assumed as beneficial for hypertrophied hearts, particularly under conditions of prolonged mechanical stress (5).

There is now a substantial evidence indicating that the rate of glycolysis is significantly increased in different models of cardiac hypertrophy (5,7,11,12). This is principally related to a simultaneous upregulation of hexokinase, phosphofructokinase and phosphorylase (5). However, according to recent quantitative assessements of rates of oxidative metabolism in pressure- and volume-overloaded hearts, this stimulation of glycolysis is not accompanied by the expected acceleration of glucose oxidation (7,13). In contrast, due to an apparent inhibition of pyruvate dehydrogenase complex, possibly related to decreased tissue levels of L-carnitine (14,15), the contribution of glucose oxidation to ATP production tends to decline (13,16). Since low tissue levels of L-carnitine further compromise long-chain fatty acid oxidation (17–19), the existence of impaired NADH delivery to the respiratory chain could be expected in mechanically overloaded hearts. The end result of this simultaneous inhibition of glucose and fatty acid oxidation might be kinetic limitation of oxidative phosphorylation (20,21). It has been speculated that, under these conditions, the energy transfer from substrates of oxidative metabolism to cytosolic adenine nucleotides could be impaired (22) so that metabolically restricted mechanically-overloaded hearts would operate at significantly lower cytosolic $\Delta G'_{ATP}$, especially at high work loads that prevail in vivo after aortic banding (23) or after aorto-caval fistula (13). Therefore, in chronically-overloaded hearts, where cytosolic ADP_f and Pi seem not to be regulatory any longer (24), the transition from compensatory cardiac hypertrophy to congestive heart failure may be accelerated.

According to combined fluorimetric NADH and ^{31}P-NMR spectrometric studies, an improved substrate delivery to the respiratory chain of intact tissues with high oxidative capacities may, per se, stimulate their oxidative phosphorylation thus maintaining cytosolic ADP_f and Pi concentrations in physiological range (21,25,26). The appropriate pharmacological interventions improving glucose or fatty acid oxidation in cardiomyopathic hearts could, therefore, avoid excessive changes in intracellular energy transfer from occurring and, thus, maintain left ventricular contractility in physiological range. It has been also speculated that the relief of the apparent metabolic privation of hypertrophied hearts may attenuate alterations in intracellular concentrations of different intermediates of energy substrate metabolism (27). Some of these latter compouds were shown to serve as ligands to different transcriptional factors involved in control of myocardial gene expression (28,29). Therefore, a possibility arises that the restoration of glucose or fatty acid utilization may reactivate the expression of genes encoding, respectively, for essential membrane proteins such as the sarcoplasmic reticulum Ca^{2+}ATPase, phospholamban and SRcalcium release channel (29,30) and the enzymes involved in control of long-chain fatty acid oxidation such as palmitoyl-CoA synthetase, carnitine palmitoyltransferase, malonyl-CoA decarboxylase, etc. (6,31). The downregulations of these latter genes, as they occur in mechanically-overloaded hearts, may be, in fact, considered as harmful misadaptations.

The aim of the present paper is to recall some of our previous data which bring an evidence that hearts of rats with chronic aorto-caval fistula are, indeed, metabolically restricted, possibly due to a significant depletion of tissue L-carnitine. This impairs their respiratory control and leads to a kinetic failure of oxidative phosphorylation. We also demonstrate that the relief of substrate limitation of oxidative phosphorylation by appropriate pharmacological interventions can be followed by the recovery of VO_{2max} and improved intracellular energy transfer in mechanically-overloaded hearts which, in turn, restores their left ventricular performance. The possibility that the reactivation of myocardial oxidative metabolism and the resulting normalization of mitochondrial respiratory control may be followed by the reversal of some of molecular manifestations of load-induced adult-to-fetal shift in myocardial gene expression is briefly discussed.

MATERIALS AND METHODS

Animals

A chronic volume overload was induced in 2-mo-old Wistar rats by surgical opening of the aorto-caval fistula. Our technique of the induction of the aorto-caval communication has been described in detail in another paper (8). Three months after surgery, the animals were sacrificed using a light ether anesthesia and their hearts were used for the in vitro perfusions. Sham-operated animals from the same litters were used as controls. A separate group of rats with the aorto-caval fistula and a group of sham-operated controls were given propionyl-L-carnitine (250 mg/kg/day, i.p.) for ten days before sacrifice (13).

Isolated heart perfusions

After excision, the hearts were rapidly fastened to the aortic cannula and perfused for 15 min via the aorta with oxygenated Krebs-Henseleit buffer containing 11 mM glucose, 2.5 mM calcium and 10 IU/l insulin, pH 7.4. After this initial period, the hearts were switched to the working mode and recirculated with the same buffer containing 11 mM glucose, insulin and 1.2 mM palmitate bound to 3 per cent bovine albumin. Separate groups of control and volume-overloaded hearts were perfused in presence of 11 mM glucose, insulin and 2.4 mM octanoate, a medium-chain fatty acid which circumvents carnitine acyltransferases of mitochondrial membranes. The perfusions were continued for 20 min under conditions of moderate workload (10 Torr preload, 70 Torr afterload). Cardiac work was then increased by clamping the aortic outflow line so that the hearts pumped for an additional 20 min period against a high resistance (high workload). The perfusion system resembled that developed by Neely et al. (32) except for the oxygenation chamber which was replaced by a hollow-fiber oxygenator. The total volume of perfusion medium recirculated was 200 ml.

Monitoring of left ventricular performance

Mechanical activity of the left ventricle was assessed throughout the experiments in terms of pressure work. The left ventricular peak systolic pressure, measured with a Millar pressure transducer in the aortic ejection line, was recorded on a Brush-Mark 440 physiograph (24). These recordings allowed instantaneous heart rates and (heart rate × peak systolic pressure) products to be determined. Aortic flow rates were measured, during the moderate workload conditions, by means of a rotameter (Manostat 36-541-12) inserted into the aortic outflow line (13).

Measurements of glucose oxidation

The rates of glycolysis and glucose oxidation were measured simultaneously according to methods developed by Lopaschuk et al. (7,16,33). In these experiments, the hearts were recirculated with the medium containing both [U-^{14}C]glucose (specific activity 400,000 dpm/ml) and [5-^{3}H]glucose (specific activity 400,000 dpm/ml). The perfusion system was closed to the ambient air. The rates of glucose oxidation were estimated from rates of $^{14}CO_2$ production from [U-^{14}C]glucose by bubbling the gas leaving the closed perfusion system through a 1 M methylbenzenthonium hydroxide (Hyamine Hydroxide) trap. The samples of the perfusion medium were also collected in 5 min intervals. They were placed without contact with the air in 25 ml stoppered flasks containing 1 ml of 1 M sodium hydroxide and, in their central wells, 1 ml of 1 M methylbenzenthonium hydroxide. The perfusate samples were then acidified by addition of 1 ml of 4.5 M H_2SO_4 and gently stirred for 2 h to determine $^{14}CO_2$ present as bicarbonate. Aliquots of Hyamine Hydroxide were diluted in Safefluor (Lumac) scintillation liquid for counting (13). The same method of $^{14}CO_2$ collection was also used, in some experiments, to quantify $^{14}CO_2$ production rates from [1-$^{14}CO_2$]octanoate and [U-$^{14}CO_2$]palmitate (8).

Measurements of rates of glycolysis

The steady-state glycolysis rates were measured by quantitative determination of the amount of $^{3}H_2O$ liberated from [5-^{3}H]glucose at the enolase level (13,16). Separation of $^{3}H_2O$ from labeled glucose was obtained by passing 200 µl samples of the perfusion medium through Dowex 1-X4 (200–400 mesh) anion exchange columns which, after elution with 800 µl of distilled water, retained about 97% of total [^{3}H/^{14}C]glucose (16). The samples were collected in vials containing the appropriate scintillation liquid and double counted. The signal obtained from the $^{3}H_2O$ eluted was corrected for the small amount of [^{3}H]glucose that was determined by measurements of the amount of [^{14}C]glucose also present in the eluent.

Measurements of palmitate oxidation

The rates of palmitate oxidation were measured in a separate group of hearts perfused under conditions identical to those of the above group. In this case, the perfusion medium contained [9,10-^{3}H]palmitate (specificity activity 160,000 dpm/ml) and the rate of $^{3}H_2O$ production was determined according to the technique described by Saddik and Lopaschuk (34). In order to separate $^{3}H_2O$ from [^{3}H]palmitate, samples of the perfusion medium (0.5 ml) were collected in 5 min intervals and treated with 1.88 ml of a 1 : 2 (vol/vol) mixture of chloroform and methanol. After a quick agitation, 625 µl of chloroform and 625 µl of 2 M KCl/HCl were added and, after the separation, the aqueous phase was extracted with a mixture of chloroform, methanol and 2 M KCl/HCl (1 : 1 : 0.9). Two 500 ml samples of the resulting aqueous phase were taken for counting (13). According to Saddik and Lopaschuk (34), this method results in a 99.7% extraction and separation of $^{3}H_2O$ from [^{3}H]palmitate.

Myocardial VO_2 measurements

The hearts used for measurements of oxygen consumption were placed in a glass vessel adapted to the support of the aortic cannula. This allowed the effluent from the pulmonary artery to be collected and transferred without contact with the ambient air to a thermostated cell with an oxygen electrode (Instech 125/05). The electrode was connected to an Instech dual channel oxygen monitor. The coronary flow rate was measured in 5 min intervals by means of a calibrated cylinder placed at the exit of oxygen electrode chamber. The calculated myocardial VO_2 rates were expressed in μmoles O_2 per min per gram dry weight (24).

Biochemical assays

The hearts were freeze-clamped by Wollenberger clamps at the end of different periods of the perfusion sequence. The frozen ventricles were freeze-dried in order to determine ventricular dry weight. The samples of lyophilized tissue were deproteinized in 0.6 N perchloric acid (4°C) and the supernatant, brought to pH 5.8, was used for biochemical assays (24,35). Tissue contents of selected metabolites were converted to concentrations with the assumption that the intracellular water space equals 2.25 ml/g dry wt (22,36).

The cytosolic phosphorylation potential (ATP/ADPf. Pi ratio) and cytosolic concentrations of unbound ADP (ADP_f) were calculated from the creatine phosphokinase equilibrium equation according to Wilson et al. (36). At 1 mM free Mg^{2+}, the pH-dependent equilibrium constant of creatine phosphokinase (K_{CPK}) equals $1.66 \times 10^9 M^{-1}$. We assume an intracellular pH of 7.0 and temperature of 37°C. The redox state of mitochondrial NAD was estimated from the glutamate dehydrogenase equation, supposed to reach equilibrium in all conditions studied. Considering the changes in the intracellular distribution of glutamate and α-ketoglutarate as negligible, we can obtain mitochondrial NAD^+/NADH ratio from the equilibrium constant for glutamate dehydrogenase (K_{GDH}) and α-KG, NH_3 and glutamate concentrations (36). The concentrations of reactants of both CPK and GDH in perchloric acid extracts of myocardial tissue were determined by spectrophotometric and fluorimetric techniques described by Williamson and Corkey (35).

Total tissue L-carnitine was assayed in samples of lyophilized tissue. The tissue was hydrolyzed at pH 12.5 and 70°C and, 1 h later, the alkaline hydrolysis was stopped by addition of 5 ml 7 N perchloric acid. The samples were then centrifuged at 10,000 rpm for 10 min. The supernatant was brought to pH 7.0 and used for carnitine assays according to radioisotopic procedure (37). This method involves the transfer of the ^{14}C-labeled acetyl moiety from [^{14}C]acetyl-CoA to L-carnitine in presence of carnitine acetyltransferase. The ^{14}C-labeled compounds ([^{14}C]acetyl CoA and [^{14}C]acetyl-carnitine) were then separated by use of an anion exchange resin (Dowex 1-X8) suspended in water. The radioactivity of the eluent reflected directly the total amount of L-carnitine present in tissue extracts (13).

Statistical analysis

Student's t test was employed to determine differences between control and volume-overloaded hearts perfused in the same conditions. The effects of propionyl-l-

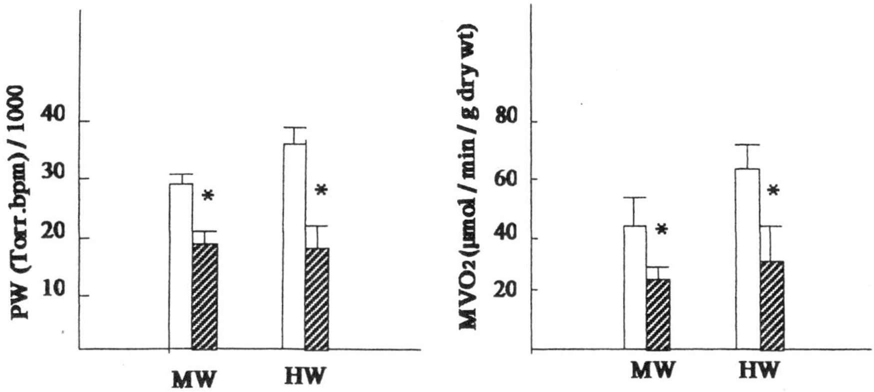

Figure 1. Pressure work (PW) and myocardial oxygen consumption (MVO_2) rates in control (open bars) and volume-overloaded (hatched bars) rat hearts perfused in presence of 10 mM glucose, insulin and 1.2 mM palmitate. MW—moderate workload, HW—high workload. Values are means ± SE for 10 hearts; *$p < 0.05$.

carnitine were assessed by analysis of variance, and the pairs of means that were not equal were compared by Fisher's protected least significant difference test.

RESULTS AND DISCUSSION

Ponderal data

In rats exposed to chronic aorto-caval fistula, heart weight was increased by about 75 per cent (268 + 17 instead of 153 + 16 mg dry wt, respectively). This difference was further accentuated when heart-to-body weight ratio was considered. The cardiac hypertrophy was bilateral and there was no apparent dilatation of the ventricles.

Effect of different lipid substrates on myocardial oxygen consumption and left ventricular performance of volume-overloaded hearts

When hearts of rats with 3-mo-old aorto-caval fistula were perfused in presence of 10 mM glucose and high (1.2 mM) concentrations of exogenous palmitate, their mechanical performance was significantly depressed both at moderate and high work loads (Figure 1a). Oxygen consumption rates recorded during these perfusions were lowered in the same proportions (Figure 1b). In contrast, when palmitate was replaced by equimolar (2.4 mM) concentrations of octanoate, no decrease in myocardial oxygen consumption and left ventricular pressure work could be detected, at least under conditions of moderate work load (Figure 2a and Figure 2b, left hand columns). After the clamp of the ejection line (high work load conditions), both MVO_2 and left ventricular pressure work were slighty depressed (Figure 2a and Figure 2b, right hand columns). However they still remained in the range of values observed in control hearts perfused with glucose alone (not shown) or with glucose

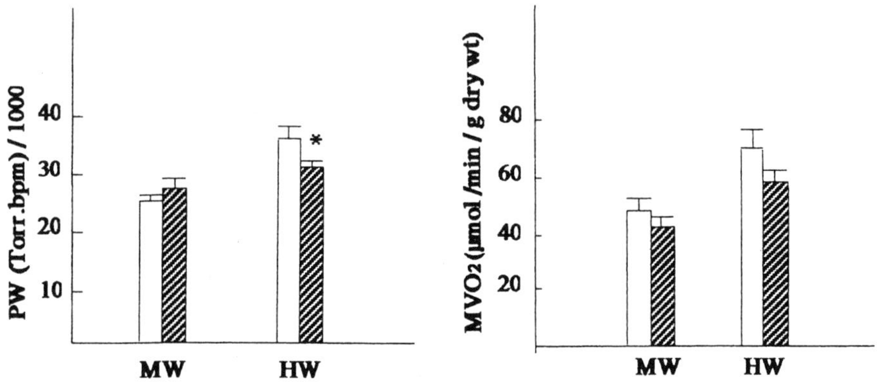

Figure 2. Pressure work (PW) and myocardial oxygen consumption (MVO_2) rates in control (open bars) and volume-overloaded (hatched bars) rat hearts perfused in presence of 10 mM glucose, insulin and 2.4 mM octanoate. MW—moderate workload, HW—high workload. Values are means ± SE for 10 hearts; *$p < 0.05$.

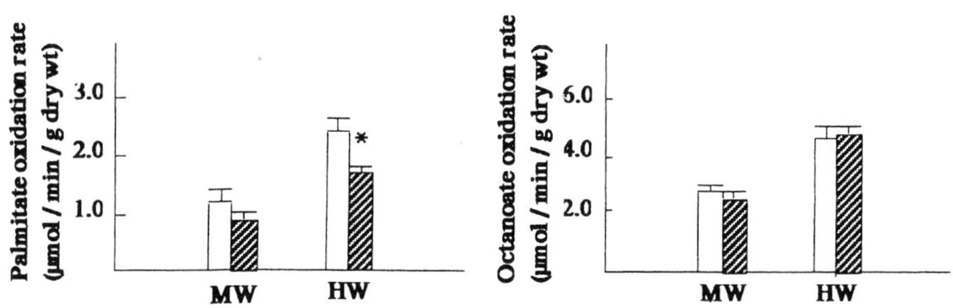

Figure 3. [U-^{14}C]palmitate and [1-^{14}C]octanoate oxidation rates in control and volume-overloaded hearts perfused at moderate (MW) and high (HW) workloads. Values are means ± SE for 10 hearts; *$p < 0.05$.

and 1.2 mM palmitate (Figure 1). These results correlated with the assessements of respective rates of $^{14}CO_2$ production from [U-^{14}C]palmitate and [1-^{14}C]octanoate which confirmed the existence of a selective inhibition of long-chain fatty acid oxidation in volume-overloaded hearts (Figure 3). Since octanoate oxidation rates remained elevated under conditions of different workloads tested, the failure of mechanically-overloaded hearts to utilize long-chain fatty acids cannot be related to tissue hypoxia but rather to a metabolic disorder interfering with their oxidation. One of the plausible candidates which can explain the limitation of the oxidative metabolim of these hearts may be the lack of tissue L-carnitine which has been reported as a constant finding in hypertrophic cardiopathies of different etiologies

(32,38–40). It has been suggested that in healthy tissues, carnitine concentrations are not found in excess but, rather at set levels appropriate for optimal substrate metabolism (41). Therefore, in pressure- or volume-overloaded hearts, where up to 40 per cent depletion of total tissue L-carnitine can occur, the estimated intracellular concentrations of free carnitine may be lower than its respective saturating concentrations for mitochondrial CPT_o (42,43). This, per se, could result in impaired kinetics of long-chain acyl transfer from CoA to L-carnitine and, thus, in decreased oxidative utilization of long-chain fatty acids (7,8). However, low tissue carnitine concentrations may also directly compromise the activities of enzymes of β-oxidation pathway, particularly that of 3-ketoacyl-CoA thiolases which are finely tuned by mitochondrial acetyl-CoA/CoA ratio (44). It has been speculated that decreased availability of L-carnitine may inhibit mitochondrial carnitine acetyltransferase and thus slow down the conversion of mitochondrial acetyl-CoA to cytosolic acetylcarnitine (45,46). As a result, mitochondrial acetyl-CoA ratio would increase resulting thereby in a feedback inhibition of 3-ketoacyl-CoA thiolase and impaired long-chain fatty acid oxidation (47). In addition, elevated mitochondrial acetyl-CoA/CoA ratio may also inhibit pyruvate dehydrogenase complex (15) and, in this way, slow down glucose oxidation rates in L-carnitine depleted hearts, particularly when high concentrations of long-chain fatty acids are also present (47,48). Therefore, a possibility arises that mechanically-overloaded hearts perfused in presence of glucose and 1.2 mM palmitate are, in fact, substrate-limited. This would explain low oxygen consumption rates and decreased left ventricular performance in volume-overloaded hearts perfused under these conditions.

Assessement of the kinetics of oxidative phosphorylation in volume-overloaded hearts; effects of different lipid substrates

In order to test this possibility, tissue contents of different chemicals involved in control of respiratory chain function were determined in control and volume-overloaded hearts perfused with 10 mM glucose and 1.2 mM palmiate or 10 mM glucose and 2.4 mM octanoate and exposed to increaseing workloads (24). Our results indicated that, in control hearts, similar metabolic profiles were observed in presence of both fatty acids at each condition tested (Langendorff, ejecting working heart, heart working against an increased aortic resistance). The only difference being a more pronounced reduction of mitochondrial pyridine nucleotides in octanoate-perfused control hearts (Table 1). Bypassing of carnitine acyltransferase with this particular substrate improved apparently mitochondrial NADH disponibility. This could contribute to an acceleration of myocardial oxygen consumption (20) but, as shown in Figure 4, respiratory rates of control hearts perfused with octanoate continued to evoluate with increased values of cytosolic phosphorylation potential (Figure 4a) and unbound ADP (Figure 4b) in a similar manner as during the perfusions with exogenous palmitate. This indicated that in control hearts, respiratory control mechanisms were not significantly affected by use of different lipid substrates. A quite different situation has been observed in mechanically overloaded hearts which, in presence of glucose and 1.2 mM palmitate, presented a pronounced

Table 1. Calculated values of parameters involved in control of oxidative phosphorylation in control and volume-overloaded hearts (effect of different lipid substrates)

	ADPf, μmol·g dry wt^{-1}	ATP/ADPf.Pi	$NAD^+/NADH$	MVO_2, μmol·min^{-1}g dry wt^{-1}
1.2 mM Palmitate				
Controls	0.092 ± 0.003	1.63 ± 0.08	4.50 ± 0.19	60.82 ± 1.50
Fistulae	0.142 ± 0.020*	0.87 ± 0.13*	8.77 ± 0.88*	30.75 ± 2.96*
2.4 mM Octanoate				
Controls	0.118 ± 0.005	1.61 ± 0.09	3.69 ± 0.26	70.45 ± 3.79
Fistulae	0.114 ± 0.014	1.53 ± 0.11	4.13 ± 0.26	59.35 ± 5.20

After 20 min of moderate workload, hearts ejected for other 15 min against an increased aortic resistance (high workload). They were then freeze-clamped for determinations of GDH and CPK reactants. Cytosolic ADPf concentrations, phosphorylation potential and mitochondrial $NAD^+/NADH$ ratio were calculated as indicated in Methods section. Values are means ± SEM for 10 hearts; *$p < 0.001$.

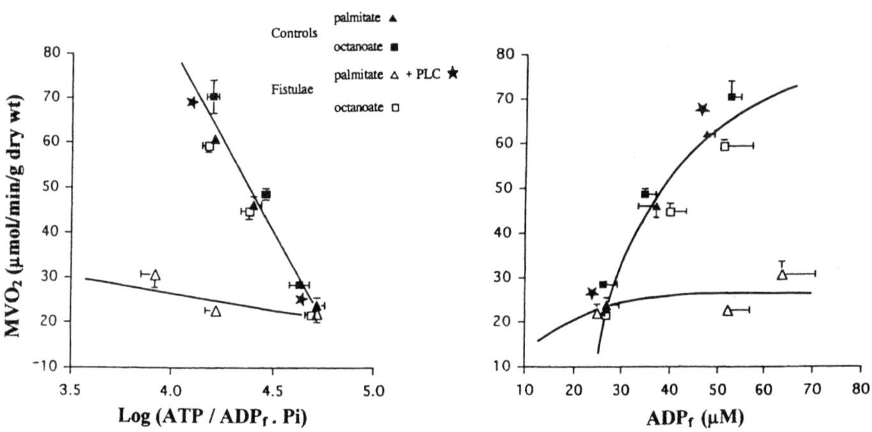

Figure 4. Control of oxidative phosphorylation by cytosolic adenylate system in control and volume-overloaded hearts perfused with glucose, insulin and different lipid substrates at increasing workloads. The effects of long-term administration of propionyl-L-carnitine are also illustrated. Figure 4a demonstrates the loss of thermodynamic control in volume-overloaded (PLC) hearts perfused with 1.2 mM palmitate (Δ). Figure 4b illustrates the kinetic limitation of oxidative phosphorylation in the same hearts (decrease of apparent VO_{2max}). The improvement of mitochondrial NADH availability by octanoate or by tissue repletion of L-carnitine restores both thermodynamic control (Figure 4a) and the VO_{2max} (Figure 4b).

oxidation of mitochondrial pyridine nucleotides and decreased MVO_2 at both moderate (not shown) and high workload conditions (Table 1). This oxidation of mitochondrial pool of pyridine nucleotides resulted in impaired respiratory control as indicated by loss of the linear relationship between cytosolic phosphorylation potential and myocardial oxygen consumption (Figure 4a). In addition, cytosolic unbound ADP was not regulatory any longer under these conditions (Figure 4b). The end result was a significant decrease in myocardial VO_{2max} (33 instead of 118 mmol/min/g

Table 2. Effect of propionyl-L-carnitine (PLC) administration on calculated values of parameters involved in control of oxidative phosphorylation in control and volume-overloaded hearts

	ADPf, μmol·g dry wt^{-1}	ATP/ADPf.Pi	$NAD^+/NADH$	MVO_2, μmol·min^{-1}g dry wt^{-1}
Untreated				
Controls	0.101 ± 0.006	1.56 ± 0.09	4.38 ± 0.63	68.86 ± 3.85
Fistulae	0.147 ± 0.019*	0.87 ± 0.14*	8.72 ± 0.29*	34.61 ± 1.70*
PLC-treated				
Controls	0.087 ± 0.005	1.49 ± 0.06	4.86 ± 0.14	79.45 ± 4.80
Fistulae	0.106 ± 0.005*†	1.26 ± 0.07†	5.19 ± 0.32†	61.25 ± 5.20†

After 20 min of moderate workload, hearts ejected for other 15 min against an increased aortic resistance (high workload). They were then freeze-clamped for determinations of GDH and CPK reactants. Cytosolic ADPf concentrations, phosphorylation potential and mitochondrial $NAD^+/NADH$ ratio were calculated as indicated in Methods section. The rats receiving propionyl-L-carnitine (PLC) were injected 250 mg/kg of the drug during 10 days prior sacrifice. Values are means ± SEM for 10 hearts; *$p < 0.05$ vs control hearts, †$p < 0.05$ vs untreated volume-overloaded hearts.

dry wt) in palmitate (and glucose) perfused volume-overloaded hearts. When palmitate was replaced by octanoate, reduction degree of mitochondrial pyridine nucleotides resembled that of control hearts (Table 1). This was accompanied by an apparent recovery of thermodynamic control (Figure 4a) and by a relief of the kinetic limitation of oxidative phosphorylation (Figure 4b).

Effects of propionyl-L carnitine on the kinetics of oxidative phosporylation in volume-overloaded hearts

Similar improvement of intracellular energy transfer also occurred in volume-overloaded hearts of rats pretreated with propionyl-L-carnitine (Table 2, Figure 4). In these hearts, tissue depletion of L-carnitine was highly attenuated (Figure 5) so that their ability to utilize long-chain fatty acids was improved, particularly at high workloads (Figure 6a). At the same time and, in accordance with data by Schonekess et al. (16), the normalization of tissue carnitine was followed by a significant improvement of glucose oxidation (Figure 6b) that may be related to a stimulation of pyruvate dehydrogenase complex (15) and improved coupling between glycolysis and glucose oxidation (46). As a result, in analogy with the effects of exogenous octanoate, the propionyl-L-carnitine-related acceleration of oxidative metabolism maintained reduction degree of mitochondrial pyridine nucleotides in a range compatible with the acceleration of respiratory chain function without any need for an excessive ADP_f accumulation (Table 2). These data are in agreement with NADH fluorimetric and ^{31}P-NMR studies by Katz et co-workers (20,25,26) according to which an enhanced mitochondrial NADH availability may, per se, stimulate oxidative phosphorylation and, thus, improve the energy transfer from substrates of cardiac metabolism to cytosolic adenine nucleotides (49,50). These observations fit with predictions of the model of integrated kinetic regulation of mitochondrial function as developed by Chance (22) and From (21) according to which the respiration of well oxygenated myocardium is under the control of three primary substrates of

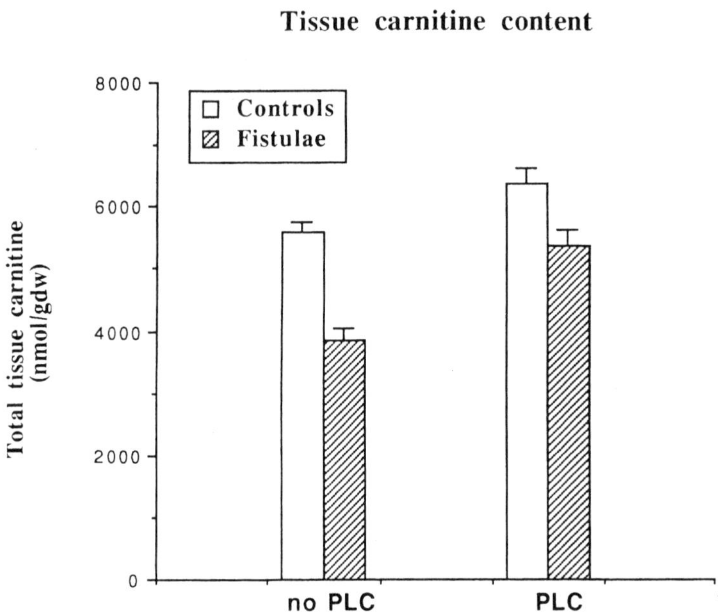

Figure 5. Total tissue L-carnitine content in control and volume-overloaded hearts: effect of propionyl-L-carnitine (PLC). Values are means ± SE for 10 hearts; *$p < 0.05$.

oxidative metabolism: NADH, ADP_f and Pi (oxygen being in excess). In this system of three substrate kinetics, it is plausible to expect load-induced changes in reaction rate to occur in absence of significant alterations of cytosolic concentrations of phosphate compounds if mitochondrial NADH concentrations are maintained saturating (22,26). This would preseve energy charge of adenylate system and ensure an appropriate ATP availability for cardiac work, even at high workloads (20,25).

Mechanisms of improved energetics in octanoate-perfused and propionyl-L-carnitine-treated hearts

While the recovery of the kinetic control of myocardial oxidative phosphorylation (increased VO_{2max}) and resulting normalization of intracellular energy charge may explain the improved work capacity of volume-overloaded hearts perfused with exogenous octanoate (22,24), the situation is possibly more complex in hearts of rats receiving propionyl-L-carnitine (13). Under conditions of moderate workloads and in presence of low (0.4 mM) concentrations of long-chain fatty acids, propionyl-L-carnitine-induced improvement in left ventricular contractility of pressure-overloaded hearts was essentially related to the stimulation of glucose oxidation (16). In contrast, in hearts of rats with chronic aorto-caval fistula, long-term administration of propionyl-L-carnitine increased the V_{max} of oxidative phosphorylation and, thus, left ventricular contractility via stimulatory effects of L-carnitine on both

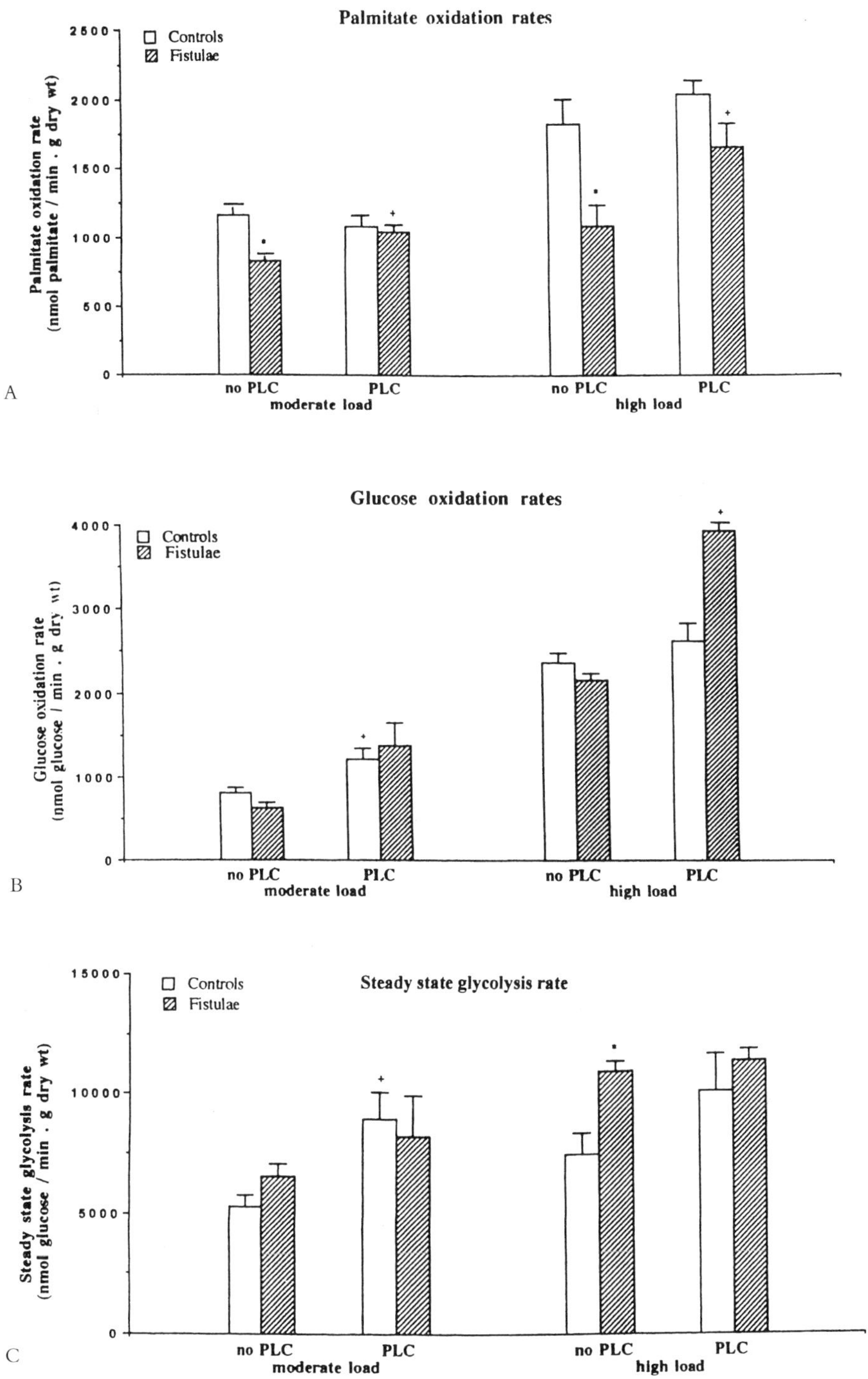

Figure 6. Steady-state [9,10-^{3}H]palmitate oxidation rates (A), [U-^{14}C]glucose oxidation rates (B) and steady-state glycolytic $^{3}H_2O$ production rates from [5-^{3}H]glucose (C) in control and volume-overloaded hearts; effect of propionyl-L-carnitine (PLC). Values are means ± SE for 6–7 hearts; $^{\star}p < 0.05$ vs control hearts, $^{+}p < 0.05$ vs untreated hearts of the same group.

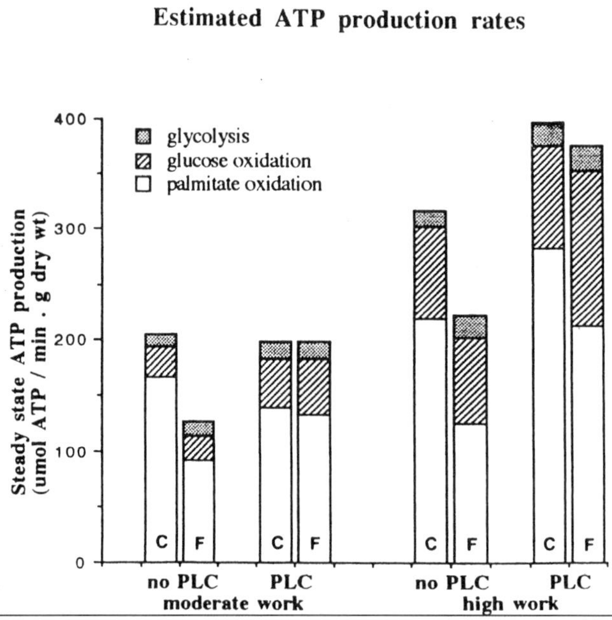

Figure 7. Steady-state ATP production rates in control (C) and volume-overloaded (F) hearts as determined from values indicated in Figure 6; effect of propionyl-L-carnitine (PLC). Respective contributions of glycolysis, glucose and palmitate oxidation are indicated considering the net gain of ATP for glycolysis as 2 mol/mol glucose. When glucose is oxidized, 36 mol of ATP are produced per mol of glucose. Oxidation of one mol of palmitate yields 129 mol ATP.

long-chain fatty acid and glucose oxidation rates (Figure 6). This may be related to the fact that, in our work, high (1.2 mM) concentrations of exogenous palmitate have been used (13). Under these conditions, mitochondrial levels of acetyl-CoA could still be elevated, so that the activity of pyruvate dehydrogenase may remain partly inhibited (51). Despite of this, propionyl-L-carnitine related acceleration of the overall ATP production rate (Figure 7) occurred sufficient for hypertrophied hearts could face elevated ATP demands without failure (13).

In addition to purely kinetic effects of propionyl-L-carnitine on myocardial energetics, another mechanism may also be considered. According to Lopaschuk's group, the amplification of the imbalance between glycolysis and glucose oxidation occurring in mechanically-overloaded hearts may have negative impact on their energetics because of an excessive H^+ production by glycolysis (7,10). In hearts of rats receiving propionyl-L-carnitine, this exagerated H^+ production may be reduced due to L-carnitine-induced stimulation of pyruvate dehydrogenase complex (46). As a result, the activities of both H^+/Na^+ and Na^+/Ca^{2+} exchangers could decrease which would futher improve cardiac energetics (51). This latter mechanism is possibly of particular importance during ischemia and early in reperfusion.

Finally, the above described stimulation of myocardial oxidative metabolism by propionyl-L-carnitine may, à la longue, modify the molecular outcome of mechanical overload to the heart. According to Micheletti et al. (52), long-term administration of propionyl-L-carnitine does not avoid myocardial hypertrophy from occurring but results in a partial repression of adult-to-fetal shift, at least at MHC level. Similar reactivation of adult genes expression was also observed after different interventions that are believed to promote carbohydrate utilization in mechanically-overloaded hearts (27,30). The effects of long-term administration of Etomoxir were studied in detail by Rupp, Dhalla and co-workers (29,30) who demonstrated that metabolic changes induced by this compound in pressure-overloaded hearts reactivate the expression of genes encoding for sarcoplasmic reticulum Ca^{2+} ATPase, phospholamban and SR calcium release channel and, at the same time, stimulate the expression of the gene encoding for fast (V_1) isoform of MHC (30). These authors suggested that pharmacological interventions improving carbohydrate utilization in hypertrophied hearts may reverse, via transcriptional mechanisms, some of the harmful molecular misadaptations that characterize adult-to-fetal shift in myocardial gene expression and, thus, delay the onset of congestive heart failure. According to data from other laboratories (6,28,31), the reactivation of genes encoding for enzymes involved in control of fatty acid metabolism (palmitoyl-CoA synthase, CPT_o, malonyl-CoA decarboxylase) by the intermediates of lipid metabolism or by long-chain fatty acids themselves may have similar effects. The resulting recovery of fatty acid oxidation rates could improve the kinetics of oxidative phosphorylation in hypertrophic hearts by simple mass action stimulation of mitochondrial respiration and, in this way, preserve their contractility (26,49). It has been also suggested that improved fatty acid availability may upregulate the expression of genes encoding for different regulatory subunits of mitochondrial F_1F_0ATP synthase (28). This further improves the intracellular energy thansfer in ventricular myocardium and other catabolic tissues supplied by appropriate exogenous substrates (20,50). Finally, it has been demonstrated that regulation of gene expression may also involve phosphorylation processes (53). Therefore a question arises whether substrate-induced alterations in the kinetics of oxidative phosphorylation and resulting changes in free energy charge of cytosolic adenine nucleotides may be directly involved in modulation of myocardial gene expression, both in health and disease.

ACKNOWLEDGMENTS

Part of this work was supported by a grant from SigmaTau S.p.a. Rome, Italy. We are particularly obliged to Pr. E. Arrigoni-Martelli. The collaboration of Pr. Zainab El Alaoui-Talibi and the constant input by Dr. Mireille Moravec are also deeply appreciated.

REFERENCES

1. Chien KR, Knowlton KU, Zhu H, Chien S. 1991. Regulation of cardiac gene expression during myocardial growth and hypertrophy. FASEB J 5:3037–3046.
2. Sadoshima J, Izumo S. 1997. The cellular and molecular response of cardiac myocytes to mechanical stress. Ann Rev Physiol 59:551–571.

3. Taegtmeyer H. 2000. Genetic Energetics: Transcriptional responses in cardiac metabolism. Ann Biomed Engineering 28:871–876.
4. Alpert NR, Mulieri LA. 1982. Increased myothermal economy of isometric force generation in compensated cardiac hypertrophy induced by pulmonary artery constriction in the rabbit. A characterization of heat liberation in normal and hypertrophied right ventricular papillary muscles. Circ Res 50:491–500.
5. Taegtmeyer H, Overturf ML. 1988. Effectss of moderate hypertension on cardiac function and metabolism in the rabbit. Hypertension 11:416–426.
6. Sack MN, Rader TA, Park S, Bastin J, McCune SA, Kelly DP. 1996. Fatty acid oxidation enzyme gene expression is downregulated in the failing heart. Circulation 94:2837–2842.
7. Allard MF, Schönekess BO, Henning SL, English DR, Lopaschuk GD. 1994. The contribution of oxidative metabolism and glycolysis to ATP production in hypertrophied heart. Am J Physiol 267:H742–H750.
8. El Alaoui-Talibi Z, Landormy S, Loireau A, Moravec J. 1992. Fatty acid oxidation and mechanical performance of volume-overloaded rat hearts. Am J Physiol 262:H1068–H1074.
9. Kobayashi K, Neely JR. 1979. Mechanism of pyruvate deshydrogenase activation by increased cardiac work. J Mol Cell Cardiol 15:369–382.
10. Schönekess BO, Allard MF, Lopaschuk GD. 1995. Propionyl-L-carnitine improvement of hyptrophied rat heart function is associated with an increase in cardiac efficiency. Eur J Pharmacol 286: 155–166.
11. Bishop SP, Altschuld RA. 1970. Increased glycolytic metabolism in cardiac hypertrophy and congestive heart failure. Am J Physiol 218:153–159.
12. Kagaya Y, Kanno Y, Takeyama D, Ishida N, Moruyama Y, Takahashi T, Iso T, Takishima T. 1990. Effects of long-term pressure overload on regional myocardial glucose and free fatty acid uptake in rats. Circulation 81:1353–1361.
13. El Alaoui-Talibi Z, Guendouz A, Moravec M, Moravec J. 1997. Control of oxidative metabolism in volume-overloaded hearts; effect of propionyl-L-carnitine. Am J Physiol 272:H1615–H1624.
14. Broderick TL, Quinney HA, Lopaschuk GD. 1992. Carnitine stimulation of glucose oxidation in fatty acid perfused isolated working rat heart. J Biol Chem 267:3758–3763.
15. Uziel G, Baravagalia B, Di Donato S. 1988. Carnitine stimulation of pyruvate deshydrogenase complex in isolated skeletal muscle mitochondria. Muscle Nerve 11:720–724.
16. Schönekess BO, Allard MF, Lopaschuk GD. 1995. Propionyl-L-carnitine improvement of hypertrophied heart function is accompanied by an increase in carbohydrate oxidation. Circ Res 77:726–734.
17. Bremer J. 1995. Carnitine-dependent pathways in the heart muscle. In: The Carnitine System. Ed. JW de Jong and R Ferrari, pp. 7–20. Dordrecht: Kluwer Academic Publishers.
18. Broderick TL, Christos SC, Wolf BA, Di Domenico D, Shug AL, Paulson DJ. 1995. Fatty acid oxidation and cardiac function in sodium pivalate model of secondary carnitine deficiency. Metabolism 44:499–505.
19. Paulson DJ. 1998. Carnitine deficiency-induced cardiomyopathy. Mol Cell Biochem 180:33–41.
20. Balaban RS. 1990. Regulation of oxidative phosphorylation in the mammalian cell. Am J Physiol 258:C377–C389.
21. Chance B, Leigh JS, Kent J, McCully K, Nioka S, Clark BJ, Harris J, Graham T. 1986. Multiple controls of oxidative phosphorylation in living tissues as studied by phosphorus magnetic resonance. Proc Natl Acad Sci USA 83:9458–9462.
22. From AHL, Zimmer SD, Michurski P, Mohanakrishnan P, Ulstad VK, Thoma WJ, Ugurbil K. 1990. Regulation of oxidative phosphorylation rate in the intact cell. Biochemistry 25:7665–7675.
23. Motterlini R, Samaja M, Tarantola M, Micheletti R, Bianchi G. 1992. Functional and metabolic effects of propionyl-L-carnitine in the isolated perfused hypertrophied rat heart. Mol Cell Biochem 116:139–145.
24. Ben Cheikh R, Guendouz A, Moravec J. 1994. Control of oxidative metabolism in volume-overloaded rat hearts: effect of different lipid substrates. Am J Physiol 266:H2090–H2097.
25. Heineman FW, Balaban RS. 1990. Control of mitochondrial respiration in the heart in vivo. Ann Rev Physiol 53:523–542.
26. Katz LA, Koretsky AP, Balaban RS. 1987. A mechanism of respiratory control in the heart: a ^{31}P NMR and NADH fluorescence study. FEBS Letters 221:270–277.
27. Rupp H, Elibman C, Dhalla NS. 1988. Succrose feeding prevents changes in myosine isozymes and sarcoplasmic reticulum Ca^{2+}-pump ATPase in pressure-loaded rat heart. Biochem Biophys Res Comm 156:917–923

28. Schwartz DA, Park EI, Visek WJ, Kaput J. 1996. The e subunit gene of murine F_1F_0-ATP synthase. J Biol Chem 271:20942–20948.
29. Zarain-Herzberg A, Rupp H. 1999. Transcriptional modulators targeted at fuel metabolism of hypertrophied heart. Am J Cardiol 83:31H–37H.
30. Zarain-Herzberg A, Rupp H, Flimban Y, Dhalla NS. 1996. Modification of sarcoplasmic reticulum gene expression in pressure overload cardiac hypertrophy by etomoxir. FASEB J 10:1303–1309.
31. Young ME, Goodwin GW, Ying J, Guthrie P, Wilson ChR, Laws FA, Taegtmeyer H. Regulation of cardiac and skeletal malonyl-CoA decarboxylase by fatty acids. Am J Physiol 280:E471–E479.
32. Vary TC, Neely JR. 1982. A mechanism for reduced myocardial carnitine content in diabetic animals. Am J Physiol 243:H154–H158.
33. Lopaschuk GD, Saddik M. 1992. The relative contributions of glucose and fatty acids to ATP production in hearts reperfused following ischemia. Mol Cell Biochem 116:111–116.
34. Saddik M, Lopaschuk GD. 1991. Myocardial triglyceride turnover and contribution to energy substrate utilization in isolated working rat hearts. J Biol Chem 266:8162–8170.
35. Williamson JR, Corkey B. 1969. Assays of intermediates of the citric acid cycle and related compounds by fluorimetric methods. In: Methods in Enzymology, vol. 13. Ed SP Colowick and NO Kaplan, pp. 439–513. New York: Academic Press.
36. Nishiki K, Erecinska M, Wilson DF. 1978. Energy relationship between cytosolic metabolism and mitochondrial respiration in the heart. Am J Physiol 234:C73–C78.
37. McGarry JD, Foster DW. 1976. An improved and simplified radioisotopic assay for the determination of free and esterified carnitine. J Lipid Res 17:277–281.
38. Reibel DK, Uboh CE, Kent RL. 1986. Altered coenzyme A and carnitine metabolism in pressure-overloaded hypertrophied hearts. Am J Physiol 244:H2090–H2097.
39. Wittels B, Spann JF. 1968. Defective lipid metabolism in the failing heart. J Clin Invest 47: 1787–1794.
40. York CM, Cantrell CR, Borum PP. 1983. Cardiac carnitine deficiency and altered carnitine transport in cardiomyopathic hamsters. Arch Biochem Biophys 221:526–533.
41. Long CS, Haller RG, Foster DW. 1982. Kinetics of carnitine dependent fatty acid oxidation: implications of tissue carnitine deficiency. Neurology 32:663–666.
42. Brunold Ch, EL Alaoui-Talibi Z, Moravec M, Moravec J. 1998. Palmitate oxidation by the mitochondria from volume-overloaded rat hearts. Mol Cell Biochem 180:117–128.
43. Fiol CJ, Kerner J, Bieber LL. 1987. Effect of malonyl-CoA on the kinetics of membrane bound carnitine palmitoyltransferase of rat heart mitochondria. Biochim Biophys Acta 916:462–492.
44. Olowe Y, Schulz H. 1980. Regulation of thiolases from pig hearts. Control of fatty acid oxidation in the heart. Eur J Biochem 109:425–429.
45. Lysiak W, Lilly K, Di Lisa F, Toth PP, Bieber LL. 1988. Quantification of the effect of L-carnitine on the levels of acid-soluble short-chain acyl-CoA and CoASH in rat heart and liver mitochondria. J Biol Chem 263:1151–1156.
46. Schönekess BO, Lopaschuk GD. 1995. The effects of carnitine on myocardial carbohydrate metabolism. In: The Carnitine System. Ed. JW de Jong and R Ferrari, pp. 39–52. Dordrecht: Kluwer Academic Publishers.
47. Schultz H. 1991. Beta-oxidation of fatty acids. Biochim Biophys Acta 1081:109–120.
48. Lopaschuk GD, Belke DD, Gamble J, Hoi T, Schönekess BO. 1994. Regulation of fatty acid oxidation in the mammalian heart in health and disease. Biochim Biophys Acta 1213:263–276.
49. From AHL, Petein MA, Michurski SP, Zimmer SD, Ugurbil K. 1986. ^{31}P-studies of mitochondrial respiration in the intact myocardium. FEBS Letters 206:257–262.
50. Matchinsky FZ. 1996. A lesson in metabolic regulation inspired by the glucose sensor paradigm. Diabetes 45:223–240.
51. Tani T, Neely JR. 1989. Role of intracellular Na^+ in Ca^{2+} overload and depressed recovery of ventricular function of reperfused rat heart. Circ Res 65:1045–1056.
52. Micheletti R, Giacalone G, Canepari M, Salardi S, Bianchi G, Reggiani C. 1994. Propionyl-L-carnitine prevents myocardial mechanical alterations due to pressure overload in rats. Am J Physiol 266:H2190–H2197.
53. Lewin B. 1984. Gene expression; Control of replication and transcription. New York: Wiley.

Frontiers in Cardiovascular Health, edited by
N.S. Dhalla, A. Chockalingam,
H.I. Berkowitz & P.K. Singal
Kluwer Academic Publishers, Boston, 2003

Conditioned Nutritional Requirements: Therapeutic Relevance to Heart Failure

Michael J. Sole and Kursheed N. Jeejeebhoy

University of Toronto, Toronto, Canada

Summary. The advent of disease, genetic predisposition or certain drug therapies may significantly alter the recommended daily intake for specific nutrients published by government agencies and established in healthy people. That is the nutritional demands of a given physiological state or pathological process such as myocardial failure may result in "conditioned nutrient requirements or deficiencies" for the affected organ—in this case the myocardium and perhaps skeletal muscle. Several specific metabolic deficiencies have been found in the failing myocardium: (1) a reduction in l-carnitine, coenzyme Q10, creatine and thiamine—nutrient co-factors important for myocardial energy production; (2) a relative deficiency of taurine, an amino acid integral to intracellular calcium homeostasis; (3) increased myocardial oxidative stress and a reduction of antioxidant defenses. Deficiencies of carnitine or taurine alone are well documented to result in dilated cardiomyopathy in animals and humans. Each of these deficiencies is amenable to restoration through dietary supplementation. A variety of nutrients have been investigated as single therapeutic agents in pharmacological fashion but there has been no broad-based approach to nutritional supplementation in CHF to correct this complex of metabolic abnormalities. We have demonstrated deficiencies in carnitine, taurine and coenzyme Q10 in cardiomyopathic hamster hearts during the late stage of the cardiomyopathy. In another study, we randomized placebo diet against a supplement containing taurine, co-enzyme Q10, carnitine, thiamine, creatine, vitamin E, C and selenium to cardiomyopathic hamsters, during the late stages of the disease. Supplementation for 3 months markedly improved myocyte sarcomeric structure, developed pressure, +dp/dt and—dp/dt measured in a Langendorff apparatus. We also documented in carnitine, taurine and coenzyme Q10 in biopsies taken from human failing hearts, the levels correlating with ven-

Corresponding Author: Michael J. Sole, MD, Rm 13-212 EN, The Toronto General Hospital, 200 Elizabeth St., Toronto, ON, Canada M5G 2C4. Voice: 1-416-340-3471, Fax: 1-416-340-4030, E-mail: michael.sole@uhn.on.ca.

tricular function. A double-blind, randomized, placebo-controlled trial of a supplement containing these nutrients, given for 30 days, restored myocardial levels and resulted in a significant decrease in left ventricular end-diastolic volume. These experiments suggest that a comprehensive restoration of adequate myocyte nutrition should be essential to any therapeutic strategy designed to benefit patients suffering from CHF. Future studies in this area are of clinical importance.

Key words: dilated cardiomyopathy, congestive heart failure, nutrition, oxidative stress, energetics, creatine, carnitine, taurine, coenzyme Q10.

The last three decades have seen remarkable progress in our understanding of the pathogenesis of congestive heart failure. This understanding has given rise to 4 conceptual models that have formed the basis of our current therapeutic approach: (1) diuretics for relief of congestion and edema, (2) positive inotropes and vasodilators to improve hemodynamic performance, (3) neurohormonal antagonists to reduce inappropriate neurohormonal stimulation, (4) the pursuit of molecular strategies to reduce progressive myocyte loss through apoptosis. In spite of our advances, no presently available therapeutic intervention has been shown to substantially improve the long-term survival of patients with dilated cardiomyopathy and congestive heart failure. The underlying heart disease is relentlessly progressive in almost all patients who develop symptoms of overt failure and mortality continues to be unacceptably high.

Several metabolic abnormalities have been found in the failing myocardium which contribute to the loss of myocytes and myocardial dysfunction. There is progressive accumulation of calcium in the failing myocyte, which in turn results in increased mitochondrial calcium. This results in decreased mitochondrial energy production with a loss of energy reserve (1), protease activation and an increase in intracellular free radical production and oxidative stress. Abnormalities in aerobic oxidation are also observed.

These processes may also adversely impact on skeletal muscle metabolism and function, which are the primary determinants of functional capacity of patients with chronic congestive heart failure (2). Indeed, muscle wasting or cachexia is common (3). A recent, randomized, controlled trial lasting 8 weeks with a protein supplement of 30g and energy supplement of 750kcals/d did not show any benefit in markers of heart failure or skeletal muscle energetics despite a marked positive energy balance (4). Thus the malnutrition in patients with congestive heart failure appears to be metabolic rather than due to protein-calorie malnutrition.

The need for increased folic acid and iron in pregnancy or calcium and vitamin D supplements in aging are well recognized. Less well understood is the concept that the advent of disease, genetic predisposition or certain drug therapies may significantly alter the recommended daily intake for specific nutrients published by government agencies and established in healthy people. That is the nutritional demands of a given physiological state or pathological process such as myocardial failure may result in "conditioned nutrient requirements or deficiencies" for the affected organ—in this case the myocardium and perhaps skeletal muscle.

CONDITIONED NUTRITIONAL REQUIREMENTS OR DEFICIENCIES

Myocardial energy production is aerobic and dependent on a continual and adequate flow of nutrients. Attainment of this metabolic need requires the assistance of a number of cofactors. Several specific metabolic deficiencies have been found in the failing myocardium—carnitine, coenzyme Q10, thiamine, creatine, taurine and antioxidant vitamins.

Carnitine is an amino acid derivative that is essential for the transport of long-chain fatty acids from the cytoplasm into the sites of beta-oxidation within the mitochondria (5). Carnitine binds acyl groups and releases free coenzyme A. This allows removal of toxic short chain acyl groups as acylcarnitines, which freely diffuse, out of the cell to be excreted in the urine. The release of free coenzyme A also activates pyruvate dehydrogenase and thus improves the coupling between glycolysis and glucose oxidation reducing the lactate and hydrogen ion burden on the myocyte (5,6). Body stores of l-carnitine are supplied by both diet and endogenous biosynthesis from trimethyllysine. Genetically determined carnitine deficiency is associated with the development of cardiac and skeletal muscle dysfunction, which can be ameliorated by L-carnitine administration (7). Carnitine deficiency may also be acquired; failing myocardium has been reported to exhibit a depletion of up to 50% (5,8).

Coenzyme Q10, or ubiquinone, plays a vital role as a rate limiting carrier for the flow of electrons through the initial portion of the mitochondrial respiratory chain (9). It is also a very important endogenous antioxidant protecting cell membranes and circulating low-density lipoprotein particles from oxidation (9). Coenzyme Q10 is actively biosynthesized within cells, particularly myocytes and neurons (10). It is also widespread throughout all food groups. Significantly reduced (up to 50%) levels of ubiquinone are well documented in the failing hearts of both animal models and humans (11).

Thiamine, or vitamin B1 functions as a coenzyme in a variety of enzyme systems, particularly those related to carbohydrate energy metabolism. Thiamine is stored in very small quantities; requirements are related to daily energy expenditure. Thiamine losses may be increased with increased urine flow following the use of diuretics (12,13). The incidence of thiamine deficiency in patients with heart failure is reported to be between 13% and 93%.

Creatine phosphate is the primary high-energy phosphate reservoir of the heart and skeletal muscle and a critical carrier of high-energy phosphate from the mitochondria to sites of utilization in the cytoplasm. Muscle creatine stores are maintained through myocardial uptake of creatine biosynthesized in the liver, pancreas and kidneys or ingested directly in the diet. Myocardial creatine depletion, with a concomitant depletion of creatine phosphate is a characteristic of failing myocardium (14,15). Such depletion appears to be a good predictor of mortality (15).

Taurine is a unique amino acid, comprising 25%–30% of the cardiomyocyte amino acid pool in humans; it does not enter into the protein synthetic or metabolic substrate pool but rather functions both as an antioxidant and the body's most important endogenous regulator of intracellular calcium homeostasis (16). Taurine is endogenously synthesized in the liver and pancreas or ingested directly through dietary sources then taken up by active transport into muscle cells. Taurine deficiency alone can produce cardiomyopathy (17). Myocardial taurine is decreased in ischemic cardiomyopathy and inadequately increased relative to the intracellular calcium burden in non-ischemic forms (16,18).

Oxidative stress is an important participant in the pathogenesis of congestive heart failure (19). Our laboratory and others have demonstrated a significant increase in free radical production and a loss of oxidative defenses such as vitamin E and selenium in both animal models and humans (19,20,21). This is not surprising because a number of factors associated with heart failure, such as the activation of the sympathetic and renin-angiotensin systems, microvascular reperfusion injury, cytokine stimulation and mitochondrial DNA mutations (particularly in complex 1), are known stimuli for free radical production and oxidative stress. Coenzyme Q10 and taurine, discussed above, are both important endogenous antioxidants.

NUTRITIONAL SUPPLEMENTATION

In each of these deficiencies restoration of a single nutrient by dietary supplementation of affected animals or humans suffering from myocardial failure has yielded mixed results. For example, we have conducted a double blind randomised, placebo controlled study of 50 patients with class II–IV heart failure. Vitamin E (1000 IU) or placebo was taken for 3 months. There was a two-fold increase in plasma vitamin E. in the active group but plasma catecholamines, ANF, TNF-alpha, and malonyldialdehyde were not affected (22). Replacement of only one nutritional constituent in the traditional pharmacological paradigm is unlikely to correct the cascade of interconnected abnormalities found in the failing myocardium. Furthermore, the need for a given nutrient may not be readily apparent, as blood levels may not reflect either deficiency or increased requirements in the diseased myocardium e.g. carnitine, creatine, taurine or Co Q10.

Therefore, we randomized a placebo diet against one containing a supplement containing taurine, coenzyme Q10, carnitine, thiaminee, creatine, vitamin E, C and selenium to cardiomyopathic Syrian hamsters during the late stages of the disease. Cardiomyopathy resulted in a depletion of myocardial vitamin E, creatine, carnitine, taurine and coenzyme Q10. Supplementation for 3 months markedly improved myocyte sarcomeric ultrastructure, developed pressure, +dp/dt, −dp/dt measured in a Langendorff apparatus (23). These deficiencies have also been documented in human failing myocardia, the deficiency correlates negatively with the grade of ventricular function. A double-blind, placebo-controlled trial of a supplement containing these nutrients for 30 days in patients with ischemic cardiomyopathy restored depleted myocardial levels of taurine, co-enzyme Q10 and carnitine and resulted in a significant decrease in left ventricular end diastolic volume (Errett et al., Am Ht J, in press).

CONCLUSIONS (24)

The population of myocytes within the failing heart is heterogeneous with respect to metabolic/biochemical composition and structure. For example, a 50% decrease in the concentration of a given factor in the whole heart reflects a distribution that includes only a minimal decrease in some cells and a profound rate-limiting decrease in others. The failing heart deteriorates over a number of years; thus only a very small minority of cells at any given time can be irreversibly injured. Hence, the vast majority of myocytes must be capable of at least partially responding to a therapeutic intervention with some recovery under appropriate conditions.

Failing myocytes are under hemodynamic, neurohormonal and cytokine stress—the targets of the contemporary treatment of heart failure. The failing myocardium exhibits both nutritional deficiencies and altered nutritional demands. These impair myocardial energy metabolism, intracellular calcium homeostasis and antioxidant defenses. It is probable that skeletal muscle nutrition is similarly impaired, but to a lesser extent. Failure to satisfy these conditioned nutritional requirements appears to be an integral contributor to the myocyte dysfunction and loss seen in heart failure. Thus, restoring adequate myocyte nutrition would seem to be essential to any therapeutic strategy designed to benefit patients with heart failure. A better recognition of the potential importance of this area and much more basic and clinical research is needed.

REFERENCES

1. Vogt AM, Kubler W. 1998. Heart failure: is there an energy deficit contributing to contractile dysfunction? Basic Res Cardiol 93:1–10.
2. Clark AL, Sparrow JL, Coates AJS. 1995. Muscle fatigue and dyspnea in chronic heart failure: two sides of the same coin? Eur Heart J 16:49–52.
3. Freeman L, Roubenoff R. 1994. The nutrition implications of cardiac cachexia. Nutr Rev 52: 340–347.
4. Broqvist M, Arnqvist H, Dahlstrom U, et al. 1994. Nutritional assessment and muscle energy metabolism in severe chronic congestive heart failure: effects of long-term dietary supplementation. Eur Heart J 15:1641–1650.
5. Arsenian MA. 1997. Carnitine and its derivatives in cardiovascular disease. Prog Cardiovasc Dis 40:265–286.
6. Schonekess BO, Allard MF, Lopaschuk GD. 1995. Proprionyl L-carnitine improvement of hypertrophied heart function is accompanied by an increase in carbohydrate oxidation. Circ Res 77:726–734.
7. Engel AG. 1986. Carnitine deficiency syndromes and lipid storage myopathies. In: Myology, Basic and Clinical. Engel AG, Banker BQ (editors) 1663–1696, Toronto: McGraw Hill Book Co.
8. Pepine CJ. 1991. The therapeutic potential of carnitine in cardiovascular disorders. Clin Ther 13: 2–18.
9. Littaru GP. 1995. Energy and Defence: Facts and Perspectives on Coenzyme Q10 in Biology and Medicien. 1–91. Rome: Casa Editrice Scientifica Internazionale.
10. Elmberger PG, Kalen A, Appelkvist EL, et al. 1987. In vitro and in vivo synthesis of dolichol and other main mevalonate products in various organs of the rat. Eur J Biochem 168:1–11.
11. Folkers K, Vadhanavikit S, Mortensen SA. 1985. Biochemical rationale and myocardial tissue data on the effective therapy of cardiomyopathy with coenzyme Q10. Proc Natl Acad Sci USA 82: 4240–4244.
12. Seligman H, Halkin H, Rauchfleisch S, et al. 1991. Thiamine deficiency in patients with congestive failure receiving long-term furosemide therapy: a pilot study. Am J Med 91:151–156.
13. Brady JA, Rock CL, Horneffer MR. 1995. Thiamine status, diuretic medications and the management of congestive heart failure. J Am Diet Assoc 95:541–544.

14. Nascimben L, Ingwall JS, Pauletto P, et al. 1996. Creatine kinase system in failing and nonfailing human myocardium. Circulation 94:1894–1901.
15. Neubauer S, Horn M, Cramer M, et al. 1997. In patients with cardiomyopathy the myocardial phosphocreatine/ATP ratio predicts mortality better than ejection fraction or NYHA class. Circulation 96:2190–2196.
16. Huxtable RJ, Chubb J, Azari J. 1980. Physiological and experimental regulation of taurine content in the heart. Fed Proc 39:2685–2690.
17. Pion PD, Kittleson MD, Rogers QR, et al. 1987. Myocardial failure in cats associated with low plasma taurine: a reversible cardiomyopathy. Science 237:764–768.
18. Azuma J, Sawamura A, Awata N. 1992. Usefulness of taurine in chronic congestive heart failure and its prospective application. Jpn Circ J 56:95–99.
19. Ball AMMM, Sole MJ. 1998. Oxidative stress and the pathogenesis of heart failure. Cardiol Clinics 16:665–675.
20. Li RK, Sole MJ, Mickle DAG, et al. 1997. Vitamin E and oxidative stress in the heart of the cardiomyopathic Syrian hamster. Free Radical Biol Med 24:252–258.
21. Keith M, Geranmayegan A, Sole MJ, et al. 1998. Increased oxidative stress in patients with congestive heart failure. J Am Coll Cardiol 31:1352–1356.
22. Keith ME, Jeejeebhoy KN, Langer A, et al. 2001. A controlled clinical trial of vitamin E supplementation in patients with congestive heart failure. Am J Clin Nutr 73: 219–224.
23. Keith ME, Ball A, Jeejeebhoy KN, et al. 2001. Conditioned nutritional deficiencies in thecardiomyopathic hamster heart. Can J Cardiol 17:449–458.
24. Sole MJ, Jeejeebhoy KN. 2000. Conditioned nutritional requirements and the pathogenesis and treatment of myocardial failure. Curr Opin Clin Nutr Metab Care 3:417–424.

Frontiers in Cardiovascular Health, edited by
N.S. Dhalla, A. Chockalingam,
H.I. Berkowitz & P.K. Singal
Kluwer Academic Publishers, Boston, 2003

Stress and Dietary Fat Influence Cell Membranes and Death Due to Ventricular Fibrillation and Heart Failure

Sigmundur Gudbjarnason and V. Edda Benediktsdottir

Science Institute, University of Iceland
Vatnsmyrarvegur 16, 101 Reykjavik
Iceland

Summary. Adaptation to chronic stress or repeated adrenergic stimulation, to dietary fat and ageing was accompanied by significant changes in fatty acyl chain profile of cell membranes in the heart. Changes in fatty acyl composition of membrane phospholipids preceded down-regulation of adrenoceptors or occurred simultaneously. Successful adaptation to stress was accompanied by a balance between 20:4n-6 and 22:6n-3 in membrane phospholipids. Increased intake of 22:6n-3 in form of cod liver oil resulted in diminished levels of 20:4n-6 in heart muscle and gastric mucosa. Reduced levels of 20:4n-6 in membrane phospholipids of both gastric mucosa and cardiac muscle increased the vulnerability of the tissue to stress induced necrosis. Sudden death in man was, on the other hand, frequently accompanied by low levels of 22:6n-3 in heart muscle and high ratio of 20:4n-6/22:6n-3. Sudden death in rats, due to ventricular fibrillation, could be significantly reduced by dietary cod liver oil and increased availability of 22:6n-3. The one factor that seems to be of major importance in stress tolerance is the cellular availability of both arachidonic acid and docosahexaenoic acid and the balance between these two competing fatty acids. The availability of these fatty acids for diverse regulatory functions can be influenced by well known risk factors of coronary artey disease such as chronic stress, dietary fat and ageing.

***Key words*:** Stress, omega-3 and omega-6 fatty acids, membrane phospholipids, adrenoceptors, heart disease.

Corresponding author: Sigmundur Gudbjarnason, Science Institute, University of Iceland, Vatnsmyrarvegur 16, 101 Reykjavik, Iceland. Tel.: 354 525 4797, Fax: 354 525 4886, E-mail: sigmgudb@raunvis.hi.is.

INTRODUCTION

Stress is considered an important environmental risk factor in development of cardiovascular diseases along with saturated dietary fat and smoking. The heart is exposed to repeated stress in every day life. The heart adapts to moderate chronic stress but failed adaptation leads to cardiovascular diseases including atherosclerosis, hypertension, spasm, cardiomyopathy and congestive heart failure. The molecular mechanisms involved in adaptation to stress are only partly understood. In this paper we describe adaptive changes in cardiac membranes during repeated moderate stress caused by adrenergic stimulation.

Stress represents the reaction of the body to stimuli (physical, chemical or psychosocial) or stressors that alter or disturb its normal equilibrium or homeostasis. The initial response to stress consists of elevated secretion of corticotrophin-releasing hormone, released mainly from the hypothalamus. It travels a short distance to the pituitary gland where it stimulates the release of adrenocorticotropic hormone, ACTH. ACTH travels the bloodstream to the adrenal gland and acts on the outer layer, cortex, leading to the release of cortisol to the bloodstream. The sympathetic nervous system is also activated to release the catecholamines epinephrine and norepinephrine. Cortisol and catecholamines are the principal stress hormones. Selye introduced the concept of biological stress and he emphasized the nonspecificity of stress etiology (1). Raab emphasized the role of emotional and sensory factors in myocardial pathology, accompanied by elevated levels of catecholamines and adrenal corticoids (2).

The term stress is also used to describe the response to heat or cold shock called heat stress. Heat shock or heat stress is characterized by an immediate increase in production of certain stress proteins or heat shock proteins (3). These stress or heat shock proteins serve to protect the cell from harm and to repair damage and the levels of such stress proteins may serve as markers for tissue and organ injury.

Another form of stress is a disruption of the cellular steady-state of prooxidants and antioxidants called oxidative stress. Oxidative stress is an imbalance in favour of prooxidants and in disfavour of antioxidants. Oxidative stress may lead to lipid peroxidation and fragmentation of lipids with damage to membranes, proteins and DNA. Oxidative stress may increase with an intake of high levels of polyunsaturated fatty acids which can result in endogenous antioxidant depletion and lipid/LDL peroxidation in vivo (4).

Adaptation to repeated adrenergic stimulation or stress is a complex process. Cell membranes are involved in cellular response to various forms of stress, modulating intracellular signalling and may act as sensors that transmit signals activating transcription (5). Membranes are dynamic structures where different lipid species are not only arranged asymmetrically across the bilayer but also organized in domains. These domains may form rafts with attached proteins and they include also clusters of sphingomyelin and cholesterol which form small cave-like structures called caveolea. Caveolea are specialized cell membrane microdomains which contain G protein-coupled receptors, G proteins and adenylyl cyclase. Caveolea serve to compartmentalize, modulate and integrate signalling events at the cell surface (6). Significant changes in the fatty acyl composition of the membrane bilayer may markedly influence the properties of proteins residing in the membrane such as hormone receptors, regulatory proteins and ion channels.

In previous studies we have shown that diverse forms of stress induced identical changes in the fatty acyl profile of cardiac membrane phospholipids. The stress induced changes in membrane lipids preceded down-regulation of adrenoceptors. Dietary fat also modified membrane lipids and adrenoceptor properties.

In this paper we examine the hypothesis that the balance between n-6 and n-3 fatty acids in membrane lipids is of major importance for successful adaptation to stress both in man and experimental animals. The balance between arachidonic acid and docosahexaenoic acid and the availability of both of these fatty acids in stress sensitive organs, such as the heart and stomach, seems to be very important.

REPEATED ADRENERGIC STIMULATION AND MEMBRANE CHANGES

Adrenergic stimulation, with epinephrine, norepinephrine or isoproterenol, modified the composition of fatty acyl chains in cell membrane phospholipids of the heart. When moderate adrenergic stimulation ceased or was stopped the membrane fatty acyl compostion returned to the previous state.

In our experimental model moderate stress was induced in male Wistar rats by repeated administration of epinephrine and more severe stress by administration of either norepinephrine or isoproterenol for 15 days, respectively. At selected time points before, during and after the repeated catecholamine administration rats were killed by decapitation, the hearts were removed quickly and extracted for lipid analysis (7,8). Sarcolemma was purified and epinephrine induced changes in membrane phospholipids were compared in sarcolemma and the heart muscle. The changes induced by epinephrine in the fatty acyl profile of phospholipids were practically identical in sarcolemma and heart muscle. Repeated administration of norepinephrine or isoproterenol caused more severe stress with mortality from 48–60%, respectively (7), and induced quantitatively greater changes in the fatty acyl profile of phospholipids than epinephrine (8).

Repeated administration of different catecholamines induced qualitatively similar changes in fatty acyl chain composition of cardiac phospholipids. The most important changes in cardiac phospholipids were about 50% lowering of linoleic acid (18:2n-6), in both phosphatidylcholine (PC) and phosphatidylethanolamine (PE) with a corresponding increase in arachidonic acid (20:4n-6) in PC and docosahexaenoic acid (22:6n-3) in PE (8,9,10). The esterified fatty acids in cell membrane phospholipids responded to catecholamines in a dynamic way and illustrate the active turnover of these lipids. The changes observed were specific for each phospholipid class, adrenergic stimulation increased, for example, the arachidonic acid level in PC but decreased the level of this fatty acid in PE. These changes reverted to control levels in 4–8 days after administration of epinephrine was stopped (9).

CHRONIC STRESS, DOWN-REGULATION OF ADRENOCEPTORS AND MEMBRANE CHANGES

Adrenergic stimulation down-regulated adrenoceptors, i.e. reduced the maximum number of binding sites, Bmax, of these receptors in heart muscle. Changes in binding properties of α_1-adrenoceptors, β-adrenoceptors and L-Ca channels in rat heart muscle were examined in sarcolemmal preparations in relation to alterations in the lipid environment within the membrane during repeated administration of epinephrine for 7 days (10). The maximum number of binding sites (Bmax) and dissociation constant (Kd) of ^{3}H-prazosin, ^{3}H-dihydroalprenolol and ^{3}H-nitrendipine binding to α_1-adrenoceptors, β-adrenoceptors and L-Ca channels, respectively, changed significantly during adrenergic stimulation. Remodeling of the cell membrane phospholipids took place before and during the down-regulation or decrease in Bmax of the adrenoceptors and L-Ca channels (10). The down-regulation of the receptors was always accompanied by replacement of 18:2n-6 by 20:4n-6 in PC and by 22:6n-3 in PE, regardless of the initial levels of these fatty acyl chains in the phospholipids.

Adaptation to daily administration of epinephrine includes down-regulation of β-adrenoceptors or decrease in Bmax. The changes in membrane phospholipids began before and continued during down-regulation of receptors. Adaptation to repeated adrenergic stimulation included thus coregulation of the lipid environment within cell membranes and the binding properties of adrenoceptors and functionally coupled proteins, such as L-Ca channels, residing in the membrane (10).

Cortisol, i.e. hydrocortisone, modified also membrane fatty acyl chains and binding properties of adrenoceptors in heart muscle. The influence of cortisol upon the binding properties of adrenoceptors and fatty acyl profile of membrane phospholipids in the rat heart was examined either alone or in combination with epinephrine. Administration of cortisol daily for 7 days decreased the affinity of α_1-adrenoceptors and decreased Bmax of β-adrenoceptors. These receptor changes were accompanied by significant alterations in the fatty acyl chain profile of membrane phospholipids which are characteristic of stress adaptation. Administration of both cortisol and epinephrine for 7 day produced severe changes both in receptor properties and fatty acyl composition (11).

PHYSIOLOGICAL STRESS AND MEMBRANE CHANGES

Physiological stress leads to alterations in myocardial membrane fatty acyl chain composition identical to those induced by repeated administration of the stress hormones, catecholamines and cortisol.

Neonatal membrane changes

The fatty acid composition of rat heart phospholipids was examined during the neonatal and postnatal period. The rats were killed on days 1, 7, 21 after birth and at the ages of 2 and 6 months. The fatty acyl chain composition of the two major phospholipids PC and PE changed significantly during the first two months (12).

The level of 20:4n-6 in PC increased rapidly during the first week of life. Blood levels of catecholamines are known to be very high during and after birth and a rapid increase in 20:4n-6 in heart muscle was observed during this period. Following the neonatal period 20:4n-6 decreased again, increasing then slowly with age. The changes in 18:2n-6 in PC were opposite to those seen in 20:4n-6. At birth the level of 18:2n-6 was low and remained low during the neonatal period increasing rapidly thereafter but decreasing then again with age. After birth the levels of 22:6n-3 in PE increased rapidly during the first two weeks of life. Neonatal stress and increased cardiac function play an important role in modification of the fatty acyl composition of cardiac phospholipids during early development (8,12). The observed alterations in fatty acyl composition of cardiac phospholipids in the neonates resemble changes induced by catecholamines and subsequent recovery. The animals respond or adapt to high levels of endogenous or exogenous catecholamines by modifying the fatty acyl chain composition of cell membranes (12,13).

Cardiac membrane changes during restricted food intake

Weight reduction due to food restriction is a common occurrence either voluntarily by overweight individuals or involuntary by populations fighting deprivation and starvation. Obese cardiac patients frequently have to restrict their food intake for the purpose of weight reduction but the effect of rapid weight loss on the heart has scarcely been examined. Food restriction has been shown to reduce the sensitivity of the rat to the cardiotoxicity of the β-adrenergic agonist isoproterenol (14). The molecular mechanisms responsible for reduced sensitivity to isoproterenol in these animals have not been elucidated.

Adult male rats weighing 500–600 g. were placed on restricted food intake, about 5 g. per day or one fourth of normal intake. After 6 days on restricted food intake the rats had lost 8.3% of body weight and after 12 days the weight loss was 12.8%. During food restriction there was progressive alteration in fatty acyl composition of PC and PE in heart muscle. In PC there was a significant increase in 20:4n-6 and stearic acid, 18:0, replacing 18:2n-6 and palmitic acid, 16:0. In PE 22:6n-3 increased significantly replacing 18:2n-6. The changes in fatty acyl composition of membrane phospholipids in the heart during restricted food intake resemble alterations induced by daily administration of catecholamines (13,14).

AGEING, MEMBRANE CHANGES AND ADRENOCEPTORS

Ageing was accompanied by changes in membrane fatty acyl chain composition and binding properties of adrenoceptors in heart muscle similar to those observed during repeated adrenergic stimulation.

The age dependence of changes in the number and affinity of adrenoceptors and alterations in their lipid environment during repeated epinephrine administration were examined in the rat heart. During ageing the level of 18:2n-6 decreased and the level of 20:4n-6 increased in PC. The level of 22:6n-3 increased with age in PE even if there were only small amounts of 22:6n-3 or fish meal in the feed (15).

Animals fed a regular, low fat feed without 22:6n-3 or fish meal did not increase their 22:6n-3 level significantly in cardiac phospholipids during ageing.

Age modified both Bmax and affinity of β-adrenoceptors. The number of binding sites decreased with age and was significantly lower in 10- and 23-months old control rats compared to 3-months old control rats (16). Simultaneously with this age dependent decrease in number of binding sites the affinity of β-adrenoceptors increased.

The down-regulation of α_1- and β-adrenoceptors following repeated epinephrine administration was not age dependent, but the alterations in affinity after epinephrine stimulation were different between age groups. The affinity of β-adrenoceptors was unchanged by epinephrine administration in the youngest age group, but in 10- and 23-months old rats it caused a significant decrease in affinity (16). Correlations were observed between specific polyunsaturated fatty acyl chains in membrane bilayers and binding parameters of β-adrenoceptors. Bmax of β-adrenoceptors was, for example, correlated positively with the level of 18:2n-6 in PC and negatively with 20:4n-6 in PC in the heart. Affinity (1/Kd) of β-adrenoceptors was negatively correlated with 22:6n-3 in both PC and PE, which means that with increasing levels of 22:6n-3 the affinity of the receptor decreased (16).

Alterations in lipid composition of cell membranes and membrane bound receptors during ageing are noteworthy because one of the striking physiological changes known to occur with age is a decline in the ability of the heart to respond to stress (17). It is reasonable to assume that older animals would be more suitable as models in studies of cardiovascular diseases since development of coronary artery disease afflicts primarily middle-aged or older individuals.

DIETARY FAT, MEMBRANE CHANGES AND ADRENOCEPTORS

The effect of adrenergic stimulation was also examined in rats fed different dietary fats and oils, i.e. diets supplemented with 10% butter, corn oil or cod liver oil.

Dietary fat influenced the affinity of both α- and β-adrenoceptors but in opposite direction in these receptors. Dietary cod liver oil increase the Kd or decreased the affinity of α- receptors and decreased the Kd, i.e. increased the affinity of β-receptors compared to the other dietary fats. The down-regulation of the receptors was always accompanied by replacement of 18:2n-6 by 20:4n-6 in PC and by 22:6n-3 in PE, regardless of the initial levels of these fatty acyl chains in the phospholipids. Adaptation to repeated adrenergic stimulation included coregulation of the lipid environment within cell membranes and regulation of the binding properties of adrenoceptors and functionally coupled proteins, such as L-Ca channels, residing in the membrane (10,13).

DIETARY FAT, ADRENERGIC STIMULATION AND VENTRICULAR FIBRILLATION

In a model of ventricular fibrillation older and heavier rats (>500 g.) were injected s.c. with isoproterenol, 1 mg/kg b.w. (14). This resulted in a transient decrease in high energy phosphates in cardiac muscle lasting 2–3 hours (18). These older rats frequently developed ventricular fibrillation during this period of energy depletion. The mortality was highest in rats fed diets supplemented with 10% butter and lowest in rats fed 10% cod liver oil (19). The cardioprotective effect of cod liver oil may be related to increased availability of 22:6n-3.

STRESS, DIETARY FAT AND TISSUE NECROSIS

a) Adrenergic overstimulation and cardiac necrosis

In a different model young rats were injected s.c. twice with large doses of isoproterenol, 40 mg/kg. b.w., the second injection 24 hours after the first one. This resulted in extended periods of diminished levels of high energy phosphates (18), development of extensive cardiac necrosis and high mortality due to congestive heart failure (20). Rats fed diets supplemented with cod liver oil had much greater mortality than control rats which may relate to lower levels of 20:4n-6 in cardiac phospholipids (20).

How could cod liver oil be cardioprotective and reduce ventricular fibrillation and sudden death in older and heavier rats but increase cardiac necrosis and mortality in the second model of overstimulation with isoproterenol in young rats? To answer that question we examined another stress sensitive organ, the stomach.

b) Emotional stress and gastric erosions

The influence of dietary fat on the stress tolerance of the stomach was also examined. Rats were fed a regular diet and diets supplemented with 10% corn oil or cod liver oil. The level of 20:4n-6 in PC and PE of gastric mucosa and the stomach wall was reduced by dietary cod liver oil to one third of control levels. The rats were then subjected to restriction stress for 18 hours when they were placed in a narrow cage where they could not move around. Gastric erosions were observed in all rats exposed to restriction stress but this form of stress induced twice the number of erosions in rats fed fish oil compared to control rats or rats fed corn oil (21). The increased incidence of gastric necrosis appears to be related to reduced availability of 20:4n-6 in mucosa but this fatty acid is known to be protective in the stomach.

The availability of arachidonic acid in membrane phospholipids seems to be critical for preservation of membrane integrity and cell survival during episodes of severe stress, both in the stomach and heart muscle.

CARDIAC MEMBRANE LIPIDS AND CORONARY ARTERY DISEASE IN MAN

Studies were also carried out on human autopsy material. The fatty acid profiles of cardiac phospholipids and nonesterified fatty acids (NEFA) were examined (22). The levels and composition of NEFA could possibly give some information about changes in release of specific fatty acids during post-mortem lipolysis indicating alterations in cardiac enzyme activities prior to death. Analyses of muscle samples from individuals that died suddenly, either in accidents or due to coronary artery disease showed reduced post mortem release of 20:4n-6 in coronary artery disease

(CAD) compared to other fatty acids. Sudden cardiac death was frequently associated with a high ratio of 20:4n-6/22:6n-3 in cardiac phospholipids (8,22). The high ratio may be due either to impaired release of 20:4n-6 or due to a decreased levels of 22:6n-3 in PE. Low levels of 22:6n-3 were frequently observed in cardiac PE. Sudden death is usually due to ventricular fibrillation which can be caused by myocardial infarction or possibly adrenergic stimulation (8,19).

The activity of hormone sensitive Plipase A2, which selectively releases 20:4n-6 seems to be impaired in patients with severe coronary artery stenosis. This may reflect chronic stress which could be due to CAD or contribute to CAD. Stress is known to increase lipocortin which inhibits Plipase A2.

DISCUSSION

Our investigation illustrates that stress induces significant changes in cell membranes of the rat heart and different forms of stress induce identical changes in the fatty acyl composition of membrane phospholipids in the heart. The observed alterations apply both to mitochondrial membranes and sarcolemma.

Several mechanisms will be considered that may aid in the understanding of the relationship between repeated adrenergic stimulation or stress and alterations in fatty acyl composition of membrane phospholipids with subsequent changes in receptor properties in heart muscle.

Adrenergic stimulation with elevated levels of catecholamines stimulates decylation or release of fatty acids from phospholipids. The phospholipids are subsequently reacylated with a new fatty acid replacing the one released during deacylation. Repeated deacylation and reacylation of the membrane phospholipids results thus in significant remodeling of the membrane phospholipids that are better suited to meet cellular requirements such as increased work load during repeated adrenergic stimulation. The stress induced changes are specific to the lipid class and are not simply dependant on availability of particular fatty acids. This is illustrated by an increase in the level of 20:4n-6 in PC whereas this fatty acid decreased in PE during stress (23).

Bilayer fatty acyl chains, cholesterol and ceramides create the microenvironment within the membrane where integral proteins; enzymes, ion channels and transmembrane receptors reside. The unsaturation and structure of these fatty acyl chains determine the fluidity and compressibility of the lipid milieu and thereby the conformation and biochemical properties of receptors, such as affinity for specific ligands and number of available binding sites. Repeated adrenergic stimulation and dietary fat have been shown to influence both fatty acyl composition of membrane phospholipids and receptor properties (10,24,25). Studies on cultured cardiac myocytes suggest also a relationship between membrane fatty acyl composition and adrenoceptor properties or receptor mediated phospholipase C activity (26–28).

Membrane phospholipids serve as substrates for synthesis of second messengers for transmembrane signal transfer. Alterations in fatty acid composition of precursor phospholipids influence the function of some of these lipids in signal transduction. Many receptor agonists use phospholipase-generated lipids as intracellular messengers. Receptor occupation stimulates, for example, the production of polyunsaturated 1,2-diacylglycerols (DAG) by phospholipase C (29). The best characterized function of receptor simulated DAG production is activation of PKCs. Polyunsaturated DAG species with 1-stearoyl-2-arachidonoylglycerol is most potent of these signalling molecules. Marked alterations in fatty acid composition of membrane phospholipids induced by stress or repeated adrenergic stimulation will thus influence the fatty acyl composition of the second messenger and thereby the function of this messenger.

Changes in fatty acid composition of phospholipids: a) alter the availability of free polyunsaturated fatty acids, released by phospholipases for synthesis of eicosanoids (30) and/or regulation of the activity of ion channels (31,32), b) may increase bilayer curvature and compressibility of the cell membrane and thereby facilitate internalization of receptors and down-regulation. Increase in unsaturation of membrane phospholipids makes the membrane more vulnerable to peroxidative damage and fragmentation of polyunsaturated fatty acids during ischemia and energy depletion caused by overstimulation with isoproterenol (20,33).

Free radicals formed during oxidation of catecholamines to corresponding aminochromes may also contribute to myocardial injury due to overstimulation with catecholamines (34,35). The free radicals increase lipid peroxidation and membrane permeability which leads to cardiac necrosis.

Cardiac necrosis observed during isoproterenol overstimulation was markedly reduced in vivo by the antioxidant α-tocopherol (20). Mortality was reduced in control animals receiving α-tocopherol from 50% to 25%. In rats fed cod liver oil cardiac membranes were enriched with the n-3 fatty acids but the level of 20:4n-6 was markedly reduced. In these animals isoproterenol induced even more extensive cardiac necrosis leading to congestive heart failure and death within 30 hours. Administration of α-tocopherol did not reduce mortality or protect these animals (20).

Increased intake of 22:6n-3 in form of cod liver oil resulted in diminished levels of 20:4n-6 in the tissues. Reduced levels of 20:4n-6 in membrane phospholipids of both gastric mucosa and cardiac muscle increased the vulnerability of the tissue to stress induced necrosis.

Sudden death in man was, on the other hand, frequently accompanied by low levels of 22:6n-3 in heart muscle and high ratio of 20:4n-6/22:6n-3. Sudden death in rats, due to ventricular fibrillation, could be significantly reduced by dietary cod liver oil and increased availability of 22:6n-3. The availability and balance of these competing fatty acids, arachidonic acid and docosahexaenoic acid, seems to be of major importance.

CONCLUSION

The one factor that seems to be of major importance in these studies is the cellular availability of both 20:4n-6 and 22:6n-3 and the balance between these two competing fatty acids. The cellular availability of these fatty acids for diverse regulatory functions can be influenced by well known risk factors of coronary artey disease such as chronic stress, dietary fat and ageing. Imbalance between these fatty acids and reduced availability of either 20:4n-6 or 22:6n-3 impairs stress tolerance.

REFERENCES

1. Selye H. 1936. A syndrome produced by diverse nocuous agents. Nature 138:32–39.
2. Raab W. 1966. Emotional and sensory stress factors in myocardial pathology. A Heart J 72:538–564.
3. Welch WJ. 1993. How cells respond to stress. Scientific Amer 34–41.
4. Stan K. 1993. Lipid oxidation products in food and atherogenesis. Nutr Rev 51:33–40.
5. Vigh L, Maresca B, Harwood JH. 1998. Does the membrane's physical state control the expression of heat shock and other genes? TIBS 23:369–374.
6. Shaul PW, Anderson RG. 1998. Role of plasmalemmal caveolea in signal transduction. Am J Physiol 275: L843–851.
7. Emilsson A, Gudbjarnason S. 1983. Reversible alterations in fatty acid profile of glycerophosphlipids in rat heart muscle induced by repeated norepinephrine administration. Biochim Biophys Acta 730:1–6.
8. Gudbjarnason S. 1989. Dynamics of n-3 and n-6 fatty acids in phospholipids of heart muscle. J Int Med 225, Suppl. 1:117–128.
9. Benediktsdottir VE, Gudbjarnason S. 1988. Reversible alterations in fatty acid composition of heart muscle membrane phospholipids induced by epinephrine in rats fed different fats. J Lipid Res 29: 765–772.
10. Gudbjarnason S, Benediktsdottir VE. 1995. Coregulation of adrenoceptors and the lipid environment in heart muscle during repeated adrenergic stimulation. J Mol Cell Cardiol 27:243–251.
11. Skuladottir G, Schiöth HB, Gudbjarnason S. 1993. Polyunsaturated fatty acids in heart muscle and α1-adrenoceptor binding properties. Biochim Biophys Acta 1178:49–54.
12. Gudmundsdottir A, Gudbjarnason S. 1983. Neonatal changes in fatty acid profile of phospholipids in rat heart muscle. Biochim Biophys Acta 752:284–290.
13. Gudbjarnason S, Benediktsdottir VE. 1996. Regulation of β-adrenoceptor properties and the lipid milieu in heart muscle during stress. Mol Cell Biochem 163/164:137–143.
14. Balazs T, Johnson G, Joseph X, Ehrreich S, Bloom S. 1983. Sensitivity and resistance of the myocardium to the toxicity of isoproterenol in rat. In: Myocardial Injury. Ed. JJ Spitzer, 563–577. New York, Plenum Publ Corp.
15. Gudbjarnason S, Benediktsdottir VE. 1989. Fatty acid composition in heart muscle modified by age, diet and stress. In: CRC Handbook of Free Radicals and Antioxidants in Medicine: Ed. J Miquel. Vol. 3:67–74. Lorida: CRC Press, Boca Raton.
16. Benediktsdottir VE, Skuladottir G, Gudbjarnason S. 1995. Effects of ageing and adrenergic stimulation on α1- and β-adrenoceptors and phospholipid fatty acids in rat heart. Eur J Pharmacol Molecular, Pharmacol Section 289:419–427.
17. Lakatta EG. 1986. Diminished beta adrenergic modulation of cardiovascular function in advanced age. Cardiol Clinics 4:185–190.
18. Fleckenstein A, Janke J, Doring HJ, Leder O. 1975. Key role of Ca in the production of noncoronarogenic myocardial necrosis. In: Pathophysiology and Morphology of Myocardial Cell Alterations, Recent Advances in Studies on Cardiac Structure and Metabolism. Ed.: A Fleckenstein and G Rona. Vol. 6:21–32. University Park Press, Baltimore, London, Tokyo.
19. Benediktsdottir VE, Gudbjarnason S. 1998. Effects of aging and dietary fat on β-adrenoceptors, L-type Ca channels, membrane fatty acids and ventricular fibrillation in rats. In: Essential Fatty Acids and Eicosanoids. Ed.: RA Riemersma, R Armstrong, RW Kelly and R Wilson, 277–279. AOCS Press, Champaign, Illinois.
20. Gudbjarnason S, Oskarsdottir G, Hallgrimsson J, Doell B. 1978. Role of myocardial lipids in development of cardiac necrosis. In: Recent Advances in Studies on Cardiac Structure and Metabolism. Heart Function and Metabolism. Ed.: T Kobayashi, T Sano, NS Dhalla. Vol. 11:571–582.
21. Olafsson OO, Hallgrimsson J, Gudbjarnason S. 2000. Dietary cod liver oil decreases arachidonic acid in rat gastric mucosa and increases stress-induced gastric erosions. Lipids 35:601–605.
22. Gudbjarnason S, Hallgrimsson J, Skuladottir G. 1983. Myocardial lipids in relation to coronary artery disease in man. In: Arterial Pollution. Ed.: H Peters, GA Gresham and R Paoletti. Plenum Publ Corp.
23. Gudbjarnason S, Benediktsdottir VE, Gudmundsdottir E. Balance between n-3 and n-6 fatty acids in heart muscle in relation to diet, stress and ageing. In: Health Effects of n-3 Polyunsaturated Fatty Acids in Seafoods. World Rev Nutr Diet, 66:292–305. Basel, Karger.

24. Wince LC, Rutledge CO. 1981. The effect of dietary lipids on the binding of (3H)dihydroalprenolol and adenylate cyclase activity in rat atria. J Pharmacol Exp Ther 219:625–631.
25. Alam SQ, Ren YF, Alam BS. 1988. (3H)Forskolin and (3H) Dihydroalprenolol binding sites and adenylate cyclase activity in heart of rats fed diets containing different oils. Lipids 23:207–213.
26. Lamers JM, Dekkers, DHW, Dejong N, Meij JTA. 1992. Modification of fatty acid composition of the phospholipids of cultured rat ventricular myocytes and the rate of phosphatidylinositol-4,5-bisphosphate hydrolysis. J Mol Cell Cardiol 24:605–618.
27. Grynberg A, Fournier A, Sergiel JP, Athias P. 1995. Effect of docosahexaenoic acid and eicosapentaenoic acid in the phospholipids of rat heart muscle cells on adrenoceptor responsiveness and mechanism. J Mol Cell Cardiol 27, 2507–2520.
28. de Jonge HW, Dekkers DHW, Bastiaanse EML, Bezstarosti K, van der Laarse A, Lamers, JMJ. Eicosapentanoic acid incorporation in membrane phospholipids modulates receptor-mediated phospholipase C and membrane fluidity in rat ventricular myocytes in culture. J Mol Cell Cardiol 28:1097–1108.
29. Hodgkin MN, Pettitt TR, Martin A, Michell RH, Pemberton AJ, Wakelam MJO. 1998. Diacylglycerols and phosphadates: which molecular species are intracellular messengers? TIBS 23:200–204.
30. Charnock JS. 1994. Lipids and cardiac arrhythmia. Prog Lipid Res 33:355–385.
31. Kang JX, Leaf A. 1996. Antiarrhythmic effect of polyunsaturated fatty acids. Recent studies. Circulation 94:1774–1780.
32. Nair SSD, Leitch JW, Falconer J, Garg ML. 1997. Prevention of cardiac arrhythmia by dietary (n-3) polyunsaturated fatty acids and their mechanism of action. J Nutr 127:383–393.
33. Lamers JM, Hartog JM, Verdouw PD, and Hulsmann WC. 1986. Dietary fatty acids and myocardial function. In: Lipid metabolism in normoxic and ischemic heart. Ed.: H Stam and GJ van der Vusse, 209–221. Steinkopff Verlag Darmstadt.
34. Dhalla NS, Yates JC, Lee SL, Singh A. 1978. Functional and subcellular changes in the isolated rat heart perfused with oxidized isoproterenol. J Mol Cell Cardiol 10:31–41.
35. Singal PK, Kapur N, Dhillon KS, Beamish RE, Dhalla NS. 1982. Role of free radicals in catecholamine-induced cardiomyopathy. Can J Physiol Pharmacol 60:1390–1397.

Frontiers in Cardiovascular Health, edited by
N.S. Dhalla, A. Chockalingam,
H.I. Berkowitz & P.K. Singal
Kluwer Academic Publishers, Boston, 2003

Pharmacotherapeutics of Diabetic Cardiomyopathy

Ramesh K. Goyal and Naranjan S. Dhalla

Institute of Cardiovascular Sciences
St. Boniface General Hospital Research Center and Department of Physiology
Faculty of Medicine, University of Manitoba
Winnipeg, Manitoba, Canada

Summary. While the prevalence of diabetes mellitus is increasing world wide, higher cardiac morbidity and mortality in diabetics remain a major concern that requires alternate strategies for the management of heart disease in patients with diabetes mellitus. At present, there is no clinically proven efficacious drug specifically designated for the treatment of diabetic cardiomyopathy; however, prevention or retardation of the progress of diabetic cardiomyopathy is considered to depend on various anti-hypertensive, anti-anginal and anti-diabetic agents. In diabetic cardiomyopathy, different neurohumoral systems such as cardiac renin angiotensin and sympathetic nervous systems are activated and these result in metabolic alterations (increased free fatty acid [FFA] beta-oxidation in heart and hyperglycemia). Such changes produce oxidative stress and alter gene expression as well as receptor sensitivity. There occurs an increase in extracellular matrix (ECM) and remodeling of the sarcolemmal (SL) and sarcoplasmic reticular (SR) membranes in the heart leading to altered signal transduction mechanisms. The increased ECM is associated with increased collagen content in the heart which leads to myocardial wall stiffness. Remodeling of the SL and SR membranes in turn causes an increase in the intracellular calcium associated with a decrease in the sensitivity of myofibrils to Ca^{2+}. Such myocardial aterations are considered to be finally responsible for the genesis of diabetic cardiomyopathy. Attempts have been made to investigate lipid lowering drugs, antioxidants as well as some trace elements for the treatment of diabetic cardiomyopathy. It is suggested that the current research may be diverted to evaluate the clinically used anti-hypertensive, anti-anginal and anti-diabetic drugs with respect to their effectiveness in retarding or preventing diabetic cardiomyopathy. In addition, newer agents like trace elements,

Address for Correspondence: Dr. Naranjan S. Dhalla, Institute of Cardiovascular Sciences, St. Boniface General Hospital Research Centre, Winnipeg, MB R2H 2A6, Canada. Tel: (204) 235-3417, Fax: (204) 233-6723, E-mail: nsdhalla@sbrc.ca.

antioxidants, anti-growth factors as well as agents acting on specific molecular or genetic targets should be discovered.

Key words: diabetic cardiomyopathy, anti-diabetics, anti-hypertensives, antioxidants.

INTRODUCTION

The evidence of increased incidences of heart failure and specific cardiomyopathy in diabetics has been reported in the early 1970s in various epidemiological (1,2), experimental (3) and clinical studies (4). During the past three decades, extensive research has been carried out to unravel the mechanisms and for providing a sequence of interrelated pathophysiological events leading to the development of diabetic cardiomyopathy (Figure 1). While the prevalence of diabetes mellitus is increasing worldwide, a significantly higher cardiac morbidity and mortality in diabetics even after the adjustment of multiple risk factors remain a major concern. The management of heart disease in a subset of patients with diabetes mellitus also needs to be improved. In this article an attempt has been made to put together different hypothesis explaining the pathophysiology of diabetic cardiomyopathy and present a picture of sequel of events that may be seen from the pharmacotherapeutics point of view.

Pathophysiology of diabetic cardiomyopathy

Earlier clinical (4,5) and experimental (6–9) results have suggested diabetic cardiomyopathy as a consequence of a direct effect of insulin deficiency on myocardial dysfunction. However, it has now been established that hypertension, hyperinsulinemia, insulin resistance and hypertriglyceridemia that cluster in the syndrome-X also lead to increased cardiovascular abnormalities in diabetes (10–12). Further, Schaffer (13) has suggested that cardiomyopathy is associated with non-insulin dependent diabetes mellitus. It is thus possible that in addition to insulin deficiency, insulin resistance that causes chronic diabetes mellitus may also initiate the development of diabetic cardiomyopathy (14). Although it has been emphasized that diabetic cardiomyopathy can occur independently of coronary artery disease (15), involvement of microangiopathy (16), macroangiopathy (4,17), autonomic neuropathy (18) and vascular endothelial dysfunction (19) can not be ruled out as all these events are major contributors for the occurrence of myocardial infarction. It should be noted that myocardial infarction has been reported to be responsible for remodeling of cardiac contractile proteins and plasma membranes leading to cardiomyopathy and cardiac dysfunction (20).

Various studies have suggested that chronic diabetes mellitus causes an activation of neurohumoral systems such as cardiac renin-angiotensin system (21–22) and sympathetic nervous systems (23–24) and produce metabolic alterations involving increased plasma lipids (25–27) and hyperglycemia (28,29). With respect to the renin-angiotensin system, an increase in mRNA levels of angiotensin II receptors in diabetics has been reported (30). The peripheral renin-angiotensin system is either downregulated or unaltered (31–33). An increase in circulating levels of plasma cat-

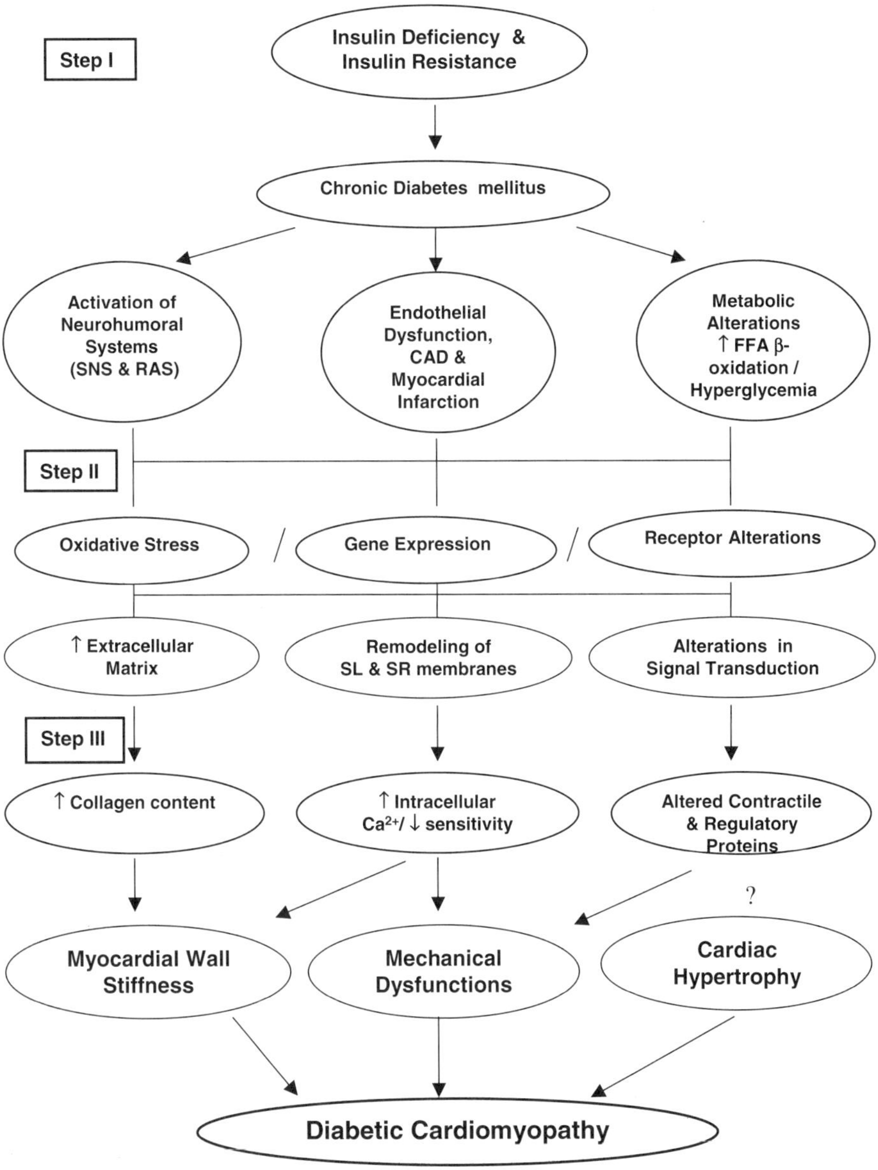

Figure 1. Sequence of pathophysiological events associated with diabetes mellitus leading to the development of cardiomyopathy. SNS—sympathetic nervous system, RAS—renin angiotensin system, CAD—coronary artery disease, SL—sarcolemma, SR—sarcoplasmic reticulum.

echolamines (34) with depressed β-adrenoceptor numbers and sensitivity (35–37) has been well documented in the diabetic heart.

In addition to neurohumoral factors, a plethora of metabolic abnormalities are triggered by diabetes in myocardium. One such abnormality is an abnormal increase in plasma lipids especially triglycerides (40) and cardiac free fatty acids (FFA) (41). High concentrations of FFA are associated with reduced contractile force and susceptibility to arrhythmias (42). Elevation of FFA in the diabetic heart may be due to increased adipocyte tissue lipolysis and lipoprotein lipase activity (43,44). Further, there is an increase in FFA oxidation by myocardium, which increases oxygen requirement and intracellular accumulation of potentially toxic intermediates of FFA metabolism such as long chain acylcarnitines and acylCo-A (45). These intermediates produce adverse electrophysiological, biochemical and mechanical effects on the heart through a cascade of events such as reduced myosin ATPase activity, decreased ability of sarcoplasmic reticulum to accumulate Ca^{2+}, depression of membrane enzymes such as Na^{+}-K^{+} ATPase and Ca^{2+}-pump ATPase (46). Like elevated lipids, hyperglycemia in diabetes also induces a bewildering list of changes in the heart that include impaired glycolysis, pyruvate oxidation, lactate uptake and non-enzymic glycation of proteins, diacylglycerol (DAG) formation, protein kinase-C (PKC) activation, aldose reductase activation and oxidative stress (47–51).

Increased sympathetic activity, activated renin-angiotensin system, myocardial ischemia, elevated levels of FFA metabolism and hyperglycemia result in oxidative stress which in turn plays a critical role in subcellular remodeling, Ca^{2+}-handling abnormalities and subsequent diabetic cardiomopathy (20,52). Precisely, there occurs impairment in sarcolemmal(SL) Na^{+}-Ca^{2+} exchange and Ca^{2+}-pump activities as well as sarcoplasmic reticular (SR) Ca^{2+}-pump activities (53–56). Further, there occurs an increase in intracellular myocardial Ca^{2+} or Ca^{2+}-overload in the heart (57). This is associated with a decrease in mitochondrial Ca^{2+}-uptake, stage-3 respiration, respiration control index and Mg^{2+} ATPase activity leading to overall decrease in calcium sensitivity (58,59). Along with alterations in Ca^{2+}-handling mechanisms in diabetes, there occurs defects in signal transduction mechanisms (51,60–63). All these mechanisms finally control the cardiac contractile (actin and myosin) as well as regulatory proteins (troponin-tropomysin) and reconstitute individual proteins of the cardiac system (64). Noticeable among these changes is a shift in cardiac myosin heavy chain (V_1–V_3) and increase in phosphorylation of myosin light chain-2 (MLC-2) and troponin I (TnI) in the diabetic heart (65–67). Diabetes also produces progressive separation of the faciae adherens, intercellular and perivascular deposition of connective tissue, thickening of the endothelial cytoplasm with pinocytotic hyperactivity and characteristic basal laminar changes (68). Collagen content of the heart is increased and it is associated with sodium and water accumulation (69); these changes contribute to myocardial wall stiffness and hence the diabetic cardiomyopathy.

Pharmacotherapeutics of diabetic cardiomyopathy

From the above mentioned discussion on the pathophysiology of diabetic cardiomyopathy, several drug targets (Figure 1) can be identified and many agents that modulate a specific enzyme or protein have been studied to prevent myocardial dysfunction. However, most of these therapeutic interventions remained at the experimental level and drugs to be prescribed specifically for the treatment of the diabetic cardiomyopathy under clinical situations are still awaited. However, commonly used drugs like anti-diabetics, anti-hypertensives and anti-anginal agents have been found to retard or partially prevent the progression of diabetic cardiomyopathy. This discussion is thus focused on reviewing the current status of these interventions with respect to their effects on myocardial function in diabetes.

Insulin

As mentioned earlier, clinical (4,5) and experimental (6–9) studies have suggested that diabetic cardiomyopathy is a consequence of a direct effect of insulin deficiency on myocardial function. Most of the studies were carried out by employing streptozotocin diabetic rats and the in vivo insulin was reported to not only prevent but also reverse the diabetes-induced myocardial alterations (70–71). There are some animal studies indicating that insulin could only partially prevent the mechanical and structural changes in diabetic rat heart (72–74). However, there are many problems with the clinical use of insulin such as the difficulty of controlling appropriate doses of insulin in patients and adverse effects like hypoglycemia and adipocyte dystrophy. In addition, development of insulin resistance in diabetic patients raises questions on the effective use of insulin as the treatment for diabetic cardiomyopathy.

Oral antidiabetics

Sulphonylurea derivatives (glibenclamide, glipizide and glyburide) and bigunides (metformin) are the most commonly used drugs for the treatment of non-insulin dependent diabetes mellitus (NIDDM). These agents reduce the glucose levels effectively and hence are expected to reduce cardiovascular mortality by adequate glycemic control. In 1970, Klimt et al. (75) reported a substantially increased cardiovascular mortality among patients taking the sulphonylurea drug, tolbutamide; this study was not supported by other, albeit smaller, studies (76,77). The discovery that sulphonylureas act by inhibiting ATP-sensitive potassium channels (78) and that these channels are present in the heart (79) again raised the question of safety of these agents for heart. Although there is no firm clinical data available to prove the deleterious effect of sulphonylureas (80), there is evidence indicating that inhibition of the ATP-sensitive potassium channels by sulphonylurea prevents ischemic preconditioning, an endogenous mechanism that protects the heart from lethal injury (81,82). Furthermore, it has been reported that treatment with glibenclamide did not prevent diabetes-induced hypertension and hyperlipidemia in rats (83). In normotensive non-insulin dependant diabetes mellitus (NIDDM) patients, treatment with glibenclamide is reported to increase the vascular resistance index (84) and prevent ventricular arrhythmias induced by transient myocardial ischemia (85).

Metformin produces hypoglycemic effect without affecting any potassium channels or insulin release but has been reported to improve cardiac function in STZ-diabetic rats (86). In normotensive NIDDM patients, metformin treatment was associated with greater reductions in body weight, total plasma cholesterol and diastolic blood pressure (84). Metformin is also appropriate in elderly obese NIDDM patients who do not have renal, liver or cardiac failure (87). Besides the above mentioned and widely prescribed antidiabetics, insulin-sensitizers like thiazolidinediones and α-glycosidase inhibitor, acarbose, have been introduced for therapy. These agents do not show any deleterious effect on heart; however, long term investigations are still warranted to evaluate the safety of these oral hypoglycemic drugs.

Anti-hypertensive drugs

It is now well recognized that both diabetes mellitus and hypertension are independent risk factors for coronary heart disease, the risk is greatly enhanced when these two diseases co-exist (88). Furthermore, it is clear that diabetes mellitus causes an activation of neurohumoral systems such as cardiac renin-angiotensin system (21,22) and sympathetic nervous systems (23,24). Rodrigues et al. (89) reported that treatment of rats with a vasodilator hydralazine prevented streptozotocin-induced cardiac dysfunctions. Later, effects of various antihypertensive agents in diabetic subjects and different animal models of diabetes mellitus were investigated by Goyal and coworkers (14). It was reported that while most of the anti-hypertensive agents used could effectively control blood pressure in different models of diabetes and hypertension as well as in diabetic patients, there were differences with respect to the effectiveness of different classes of drugs on cardiovascular metabolic and functional alterations induced by diabetes and/or hypertension. Besides hydralazine, prazosin (90), angiotensin converting enzyme (ACE) inhibitors enalapril (91), lisinopril (92), spirapril (93); Ca^{2+}-channel blockers like nifedipine (94) and amlodipine (95,96) and α_2-adrenoceptor agonist clonidine (97) were shown to prevent STZ-induced cardiomyopathy, cardiac dysfunction and hyperlipidemias. These investigators also reported that cardioselective β-adrenoceptor blockers atenolol (98), ramipril (99), and nitrendipine (100) did not improve diabetes-induced cardiac dysfunctions, cardiomyopathy, and hyperlipidemia. Extension of the studies to clinical situations supported the beneficial effects of enalapril, nifedipine and clonidine especially in lowering lipid levels in diabetic patients (101–103). Suitability of ACE inhibitors and calcium channel blockers has also been reviewed by others (104,105). Beneficial effects have also been reported for beraprost sodium (106), diltiazem (107,108) and captopril in diabetic animals (109) and patients (110). Veraparmil has also been reported to attenuate diabetes-induced changes in heart function, metabolism and ultrastructure in rats (111,112). Clinical studies are required, however, to evaluate the effectiveness of various anti-hypertensives in improving cardiac function of diabetic patients.

Drugs affecting lipid metabolism

The unexpected finding that hydralazine not only prevented the streptozotocin-induced cardiac dysfunction but also the elevated lipid levels (89) provoked a series of investigations for examining the effect of drugs that affect lipid metabolism by McNeill and his coworkers (46). Methionine and choline are lipotropic agents that are involved in the synthesis of phosphatidylcholine (which is an integral part of the structural and assembly system of lipoproteins) and bile salt micels (which play a strategic role in cholesterol transport). These agents were found to lower plasma and myocardial lipid content along with improvement of cardiac functions (113). Other treatments that were found to be effective in streptozotocin diabetic rats through modulation of lipid metabolism are intraperitoneally administered carnitine (114), omega-3-fatty acids supplementation in food (115), and myoinositol (116). It is however, a paradox that the classical lipid lowering drugs that are used in clinical practice like clofibrate (117) was not found to improve the depressed cardiac function in streptozotocin diabetic rats. Later, an association with decreased cardiac glucose metabolism resulting from increased utilization of fatty acid metabolism in the diabetic heart was considered to be an important factor in the depression of cardiac function. Drugs like phenylalkyloxiranecarboxylic acid (118), etomoxir (119), or methylpalmoxirate (120) (inhibitor of carnitine palmitoyltransferase) and dichloroacetate (121) that stimulate glucose oxidation were reported to improve cardiac function along with reduction in lipid levels. Probucol, a lipid lowering drug, could not decrease the myocardial oxyterol content (122). However, it is reported to reverse cardiac dysfunction in diabetic rats and was associated with antioxidant effect of probucol (123,124). Recently it has been reported that there is a decrease in coenzyme Q10 levels in NIDDM patients and the treatment with 3-hydroxy-3 methylglutaryl coenzyme A (HMG Co-A) inhibitors like simvastatin produce beneficial effect in diabetic cardiomyopathy (125). Although the significance of lipid and glucose metabolism in chronic diabetes and subsequently cardiomyopathy can not be challenged, it is still a long way to get a drug that can prevent or reverse the diabetic cardiomyopathy by directly affecting lipid metabolism.

Antioxidants

As mentioned earlier, probucol produces beneficial effects in diabetic cardiomyopathy by virtue of its antioxidative mechanism. There is, however, enough evidence that indicates the effectiveness of antioxidants in diabetic cardiomyopathy. Increase in lipid peroxidases, thiobarbituric acid reactive substances and isoprostanes, such as 8-epi-isoprostaglandin F_{2a}, have been reported to be elevated in diabetic heart (126–128). There is also a decrease in vitamin E, intracellular tocopherol and glutathione concentration in patients with NIDDM (129,130). Supplementation with vitamin E or alpha-tocopherol has been reported to prevent this depression and produce adequate glycemic control. However, studies are scanty to illustrate the effects of these supplementation on cardiac function in animal models of diabetes mellitus or NIDDM patients. Ascorbic acid (131) and probucol (123) and Ginkgo biloba extract Egb 761 (130) have been reported to produce favorable effects in cardiac function with reduction in oxidative stress. Recently, it has been shown that high glucose induces generation of superoxide anions and to thereby activation of transcription factors such as NF-κB proteins including gene encoding TNF-α, interleukins-I (133). Once again several therapeutic strategies have been suggested to reduce cardiac contractile depression through factors like TNF-α (134) but studies are warranted in relation to their beneficial effects in preventing diabetic cardiomyopathy.

Trace elements and their complexes

In 1985, Heyliger et al. (135) first reported that oral administration of sodium orthovanadate produced not only euglycemia but also prevented decrease in cardiac functions in streptozotocin-induced diabetic rats. This was subsequently confirmed by other studies using metavanadate (136), vanadyl sulphate (137), and bis(maltolato)oxovanadium(IV) (BMOV) (138,139). BMOV has also been shown to attenuate hyperinsulinemia and hypertension in spontaneously diabetic (BB) rats (140), insulin resistant spontaneously hypertensive rats (141), insulin-resistant Zucker *fa/fa* rats (142) and in human trials (143). Thus, vanadium or its complexes may have a potential for the treatment of not only diabetes but also the associated cardiovascular complications. However, there have been scanty toxicological studies to evaluate the safety of these complexes. Dai et al. (144) reported that vanadyl sulphate is devoid of any serious toxic effects after one year of treatment in rats. Although vanadium has recently been introduced as a food supplement in some parts of the world, its effectiveness and toxicological profile in patients with cardiac problems has not yet been obtained. Besides vanadium, other trace elements have been reported effective in diabetes mellitus. They include selenium (145), chromium (146), zinc (147), copper and magnesium (148). Their effectiveness in cardiac dysfunctions has not been studied except for a few agents like selenium (145) and magnesium (149). Considering the success of vanadium, trace elements can be considered as potential therapeutic agents for the treatment of diabetic cardiomyopathy.

Miscellaneous agents

With the understanding of various defects in SL and SR membrane proteins and signal transduction mechanisms, several other agents have been studied in diabetic cardiomyopathy in streptozotocin-diabetic rat models. These include L-propionyl-carnitine (150), carnitine palmitoyl-transferase inhibitor I inhibitor, etomoxir (151), PKC β-selective inhibitor LY333531 (51), thiotic acid (152), prostacyclin analogue, beraprost (106) and collagen content reducer, L-arginine (153). All of these agents are experimental drugs only and thus should be exploited for clinical trials. In addition there are several targets like 5-hydroxytryptamine (5-HT_{2A}) receptors and growth factors that have proven to be effective in improving cardiac conditions like myocardial ischemia, volume-overload and myocardial infarction in non-diabetic situation. These targets may also be considered as potential for diabetic cardiomyopathy and there is a need to investigate these in the diabetic state in animal models and clinical situations.

CONCLUDING REMARKS

Cellular mechanisms involved in the pathogenesis of diabetic cardiomyopathy appear to be relatively clear and it has opened up several drug targets for the treatment of this disease. At present, there is no clinically proven efficacious drug specifically designated for the treatment of diabetic cardiomyopathy. Prevention or retardation of the progress of diabetic cardiomyopathy still depends on various anti-hypertensive and anti-diabetic agents. Lipid lowering drugs, antioxidants as well as some trace elements and their complexes have been investigated for their effectiveness in preventing or retarding the progression of diabetic cardiomyopathy. However, extensive clinical studies are required to be carried out in this direction. Antioxidants, trace metals and agents acting on specific molecular or genetic targets are being used as the experimental tools only. It can be suggested, that the current research may be diverted to evaluate the clinically used antihypertensive and antidiabetic drugs from the view point of their effectiveness in retarding or preventing diabetic cardiomyopathy, in addition to a search for newer agents like trace elements, antioxidants and anti-growth factors.

ACKNOWLEDGEMENTS

The research reported in this article was supported by a grant from Canadian Institutes of Health Research (CIHR) Group in Experimental Cardiology. NSD holds a CIHR/Pharmaceutical Research and Development Chair in Cardiovascular Sciences supported by Merck Frosst Canada. RKG was a Visiting Professor from L.M. College of Pharmacy, Ahmedabad, India.

REFERENCES

1. Ahmed SS, Jaferi G, Narang RM, Regan TJ. 1975. Preclinical abnormality of left ventricular function in diabetes mellitus. Am Heart J 89:153–158.
2. Kannel WB, McGee DL. 1979. Diabetes and cardiovascular disease: The Framingham study. JAMA 241:2035–2038.
3. Hamby RI, Zoneraich S, Sherman L. 1974. Diabetic cardiomyopathy. JAMA 229:1749–1754.
4. Ledet T, Neubauer B, Christensen NJ, Lundbaek K. 1979. Diabetes cardiopathy. Diabetologia 16:207–209.
5. Fein FS, Sonnenblick EH. 1985. Diabetic cardiomyopathy. Prog Cardiovasc Res 27:255–270.
6. Regan TJ, Wu CF, Yeh CK, Oldewurtel HA, Haider B. 1981. Myocardial composition and function in diabetes: the effects of chronic insulin use. Circ Res 49:1268–1277.
7. Miller TB Jr. 1979. Cardiac performance of isolated perfused hearts from alloxan diabetic rats. Am J Physiol 236:808–812.
8. Vadlamudi RVSV, Rodgers RL, McNeill JH. 1982. The effect of chronic alloxan- and streptozotocin-induced diabetes on isolated rat heart performance. Can J Physiol Pharmacol 60:902–911.
9. Fein FS, Kornstein LB, Strobeck JE, Capasso JM, Sonnenblick EH. 1980. Altered myocardial mechanics in diabetic rats. Circ Res 47:922–933.
10. Factor SM, Minase T, Sonnenblick EH. 1980. Clinical and morphological features of human hypertensive-diabetic cardiomyopathy. Am Heart J 99:446–458.
11. Reaven GM. 1988. Role of insulin resistance in human disease. Diabetes 37:1595–1607.
12. Reaven GM, Lithell H, Landsberg L. 1996. Hypertension and associated metabolic abnormalities—the role of insulin resistance and the sympathoadrenal system. New Engl J Med 334:374–381.
13. Schaffer SW. 1991. Cardiomyopathy associated with non-insulin-dependent diabetes. Mol Cell Biochem 107:1–20.

14. Goyal RK. 1999. Hyperinsulinemia and insulin resistance in hypertension: Differential effects of antihypertensive agents. Clin Exptl Hyperten 21:167–179.
15. Regan TJ. 1983. Congestive heart failure in diabetics. Ann Rev Med 34:161–168.
16. Geer JC, Bishop SP, James TN. 1979. Pathology of small intramural coronary arteries. Pathol Annu 28:125–154.
17. Squadrito G, Cucinotta D. 1991. The late complications of diabetes mellitus. Ann Ital Med Int 6:126–136.
18. Page MM, Watkins PJ. 1977. The heart in diabetes: autonomic neuropathy and cardiomyopathy. Clin Endocrinol Metabol 6:377–388.
19. Pinkney JH, Stehouwer CD, Coppack SW, Yudkin JS. 1998. Endothelial dysfunction: Cause of the insulin resistance syndrome. Diabetes 46:S9–S13.
20. Liu X, Wang J, Takeda N, Binaglia L, Panagia V, Dhalla NS. 1998. Subcellular remodeling and heart dysfunction in chronic diabetes. Cardiovasc Res 40:239–247.
21. Christlieb AR, Underwood L. 1979. Renin-angiotensin-aldosterone system, electrolyte homeostasis and blood pressure in alloxan diabetics. Am J Med Sci 277:295–303.
22. Sechi A, Griffin CA, Shambelan M. 1994. The cardiac renin-angiotensin system in STZ-induced diabetes. Diabetes 43:1180–1184.
23. Dhalla NS, Pierce GN, Innes IR, Beamish RE. 1985. Pathogenesis of cardiac dysfuncion in diabetes mellitus. Can J Cardiol 1:263–281.
24. Kaul CL. 1999. Role of sympathetic nervous system in experimental hypertension and diabetes mellitus. Clin Exptl Hypertens 21:95–112.
25. Opie LH, Tansey MJ, Kennelly BM. 1979. The heart in diabetes mellitus. Part I Biochemical basis of myocardial dysfunction. S Afr Med J 56:207–211.
26. Dhalla NS, Elimban V, Rupp H. 1992. Paradoxical role of lipid metabolism in heart function. Mol Cell Biochem 116:3–9.
27. Rodrigues B, McNeill JH. 1992. The diabetic heart: metabolic causes for the development of cardiomyopathy. Cardiovasc Res 26:913–922.
28. Brownlee M, Cerami A, Vlassara H. 1988. Advanced glycosylation end products in tissue and the biochemical basis of diabetic complications. N Eng J Med 117:1315–1321.
29. Willamson JR, Chang K, Frangos M, Hasan KS, Ido Y, Kawamura T, Nyengaard JR, van den Enden M, Kilo C, Tilton RG. 1993. Hyperglycemic pseudohypoxia and diabetic complications. Diabetes 42:801–813.
30. Khattar JC, Sadi P, Zhang M, Hoeschen RJ. 1996. Myocardial angiotensin II (Ang II) receptors in diabetes. Ann NY Acad Sci 793:466–472.
31. Classis LA. 1992. Down regulation of renin-angiotensin system in STZ-diabetic rats. Am J Physiol 262:E105–E109.
32. Christlieb AR. 1974. Renin angiotensin and NE in alloxan diabetes. Diabetes 23:962–970.
33. Rett K, Janch KW, Wicklmayr M, Dietze G, Fink E, Mehnert H. 1996. Angiotensin converting enzyme inhibitors in diabetes: experimental and human experience. Postgrad Med J 62:59–64.
34. Ganguly PK, Dhalla KS, Innes IR, Beamish RE, Dhalla NS. 1985. Altered norepinephrine turnover and metabolism in diabetic cardiomyopathy. Circ Res 59:684–693.
35. Gotzsche O. 1983. The adrenergic β-receptor adenylate cyclase system in heart and lymphocytes from streptozotocin-induced diabetic cardiomyopathy. Diabetes 32:1110–1116.
36. Smith CE, Pierce GN, Dhalla NS. 1984. Alterations in adenylate cyclase activity due to streptozotocin-induced diabetic cardiomyopathy. Life Sci 34:1223–1230.
37. Ingerbretsen CG, Hawelu-Johnson C, Ingerbretsen WR. 1983. Alloxan-induced diabetes reduces β-adrenergic number without affecting adenylate cyclase in rat ventricular membranes. J Cardiovasc Pharmacol 5:454–461.
38. Dillmann WH. 1989. Diabetes and thyroid hormone-induced changes in cardiac function and their molecular basis. Ann Rev Med 40:373–394.
39. Goyal RK, Rodrigues B, McNeill JH. 1987. Effect of tri-iodothyronine on cardiac responses to adrenergic-agonists in STZ-induced diabetic rats. Gen Pharmacol 18:357–362.
40. Rodrigues B, McNeill JH. 1992. The diabetic heart: Metabolic causes for the development of a cardiomyopathy. Cardiovasc Res 26:913–922.
41. Rodrigues B, Cam MC, McNeill JH. 1995. Myocardial substrate metabolism: Implications for diabetic cardiomyopathy. J Mol Cell Cardiol 27:169–179.
42. Opie LH. 1970. Effect of fatty acid on contractility and rhythm of the heart. Nature 227: 1055–1056.

43. Rodrigues B, Braun JE, Spooner M, Severson DL. 1992. Regulation of lipoprotein lipase activity in cardiac myocytes from control and diabetic rats by plasma lipids. Can J Physiol Pharmacol 70:1271–1279.
44. Rodrigues B, Cam MC, Jian K, Lim F, Sambandam N, Sherpherd G. 1997. Differential effects of streptozotocin-induced diabetes on cardiac lipoprotein lipase activity. Diabetes 46:1346–1353.
45. Rodrigues B, Cam MC, McNeill JH. 1998. Metabolic disturbances in diabetic cardiomyopathy. Mol Cell Biochem 180:53–57.
46. McNeill JH. 1996. Role of elevated lipids in diabetic cardiomyopathy. Diab Res Clin Pract 31: S67–S71.
47. Chatham JC, Foder JR. 1993. A ^{13}C-NMR study of glucose oxidation in the intact functions of rat heart following diabetes-induced cardiomyopathy. J Mol Cell Cardiol 25:1203–1213.
48. Gamble J, Lopaschuk GD. 1994. Glycolysis and glucose oxidation during reperfusion of aschemic hearts from diabetic rats. Biochim Biophys Acta 1225:191–199.
49. Stanley WC, Lopaschuk GD, McCormak JG. 1997. Regulation of energy substrate metabolism in the diabetic heart. Cardiovasc Res 34:25–33.
50. Banes JW. 1991. Role of oxidative stress in the development of complications in diabetes. Diabetes 40:405–412.
51. Koya D, King GL. 1998. Protein kinase-C activation and the development of diabetic complications. Diabetes 47:859–866.
52. Baynes JW. 1991. Role of oxidative stress in development of complications in diabetes. Diabetes 40:405–412.
53. Russ M, Reinauer H, Eckel J. 1991. Diabetes-induced decrease in the mRNA coding for sarcoplasmic reticulum Ca^{2+} ATPase in adult rat cardiomyocytes. Biochim Biophys Res Commun 178:906–912.
54. Zarain-Herzberg A, Yano K, Elimban V, Dhalla NS. 1994. Cardiac sarcoplasmic reticulum Ca^{2+} ATPase expression in streptozotocin-induced diabetes. Biochim Biophys Res Commun 203:113–120.
55. Xu YJ, Elimban V, Takeda S, Ren B, Takeda N, Dhalla NS. 1996. Cardiac sarcoplasmic reticulum function and gene expression in chronic diabetes. Cardiovasc Pathobiol 1:89–96.
56. Pierce GN, Dhalla NS. 1987. Sarcolemmal Na^+-K^+ ATPase activity in diabetic rat heart. Am J Physiol 245:C241–C247.
57. Dhalla NS, Pierce GN, Panagia V, Singal PK, Beamish RE. 1982. Calcium movements in relation to heart function. Basic Res Cardiol 77:117–139.
58. Pierce GN, Dhalla NS. 1985. Heart mitochondrial function in chronic experimental diabetes in rats. Can J Cardiol 1:48–54.
60. Ziegelhoffer A, Ravingerova T, Styk J, Sebokova J, Waczulikova I, Breier A, Dzurba A, Volkovova K, Carsky J, Turecky L. 1997. Mechanisms that may be involved in calcium tolerance of diabetic heart. Mol Cell Biochem 176:191–198.
61. Okumura K, Akiyama N, Hashimoto H, Ogawa K, Satake T. 1988. Alteration of 1,2-diacylglycerol content in myocardium from diabetic rats. Diabetes 37:1168–1172.
62. Xiang H, McNeill JH. 1991. α-Adrenoceptor-mediated phosphoinoside breakdown and inotropic responses in diabetic hearts. Am J Physiol 260:H557–H562.
63. Tanaka Y, Kashiwagi A, Saeki Y, Shigeta Y. 1992. Abnormalities in cardiac α_1-adrenoceptor and its signal transduction in streptozotocin-induced diabetic rats. Am J Physiol 263:E425–E429.
64. Williams SA, Tappia PS, Yu CH, Bibeau M, Panagia V. 1998. Impairment of the sarcolemmal phospholipase D-phosphatidate phosphohydrolase pathway in diabetic cardiomyopathy. J Mol Cell Cardiol 30:109–118.
65. Malhotra A, Sanghi V. 1997. Regulation of contractile proteins in diabetic heart. Cardiovasc Res 34: 34–40.
66. Dillmann WH. 1980. Diabetes mellitus induces changes in cardiac myosin of the rat. Diabetes 29: 579–582.
67. Liu X, Takeda N, Dhalla NS. 1996. Troponin I phosphorylation in heart homogenate from diabetic rat. Biochim Biophys Acta 1316:78–84.
68. Thompson EW. 1988. Structural manifestations of diabetic cardiomyopathy in the rats and its reversal by insulin treatment. Am J Anat 182:270–282.
69. Regan TJ, Wu CF, Yeh CK, Odewurtel HA, Haider B. 1981. Myocardial composition and function in diabetics. The effects of chronic insulin use. Circ Res 49:1268–1277.

70. McNeill JH, Tahiliani AG. 1986. Diabetes-induced cardiac changes. Trend Pharmacol Sci 7: 364–367.
71. Fein FS, Strobeck JE, Malhotra A, Scheuer J, Sonnenblick EH. 1981. Reversibility of diabetic cardiomyopathy with insulin in rats. Circ Res 49:1268–1277.
72. Fein FS, Malhotra A, Miller-Green B, Scheuer J, Sonnenblick EH. 1984. Diabetic cardiomyopathy in rats: Mechanical and biochemical response to different insulin doses. Am J Physiol 247:H817–H823.
73. Hockaday TD. 1987. Serum insulin concentrations and anticipatory factors of cardiomyopathy in NIDDM. Diabetes Metab 13:354–358.
74. Thompson EW. 1994. Quantitative analysis of myocardial structure in insulin-dependent diabetes mellitus: Effects of immediate and delayed insulin replacement. Proc Soc Exp Biol Med 205:294–305.
75. Meinert CL, Knatterud GL, Prout TE, Klimt C. 1970. A study of the effects of hypoglycemic agents on vascular complications in patients with adult-onset diabetes. II. Mortality results. Diabetes 19:747–830.
76. Pasikivi J. 1970. Long term tolbutamide treatment after myocardial infarction: a clinical and biochemical study of 178 patients without overt diabetes. Acta Med Scand 507:1–82.
77. Seltzer H. 1972. A summary of criticisms of the findings and conclusions of the University Group Diabetes Program (UGDP). Diabetes 21:4–11.
78. Ashcroft S, Ashcroft FM. 1992. The sulphonylurea receptor. Biochim Biophys Acta 1175:45–59.
79. Fosset M, De Weille JR, Green RD, Schmid-Antomarchi H, Lazdunski M. 1988. Antidiabetic sulphonyureas control action potential properties in heart cells via high affinity receptors that are linked to ATP-dependent K^+ channels. J Bio Chem 263:7933–7936.
80. Schotborgh CE, Wilde AAM. 1997. Sulphonyurea derivatives in cardiovascular research and in cardiovascular patients. Circ Res 34:73–80.
81. Engler RL, Yellon DM. 1996. Sulphonylurea K_{ATP} blockade in type II diabetes and preconditioning in cardiovascular disease: time for reconsideration. Circulation 94:2297–2301.
82. Brady PA, Terzic A. 1998. The sulphonylurea controversy: More questions from the heart. J Am Coll Cardiol 31:950–956.
83. Kulkarni JS, Mehta AA, Santani DD, Goyal RK. 2002. Effect of chronic treatment with cromakalim and glibenclamide in alloxan diabetic rats. Pharmacol Res 46:101–105.
84. Chan JC, Tomlinson B, Critchley JA, Cockran CS, Walden RJ. 1993. Metabolic and hemodynamic effects of metformin and glibenclamide in normotensive NIDDM patients. Diabetes Care 16:1035–1038.
85. Cacciapuoti F, Spiezia R, Bianchi U, Lama D, D'Avino M, Varricchio M. 1991. Effectiveness of glibenclamide on myocardial ventricular arrhythmias in non-insulin dependent diabetes mellitus. Am J Cardiol 67:843–847.
86. Verma S, McNeill JH. 1994. Metformin improves cardiac function in isolated streptozotocin-diabetic rat hearts. Am J Physiol 266:714–719.
87. Jennings PE. 1997. Oral antihyperglycemics. Considerations in older patients with non-insulin dependent diabetes mellitus. Drugs Aging 10:323–331.
88. MacMohan S, Peto R, Cutler J, Collins R, Sorlie P, Neaton J, Abbott R, Godwin J, Dyer A, Stamler J. 1990. Blood pressure, stroke and coronary heart disease. Lancet 335:765–774.
89. Rodrigues B, Goyal RK, McNeill JH. 1986. Effects of hydralazine on STZ induced diabetic rats: Prevention of hyperlipidemia and improvement in cardiac function. J Pharmacol Exptl Therap 237:299–307.
90. Bangaru RA, Lakkad NB, Goyal RK. 1996. Effect of chronic atenolol and prazosin treatment on diabetes induced cardiac depression and other complications. Ind J Physiol Pharmac 40:220–224.
91. Goyal RK, Lakkad NB, Bangaru RA Rao MV. 1997. Effects of chronic treatment with enalapril on streptozotocin-induced diabetic rats. Pharmacol Rev Commun 9:133–139.
92. Sevak AR, Goyal RK. 1996. Effect of chronic treatment with lisinopril on cardiovascular complications in streptozotocin diabetic and DOCA hypertensive rats. Pharmacol Res 34:201–209.
93. Parulekar AA, Srinivasan PS, Hakim ZS, Santani DD, Goyal RK. 1996. Spirapril attenuates hyperinsulinemia and hypertension in spontaneously hypertensive rats. Ind J Hypertens 1:8–10.
94. Shah TS, Bangaru RA, Goyal RK. 1995. Effect of chronic treatment with nifedipine on diabetes induced cardiac dysfunction and other complication. J Cardiovasc Pharmacol 26:6–12.
95. Srinivasan PS, Hakim ZS, Santani DD, Goyal RK. 1997. Effects of chronic treatment with amlodipine in streptozotocin-diabetic and spontaneously hypertensive rats. Pharmacol Res 35:423–428.

96. Gokhale MS, Shah DH, Hakim ZS, Santani DD, Goyal RK. 1998. Effect of chronic treatment with amlodipine on insulin sensitivity in NIDDM-diabetic rats. Pharmacol Res 37:455–459.
97. Damani RC, Satia MC, Goyal RK. 1997. Beneficial effects of clonidine in streptozotocin induced diabetes and DOCA hypertensive rats. J Pharm Pharmacol 49:1030–1035.
98. Bangaru, RA, Lakkad NB, Goyal RK. 1996. Effect of chronic atenolol treatment on diabetes induced cardiac depression and other complications. Ind J Physiol Pharmacol 40:220–224.
99. Hakim ZS, Patel BK, Goyal RK. 1997. Effect of chronic ramipril treatment in streptozotocin-induced diabetic rats. Ind J Physiol Pharmacol 41:353–360.
100. Joshi SS, Shah TS, Goyal RK. 1996. Effect of chronic treatment with nitrendipine in streptozotocin induced diabetic rats. Ind J Pharm Sci 58:100–105.
101. Satia MC, Shukla ML, Goyal RK. 1995. Comparative effects of atenolol versus nifedipine on serum lipids and other biochemical parameters in diabetic and non-diabetic hypertensive subjects. Ind J Physiol Pharmacol 39:237–241.
102. Satia MC, Shukla ML, Goyal RK. 1996. Effects of enalapril on lipids profile in diabetic and non-diabetic essential hypertensive patients. Ind J Physiol Pharmacol 40:83–86.
103. Satia MC, Shukla ML, Gandhi TP, Goyal RK. 1997. Prevalence of hypertension and comparative evaluation of four antihypertensive monotherapy in Indian NIDDM hypertensive patients. Ind J Hypertens 2:17–27.
104. Mahgoub MA, Abd-Elfattch AS. 1998. Diabetes mellitus and cardiac function. Mol Cell Biochem 180:59–64.
105. Moser M. 1997. Angiotensin converting enzyme inhibitors, angiotensin II receptor antagonists and calcium channel blocking agents: a review of potential benefits and possible adverse reactions. J Am Coll Cardiol 29:1414–1421.
106. Ueno Y, Koike H, Nishio S. 1995. Beneficial effects of beraprost sodium, a stable prostacyclin analogue in diabetic cardiomyopathy. J Cardiovasc Pharmacol 26:605–607.
107. Shimoda T. 1993. Correlation between metabolic and histopathological changes in the myocardium of the KK mouse. Effect of diltiazem on the diabetic heart. Jpn Heart J 34:617–626.
108. Fein FS, Cho S, Malhotra A, Akella J, van Hoeven KH, Sonnenblick EH, Factor SM. 1991. Beneficial effects of diltiazem on the natural history of hypertensive diabetic cardiomyopathy in rats. J Am Coll Cardiol 18:1406–1417.
109. Rosen R, Romp AF, Rosen P. 1995. The ACE inhibitor captopril improves myocardial performence in spontaneously diabetic (BB) rats. Diabetologia 38:509–517.
110. Risler T, Braun U, Klarner HG, Muller-Schauenburg W, Heitkamp HC, Brilla GG, Kramer BK, Seipel L. 1991. Comparison of lisinopril and captopril in the treatment of severe heart failure (NYHA III–IV) in high risk patients. Preliminary results of the trial. Z Kardil 80:40–43.
111. Afzal N, Ganguly PK, Dhalla KS, Pierce GN, Singal PK, Dhalla NS. 1988. Beneficial effects of verapamil in diabetic cardiomyopathy. Diabetes 37:936–942.
112. Afzal N, Pierce GN, Elimban V, Beamish RE, Dhalla NS. 1989. Influence of verapamil on some subcellular defects in diabetic cardiomyopathy. Am J Physiol 256:453–458.
113. Heyliger CE, Rodrigues B, McNeill JH. 1986. Effect of choline and methionine treatment on cardiac dysfunction of diabetic rats. Diabetes 35:1152–1157.
114. Rodrigues B, Xiang H, McNeill JH. 1988. Effect of L-carnitine treatment on lipid metabolism and cardiac function in chronically diabetic rats. Diabetes 37:1358–1364.
115. Black SC, Katz S, McNeill JH. 1989. Cardiac performance and plasma lipids of omega-3-fatty acid treated streptozotocin-induced diabetic rats. Diabetes 38:969–974.
116. Xiang H, Heyliger CE, McNeill JH. 1988. Effect of myo-inositol and T_3 on myocardial lipids and cardiac function in streptozotocin-induced diabetic rats. Diabetes 37:1542–1547.
117. Rodrigues B, Grassby PF, Battel ML, Lee SY, McNeill JH. 1992. Hypertriglyceridemia in experimental diabetes: relationship to cardiac dysfunction. Can J Physiol Pharmacol 72:447–455.
118. Rosen P, Reinauer H. 1984. Inhibition of carnitine palmitoyltransferase I by phenylalkyloxirane-carboxylic acid and its influence on lipolysis and glucose metabolism in isolated, perfused hearts of streptozotocin-diabetic rats. Metabolism 22:177–185.
119. Schmitz FJ, Rosen P, Reinauer H. 1995. Improvement of myocardial function and metabolism in diabetic rats by the carnitine palmitoyltransferase inhibitor etomoxir. Horm Metab Res 27:515–522.
120. Tahiliani AG, McNeill JH. 1985. Prevention of diabetes-induced myocardial dysfunction in rats by methylpalmoxirate and triiodothyronine treatment. Can J Physiol Pharmacol 63:925–931.
121. Nicholl TA, Lopaschuk GD, McNeill JH. 1991. Effect of free fatty acids and dichloroacetate on isolated working diabetic rat heart. Am J Physiol 261:H1053–H1059.

122. Matsui H, Okumura K, Mukawa H, Hibino M, Toki Y, Ito T. 1997. Increased oxysterol contents in diabetic rat hearts: Their involvement in diabetic cardiomyopathy. Can J Cardiol 13:373–379.
123. Tada H, Oida K, Kutsumi Y, Shimada Y, Nakai T, Miyabo S. 1992. Effect of probucol on impaired cardiac performance and lipid metabolism in streptozotocin-induced diabetic rats. J Cardiovasc Pharmaciol 20:179–186.
124. Kaul N, Siveski-Iliskovic N, Hill M, Khaper N, Seneviratne C, Singal PK. 1996. Probucol treatment reverses antioxidant and functional deficit in diabetic cardiomyopathy. Mol Cell Biochem 160:283–288.
125. Miyake Y, Shouzu A, Nishikawa M, Yonemoto T, Shimizu H, Omoto S, Hayakawa T, Inada M. 1999. Effect of treatment with 3-hydroxy-3-methylglutaryl coenzyme A reductase inhibitors on serum coenzyme Q 10 in diabetic patients. Arzen Forsch 49:324–329.
126. Nishigaki I, Hagihara M, Tsunekawa H, Maseki M, Yagi K. 1981. Lipid peroxidase levels of serum lipoprotein fractions of diabetic patients. Biochem Med 25:373–378.
127. Rosen P, Du X, Tschope D. 1998. Role of oxygen derived radicals for vascular dysfunction in the diabetic heart: prevention by alpha-tochopherol? Mol Cell Biochem 188:103–111.
128. Gopaul NK, Anggard EE, Mallet AI. 1995. Plasma 8-epi-$PGF_{2\alpha}$ levels are elevated in individuals with NIDDM. FEBS Lett 368:225–229.
129. Bellomo G, Maggi E, Palladini G, Perugini, Seccia M. 1997. Oxidation of low density lipoproteins and vitamin E status in non insulin dependent diabetes melllitus (NIDDM). Diabetes & Stoffw 6(Suppl 2):29–33.
130. Simon-Schnass I, Rosak CH, Tritschler HJ, Rosen P. 1997. Alpha-tochoperolaufnahme und-zufur bei Typ II Diabetikern. Diabetes & Stoffw 6(Suppl 2):16–19.
131. Dai S, McNeill JH. 1995. Ascorbic acid supplementation prevents hyperlipidemia and improves myocardial performance in streptozotocin-induced diabetic rats. Diabetes Res Clin Pract 27:11–18.
132. Welt K, Weiss J, Koch S, Fitzl G. 1999. Protective effects of Ginkgo biloba extract EGB 761 on the myocardium of experimentally diabetic rats. Ultrastructural and imunohistochemical investigation on microvessels and interstitium. Exp Toxicol Pathol 51:213–222.
133. Brand K, Page S, Rogler G. 1996. Activated transcription factor nuclear factor kappa B is present in atherosclerotic lesion. J Clin Invest 97:1715–1722.
134. Cain BS, Harken AH, Meldrum DR. 1999. Therapeutic strategies to reduce TNF-α mediated cardiac contractile depression following ischemia and reperfusion. J Mol Cell Cardiol 31:931–947.
135. Heyliger CE, Tahiliani AG, McNeill JH. 1985. Effect of vanadate on elevated blood glucose and depressed cardiac performance of diabetic rats. Science 227:1474–1477.
136. Meryerovitch J, Farfel Z, Sack J, Shechter Y. 1987. Oral administration of vanadate normalizes blood glucose leves in streptozotocin-treated rats. Characterization and mode of action. J Biol Chem 262:6658–6662.
137. Ramanadhan S, Mongold JJ, Brownsey RW, Cros GH, McNeill JH. 1989. Oral vanadyl sulphate treatment of diabetes in rats. Am J Physiol 257:H904–H911.
138. McNeill JH, Yuen VG, Hoveyda HR, Orvig C. 1992. Bis(maltolato)oxovanadium(IV) is a potent insulin mimic. J Med Chem 35:1489–1491.
139. Yuen VG, Orvig C, McNeill JH. 1997. Effects of bis(maltolato)oxovanadium(IV) are distinct from food restriction in STZ-diabetic rats. Endocrinol Metab 272:E30–E35.
140. Battel ML, Yuen VG, McNeill JH. 1992. Treatment of BB rats with vanadyl sulphate. Pharmacol Commun 1:291–301.
141. Bhanot S, BryerAsh M, Chenung A, McNeill JH. 1994. Bis(maltolato)oxovanadium (IV) attenuates hyperinsulinaemia and hypertension in spontaneously hypertensive rats. Diabetes 43:857–861.
142. Brichard SM, Poitier AM, Henquin JC. 1989. Long term improvement of glucose homeostasis by vanadate in obese hyperinsulinemic fa/fa rats. Endocrinology 125:2510–2516.
143. Cohen N, Halberstam M, Shimovich P. 1995. Oral vanadyl sulphate improves hepatic and peripheral insulin sensitivity in patients with non-insulin dependent diabetes mellitus. J Clin Invest 95: 2501–2509.
144. Dai S, McNeill JH. 1994. Toxicity studies on one year treatment of non-diabetic and streptozotocin-diabetic rats with vanadyl sulphate. Pharmacol Toxicol 75:265–273.
145. Battel ML, Delgatty HL, McNeill JH. 1998. Sodium selenate corrects glucose tolerance and heart function in STZ diabetic rats. Mol Cell Biochem 179:27–34.
146. Ravina A, Slezak L, Mirsky N, Bryden NA, Anderson RA. 1999. Reversal of corticosteroid-induced diabetes mellitus with supplemental chromium. Diabet Med 16:164–167.

147. Brando-Neto J, daSilva CA, Figueiredo NB, Shuhama T, Holanda MB, Diniz JM. 1999. Lack of acute zinc effect in glucose metabolism in healthy and insulin-dependent diabetes mellitus patients. Biometals 12:161–165.
148. Zargar AH, Shah NA, Masoodi SR, Laway BA, Dar FA, Khan AR, Sofi FA, Wani AI. 1998. Copper, zinc and magnesium levels in non-insulin dependent diabetes mellitus. Postgraduate Med J 74: 665–668.
149. Tosaki A, Engelman DT, Engelman RM, Das DK. 1996. The evolution of diabetic response to ischemia/reperfusion and preconditioning in isolated working rat hearts. Cardiovasc Res 31:526–536.
150. Pasini E, Comini L, Ferrari R, de Giuli F, Menotti A, Dhalla NS. 1992. Effect of propionyl-L-carnitine on experimental induced cardiomyopathy in rats. Am J Cardiovasc Pathol 4:216–222.
151. Kato K, Chapman DC, Rupp H, Lukas A, Dhalla NS. 1999. Alterations of heart function and Na^+-K^+ ATPase activity by etomoxir in diabetic rats. J Appl Physiol 86:812–818.
152. Strodter D, Lehmann E, Lehmann U, Tritschler HJ, Bretzel RG, Federlin K. 1995. The influence of thioctic acid on metabolism and function of the diabetic heart. Diabetes Res Clin Pract 29:19–26.
153. Khaidar A, Marx M, Lubec B, Lubec G. 1994. L-arginine reduces heart collagen accumulation in the diabetic db/db mouse. Circulation 90:479–483.

Frontiers in Cardiovascular Health, edited by
N.S. Dhalla, A. Chockalingam,
H.I. Berkowitz & P.K. Singal
Kluwer Academic Publishers, Boston, 2003

Atherosclerotic Regression— A Myth or Reality

Adarsh Kumar, Harharpreet Kaur, Pushpa Devi, and Varun Mohan

Govt. Medical College, Amritsar (India)

Summary. The results of various trials aided by newer modalities to study the atherosclerotic process provide ample evidence that it is not only possible to halt the relentless process of atherosclerosis but also to induce regression. Thus regression of atherosclerotic process is no longer a myth but a well-accepted reality, even though its extent is not very large. This reality has been elegantly articulated by William Roberts "If the serum cholesterol can be prevented from rising above 150 mg/dl, plaques are not laid down, if elevated levels are lowered to 150 mg/dl, further plaques do not form and part of those present may vanish". The process can be modified favorably not only in case of chronic, but also in case of acute atherosclerosis. Besides statins and ACE inhibitors, multitudes of novel therapies are being tested and hold promise in future. Even though the success achieved in inducing regression of atherosclerotic lesions has been modest, it is a step in the right direction. No doubt further exciting research and prospects lie ahead in this field.

***Key words*:** atherosclerosis, regression, coronary artery disease, statins, evidence.

INTRODUCTION

The process of atherosclerosis continues to generate keen interest among the research workers and clinicians of the new millenium due to the increasing incidence of atherosclerotic cardiovascular disease worldwide. The past decade witnessed dramatic improvements in the management of coronary artery disease (CAD). The CRVP (coronary revascularization procedures) though highly effective in relieving angina do not reduce the subsequent risk of MACE (major acute coronary events) as they have no impact on the natural history of CAD (1) and therefore cannot be the

Address for correspondence: Dr. Adarsh Kumar MD, DM., Professor and Head, Department of Cardiology, Govt. Medical College, Amritsar 2121-C, Ranjit Avenue, Amritsar—143001—India. Ph: 91-183-502855, Fax: 91-183-500707, E-mail: adarshk@jla.vsnl.net.in.

answer to tackle this massive global problem. A major shift to expand the treatment of CAD beyond relief of severe symptomatic obstruction towards a more comprehensive therapy aimed at treatment of underlying disease process is necessary (2). But whether it is really possible to alter the history of CAD, slowing, arresting, curbing or even reversing the inexorable atherosclerotic process has been the subject of hottest debate amongst cardiologists of the whole world.

An attempt to understand the basic pathology and the factors that influence the evolution of the atheromatous plaque causing the coronary event has in the recent years shed new light on the subject of plaque regression and stability. With the results of the several large scale trials and advent of new promising techniques to visualize the plaque, the mysteries of atherosclerosis have begun to unfold and have ushered in an era of preventive, rather than just palliative cardiology.

A few years ago there was a genuine doubt as to whether it is possible either to prevent progression of atheromatous lesions in man or to induce partial regression even though both phenomenon had been demonstrated in animals (3) but the studies in recent years have laid this controversy to rest.

PATHOPHYSIOLOGY OF ATHEROSCLEROTIC REGRESSION (Figures 1 & 2)

The knowledge of latest concepts in the pathogenesis of atherosclerosis is essential in order to understand the mechanism of plaque regression and stabilization. Atherosclerosis is a disease with both chronic and acute manifestations. The process begins with the infiltration of LDL-C particles through the endothelium into the intimal layer of arterial wall where they are thought to be oxidized. This is associated with endothelial dysfunction. Activated endothelial cells express adhesion molecules and recruit inflammatory cells predominantly monocytes. Adherence and entrance of monocytes in the subendothelial tissues initiates the vicious cycle.

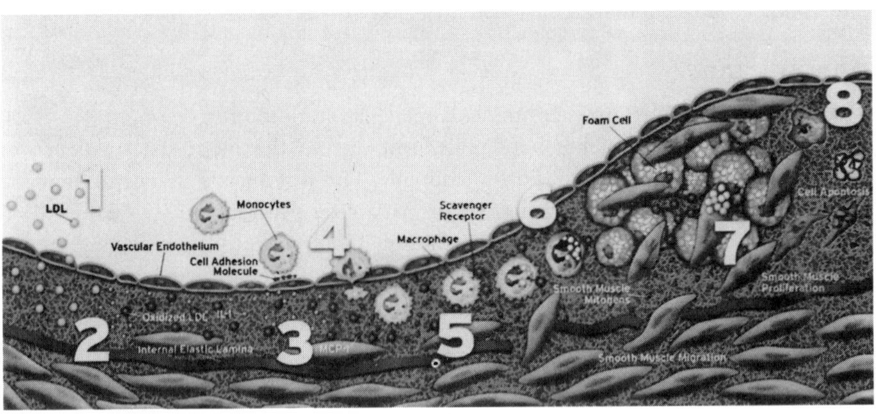

Figure 1. Step wise schematic evolution of the atherosclerotic plaque.

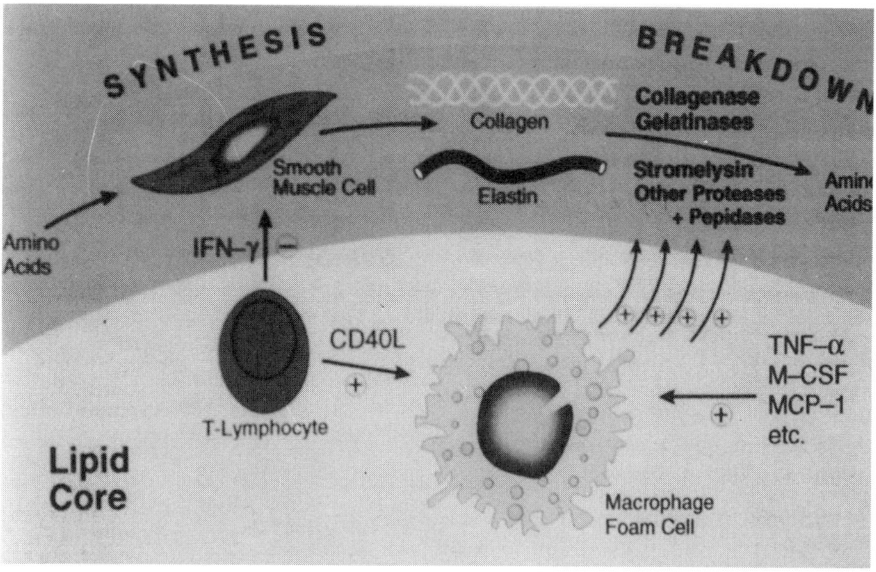

Figure 2. Relationship of extracellular matrix metabolism to intimal inflammation during atherogenesis.

The monocyte imbibes the lipid and becomes a foam cell or a lipid laden macrophage (4), a process which also depends on the LDL receptors (the susceptible persons appear to have "Scavenger" receptors rather than the classical LDL receptors) (5) which mediate excessive lipid uptake characteristic of foam cell formation. Cytokines and growth factors produced by activated macrophages induce smooth muscle cell migration into the intima forming a more complex atheroma (6). There also occurs neovascularization (7). A core of extracellular lipid with an overlying fibrous collagen rich cap characterizes the stable plaque. The vulnerable plaque is rich in lipids, has high macrophage density, a thin fibrous cap and a low content of smooth muscle cells (SMC). The large size, soft consistency and the temperature of the core makes it more prone to rupture. A vulnerable plaque, which can be identified by newer modalities, can be stabilized by intensive therapy so as to prevent an acute event. Activated macrophages induce intimal smooth muscle death and weaken the cap by secretion of enzymes of metalloproteinase family (8), causing erosion and disruption of the plaque and triggers platelet aggregation and atherothrombosis which thus causes transition from chronic to acute atherosclerosis. Certain mediators released from degranulating platelets can increase smooth muscle collagen synthesis and repair of the fibrous cap (PDGF, TGF-β) (9). It has been reported that some smooth muscle cell properties associated with atherogenesis are favorably affected by lipid lowering drugs (10). The success of lipid lowering therapy results not only from reducing lipid accumulation but also by a decrease in the inflammatory process. The recent advances in pathophysiology opens up new avenues for regression of atherosclerosis.

Role of HDL

HDL is thought to have the ability to remove cholesterol from macrophages thus preventing formation of foam cells. Apolipoprotein-A1 present on its surface correlates with HDL-C levels. Tangrila et al. reported that increased levels of Apo-AI can induce atherosclerotic regression (11). Drugs that increase HDL like niacin, estrogens and to some extent statins etc have been tried for atherosclerotic regression. Cholesterol efflux is mediated by the ATP binding cassette A^1 transporter ($ABCA^1$), the rate limiting step in the production of HDL. The results of a study (12) showed a direct relation between $ABCA^1$ mediated cellular cholesterol efflux and arterial wall thickness, which suggests that increasing efflux could inhibit atherosclerosis progression before the manifestations of symptomatic cardiovascular disease.

ROLE OF STATINS

Although vascular remodeling occurs naturally in the course of atherosclerosis, it was hypothesized that the introduction of cholesterol lowering therapy would promote regression and/or retard the progression of atheroma (13). There is increasing evidence that atherosclerotic regression does occur with lipid lowering therapy (14) though the extent to which it has been observed so far is not very impressive.

Regression studies directly assess changes in arterial wall thickness or luminal diameter in high risk patients or those with established CAD, by imaging techniques such as angiography (Figure 3) or B mode ultrasound (Figure 6). There have been several published studies that have explored progression, stabilization and regression of coronary artery lesions during aggressive risk factor modification, most notably lipid lowering therapy (Table III). Data from these studies indicate that statins slow the progression of atherosclerosis in both coronary and carotid arteries. These studies demonstrate that plaque progression is common without therapy in 40–50% of the patients and is reduced by more than one third with statin therapy. Although clear plaque regression is uncommon without therapy the frequency of regression more than doubles with statins (15).

ANGIOGRAPHIC STUDIES WITH STATINS

Although the placebo controlled angiographic studies used different patient selection criteria and different baseline cholesterol levels and variable doses and duration of statin therapy, they uniformly demonstrated benefit in altering the course of atherosclerosis (Tables 1 & 2).

The MASS (16) trial was an angiographic trial that analyzed the effect of diet plus either Simvastatin or placebo in subjects with documented CAD. Quantitative angiographic analysis using computer assisted cardiovascular angiographic analysis system (CAAS) was performed to determine the mean luminal diameter of angiographically diseased segments, minimum lumen diameter, reference diameter and

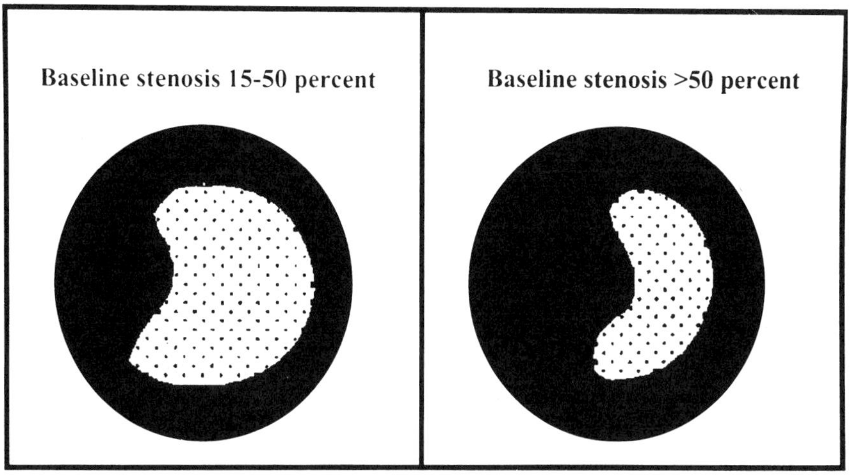

Figure 3. A carton representing the approximate extent of regression (black area) which has been recorded in quantitative angiographic trials of cholesterol lowering by statins (The spotted area represents the lumen)

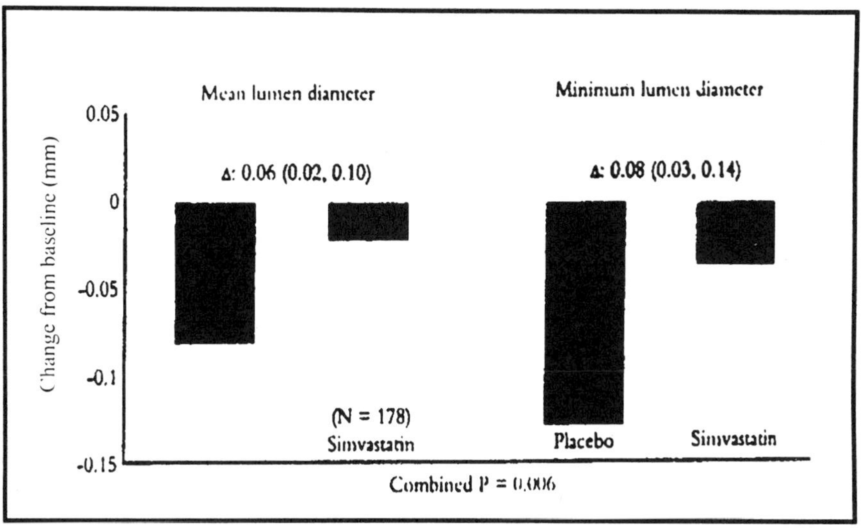

Figure 4. The differences in mean and minimum lumen diameter in the MAAS trial after four years of simvastatin treatment

percent diameter stenosis. Mean arterial diameter needs to be judged in the context that a 50 percent arterial occlusion equals about 2-mm intrusion into the lumen (Figure 3). Simvastatin therapy resulted in a beneficial alteration of the mean lumen diameter, minimum lumen diameter and diameter stenosis when compared with diet and placebo alone (Figure 4). Progression was the predominant angiographic picture

Table 1. Summary of major angiographic trials of the effects of statins on coronary artery disease

Study	Study Description	Duration (yrs)	% Red LCL-C	Control	Treatment	Clinical events
FATS	146 pts. Lovastatin 40–80 mg/d (+colestipol)	2.5	46	46% Prog 11% Regr	21% Prog 32% Regr	Decreased
MARS	270 pts Lovastatin 40 mg bid	2.2	38	41% Prog 12% Regr	29% Prog 23% Regr	NS Reduction
CCAIT	331 pts Lovastatin 20–80 mg/d	2	29	50% Prog 7% Regr	33% Prog 10% Regr	NS Reduction
MASS	381 pts Simvastatin 20 mg/d	4	31.4	32% Prog 12% Regr	23% Prog 18% Regr	NS reduction
REGRESS	885 pts Pravastatin 40 mg/d	2	29	NA	NA	Decreased
PLAC-1	408 pts Pravastatin 40 mg/d	3	28	50% Prog 15% Regr	37% Prog 21% Regr	Decreased
CIS	254 pts Simvastatin 40 mg/d	2.3	35	53.5% Prog 12.9% Regr	34.6% Prog 18.3% Regr	No difference
LCAS	340 pts Fluvastatin 20 mg bid	2.5	23.9	39.1% Prog 8.3% Regr	28.7% Prog 14.6% Regr	NS reduction

Prog: Progression; Regr: Regression; NS = Non-significant; NA: Not available.

Table 2. Angiographic studies of statin monotherapy: modest vascular changes are associated with disproportionate event reductions

Trial (intervention)	% LDL-C reduction Rx-Pbo	MLD $Rx_{final} - RX_{baseline}$	Coronary event reduction (p value)
PLAC (pravastatin)	29	−0.03	60% (p = 0.05)
CCAIT (lovastatin)	27.4	−0.02	22% (NS)
MAAS (simvastatin)	31.4	−0.02 (diffuse disease)	22% (NS)
LCAS (fluvastatin)	26.5	−0.03	24% (NS)

in 54 patients randomized to placebo compared with 41 randomized to simvastatin. In the simvastatin group 33 patients were classified as having undergone angiographic regression as compared with 20 in the placebo group. Thus simvastatin therapy resulted in fewer patients experiencing angiographic progression and a higher proportion who demonstrated actual regression ($p = 0.02$). Angiographic benefit was least evident in current smokers, who accounted for less than 25 percent of both treatment groups. Plaque stability was observed in 94 patients of Simvas-

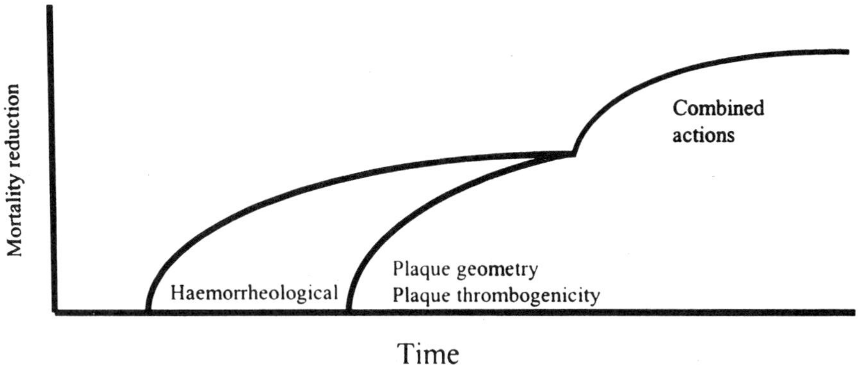

Figure 5. Time courses of putative beneficial effects of statins

tatin compared with 72 randomized to placebo. Fewer lesions and complete occlusions developed in the simvastatin treatment group. The MAAS trial was interpreted as demonstrating that Simvastatin could induce improvements in both focal and diffuse atherosclerosis. Although the angiographic differences between the treatment and control groups were small in absolute terms, the results were consistent with other long-term angiographic trials (Table 1).

Multicentre Coronary Intervention Study (CIS TRIAL) (17)

The mean global change score was +0.2 in the simvastatin group and +0.58 in the placebo group representing a statistically significant decrease in the rate of progression in the group randomized to drug therapy (p 0.02). The mean quantitative change in minimum lumen diameter stenosis was −0.02 mm in the simvastatin group and −0.10 mm in the placebo group again showing a statistically significant slowing of progression ($p = 0.002$) in treatment group as compared to placebo, although there was no difference in clinical events (Table 1).

Canadian Coronary Atherosclerosis Intervention Trial (CCAIT TRIAL) (18)

In this landmark study, progression of atherosclerosis was significantly reduced by Lovastatin therapy. M.L.D. (minimum lumen diameter) decreased by 0.05 mm in lovastatin group and 0.09 mm in the placebo group. Percent diameter stenosis was also increased to a lesser degree with lovastatin (1.66 percent increase with lovastatin compared with 2.89 percent increase with placebo). Lovastatin also significantly reduced the development of new lesions (16% with treated group versus 32% in placebo patients). Anatomical regression could not be demonstrated (Tables 1 & 2).

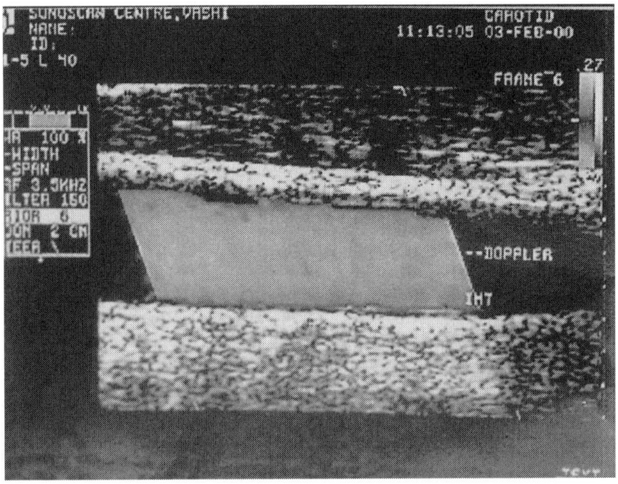

Figure 6. Colour Doppler flow with intima-modia thickness in common arotid

Regression Growth Evaluation Statin Study (REGRESS) (19)

It evaluated a patient cohort with CAD and lipid levels that approximated the distribution of general population. The beneficial changes in the lipid profile by pravastatin therapy could be correlated with improvement in the angiographic parameters. There was also a reduction of risk for clinical events (Table 1).

Monitored Atherosclerosis Regression Study (MARS STUDY) (20)

On analysis of angiographically significant lesions (>50% luminal impingement), in placebo patients average diameter stenosis was increased by 9 percent and decreased by 4.1% in lovastatin recipients indicating highly statistically significant regression ($p = 0.005$) (Table 1).

LCAS (21) and FATS (22) were other such studies demonstrating significant regression of atherosclerosis with lipid lowering therapy versus placebo (Table 1).

B-mode ultrasound atherosclerotic regression trials (Figure 6)

Mention needs to be made of the carotid ultrasound measurements of Intima-media thickness (IMT) which is a validated surrogate marker for atherosclerosis (23). The rate of change of IMT with age has been calculated to be about 0.01 mm/year in general population and 0.03–0.06 mm/year in patients with IHD. In cross-sectional and prospective studies, this variable has emerged as a predictor of future end points for CAD and assessment of carotid IMT changes over time is increasingly used to assess effect of intervention strategies in the cardiovascular disease. The Carotid Atherosclerosis Italian Ultrasound Study (CAIUS) (24) study performed in 805

Table 3. Summary of major clinical intervention trials of the effects of statins on coronary events and stroke

Trial	Study Description	Reduction				
		Duration (yrs)	LDL-C (%)	Mortality (%)	CAD Death (%)	Stroke (%)
4S	4444 pts, HC, CAD, Simvastatin 10–40 mg/d	5.0	35	30	42	30
WOSCOPS	6595 pts, HC, No CAD Pravastatin 40 mg/d	4.9	26	22 (NS)	33	11 (NS)
CARE	4159 pts, NC, CAD Pravastatin 40 mg/d	5.0	28	8 (NS)	19	31
AFCAPS/Tex CAPS	6605 pts, NC, No CAD Lovastatin 20–40 mg/d	5.2	25	NA	36	NA
LIPID	9014 pts, NC, CAD Pravastatin 40 mg/d	6.1	25	22	24	19

HC: Hypercholesterolemia; NC: Normocholesterolemia; CAD: Coronary artery disease; NS: Not significant; NA: Not available.

asymptomatic patients with hypercholestrolemia showed that pravastatin stopped the progression of carotid IMT as against the placebo group.

ACAPS (25) study included patients with moderately raised cholesterol. There was small but significant decrease in IMT (0.009 mm yearly) in ACAPS trial. The changes in the intima-media thickness were similar to changes in luminal diameter that had been reported in lipid lowering angiographic trials. The ASAP (26) study showed that aggressive approach to lipid lowering with statins is more beneficial than the more conventional one. In the ASAP trial true regression of carotid atherosclerosis was seen in two third of the atorvastatin treated patients in whom LDL-cholesterol was reduced by half. The mean change in overall IMT thickness after 2 years was −0.031 mm in atorvastatin group.

EBCT (Electron Beam Computed Tomography) (27)

It offers potential to follow disease progression, stabilization and possible regression through serial imaging. Limited data, which is available, gives encouraging results. In addition, quantification of plaque calcium, which may be a predictor of future cardiovascular events, can be done by this method. Statins have recently been shown to reduce the volume of calcium in coronary arteries in 12 months.

All the above mentioned study trials have demonstrated that statins reduce CAD morbidity and mortality and increase survival in the setting of both hypercholesterolemia or normocholesterolemia and improve the arterial topographical morphology that occurs slowly and to a small extent, which is significantly less than the clinical benefits noted. One to two percent regression in lesion severity was associated with a surprisingly high 40–80 percent reduction in MACE (28) (Table 2, Figure 5) much before anatomical regression could occur. The statin therapy may cause regression of lipid rich lesions prone to rupture and/or modulates atherosclerosis through mechanisms independent of anatomical regression. It is the composition of the plaque rather than the severity of stenosis that determine the development of MI (rupture of plaque) and acute clinical events (29). Lesions that cause less than 75% stenosis can be effectively stabilized by lipid lowering therapy.

Mechanisms of atherosclerotic regression by Statins (30)

- Significantly lowering LDL
- Mild lowering of triglycerides
- Mild elevation of HDL
- Reduction in PAI levels
- Reduction of matrix metalloproteinase 9 secretion by macrophages
- stabilization of the vulnerable plaque
- antithrombotic and antiplatelet action
- anti-inflammatory action
- antioxidant effect
- restoration of endothelial function
- anti-ischemic effect

NEWER TECHNIQUES TO DOCUMENT REGRESSION (31)

Modalities capable of characterizing the tissue of the atherosclerotic lesions may help to understand its natural history and detect lesions with high risk for acute events.

(i) Intravascular ultrasound (IVUS)

It is a catheter based imaging technique that provides two-dimensional cross sectional tomographic images of the arterial wall. Currently it is the only imaging modality that provides images in which variations in arterial geometry and atherosclerotic plaque along with the artery can be studied in vivo. In the ongoing REVERSAL trial comprising of 600 patients, the end point is change in plaque volume by IVUS with the use of atorvastatin 80 mg and pravastatin 40 mg (32).

(ii) IVUS elastography

It is a new method that can discriminate lipid rich regions from fibrous regions within the atherosclerotic plaque.

(iii) Coronary angioscopy

It allows visualization of the plaque with high sensitivity. We can see the plaque color, rupture and thrombosis.

(iv) Magnetic resonance imaging

It can visualize the blood flow and thus the lumen boundaries. MRI studies are currently being done to study the progression and regression of atherosclerotic plaques over time. It is the first noninvasive imaging technique that allows discrimination of lipid and fibrous tissue and theoretically a promising tool for detecting the unstable plaque. With improved resolution, MRI technique shows about 80% agreement with histopathology. It can analyze intimal thickness and plaque size accurately.

(v) Nuclear scintigraphic imaging techniques

It is based on the specific binding of radioactive labeled molecules to the target tissue, in this case the atherosclerotic prone lesion.

(vi) Thermometry

It provides a measure of inflammation within the vessel wall.

(vii) Optical coherance tomography

It uses a beam of infrared laser light rather than sound for imaging the atherosclerotic lesion.

(viii) Raman spectroscopy

It identifies gross chemical changes in the tissue and has potential to identify the lipid rich calcified and fibrotic plaque.

Imaging modalities aim to detect the vulnerable plaque, to identify the thickness of the fibrous cap, the extent of atheromatous core and local inflammation. The highest resolutions are achieved by catheter based techniques. These techniques may provide new insights into the etiology of sudden progression of atherosclerotic disease or acute events.

EFFECT OF LIFE STYLE MODIFICATION AND DIET ON ATHEROSCLEROTIC REGRESSION

Many studies have shown that the behavioral modification and yogic exercises etc may help in regression. In the **Life Style Heart Trial** (33), life style changes that included a diet containing 10% fat, stress management, regular exercise (at least 3 hours per week of aerobic exercise and group psychosocial support), at the end of one year showed a mean regression of 16.5% of the coronary artery lesions. However regression was more prevalent in those who were most adherent to the programme. In the **Stanford Coronary Risk Intervention Project (SCRIP) study** (34), 300 patients with angiographically proven CAD were randomly assigned to receive usual care and multifactorial risk reduction including LDL reduction. At 4 years, when patients again underwent angiography, the researchers found that the coronary artery lesions progressed in both groups but only by approximately half in the intervention group (0.024 vs. 0.045 mm/year); $p < 0.01$).

Life style studies are also being done to examine the combined influence of workplace demands and changes in blood pressure induced by stress (chronobiological basis) on the progression of atherosclerosis and show that behaviorally evoked cardiovascular reactivity may have a role in atherogenesis (35).

Role of diet and vitamins

Diet plays an important role in the genesis of atherosclerosis. In one ongoing trial, the effect of diet and OMEGA 3 PUFA on the atherosclerosis by measurement of intima media thickness of carotid arteries, clinical endpoints and biochemical markers is being studied (36). Increased levels of homocysteine cause vascular dysfunction that has been shown to be an early manifestation of atherosclerosis. Supplementation of vitamin B_1 and folate has been found to be useful (37).

Role of antioxidants

Oxidative stress is increased and antioxidant levels are decreased in angiographically proven cases of coronary artery disease (38), with lipid peroxidation (oxidized LDL) playing a crucial role in atherogenesis. The antioxidants vitamin E, C, carotene either in dietary form or supplements have been found to have beneficial effects. Vitamin E when tested in SECURE (39) and HOPE trials did not show any beneficial effect on the progression of atherosclerosis. However, in the CHAOS study (40) it was seen to have significant benefit. A new novel vitamin E derivative TMG has recently been evaluated and has experimentally been found to inhibit development of atherosclerosis even in a very low concentration (41).

The HDL Atherosclerosis Treatment Study (HATS) (42) observed the effect of simvastatin-niacin combination and/or antioxidants on angiographic stenoses and cardiovascular events. The average stenosis progressed by 3.9% in the placebo group, 1.8% in the antioxidant group, 0.7% in the simvastatin, niacin, antioxidant group and regressed by 0.4% in the simvastatin-niacin group. The clinical endpoint or cardiovascular events occurred in 24%, 21%, 14% and 3% respectively. Thus antioxidants had important role in decreasing progression and cardiovascular events in this study.

Drugs like probucol have far greater antioxidant properties and inhibit atherosclerosis much more than vitamin E but inspite of this evidence, in Probucol Quantitative Regression Swedish Trial (43), the addition of probucol to low cholesterol diet with cholestyramine was no better than placebo in reducing atherosclerotic lesions in femoral artery. Thus the clear role of antioxidants in atherosclerotic regression is yet to be established.

Role of trace elements

Available information indicates that magnesium and selenium regress atherosclerosis by influencing lipid and lipoprotein levels and antioxidant defence mechanisms (44).

Role of ACE inhibitors

It is known that angiotensin II can stimulate superoxide anion formation and promote adhesions of monocytes on the endothelium, which is one process integral to the initiation of the atherogenic cascade. ACE inhibitors decrease the cellularity of the plaque and stabilize them. The SECURE TRIAL (37) which was a randomized double blind placebo controlled clinical trial that revealed significant reduction in progression of atherosclerosis with Ramipril compared with placebo ($p = 0.028$) as assessed by quantitative B mode carotid ultrasound. PROTECT trial (45) (Perindopril Regression of Vascular Thickening European Community Trial) aimed to compare slowing or reversing effects of Perindopril and hydrochlorothiazide on the vascular thickening of carotid and femoral arteries in hypertensive patients.

ROLE OF CALCIUM CHANNEL BLOCKERS

In International Nifedipine Trial on antiatherosclerotic therapy (INTACT) (46) study in 1990's, nifedipine treatment over 6 years confirmed the antiatherosclerotic effects and demonstrated a significant 28% reduction in angiographically new lesions in CAD compared to placebo. It reverses endothelium dysfunction by improvement of endothelial NO availability. REGRESS TRIAL (47) showed that concomitant use of calcium channel blockers with lipid lowering agents appears to have synergistic effect in slowing the progression of coronary atherosclerosis. In this study fewer subjects who received combination therapy developed new lesions. The emerging evidence suggests that their antiatherosclerotic action can be demonstrated in patients but the extent and clinical importance of this effect have yet to be fully established.

ROLE OF INFECTIONS

Many studies indicate that infections may contribute to atherogenesis and atherothrombotic acute plaque rupture especially the C. pneumonae, H. pylori, cytomegalovirus etc. Treatment with antibiotics like azithromycin and roxithromycin has been tested in trials like ROXIS (48) ACADEMIC (49) and WIZARD trials. All the trials do not uniformly show beneficial effects. The macrolides may have direct plaque stabilizing effects also. The results of ongoing trials like MARBLE (Might Azithromycin Reduce Bypass List Events) and others are expected from the year 2003 onwards. As at present, regular use of antibiotics for atherosclerotic regression or plaque stabilization in acute coronary syndrome is not recommended till the larger ongoing trials clarify their status.

HORMONAL REPLACEMENT THERAPY

Estrogens influence oxidative stress, lipid metabolism, coagulation, intimal hyperplasia, blood flow and arterial tone. Hormone replacement therapy is associated with reduced risk of coronary artery disease in post-menopausal women. Animal studies have shown alterations in atherosclerotic plaque. Whereas NURSES HEALTH STUDY (50) showed beneficial effects, HERS (51) (Heart Oestrogen Progestone Replacement Study) trial did not show benefits of HRT.

The BELLE trial (32) (Beyond Endorsed Lipid Levels Evaluation Study) with the primary efficacy parameters as change in plaque volume measured by EBCT studies and the effect of lipid lowering therapy in post-menopausal women is underway and the results are awaited. The ongoing WELL-HART (52) study aims to determine the effect of hormone replacement on regression of atherosclerosis by carotid IMT measurement.

GENE THERAPY (53)

Genetic factors may also influence the likelihood of atherosclerotic regression and plaque rupture. The rate of atherosclerotic progression can be slowed and some degree of regression is possible. However the same treatment may not be correct for all the patients as some genes respond to nutritional modulation. This new field is generating lot of interest.

NEWER THERAPIES

LDL APHRESIS AND VASOCARE THERAPY (54) have been reported to have beneficial effects on atherosclerosis. The experimental drug ENDOSTATIN (55) is also being tested for its effect on atherosclerosis (It is being developed for its ability to shrink cancerous tumors by inhibition of development of new blood vessels).

The problem of **restenosis** after angioplasty represents a special form of atherosclerosis, with the role of PGDF and fibroblast growth factors in triggering smooth muscle proliferation along with adventitial inflammation with scar formation and wound contraction and myxomatous tissue deposition as its likely mechanisms. Significant regression in this set up may be achieved by stent implantation, radiation therapy and drugs like Trapidil as shown in STARC trial (56).

The other special form of atherosclerosis pertains to **cardiac transplantation**. This form is mostly immunological based without much of lipid core, and produces diffuse concentric lesions (57). It responds well to immunosuppressant drugs like cyclosporin alone or with other immunosuppressive agents to suppress the endothelial allogenic response.

REFERENCES

1. Forrester JS, Shah P. 1997. Lipid lowering versus revascularization. An idea whose time for testing has come. Circulation 96:1360–1362.
2. Enas EA, Jacob S, Joseph AK. 2000. Paradigm change from palliative to preventive cardiology: A critical review of mechanical coronary interventions versus comprehensive medical management. Asian J Clinical Card 3:21–52.
3. Oliver MF. 1992. Perspective of trials of regression of coronary atherosclerosis. Cardiovas. Risk Factors 2:234–248.
4. Anitschkow N, Chalatow S. 1983. On experimental cholesterin steatosis and its significance in the origin of some pathological processes, 1913. Reprinted in Arteriosclerosis 3:178–182.
5. Krieger H. 1997. The other side of scavenger receptors: pattern recognition for host defenses. Curr Opin Lipidol 8:275–280.
6. Stary HC, Chandler AB, Diusmore RE, et al. 1995. A definition of advanced types of atherosclerotic lesions and a histological classification of atherosclerosis: A report from the committee on vascular lesions of the council on arteriosclerosis. American Heart Association. Circulation 92:1355–1374.
7. O'Brien, Garvin MR, Dev R, Stewart DK, Hinohara T, Simpson JB, Schwartz SM. 1994. Angiogenesis in human coronary atherosclerotic plaques. Am J Pathol 145:883–894.

8. Dollery CH, McEwan JR, Henney AM. 1995. Matrix mettaloproteinases and cardiovascular disease. Cir Res 77:863–868.
9. Amento EP, Ehsani N, Palmer H, Libby P. 1991. Arteriosclerosis and Thrombosis. Cytokines positively and negatively regulate interstitial collagen gene expression in human vascular smooth muscle cells. Arteriosclerosis 11:1223–1230.
10. Nigro J, Dilley RJ, Little PJ. 2002. Differential effects of gemfibrozil on migration, proliferation and proteoglycan production in human vascular smooth muscle cells (abstract). Elsevier Medical Journals. www.cardiosource.com.
11. Tangirala RK, Tsukamoto K, Chun SH, Usher D, Pure E, Rader DJ. 1999. Regression of atherosclerosis induced by Liver—directed gene transfer of apolipoprotein-A. Circulation 100:1816–1822.
12. Marjel J van Dam, Eric de Groot, Susanne M Clee, G Kess Hovingh, Roosje Roelants, Angie Brooks-Wilson, Aeiko H Zwinderman, Andries J Smit, August HM Smelt, Albert K Groen, Michael R Hayden, John JP Kastelein. 2002. Association between increased arterial wall thickness and impairment in ABCA[1]-driven cholesterol efflux: an observational study. Lancet 359:37–41.
13. Lipid Research Clinics Programme. 1984. The Lipid Research Clinics Coronary Primary Prevention Trial Results: I. Reduction in the incidence of coronary artery disease. JAMA 251:351–364.
14. Schedit S. 1992. Prevention of coronary artery disease: control of risk factors, potential new therapies and an update on regression CVR & R; 60–69.
15. Carl J Vaughan. 2000. The evolving role of statins in management of atherosclerosis. JACC 35(1):7–10.
16. MAAS Investigators. 1994. Effects of simvastatin on coronary Atheroma a Multicentric Antiatheroma Study. Lancet 344:633–638.
17. Bestohorn HP, Rewing UF, Roskanmutt, et al. 1997. The effect of simvastatin on coronary atheroma. Progression of coronary artery disease. The Multicentre Coronary Intervention Study (CIS). Eur Heart J 18:226–234.
18. Waters D, Higginson L, Gladstore P, et al. 1994. Effects of monotherapy with an HMG-CoA reductase inhibitor on the progression of coronary atherosclerosis as assessed by serial quantitative arteriography. The Canadian Coronary Atherosclerotic International Trial. Circulation 89:959–968.
19. Jukema JW, Brusdike AVG, Van Boren AJ, et al. 1995. On behalf of the regress study group. Effects of lipid lowering by pravastatin on progression and regression of coronary artery disease in symptomatic men with normal to moderately elevated serum cholesterol levels. The Regression Growth Evaluation Statin Study. Regress Circulation 91:2528–2540.
20. Blankenhorn DIL, Azen SP, Krosch DM, et al. and the MARS Research group. 1993. Coronary angiographic changes with lovastatin therapy. The Monitored Atherosclerosis Regression Study (MARS). Ann Int Med 179:969–976.
21. Herd JA, Ballantyne CH, Farmer JA, et al. 1997. For the LCAS investigators. Effects of flurastatin on coronary atherosclerosis in mild and moderate cholesterol elevations (Lipoprotein and Coronary Atherosclerosis) Study (LCAS). Am J Cardiology 80:278–286.
22. Brown G, Albers JJ, Fisher LD, Schaefer SM, Lin JT, Kaplan C, Zhao XQ, Bisson BD, Fitzpatrick VF, Dodge HT. 1990. Regression of coronary artery disease as a result of intensive lipid lowering therapy in men with high levels of apolipoprotein B N Engl J Med 323:1289–1298.
23. Pignoli P, Iremoli E, Poli A, Oreste P, Paoletti R. 1986. Intimal plus medial thickening of the arterial wall: A direct measurement with ultrasound imaging. Circulation 14:1399–1406.
24. Mercuri H. 1996. Pravastatin reduces carotid intima media thickness progression in asymptomatic hypercholesterolemic midterm population. The CAIUS American Journal of Medicine 101(6): 627–634.
25. Furberg CD, Adams HP Jr, Applegate WB, et al. 1994. For the Asymptomatic Carotid. Artery Progression Study (ACAPS) Research Group. Effect of lovastatin on early carotid atherosclerosis and cardiovascular events. Circulation 90:1679–1687.
26. Smilde TJ, Van Wissen, Wolesteim H, et al. 2001. Effect of aggressive versus conventional lipid lowering on atherosclerosis progression in familial hypercholesterolemia (ASAP): a prospective randomized double blind trial. Lancet 357:577–581.
27. Robert A O'Rourke, Bruce H Brundage, Victor F Froelicher, Philip Greenland, Scott M Grundy, Rory Hachamovitch, Gerald M Pohost, Leslee J Shaw, William S Weintraub, William L Winters. 2000. Electron beam computed tomography. Assessment of Progression or Regression of CHD by EBCT. JACC June, pp. 337–338.
28. Superko HR. 1996. Surprising clinical lessons from the regression trials. 21st Annual Tutorials in Teton. Educational Highlights of Am J Cardiology 11:1–4.

29. Little WC, Constantinescu M, Applegate RJ, Kutcher MA, Burrows MT, Kahl FR, Santamore WP. 1988. Can coronary angiography predict the site of a subsequent myocardial infarction in patients with mild to moderate coronary artery disease? Circulation 78:1157–1166.
30. Rosenson RS, Tanghey CC. 1998. Antiatherothrombotic properties of statins: implications for cardiovascular event reduction. JAMA 29:1643–1650.
31. Gerard Paster Kamp, Erling Falk, Hein Woutman, Cornelius Borst. 2000. Techniques characterizing the coronary atherosclerotic plaque. Influence on clinical decision making? Visualization of the vulnerable plaque. JACC 36(1):13–21.
32. Daniell Pella. 2002. 2nd International Congress on Cardiovascular Diseases. PJ Safarik, University of Kosice, Slowakia). REVERSAL TRIAL Plaque Stability Role of Statins (Symposium).
33. Ornish D, Brown S, Scherwitz L, et al. 1990. Can lifestyle changes reverse coronary heart disease? The Life Style Heart Trial. Lancet 336:129–133.
34. Haskell WL, Aldesman EI, Fair JM, et al. 1994. Effects of intensive multiple risk factor reduction in coronary atherosclerosis and clinical cardiac events in men and women with coronary artery disease. The Stanford Coronary Risk Intervention project (SCRIP). Circulation 89:975–990.
35. Susan A Everson, John W Lynch, Margaret A Chesney, George A Kaplan, Debbie E Goldberg, Starley B Shade, Richard D Cohen, Riitta Salonen, Jukka T Salonen. 1997. Interaction of workplace demands and cardiovascular reactivity in progress of carotid atherosclerosis: population based study. BMJ 314:553.
36. Eisa N Hjerkin. 2002. Anticipated first presentation. Diet and/or Omega 3 PUFA intervention trial on atherosclerosis. Ullevaal University Hospital Oslo, 0407 Norway. Elsevier Medical Journals. www.cardiosource.com.
37. Kam S Woo FRACP, FACC MD, Ping Chook MD, Yvette I Lolin PhD, John E Sanderson FACC MD, Con Metreweli FRCR MD, David S Celermajer FRACP PhD. 1999. Folic acid improves arterial endothelial function in adults with hyperhomocystenemia. J Am Coll Cardiol 34:2002–2006.
38. Sainani GS, Oxidative stress. 1997. A key factor in pathogenesis of chronic diseases. Medicine Update edited by YP Munjhal 7:1–10.
39. Eva M Lonn, Salim Yusuf, Vladimir Dzavik, C Ian Doris, Qlong Yi, Sandra Smith, Annie Moorelox, Jackie Bosh, Ward A Riby Koon K Teo, for Secure investigators. 2001. The Study to Evaluate Carotid Ultrasound Changes in Patients Treated with Ramipiril and Vitamin E (SECURE) for Secure investigators. Circulation 103:919–925.
40. Stephens WG, Garsons A, Schofield PM, et al. 1996. Randomized control trial of vitamin E in patients with coronary disease. Coronary Heart Antioxidative Study (CHAOS). Lancet 347:781–786.
41. Normasa Yoshida. 2002. Inhibitory effect of a novel water soluble vitamin E derivative on atherosclerosis in rabbits (TMG) (Abstract) Elsevier Medical Journals www.cardiosource.com. Elsevier Science Ireland.
42. B Greg Brown MD, PhD, Xue-Qiao Zhao MD, Alan Chait MD, Lloyd D Fisher PhD, Marian C. Cheung PhD, Josh S Morse BS, Alice A Dowdy RD, Emily K Marino MS, Edward L Bolson MS, Petar Alaupovic PhD, Jiri Frohlich MD, Leny Serafini BS, Ellen Huss-Frechette BS, Shari Wang BS, Debbie DeAngelis RT, Arthur Dodek MD, John J Albers PhD. 2001. The HDL Atherosclerosis Treatment Study (HATS) (Simvastatin and Niacin, Antioxidant Vitamins, or the Combination for the Prevention of Coronary Disease). New Eng J Med 345:1583–1592 (Medline).
43. O'Wallidius, Q Erikson, U Olsson AG, et al. 1994. The effect of probucol on femoral atherosclerosis. The PQRST (Probucol Qualitative Regression Sweedish Trial). Am J Cardiol 74:875–883.
44. Nave J. 1996. Selenium as a factor for cardiovascular disease. J Cardiovas Dis 3(1):42–47.
45. Klaus O Stumpe. 1993. PROTECT (Perindopril Regression of Vascular Thickening European Community Journal). J Hypertens 11(Suppl 5):S316–S317 (Medline). Am J Cardiol 1995;76:50E–54E (Medline).
46. Lichtlen PR, Hugenholtz PG, Raltlenbeul W, Hecker H, Jost S, Nikutta P, Deckers JW. 1996. Retardation of coronary artery disease in humans by the calcium channel blocker nifedipine: results of the INTACT study. International Nifedipine Trial on Antiatherosclerotic Therapy. Cardiovasc. Drugs Ther Aug 4(Suppl 5):1047–1068.
47. Jukema JW, Zwinderman AH, Van Boven AJ, Reiber JH, Van der Laarse A, Lie KI, Brusdhke AV. 1996. Evidence for a synergistic effect of calcium channel blockers with lipid lowering therapy in retarding progression of coronary atherosclerosis in symptomatic patients with normal to moderately raised cholsterol levels. The Regress study group. Arterioscles Thromb Vas Biol 16:426–450. Elsevier Medical Journal. www.cardiosource.com.
48. Roxis—Gurfinkel E, Bozovicu G, Doraco A, et al. 1991. Randomized trial of roxithromycin or non-Q wave coronary syndrome. Roxis Pilot study. Lancet 350:404–417.

49. Mahlestein IB, Anderson JL, Cardquiet JF, et al. 2000. Randomized prevention trial of azithromycin in patients of coronary artery disease. Primary clinical results of the academic study. Circulation 102:1755–1760.
50. Stampfer MJ, Colditz GA, Willet WL, et al. 1991. Post-menopausal oestrogen therapy and cardiovascular disease. Ten year follow up from the Nurses Health Study. N Eng J Med 325:756.
51. Hulley S, Grady D, Bush T, et al. 1998. Randomized trial of oestrogen plus progestin for secondary prevention of coronary artery disease in post menopausal women. JAMA 280:605–613.
52. WELL-HART study (Women Estrogen Progestin Lipid Lowering Harmone Atherosclerosis Regression Study): Contacts Dr. Howard HODS 2250 Alxzar St CSC 132, Los Angles, California. watcher@hsc.uscedu. Elsevier Medical Journal. www.cardiosource.com.
53. Aggarwal KK. 2001. Asian Journal of Cardiology, 4(2) (Editorial).
54. Saeid Babaei, Duncan J Stewart, Pierre Picard, Juan Carlos Monge. 2002. Effects of vasocare™ therapy on the initiation and progression of atherosclerosis. Elsevier Medical Journals, www.cardiosource.com.
55. Scott Gottlieb. 1999. Endostatin may stop the progression of atherosclerosis. BMJ 318:1030.
56. Maresta A, Balducall M, Cantini L, et al. 1994. For the STARC investigators, irazolopyremedine a platelet derived growth factor antagonist, reduces restenosis after PTCA. Circulation 90:2710–2715.
57. Billingham ME. 1992. Histopathology of graft coronary disease. J Heart Lung Transplant 11:338–344.

Frontiers in Cardiovascular Health, edited by
N.S. Dhalla, A. Chockalingam,
H.I. Berkowitz & P.K. Singal
Kluwer Academic Publishers, Boston, 2003

Monolayers of Apolipoprotein AII at the Air/Water Interface

J. Mas-Oliva,[1] A Moreno,[2] S. Ramos,[3] J. Xicohtencatl-Cortes,[1]
J. Campos,[3] and R. Castillo[3]

[1] *Instituto de Fisiología Celular, UNAM, P.O. Box 70–243, México. D.F. 04510*
[2] *Instituto de Química, UNAM, México, D.F. 04510*
[3] *Instituto de Física, UNAM, P.O. Box 20–364, D.F. 04510*

Summary. Lipoproteins in plasma present the property to exchange lipids between themselves and also with different types of cells. Associated proteins known as apolipoproteins give these particles their lipid exchange characteristics, and also provide a way to control their directionality and ability to interact with receptors located at the surface of cells. In order to provide information on the three dimensional structure of apolipoprotein AII (apoAII), an important constituent of high density lipoprotein particles (HDL), we have studied monolayers of this apolipoproteins combining Langmuir techniques with Brewster Angle Microscopy and Atomic Force Microscopy. We describe the gas/liquid-phase transition in this protein and a phase transition between two condensed phases at high lateral pressures. This transition corresponds to a conformational change of the protein due to the desorption of one of its α-helix segments from the subphase. This result suggests that changes in lateral pressure along changes in shape, size, and composition of HDL particles, might affect the conformation of apolipoproteins including apoAII interacting with the surface of the lipoprotein. This type of conformational change in apoAII might be involved with the exchangeability process as observed with this class of apolipoproteins, as well as with protein recognition by specific receptors at the cell surface.

Key words: Apolipoprotein AII, Protein Monolayers, and HDL.

1. INTRODUCTION

Important molecules such as cholesterol, triglycerides and phospholipids that are mostly water insoluble, are transported in plasma and mobilized to and from cells

Corresponding author: J. Mas-Oliva, E-mail: jmas@ifisiol.unam.mx.

in the form of lipoprotein particles. Together with these lipids, associated proteins known as apolipoproteins represent the molecules that apparently give lipoproteins directionality and the ability to interact with receptors in the surface of cells (1,2). Several of these apolipoproteins present the property to exchange between the different classes of lipoproteins (apoAI, AII, AIII, CI, CII, CIII and E), while others form part of the particle as fixed proteins (apoB48 and B100) (3,4). Although this characteristic is well documented, the specific circumstances that define this behavior are still not well understood.

Since apolipoprotein transfer between lipoprotein particles can critically modify their metabolism, and therefore their fate, the way lipid molecules might get absorbed or released from cells, as well as the chemical and physical properties that control this transfer have become critical in understanding lipoprotein metabolism. In general terms, while low density lipoprotein particles (LDL) and very low density lipoproteins (VLDL) have been given a pro-atherogenic role, high density lipoproteins (HDL) have been recognized as an anti-atherogenic factor (5). Although this characteristic behavior has been recognized for some time, the molecular explanation to this phenomenon is still lacking. Most probably its explanation resides in the way the different apolipoproteins are structured when associated to the surface of lipoprotein particles (6–8). As an example of this behavior, we can examine the change in size and shape of HDL particles from the time these are formed as nascent flat-discoidal particles; to the time they reach maturity as spherical particles (9). In the latest stage, HDL particles mainly containing apoAI, apoAII and apoCI, have been loaded with cholesterol mostly from endothelial cells. After the intervention of a good number of several plasma factors, HDL particles only in the spherical and not in the discoidal form get ready to be taken up by the liver and adrenal glands for bile acid and steroid hormone synthesis respectively (5). Therefore, what is the signal employed by the system that allows only spherical HDL particles to be recognized by the putative receptor and taken up by the liver cells? Although changes in size and shape that dramatically might affect apolipoprotein conformation have remained a key feature for understanding recognition of HDL particles by the liver, the experimental approach to study this phenomenon is just emerging. Recently, our group has started to study the surface properties of the exchangeable family of apolipoproteins measuring as monolayers, their surface pressure and adsorption isotherms at the air/water interface (10–12).

To provide information on the three-dimensional structure of exchangeable apolipoproteins in the form of monolayers, we have combined Langmuir Techniques with Brewster Angle Microscopy (BAM) and Atomic Force Microscopy (AFM). Our studies have focused on the structural changes observed during lateral compression and decompression of apoAII monolayers, trying to mimic what it might be happening at the surface of HDL particles, from the time of synthesis as discoidal nascent particles to the time of uptake by the liver and adrenal glands as spherical particles. The result of our studies suggests that changes in lateral pressure correlated to changes in shape, size and composition of HDL particles, might affect the conformation of apolipoproteins interacting with the lipoprotein surface. We propose that specific conformational states associated with the absorption or desorption of a segment of these apolipoproteins at the surface of HDL particles, might be involved in the exchangeability process as well as in molecule recognition by specific receptors at the surface of cells specialized in taking up these type of mature HDL particles.

2. METHODS

Lyophilized apoAII isolated from its natural source, was purchased from Sigma Chem. Co. (San Louis, MO). Protein solutions were always filtered using 0.22 μm membrane filters before carrying out the experiments The protein concentration was determined according to the equation: $A = \varepsilon\, l\, C$. Here, A is sample absorbance; l is the path length; ε is the molar absorption coefficient and C = protein concentration. ε at *280 nm* was obtained according to the procedure described by Pace (13).

ApoAII was solubilized in a buffered solution, and spread onto a subphase of a phosphate buffered solution (20 mM, pH 8.0) prepared with ultrapure water (Nanopure-UV) containing 3.5 *M* KCl (Baker, Mexico). The different apolipoprotein spreading solutions were diluted to a final concentration ca. 0.2 mg/ml. It is important to note that before preparing the KCl solution, the KCl salt was heated for *4* hours at *300°C* to prevent spurious organic compounds in the surface of the subphase. Monolayers were prepared on a computerized Nima Langmuir-Blodgett trough (TKB *2410A*, Nima Technology Ltd., England) using a Wilhelmy plate to measure the surface pressure, $\Pi = \gamma_0 - \gamma$, i.e., the surface tension difference of the clean subphase and that of the protein covered subphase. The cleanliness of the subphase can be assured making a compression of the barriers without protein and obtaining a negligible pressure rise ($\Pi < 0.1\,mN/m$).

The trough was isolated from vibrations using a pneumatic tube incorporated into a steel base. The barriers are made of PTFE fitted with stiffening bars defining a working circular area, starting at *1000 cm²*. All experiments were carried out in a dust-free environment at *25°C*. Temperature in the trough was kept constant at 25°C with the aid of a water circulation bath. The speed of compression was in the order of 50 cm^2/min. This compression rate corresponds to 145, $\AA^2/molec.\,min.$, for apoAII.

BAM observations were performed in a BAM1 Plus (Nanofilm Technologie GmbH, Germany), with a spatial resolution ca. *4* μm. Here, the interface is illuminated at the Brewster incidence (~53°) with a polarized laser beam from a He-Ne laser. A microscope receives the reflected beam that is analyzed by a polarization analyzer, and the signal is received by a CCD video camera to develop an image of the monolayer.

For secondary structure predictions, the computer program employed was based on the Profile Network Prediction Heidelberg method (PHD version 5.94-317, Heidelberg). This program consist of a neural network approach that averages several independently trained networks before making the final assessment with an average for successful prediction above 72%.

Mica surfaces were made hydrophobic with a Langmuir-Blodgett deposit of octadeciltriethoxisilane (OTE) according to the procedure developed by Wood and Sharma (14,15). A film of prepolymerized OTE was spread onto a water subphase, acidified with HCl to obtain *pH 2*. After spreading the OTE solution, we waited until the pressure drop was negligible; typical waiting times were in the range of *15 min*. The degree of polymerization of the monolayer was observed with the BAM. We compressed and deposited the film on mica, at a constant lateral pressure at *20–25 mN/m* ($T = 23°C$). The mica was previously activated by a radio frequency-generated Air/H_2O plasma (*2 min.* at ~*30 W*, *100 mTorr*, in a Harrick Plasma Cleaner, PDC-23G, New York). After deposition, the hydrophobic mica surfaces were baked and annealed for *2* hours in a vacuum oven (*120°C*, *100 mTorr*) before use.

The transferred protein monolayers were scanned with a NanoScope IIIa SFA (Digital Instruments, California, USA.) using a $15 \times 15 \mu m^2$ scanner. Preliminary scanning measurements in contact mode and deflection mode were made at *2.5 Hz* using Si_3N_4 tips using a typical force constant of $0.3\, Nm^{-1}$. The contact atoms mode was used in flat regions of the covered mica in order to improve data and image acquisition using reduced scan rates of *1 Hz*. All images were analyzed with the Digital Instruments software.

3. RESULTS AND DISCUSSION

As an example of an apolipoprotein that forms an important part of HDL particles and therefore plays a significant role in HDL metabolism, we shall concentrate with our findings related to the study of apoAII. Although apoAII is considered a pro-atherogenic molecule since displaces apoAI from the surface of HDL particles, the mechanisms that control and modulate this process are still unknown. ApoAII is composed by 77 aminoacids and present two well defined amphipathic α-helices between residues 7–27 and 32–67 (Figure 1). Both α-helix residues present high hydrophobic moment (μH) values with 0.49 and 0.34 kcal/mol residue respectively. These values give us a good idea of the amphipathicity of both regions, since values above 0.20 kcal/mol residue are considered good candidates to form amphipathic helices (16). The primary structure of apoAII has also shown a high homology (55%)

Apo AII

```
                10           20           30
QAKEPC VES LVS QYFQT VTDYGKDLMEKVKSP EL QAEA
L LL L . L HHHHHHHHHHHHHHH . HHHHH . . L LHHHHHHH

 40             50             60           70
KSY FE KSKE QLTPL I KKAGT ELV NFLS YFVELGTQPATQ
HHHHHHHHH . H .HHHHHH . HHHHHHHHHH . . . L LL LLLL
```

Figure 1. Secondary structure prediction of apoAII according the PHD method. H = α-helix, L = loop, and . = no prediction for the segment.

with the murine senile amyloid protein (ASsam). Since it has been reported that apoAII might be considered a putative precursor of ASsam, it has been suggested that apoAII might be also involved in amyloidogenic processes such as in Alzheimer disease (17). Therefore, in biomedicine it has become crucial to understand the way apolipoproteins change their structure, and as a physiological response regulate not only lipoprotein metabolism, but also the fate of related proteins associated for instance to the physiopathology of the central nervous system.

As recently confirmed for the human apoCI (10–12), apoAII although freely soluble in water, remains at the air/water interfase in a Langmuir trough when spread directly onto a 3.5 M KCl subphase solution. As shown in figure 2, an isotherm obtained at 25°C and pH 8.0 shows several well defined features: a) starting at a very low surface area density, a region of $\pi \sim 0$ mN/m is found. This region ends at approximately a = 5000 Å^2/molecule. Although BAM observations could not show domains of condensed phase, this behavior corresponds to a gas/condensed phase transition (Figure 3). b) After lateral pressure increases, a typical low compressibility phase appears (Figure 2). During this period of low compressibility, BAM observations did not show any well defined domains. Nevertheless, we could immediately notice that defects on the monolayers move at a slower pace than the ones found in the gas/condensed phase coexistence. c) As pressure continues to build up, the apoAII monolayer presents a second phase transition just before it collapses at $\pi \sim 32$ mN/m (Figure 4). When the condensed phase (L_1) is compressed, a wide kink is found around $\pi \sim 30$–35 mN/m and a ~1000–2500 Å^2/molecule. This phenomenon exemplifies the classical behavior of a phase transition between two condensed phases (L_1/L_2). Furthermore, it was confirmed that this phase transition is reversible, since several compression/decompression cycles showed negligible changes in π. In the same way, when the monolayers were left untouched at $\pi \sim$ 30 mN/m for an hour, changes in lateral pressure were not modified over 3 mN/m. Although the different compression/decompression assays did not exactly retrace on top of each other, after each decompression, the isotherm presented the same characteristics as the very first one obtained. The small loss in area could be explained in a negligible fashion as a very small loss of protein from the surface. BAM observations showed that under these conditions, the monolayer changed from a tenuous gray to a bright gray covering big domains and some times the entire field of view. The monolayer collapses at the end of the compression at $\pi \sim 47$ mN/m and a ~500 Å^2/molecule (Figure 5).

AFM is an emerging technology that can be used for sizing of protein to a surface. In the optimal condition, the AFM resolves single atoms (0.2 nm resolution) (18,19), nevertheless under more usual conditions; the resolution could be 2–25 nm. The extremely good signal-to-noise ratio for the AFM allows direct visualization of single protein molecules without the use of contrast enhancing agents (20,21). Therefore, we have developed a method to study apolipoprotein monolayers in Langmuir-Blodgett arrays by AFM. ApoAII monolayers were transferred on mica at a low speed (1.0 mm min^{-1}) and scanned in the contact mode at 2.5 Hz using Si_3N_4 tips with a constant force of 0.3 Nm min^{-1}. Monolayers were initially transferred in the

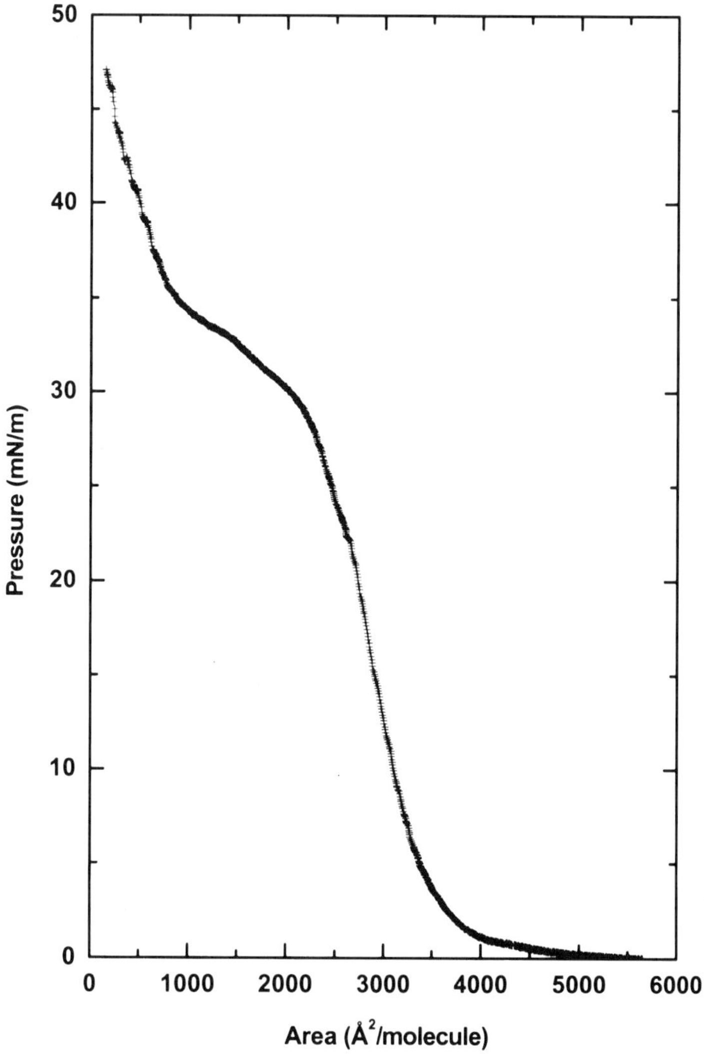

Figure 2. Typical isotherm of apoAII. The assays were performed al 25°C, a protein concentration of 0.3 mg/ml and a compression speed of $50\,cm^2/min$.

liquid (L_1) phase at $\pi \sim 20\,mN/m$ far from the pressure at which the phase transition takes place (Figure 6). The image shows an arrangement of molecules in the form of rows. The average width for these rows corresponds to 17 Å, measurement that correlates well with the width of apoAII in a dimeric form. These rows present a continuous image that is in agreement with the molecule entirely lying on the

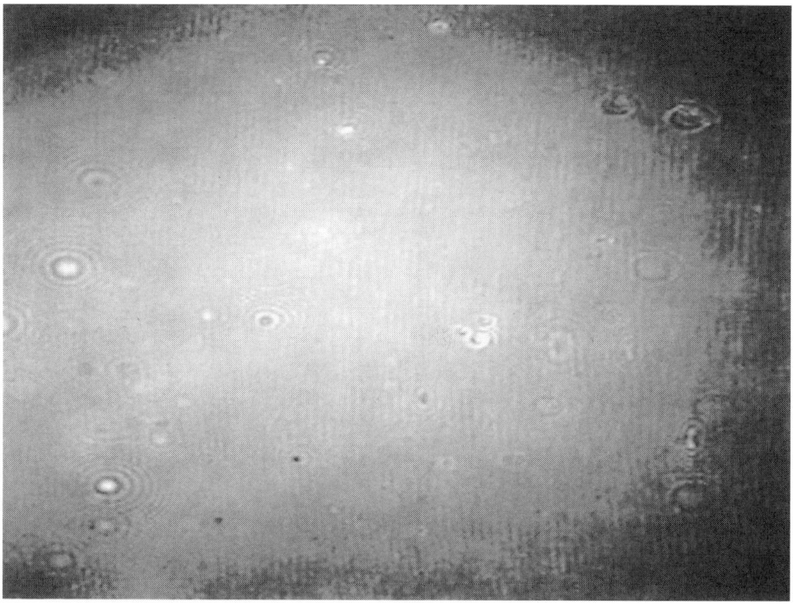

Figure 3. BAM image of the apoAII monolayer just before the L_1/L_2 transition.

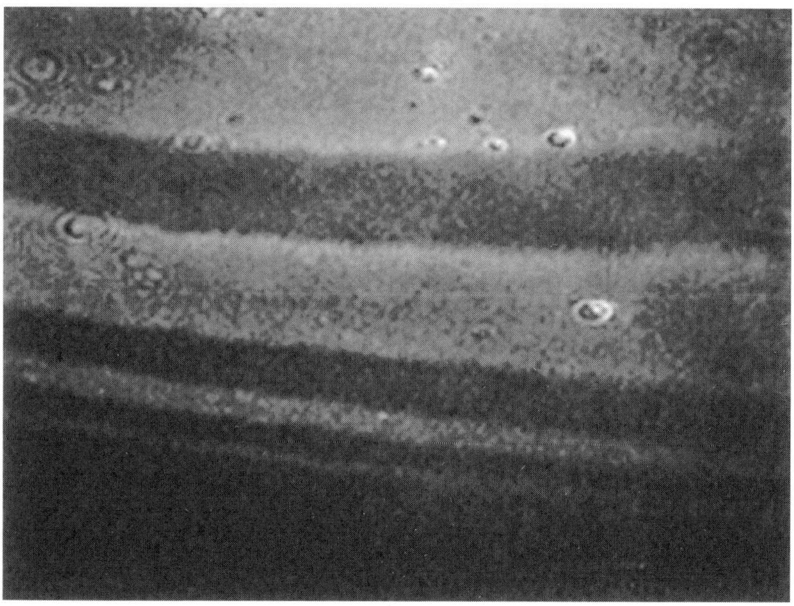

Figure 4. BAM image of the apoAII monolayer at $\Pi \sim 30\text{–}35\,mN/m$ and an area of ~1000–2000 Å^2/molec.

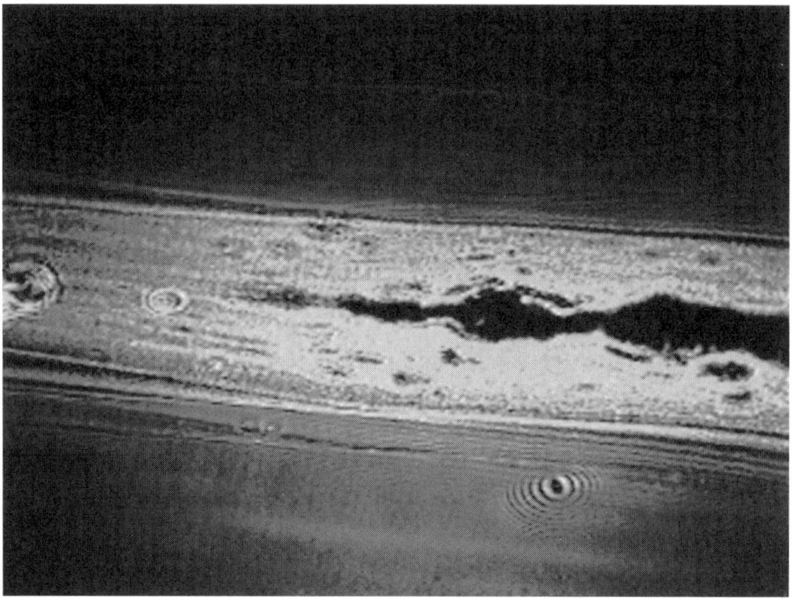

Figure 5. BAM image of the apoAII collapsed monolayer at $\Pi \sim 47\,mN/m$ and an area of $\sim 500\,Å^2/molec$.

surface of the interface. In contrast, if the monolayers are transferred to mica in the liquid-crystalline (LC) phase at $\pi \sim 33\,mN/m$, just before the phase transition shown in the isotherms takes place, the images appear to be quite different. Here, elongated domains with high contrast are observed (Figure 7). In accordance to our measurements, these domains that get lifted from the background correspond to one of the α-helix segments of apoAII arranged as a dimer.

Since we wanted to explore the behavior of apoAII when placed on a hydrophobic surface, apoAII monolayers were transferred in the L_1 phase on mica pre-treated with OTE. AFM images show that under these conditions the moithinules also organize themselves in rows with measurements consistent with the width of single α-helices (5–7 Å) (Figure 8). Under these conditions, when placed on hydrophobic surfaces, apoAII appears to separate well both α-helices forming the dimer. Since apoAII corresponds to a dimer bonded by a disulfide bonds at position 6 of both amino ends of the molecule, the image also appears to show such bonding. Although the arrangement between molecules seems to be more disordered than images obtained from hydrophilic surfaces, employing hydrophobic surfaces, the molecules arrange between themselves in parallel rows. These monolayers placed on OTE covered mica were transferred at 20–25 mN/m. Since the hydrophobic halves of apoAII in this condition most probably are facing the mica surface, it was not possible to perform experiments increasing the surface pressure. This is based on the

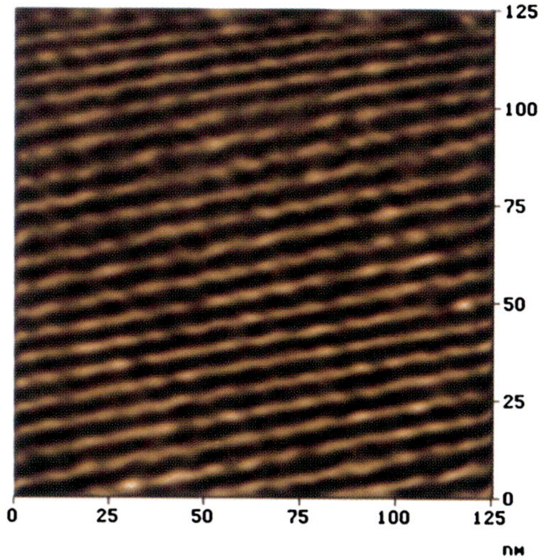

Figure 6. Atomic Force Microscopy image of an apoAII monolayer transferred to the hydrophilic surface of mica. A transfer speed of 1 mm/min was employed and $\Pi \sim 20$ mN/m.

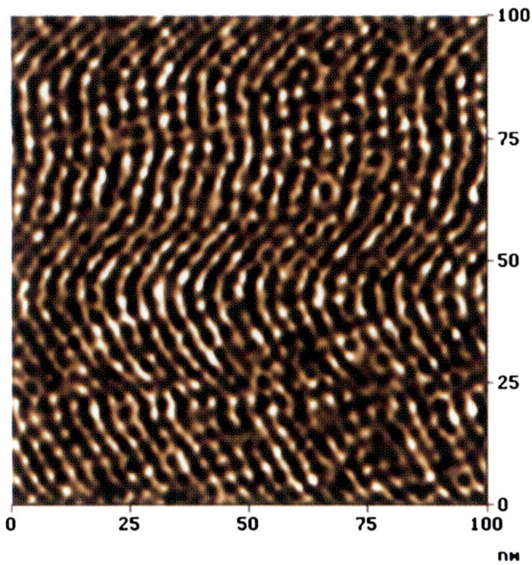

Figure 7. Atomic Force Microscopy image of an apoAII monolayer transferred to the hydrophilic surface of mica. A transfer speed of 1 mm/min was employed and $\Pi \sim 33.7$ mN/m.

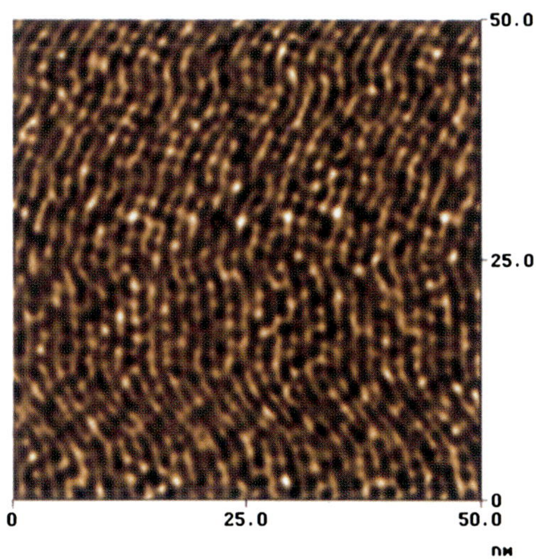

Figure 8. Atomic Force Microscopy image of an apoAII monolayer transferred to the hydrophobic surface of mica covered with octadeciltriethoxilane (OTE). The transfer speed of OTE to cover freshly cleaved mica was carried out at 1 mm/min and $\Pi \sim 25$ mN/m. The transfer speed for the protein on mica previously covered with OTE corresponded also to 1 mm/min and $\pi \sim 20$ mM/m.

apoAII in this condition most probably are facing the mica surface, it was not possible to perform experiments increasing the surface pressure. This is based on the conformational arrangements described above using hydrophilic surfaces that would destroy these monolayers when placed on a hydrophobic surface. Nevertheless, our model having the two alpha helices laying down parallel to the water surface has been confirmed.

Since the way these exchangeable apolipoprotein molecules move between lipoprotein particles has remained an open question, based in our past and present observations, a proposal can be made. This proposal is based on the physicochemical properties of amphipathic α-helices, the number of apolipoprotein copies present on the surface of lipoproteins, and a theoretical decrease in lateral surface pressure given by changes in volume and/or shape of lipoproteins. First of all, HDL particles synthesized by hepatocytes and enterocytes as small disk-shaped particles, contain relatively low amounts of free cholesterol, no cholesterol esters, and appear to be rich in apolipoproteins. These apo proteins making up to 55%of the total mass of these particles, contain at their surface a mixture of apolipoproteins (CI, CII, CIII, AI; AII, D and E), as well as the cholesterol esters transfer protein (CETP) and the enzyme lecithin-cholesterol-acyl-transferase (LCAT). This latest enzyme located at the surface of nascent discoidal HDL particles converts cholesterol and lecithin taken up from chylomicron and very low density lipoprotein remnants (remnant VLDL), to cholesteryl esters. Therefore, they begin to form a core, transforming the disk-shaped nascent HDL to a mature spherical HDL particle. In such a case, due to the size and rich protein composition of nascent HDL particles, lateral pressure between the different apolipoproteins and accessory proteins could be thought to be high, and only decreases in parallel to changes in size and form that take place during the permanence of HDL in circulation as spherical particles. Theoretical calculations employed to measure the difference in size of nascent and mature particles, together with the area values obtained from the shadows of α-helices contained in the different apolipoproteins projected at the surface of HDL, allow us to speculate that lateral pressure between proteins at the surface of HDL particles might be very different in both conditions. Such a proposal could be related to the one suggested for apoAI during its interaction with discoidal or spheroidal HDL particles (22), or when apoCI modulates the interaction of apoE with β-migrating VLDL particles (23).

From our study it can be concluded that adsorption of apolipoproteins onto a monolayer is of interest; first as an approach to study protein/protein interactions, and second to analyze their behavior as exchangeable proteins. Based on the concept that the presence of amphipathic α-helices might be considered a key factor in defining the physiological behavior of exchangeable apolipoproteins, we could start to have a clearer picture of the mechanisms that facilitate the exchange of these proteins between lipoproteins, as well as the structural changes related to their physiological function. Since there is still a limited knowledge about the molecular forces and interactions that determine the surface properties of exchangeable apolipoproteins, one of our next goals will be to study the surface pressure of both disk-shaped spheroidal HDL particles (22), or when apoCI modulates the interaction of apoE with β-migrating VLDL particles (23).

From our study it can be concluded that adsorption of apolipoproteins onto a monolayer is of interest; first as an approach to study protein/protein interactions, and second to analyze their behavior as exchangeable proteins. Based on the concept that the presence of amphipathic α-helices might be considered a key factor in defining the physiological behavior of exchangeable apolipoproteins, we could start to have a clearer picture of the mechanisms that facilitate the exchange of these proteins between lipoproteins, as well as the structural changes related to their physiological function. Since there is still a limited knowledge about the molecular forces and interactions that determine the surface properties of exchangeable apolipoproteins, one of our next goals will be to study the surface pressure of both disk-shaped HDL particles and spherical HDL particles in order to better correlate the results here obtained with their actual physiological implications here also proposed.

ACKNOWLEDGMENTS

We acknowledge financial support from CONACyT (Mex), and DGAPAUNAM (Mex). The technical assistance of biologist Blanca Delgado and the secretarial help of Mrs. Ma. Elena Gutiérrez are gratefully acknowledged.

REFERENCES

1. Fielding PE, Fielding CJ. 1996. Dynamics of Lipoprotein Transport in the Circulatory System. In: Biochemistry of Lipid, Lipoproteins and Membranes (Vance DE, Vance J eds.) pp. 427–458.
2. Eisenberg S. 1990. Metabolism of apolipoproteins and lipoproteins. Curr Opinion Lipidol. 1:205–215.
3. Weisgraber KH, Pitas RE, Mahley RW. 1995. In: Atherosclerosis (Wodford FD, Davignon J , and A Snideerman eds. Elsevier Science, pp. 670–674.
4. Purcell-Huynh DA, Farese RV, Johnson DF, Flynn LM, Pieroti V, Newland DL, Linton MF, Sanan DA, Young SG. 1995. Transgenic mice expressing high levels of human apolipoprotein-B develop severe atherosclerotic lesions in response to a hight fat diet. J Clin Inv 95:2246–2257.
5. Maiorano JN, Davidson WS. 2000. The orientation of helix 4 in apolipoprotein A-I-containing reconstituted high density lipoproteins. J Biol Chem 275:(23) 17374–17380.
6. Wlodawer A, Segrest JP, Chung BH, Chiovetti RJ, Weinstein JN. 1979. High-density lipoprotein recombinants: evidence for a bicycle tire micelle structure obtained by neutron scattering and electron microscopy. FEBS Lett 104:231–235.
7. Tall AR, Small DM, Deckelbaum RJ, Shipley GG. 1977. Structure and thermodynamic properties of high density lipoprotein recombinants. J Biol Chem 252:4701–4711.
8. Segrest JP, Joanes MK, Klon AE, Sheldahl CJ, Hellinger M, De Loof H, Harvey SC. 1999. A detailed molecular belt model for apolipoprotein A-I in discoidal high density lipoprotein. J Biol Chem 274:31755–31758.
9. Rye KA, Clay MA, Barter PJ. 1999. Remodelling of high density lipoproteins by plasma factors. Atherosclerosis 145(2):227–238.
10. Bolaños-García V, Mas-Oliva J, Ramos S, Castillo R. 1999. Phase transitions in monolayers of human apolipoprotein CI. J Phys Chem B 103:6236–6242.
11. Bolaños-García V, Ramos S, Castillo R, Xicohtencatl-Cortes J, Mas-Oliva J. 2001. Monolayers of apolipoproteins at the air/water interface. J Phys Chem B 105:5757–5765.
12. Ruíz-García J, Moreno A, Brezesinski G, Möhwald H, Mas-Oliva J, Castillo R. (Submitted).
13. Pace CN, Vajdos F, Fee L, Grimsley G, Gray T. 1995. How to measure and predict the molar absorption coefficient of a protein. Prot Sci 4:2411–2423.

14. Wood J, Sharma R. 1994. Preparation of a robust hydrophobic monolayer on mica. Langmuir 10:2307–2310.
15. Wood J, Sharma R, 1995. How long is the long-range hydrophobic attraction? Langmuir 11(12): 4797–4802.
16. Bolaños-García V, Soriano-García M, Mas-Oliva J. 1997. CETP and Exchangeable Apoproteins. Common Features in Lipid Binding Activity. Mol and Cell Biochem 175:1–10.
17. Yonezu T, Higuchi K, Tsunasawa S, Takagi S, Sakiyama F, Takeda T. 1986. High homology is present in the primary structures between murine senile amyloid (AS_{SAM}) and human apolipoprotein A-II. FEBS Lett 203:149–152.
18. Glass C, Pittman RC, Civen M., Steinberg D. 1985. Uptake of high-density lipoprotein-associated apoprotein A-I and cholesterol esters by 16 tissues of the rat in vivo and by adrenal cells and hepatocytes in vitro. J Biol Chem 260:744–750.
19. Muller DJ, Heyman JB, Oesterhelt F, Moller C, Gaub H, Buldt G, Engel A. 2000. Atomic force microscopy of native purple membrane Biochim Biophys Acta 1460:27–38.
20. Giessibl FJ. Atomic resolution of the silicon (III)-(7X/) surface by atomic force microscopy. Science 267:68–71.
21. Shao Z, Mou J, Czajkowski DM, Yang J, Yuan J-Y. 1996. Biological atomic force microscopy: What is achieved and what is needed. Adv Phys 45:1–86.
22. Fielding CJ, Fielding PE. 1995. Molecular physiology of reverse cholesterol transport. J Lipid Res 36:211–228.
23. Weisgraber KH, Mahley RW, Kowal RC, Herz J, Goldstein JL, Brown MS. 1990. Apolipoprotein C-I modulates the interaction of apolipoprotein E with β-migrating very low density lipoproteins (β-VLDL) and inhibits binding of βVLDL to low density lipoprotein receptor-related protein. J Biol Chem 265:22453–22459.

Frontiers in Cardiovascular Health, edited by
N.S. Dhalla, A. Chockalingam,
H.I. Berkowitz & P.K. Singal
Kluwer Academic Publishers, Boston, 2003

Changing Partially Hydrogenated Fat for Palmitic Acid in the Diet Increases LDL-Cholesterol and Endogenous Cholesterol Synthesis in Normocholesterolemic Women

Margaret A. French,[1] Kalyana Sundram,[2] and M. Thomas Clandinin[1]

[1] *Nutrition and Metabolism Research Group*
Department of Agricultural, Food and Nutritional Science and Department of Medicine
University of Alberta, Edmonton Canada
and [2] *Malaysian Palm Oil Board*
Selangor, Malaysia

Summary. The present studies assessed the effect of dietary intake of high versus low palmitic acid and the effect of exchanging palmitic acid for *trans* fatty acids on plasma lipoprotein cholesterol levels and on rates for endogenous synthesis of cholesterol in normal and hyperlipidemic subjects. Healthy subjects received each of the diet treatments for 21 days, followed by washout periods of 21 days. On day 20 of each diet treatment, a priming dose of deuterium was consumed and was used to determine incorporation of deuterium into the newly synthesized cholesterol molecule, and fractional synthetic rates were calculated. The high level of 16:0 did not significantly affect serum total cholesterol and LDL-cholesterol when diets also contained a high level of 18:2n-6. The results indicate that 16:0 has no effect on serum lipoprotein profiles in the presence of recommended intakes for 18:2n-6. When the diet contained *trans* fatty acids total and LDL-cholesterol increased and cholesterol synthesis increased with a decrease in HDL-cholesterol.

***Key words*:** palmitic acid, trans fatty acids, deuterium, cholesterol.

Corresponding Author: Dr. M.T. Clandinin, Department of Agricultural, Food and Nutritional Science, 4-10 Agriculture/Forestry Centre, University of Alberta, Edmonton, Alberta, Canada, T6G 2P5. Phone: (780) 492-5188, Fax: (780) 492-8855, E-mail: tom.clandinin@ualberta.ca.

INTRODUCTION

Saturated fatty acids and hydrogenated oils are common components of margarines and prepared foods. Specific dietary saturated fatty acids may raise total cholesterol levels and LDL-cholesterol levels. Understanding of the effects of individual saturated fatty acids is complicated by evidence showing that all saturated fats do not affect lipoprotein profiles equally (1–3). Stearic acid (18:0) has little effect on lipid levels, similar to that of some monounsaturates, while lauric (12:0) and myristic (14:0) acids have potent cholesterol-raising effects (4–6). According to the original Keys hypothesis (1,7), palmitic acid (16:0) should increase blood cholesterol levels but these commonly cited equations fail to separate the effect of three saturated fatty acids (12:0, 14:0 and 16:0), defining each as equally hypercholesterolemic. When the Keys equation is modified to treat palmitic acid as neutral (similar to stearic acid), the equation is a better predictor of changes observed in serum cholesterol levels (8). In a study, which exchanged 5% of energy from 12:0 plus 14:0 for 16:0 in healthy young men consuming a low cholesterol diet, the dietary combination of 12:0 plus 14:0 produced significantly higher serum cholesterol levels than 16:0 (9). Other studies have failed to demonstrate elevated plasma cholesterol following palmitic acid consumption (10). Ng et al. compared the effects of palmitic acid and oleic acid in normolipemic subjects (10). Exchanging 7% of energy between palm oil and olive oil produced identical lipoprotein profiles suggesting that in healthy humans, exchanging dietary palmitic acid for oleic acid within the normally present range of these fatty acids would not affect serum cholesterol concentration.

Partial hydrogenation of oils is widely used to produce edible fat products having specific physical and textural properties. This process results in conversion of the *cis* bond to *cis* or *trans* configurations at a variety of positions along the fatty acid chain. Clinical (11) and epidemiological (12) studies have suggested that hydrogenated fats containing *trans* fatty acids increase plasma total cholesterol, LDL-cholesterol and lipoprotein Lp(a) while depressing HDL-cholesterol levels. The metabolic basis for these observations is unknown but these metabolic effects will tend to increase risk of cardiovascular disease (13) particularly if dietary *trans* fatty acids increase endogenous rates of cholesterol synthesis.

The first study was designed to assess the effect of high versus low palmitic acid intakes in combination with high and low linoleic acid (18:2n-6) levels on plasma lipoprotein cholesterol levels and on rates of endogenous synthesis of cholesterol in normal and hyperlipidemic subjects. A second study was designed to determine if substitution of palmitic acid for hydrogenated fat containing *trans* fatty acids at a usual level of linoleic acid intake (6% of energy) would mitigate the hypercholesterolemic effects of dietary *trans* fatty acids.

MATERIALS AND METHODS

The Faculty of Agriculture, Forestry and Home Economics Human Ethics Review Committee (Study 1) and the Malaysian Palm Oil Board Ethical Committee (Study

Table 1. Descriptive characteristics of subjects

Demographic parameters	Normal Subjects	Hypercholesterolemic Subjects
Study 1		
Age (years)	24.0 ± 4.7	45.2 ± 4.2
Body Weight (kg)	77.8 ± 17.6	74.5 ± 4.9
Height (cm)	182.4 ± 4.4	169 ± 3.3
BMI	23.4 ± 3.5	25.9 ± 1.4
Initial TC[1] (mmol/L)	N/A	6.07 ± 0.34
Study 2		
Age (years)		
Body Weight (kg)	56.86 ± 2.41	
Height (cm)	154.2 ± 1.9	
BMI	23.88 ± 0.80	
Initial TC (mmol/L)	5.37 ± 0.35	

[1] TC—Total cholesterol.

2) approved all procedures. Subjects gave informed written consent. An in-depth questionnaire was completed by all subjects to screen for medical problems known to affect lipoprotein levels, and to characterize the subjects' activity levels and sleep patterns. Subjects were nonsmokers and were not taking any medication or vitamin supplements during the study.

Subjects and diets

In the first study normal male (n = 6) and moderately hyperlipidemic male and female subjects (n = 6) were recruited (Table 1). Caloric requirements were determined and maintained as described earlier (14). The study consisted of four 21-day treatments, each consisting of a three-day rotational menu partitioned into three isocaloric meals. All meals were prepared in the Metabolic Research kitchen and consumed at fixed times. For female subjects, diet treatments were coordinated with their menstrual cycles such that cholesterol synthesis and lipogenesis were measured during the luteal phase in order to be comparable to rates measured in male subjects (15). Diets were formulated using published nutrition composition tables (16) to contain an average of 28.9 ± 1.6% of energy from fat, 56.2 ± 1.9% of energy from CHO, and 16.3 ± 0.5% energy from protein. Each diet treatment was balanced for n-3 fatty acid, cholesterol and fibre content. The four diets were designed to provide low (~3% energy) or high (~10–12% energy) combinations of 16:0 (palmitic acid) in relation to 18:2n-6 (linoleic acid) (Table 2).

The second study was conducted with ten normolipemic female Malaysian subjects described in Table 1. The subjects began the study after a three-week control period that represented the habitual Malaysian diet normally consumed by these volunteers (Table 3). The habitual diet, containing 29% of energy as fat incorporated typical local Malaysian recipes and nutrient content (17). A mixture of palm olein and coconut oil in the approximate ratio of 90:10 represented the fat blend

Table 2. Analyzed composition of diets for study 1*

% Energy	Low 16:0/Low 18:2	Low 16:0/High 18:2	High 16:0/Low 18:2	High 16:0/High 18:2
Calories (kcal)	3074 ± 158	2991 ± 268	3028 ± 32	2988 ± 228
Protein	15.7 ± 3.1	16.9 ± 2.3	16.3 ± 0.4	16.1 ± 2.1
Carbohydrate	56.5 ± 4.8	57.0 ± 3.3	57.8 ± 0.8	53.5 ± 2.6
Total fat	29.3 ± 2.1	27.0 ± 1.8	28.0 ± 3.4	31.9 ± 2.1
16:0	3.6 ± 0.2	2.2 ± 0.2	7.7 ± 0.6	8.7 ± 0.4
18:0	0.7 ± 0.2	1.6 ± 0.1	1.5 ± 0.1	1.1 ± 0.1
18:1	14.8 ± 1.4	6.2 ± 1.1	6.7 ± 0.8	7.7 ± 0.7
18:2n-6	3.3 ± 0.2	9.8 ± 0.9	1.6 ± 0.2	10.1 ± 0.5
18:3n-3	0.2 ± 0.0	0.3 ± 0.0	0.2 ± 0.0	0.1 ± 0.0
20:5n-3	0.05 ± 0.05	0.01 ± 0.01	0.01 ± 0.01	0.01 ± 0.01
22:6n-3	0.06 ± 0.06	0.03 ± 0.02	0.01 ± 0.01	0.01 ± 0.02

*Diets were formulated using Food Processor II nutrient analysis software (Esha Research, Salem, Oregon). Meals were analyzed in duplicate and values pooled to obtain per day values (means ± SD). Fatty acids were analyzed in duplicate portions of food as methyl esters by gas-liquid chromatography. Analyzed values are calculated means ± SD of 3-day menu in duplicate (n = 6) and are expressed as % energy.

Table 3. Nutrient intake per day (% energy) in study 2*

	Baseline	High saturated fat	High *Trans* fat
Total energy (kcal)	2112 ± 496.9	2140 ± 166.4	2070 ± 293.0
Total fat	29.3 ± 3.90	30.5 ± 1.59	29.9 ± 3.03
Protein	17.2 ± 2.90	14.5 ± 1.04	14.3 ± 2.91
Carbohydrate	53.4 ± 4.20	55.5 ± 2.24	55.7 ± 3.68
SFA	13.20 ± 2.34	13.0 ± 1.75	8.14 ± 1.11
10:0	0.15 ± 0.18	n.d.	0.08 ± 0.07
12:0	1.16 ± 1.08	0.47 ± 0.42	0.86 ± 0.39
14:0	0.70 ± 0.41	0.46 ± 0.15	0.48 ± 0.15
16:0	9.77 ± 1.65	10.6 ± 1.51	4.54 ± 0.60
18:0	1.35 ± 0.25	1.31 ± 0.16	2.06 ± 0.33
MUFA	11.85 ± 1.97	12.9 ± 1.45	8.00 ± 0.94
16:1 (n-9)	0.43 ± 0.40	0.23 ± 0.09	0.25 ± 0.15
18:1 (n-9)	11.42 ± 1.79	12.7 ± 1.45	7.75 ± 0.92
PUFA	3.41 ± 0.63	3.80 ± 0.47	6.54 ± 1.12
18:2 (n-6)	3.20 ± 0.58	3.54 ± 0.46	5.80 ± 1.11
18:3 (n-3)	0.14 ± 0.04	0.11 ± 0.08	0.49 ± 0.27
22:6 (n-3)	0.08 ± 0.12	0.14 ± 0.16	0.25 ± 0.17
Trans FA	n.d.	n.d.	5.59 ± 1.12
18:1 te	n.d.	n.d.	3.13 ± 0.67
18:1 (n-11t)	n.d.	n.d.	0.66 ± 0.20
18:1 (n-13t)	n.d.	n.d.	1.14 ± 0.40
18:2 (n-6tt)	n.d.	n.d.	1.60 ± 0.10
18:2 (n-6tc)	n.d.	n.d.	0.25 ± 0.06
P/S ratio	0.26 ± 0.04	0.30 ± 0.04	0.82 ± 0.18

*Nutrients analyzed from double portions of food consumed by volunteers (n = 10). 18:1 te = *trans* elaidic acid, t = *trans*, tt = *trans trans*, tc = *trans cis*, n.d. = not detectable.

during this habitual diet. At the end of the control period subjects were randomly assigned to one of two dietary test periods in which a minimum of two-thirds of the fat energy was replaced by a test fat. Energy requirements were determined to maintain the subjects' current weight (14). Subjects were weighed weekly to verify maintenance of body weight. Subjects consumed each of the two diets containing 30% of energy as fat for a 30 d period. The high saturated fat diet was high in palmitic acid (10.6% of energy) and the other diet, high *trans* fat, exchanged 5.6% of energy as *trans* fatty acids for palmitic acid. This partially hydrogenated diet fat treatment provided 3.1% of energy as elaidic acid and 2.6% as other *trans* isomers. The dietary design reflects a real life situation wherein consumers purchase high linoleic acid products containing hydrogenated fatty acids. Using a 6-day rotating menu, subjects were provided with three meals (breakfast, lunch and high tea), which were prepared fresh each day in a central laboratory kitchen by a trained caterer. Meals were provided from Monday to Saturday of each week. To further enhance compliance the test oils were provided to the volunteers' families for preparation of dinner and all meals on Sunday.

Experimental design

In the first study subjects were fed the diets for 21 days with a washout period of 21 days between diet treatments. On day 21 of each treatment, a fasting blood sample (30 mL) was taken. Subjects then consumed a priming dose of deuterium oxide and a maintenance dose over the next 24 hours (18). Exactly 24 hours later (day 22), a second fasting blood sample (30 mL) was collected.

Subjects in the second study were fed either the high saturated fat or the high *trans* fat diet for 30 d separated by a washout period of four weeks. The deuterium administration protocol was exactly the same as Study 1.

Serum was analyzed for lipoprotein cholesterol levels. The remaining blood from day 21 and 22 was centrifuged at 3000 rpm for 15 min. at 4°C (Jouan refrigerated centrifuge, CR 4.11, Sainte Nazaire, France) to obtain plasma. Day 21 plasma was used to determine background deuterium enrichment and Day 22 plasma was used to measure deuterium enrichment at 24 hours in cholesterol, cholesteryl ester and plasma water.

RESULTS

Study 1

Subject compliance in consuming all food provided from the metabolic research kitchen was high. Weight changes were minimal throughout the study period. There were no significant differences between diets in regard to total fat intake. The analyzed 16:0 content of the diet varied little from formulated values. There were no significant differences between diet treatments in regard to dietary fiber (22.9 ± 2.8 g), n-3 fatty acid (1.54 ± 1.16 mg and cholesterol 183 ± 26 mg) content. The arachidonic acid, eicosapentaenoic acid and docosahexaenoic acid in each of the diet treatments was 0.02 ± 0.01%, 0.002 ± 0.012%, and 0.30 ± 0.01% of fatty acids, respectively. The analyzed fat content of meals in each diet treatment was close to the values formulated, and was consistent within each diet treatment.

Total cholesterol

During the entire study period, total cholesterol values were between 3.17 and 4.02 mmol/L in normal subjects (Figure 1). Feeding a high 16:0 diet increased levels of total cholesterol from 3.30 to 3.61 mmol/L ($p < 0.0001$) when the diet was low in 18:2n-6. When the diet was high in 18:2n-6 raising the level of 16:0 did not have a significant effect on total plasma cholesterol level, in normal or hypercholesterolemic subjects.

LDL-cholesterol

LDL-cholesterol values ranged from 1.76 to 2.48 mmol/L in normal subjects; within the low range of normal (Figure 1). Plasma LDL-cholesterol level was higher ($p < 0.0001$) when subjects consumed the higher level of 16:0 (2.18 mmol/l) at the low 18:2n-6 intake level. LDL-cholesterol levels decreased ($p < 0.01$) at the high level of 18:2n-6 consumption (1.92 mmol/L) compared to the lower level of 18:2n-6 (2.12 mmol/L). Similar to the total cholesterol response, when the diet was high in 18:2n-6, raising the level of 16:0 did not have a significant effect on plasma LDL-cholesterol level in normal or hypercholesterolemic subjects.

HDL-cholesterol

Throughout the study HDL-cholesterol values varied only minimally, ranging from 1.08 to 1.24 mmol/L (Figure 1) in normal subjects. No significant main effects of diet on HDL-cholesterol levels were observed in hypercholesterolemic subjects. At high levels of 18:2n-6, a high 16:0 intake lead to significant reductions in HDL-cholesterol levels (1.21 mmol/L vs. 1.08 mmol/L) ($p < 0.003$) in normal subjects.

Study 2

Total cholesterol

Mean level of total cholesterol for the subjects after consuming the baseline diet was 5.37 ± 0.35 mmol/L. After consuming the high saturated fat diet the mean total cholesterol level dropped to 5.28 mmol/L compared to the baseline diet. Mean total cholesterol increased significantly by 6.6% ($p < 0.05$) when the *trans* fatty acid diet was fed compared to the high saturated fat diet (Figure 2). Total cholesterol values for eight out of ten subjects increased and one remained unchanged after the high *trans* fat diet was consumed relative to the high saturated fat.

LDL-cholesterol

The mean LDL-cholesterol after the baseline diet was 3.35 ± 0.27 mmol/L. LDL-cholesterol decreased marginally to 3.23 ± 0.17 mmol/L when the high saturated fat diet was fed. When the *trans* fatty acid diet was ingested, mean LDL-cholesterol

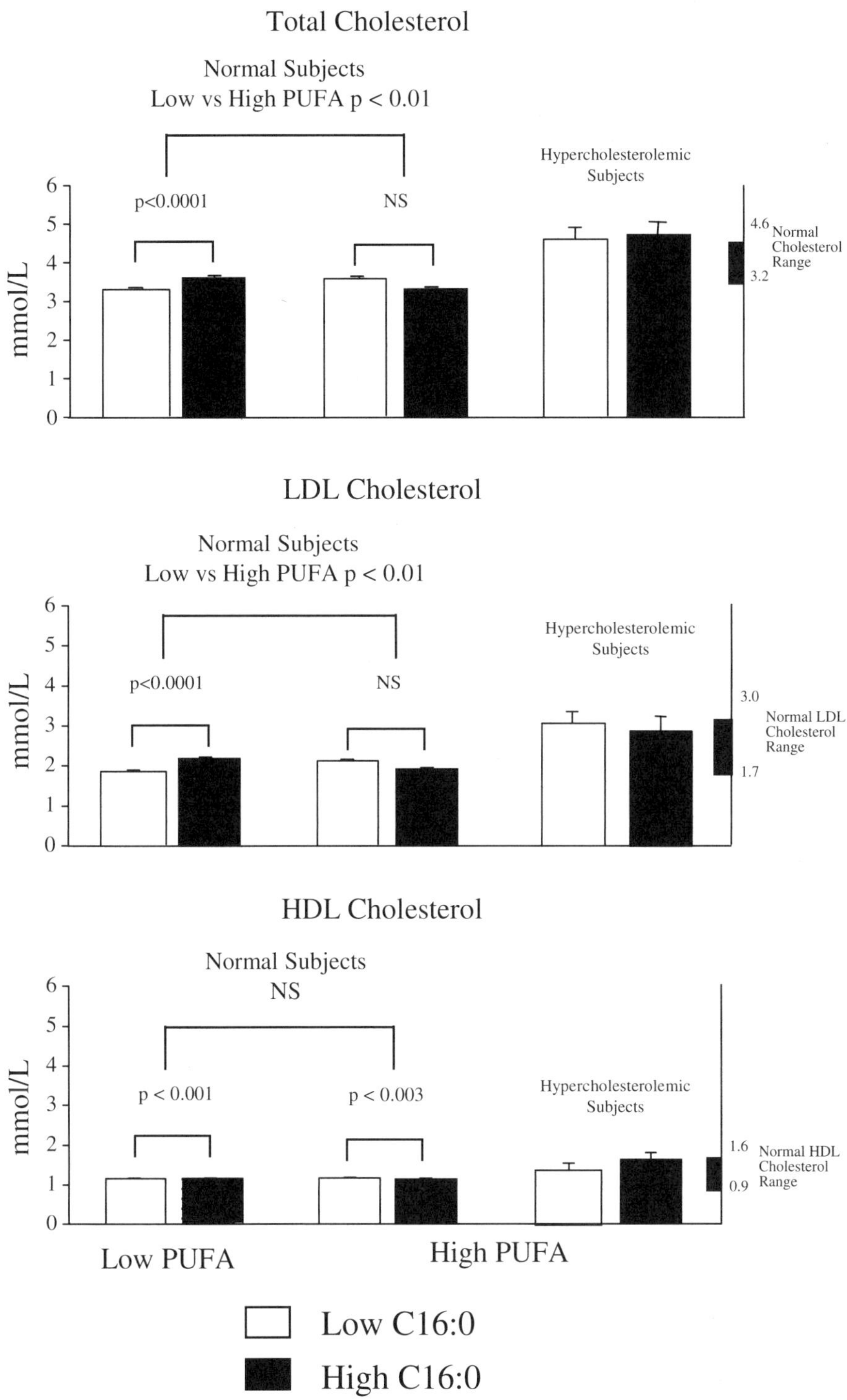

Figure 1. The effect of palmitic acid on plasma lipoprotein cholesterol values in subjects consuming diets high or low in linoleic acid (Study 1). The panels show total cholesterol, LDL-cholesterol and HDL-cholesterol for subjects. Values represent means ± SEM for 6 normocholesterolemic men and for 6 moderately hypercholesterolemic subjects. NS indicates non-significant ($P > 0.05$).

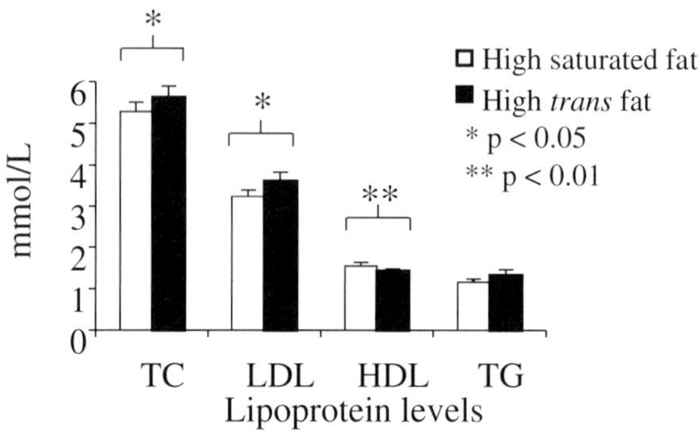

Figure 2. The effect of consuming high saturated fat and high *trans* fat diets on plasma lipoprotein cholesterol levels (n = 10). Values represent means ± SEM.

levels increased by 11.5% over the high saturated fat diet ($p < 0.05$) (Figure 2). A similar pattern for individual subjects was observed for the LDL-cholesterol as with total cholesterol levels.

HDL-cholesterol

HDL-cholesterol of the subjects averaged 1.44 ± 0.09 mmol/L after consuming the baseline diet, which increased to 1.55 ± 0.08 mmol/L after the high saturated fat diet was fed. Mean HDL levels fell back close to the baseline diet when the high *trans* fat diet was consumed (Figure 2). The mean HDL-cholesterol of the subjects decreased by 7.7% ($p < 0.01$) when the high *trans* fat diet was fed compared to a high saturated fat diet. The HDL-cholesterol levels of all subjects decreased when a high *trans* fat diet was fed. When the high saturated fat diet was fed the LDL/HDL ratio averaged 2.12 ± 0.11 but increased to 2.58 ± 0.20 when the fat source was the high *trans* fat diet ($p < 0.01$).

Cholesterol fractional synthetic rate

The deuterium uptake method determines the short-term cholesterol synthesis in humans by measuring the rate of D_2O uptake from the body water pool into newly synthesized cholesterol molecule relative to the initial cholesterol enrichment. In the first experiment values for FSR were not significantly affected by either 16:0 or 18:2n-6 content of the diet for either normal or hypercholesterolemic subjects.

In the second experiment, the total cholesterol synthetic rate (FSRtot) was measured to be 0.020 ± 0.005 when the high saturated fat diet was fed and 0.026 ± 0.004 when the high *trans* fat diet was consumed (Figure 3). However, when free cholesterol and cholesterol ester fractions were considered separately, the FSR of the free cholesterol fraction was significantly greater (FSR of 0.046 ± 0.006) when the high *trans* fat diet was consumed compared to the high saturated fat diet (FSR of

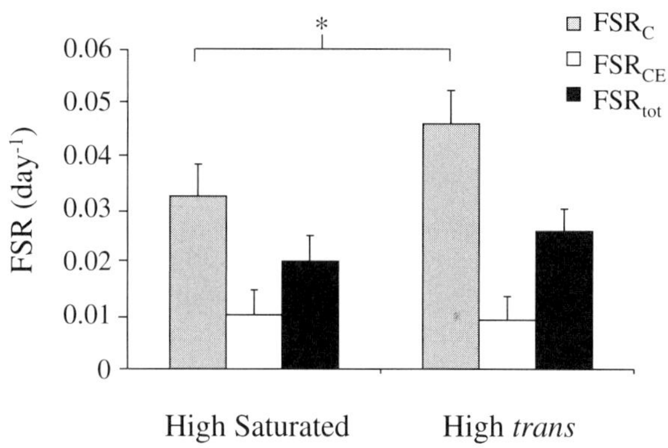

Figure 3. Effect of diet treatment on mean FSR for free cholesterol, cholesteryl ester and total cholesterol. The fractional synthetic rate of free cholesterol increases significantly when a high *trans* fat diet is consumed ($p < 0.05$).

0.032 ± 0.006). Eight out of ten subjects increased their FSRtot when a high *trans* fat diet was fed but this did not attain significance compared to the high saturated fat diet.

DISCUSSION

In North America, palmitic acid is the predominant saturated fatty acid in the diet, contributing approximately 7–8% of the total energy intake. The results from the first study support the hypothesis that increasing levels of 18:2n-6 in the diet will result in a decrease in both the total and LDL-cholesterol levels. The reduction in these lipoprotein subfractions was maintained and even enhanced in the majority of subjects as the level of palmitic acid was increased from 3% to 10% of total energy. Conversely at low levels of dietary 18:2n-6 (3% energy) increasing the content of palmitic acid resulted in significant increases in both total and LDL-cholesterol. These data lend support to previous research suggesting that palmitic acid is "conditionally" hypercholesterolemic (19,20).

Current dietary recommendations suggest that no more than 30% of the total energy be derived from fat. Of this one third, or 10% of energy should be obtained from polyunsaturated fatty acids such as 18:2n-6. The diets in this study designated as high in linoleic acid, contained 18:2n-6 at levels consistent with those recommended. The addition of linoleic acid in the high 16:0, high 18:2n-6 diet may have resulted in a more favorable polyunsaturated fatty acid to saturated fatty acid ratio (P/S). For example, in the high 16:0, low 18:2n-6, the P/S ratio was 0.14 and the resultant total cholesterol level observed was 4.02 ± 0.08 mmol/L. In contrast, the P/S ratio of the high 16:0, high 18:2n-6 diet was 1.19 (very close to the recommended 1.0 ratio) and the corresponding total cholesterol dropped to 3.20 ±

0.08 mmol/L. This rationale also supports the requirement of adequate amounts of dietary saturated fat because the diet low in 16:0 and high in 18:2n-6 (P/S = 2.55) resulted in the second highest total cholesterol response (3.42 ± 0.08 mmol/L), providing evidence that, at some point, the intake of saturated fat may become suboptimal. It has been suggested that 18:2n-6 stimulates LDL-receptor activity, which is enhanced in the presence of saturated fat (21). This concept is based on the premise that for maximal up-regulation of LDL-receptor activity, and consequent removal of LDL, a threshold intake of both 18:2n-6 and saturated fatty acid is required. Although previous researchers have not identified at what levels such up-regulation occurs, it is apparent from the data presented here that 18:2n-6 at 3% energy (i.e., the high 16:0, low 18:2n-6 diet) was not sufficient to up-regulate LDL-receptor activity. However, the 18:2n-6 content of the high 16:0, high 18:2n-6 diet (10% energy) was adequate to promote decreased LDL levels. Clearly, further research is required to establish at what combination of 18:2n-6 and saturated fat this beneficial effect occurs.

The data suggest that for subjects who have cholesterol values within the normal range, palmitic acid does not influence endogenous cholesterol synthesis. While no significant differences occur in the FSR for cholesterol, it appears that larger FSR values occur in the individual subjects who exhibit a greater change in serum cholesterol values in response to diet treatment. This relationship, unlike that of the lipoprotein response, appears to be independent of the dietary linoleic acid level. Clearly, the presence of adequate linoleic acid is of primary importance and cannot be overlooked. The finding that palmitic acid does not exert a cholesterol-raising effect in the presence of adequate linoleic acid has practical applications to the food industry as well as to nutritionists.

In the second study, the current results extend previous findings that moderate intake of *trans* fatty acids increase the LDL/HDL-cholesterol ratio. Subjects consuming high saturated or high *trans* fat diets had similar energy intakes, which consequently cannot explain the changes in LDL-cholesterol or rates of endogenous cholesterol synthesis observed (20).

Elevated total cholesterol and LDL-cholesterol levels and low HDL-cholesterol levels are associated with increased risk of cardiovascular disease. It is commonly accepted that diets high in saturated fat raise plasma total cholesterol and LDL-cholesterol. However, recent studies suggest that the saturated fatty acids are not uniformly cholesterolemic, with stearic acid being described as neutral (21), while myristic acid has been assigned the highest cholesterol-raising potency (22). It was found in the first experiment that diets high in palmitic acid are cholesterol-raising unless they are accompanied by sufficient levels of linoleic acid.

It should be noted that in the present study the level of linoleic acid in the high *trans* fat diet was higher than in the high saturated fat diet. Linoleic acid appears not to have the same hypocholesterolemic effect when consumed in conjunction with *trans* fatty acids as with palmitic acid. This observation is also supported by data from Mattan et al. (23).

Judd et al. (24) reported the relative effect of different fatty acids on total cholesterol and LDL-cholesterol levels to be oleic acid < moderate *trans* < high *trans* < saturated fats. The linoleic acid content was kept constant at 6% of energy through all of the diet treatments. In the present study, the order of the cholesterolemic effect of high *trans* vs. high saturated fat was opposite to that observed by Judd et al. the amount of linoleic acid was 3.5% of total energy in the high saturated fat diet and the mean total cholesterol was 6.6% lower than that observed with a high *trans* diet containing 5.8% of energy of linoleic acid. There are instances where saturated fats resulted in lower cholesterol levels than trans fatty acids. Sundram et al. (17) compared the effects of exchanging *cis* 18:1, 16:0 or 12:0 + 14:0 for *trans* elaidic acid in humans. The *trans*-rich diet significantly elevated total and LDL-cholesterol levels relative to the 16:0 and 18:1-rich fat but attained no significance compared to the saturated 12:0 + 14:0-rich dietary fat. However, the *trans* diet uniquely lowered HDL-cholesterol and elevated Lp(a) relative to all other dietary treatments. These effects were apparent despite the fact that linoleic acid content in the *trans*-rich diet was significantly higher than *cis* 18:1 and saturated 16:0-rich diets. Therefore in the present study linoleic acid content is not responsible for the higher cholesterolemic effect of *trans* fat compared to saturated fat.

Trans fatty acids decrease HDL-cholesterol, and this is currently viewed as a major public health concern (25). Saturates, in addition to raising total and LDL-cholesterol, do not appear to affect HDL-cholesterol levels to the same extent (26) or are even capable of raising the beneficial HDL-cholesterol (27). The effect of *trans* fatty acids in elevating LDL-cholesterol levels and depressing HDL-cholesterol can have a large effect on the LDL/HDL ratio which is used to assess risk of cardiovascular disease. Thus the resulting LDL/HDL–cholesterol ratio is significantly lowered by *trans*-rich diets (25,26).

Cholesterol ester transfer protein (CETP) activity has been postulated as a possible mechanism, i.e. enhanced transfer of cholesteryl ester (CE) from HDL to LDL, to explain the observed shifts in the LDL/HDL ratio (28). In individuals whose LDL-receptors are down regulated, increased CE transfer from HDL could be expected to diminish the HDL-CE pool and overload the LDL-CE pool when LDL clearance is impaired. This was demonstrated in *Cebus* monkeys whose LDL-receptor activity and clearance of LDL are highly efficient. When fed an elaidic-rich *trans* diet, these monkeys were found to have elevated CETP activity and depressed HDL levels without affecting the LDL-pool size or LDL-clearance rate (29).

The effect of linoleic acid level in different diet treatments may also affect endogenous cholesterol synthesis. In a study using various levels of hydrogenated fat in different margarines Matthan et al. (23) found that as the degree of *trans* fatty acids in the diet increased, the FSR_{FC} decreased. This is opposite to the effect that was found in the present study. In Matthan's study the linoleic acid decreased gradually as the *trans* fatty acid content increased, whereas in the present study *trans* fatty acids were accompanied by a higher level of linoleic acid than the high saturated fat diet. High levels of polyunsaturated fats have been shown to increase cholesterol synthesis (24) so it is difficult to attribute the observed increase in cholesterol synthesis to either increased linoleic or increased *trans* fatty acids. High levels of linoleic acid appear not to have the hypocholesterolemic effect observed when consumed in conjunction with high palmitic acid levels. Therefore, increasing *trans* fatty acids in the diet promotes increased LDL-cholesterol by increasing endogenous cholesterol synthesis.

It is well accepted that *trans* fatty acids raise total and LDL-cholesterol levels. Food manufacturers need to find a healthy alternative in the production of processed food requiring a solid fat. Saturated fat containing high amounts of palmitic acid but not lauric or myristic acid could fill this void. Separate identification of saturated and *trans* fat content in food labeling currently appears pertinent so that it would enable the consumer to make a choice between these two fat sources. This study has shown that substitution of palmitic acid for hydrogenated fat containing *trans* fatty acids at a usual level of linoleic acid intake (6% of energy) mitigates the hypercholesterolemic effects of dietary *trans* fatty acids.

It is concluded for normolipemic and mildly cholesterolemic subjects who typically consume a relatively low fat diet (30% energy) from fat containing the recommended intake of n-6 polyunsaturated fat, it is unlikely that consumption of palmitic acid will have an appreciable effect on lipoprotein profiles. Furthermore, it can be inferred that an adequate amount of palmitic acid is necessary to promote a more favorable serum cholesterol response. Selected epidemiological data suggests that as intake of saturated fatty acids is decreased to about 10% of energy, there is a progressive fall in mortality due to cardiovascular disease. Contradictory population studies have also been reported. Evidence for lowering the level of saturated fat in the diet below this 10% of energy level is lacking, leading one to question the benefit of reductions beyond this point. This finding may be of particular importance as low and even negligible levels of dietary saturated fat are frequently recommended by health professionals to promote lowered lipid levels. Because palmitic acid is an abundant fatty acid in palm oil, meat and dairy products, food items also high in nutritive value in other ways, re-evaluation of the recommendations to limit consumption of these food items is warranted.

AKNOWLEDGEMENTS

The authors gratefully appreciate the cooperation of study subjects and acknowledge the excellent technical assistance of H. Podjarkowski, A.A. Wierzbicki and S. Vichnevskaia. The study was supported by grants from the Natural Science and Engineering Research Council of Canada, the Dairy Farmers of Canada, the Malaysian Palm Oil Board and The Alberta Agricultural Research Institute.

REFERENCES

1. Hegsted PM, McGandy RB, Meyers ML, Stare FJ. 1965. Quantitative effects of dietary fat on serum cholesterol in man. Am J Clin Nutri 17:281–295.
2. Cox C, Mann J, Sutherland W, Chisholm A, Skeaff M. 1995. Effects of coconut oil, butter and safflower oil on lipids and lipoproteins in persons with moderately elevated cholesterol levels. 36:1787–1796.
3. Zock PL, de Vries J, Katan MB. 1994. Impact of myristic acid versus palmitic acid on serum lipid and lipoprotein levels in healthy women and men. 14:567–575.

4. Bonanome A, Grundy SM. 1988. Effect of dietary stearic acid on plasma cholesterol and lipoprotein levels. N Engl J Med 318:1244–1248.
5. Grundy SM. 1994. Influence of stearic acid on cholesterol metabolism relative to other long-chain fatty acids. Am J Clin Nutr 60(suppl):986S–990S.
6. Grundy SM, Denke MA. 1990. Dietary influences on serum lipids and lipoproteins. J Lipid Res 31:1149–1168.
7. Keys A, Anderson JT, Grande F. 1957. Prediction of serum cholesterol responses of man to changes in fats in the diet. Lancet 2:959–966.
8. Hayes KC, Pronczuk A, Lindsey S, Diersen-Schade D. 1991. Dietary saturated fatty acids (12:0, 14:0, 16:0) differ in their impact on plasma cholesterol and lipoproteins in nonhuman primates. Am J Clin Nutr 53:491–498.
9. Sundram K, Hayes KC, Siru OH. 1994. Dietary palmitic acid results in lower serum cholesterol than does a lauric-myristic combination in normolipidemic humans. Am J Clin Nutr 59:841–846.
10. Ng TKW, Hayes KC, Dewitt GF, Jegthesan M, Satgunasigam N, Ong AS, Tan D. 1992. Dietary palmitic and oleic acid exert similar effects on serum cholesterol and lipoprotein profiles in normocholesterolemic men and women. Am J Coll Nutr 11:383–390.
11. Katan MB, Zock PL, Mensink RP. 1995. *Trans* fatty acids and their effects on lipoproteins in humans. Ann Rev Nutr 15:473–493.
12. Ascherio A, Willett WC. 1995. Metabolic and atherogenic effects of *trans* fatty acids. J Internal Med 238:93–96.
13. Willett WC, Stampfer MJ, Manson JE, et al. 1993. Intake of *trans* fatty acids and risk of coronary heart disease among women. Lancet 341:581–585.
14. Bell L, Jones PJH, Telch J, Clandinin MT. 1985. Prediction of energy needs for clinical studies. Nutr Res 5:123–129.
15. Faix D, Neese R, Kletke C, Wolden S, Cesar D, Coutlangus M, Shackleton CHL, Hellerstein MK. 1993. Quantification of menstrual and diurnal periodicities in rates of cholesterol and fat synthesis in humans. J Lipid Res 34:2063–2075.
16. US Department of Agriculture. 1976. Agriculture Handbook 8-1 to 8-12.
17. Sundram K, Ismail A, Hayes KC, Jeyamalar R, Pathmanathan R. 1997. Trans (elaidic) fatty acids adversely affect the lipoprotein profile relative to specific saturated fatty acids in humans. J Nutr 127:S514–S520.
18. Jones PJH, Leitch CA, Li Z-C, Connor WE. 1993. Human cholesterol synthesis measurements using deuterated water. Theoretical and procedural considerations. Arterioscler Thromb 13:247–253.
19. Choudhury N, Tan L, Truswell AS. 1995. Comparison of palmolein and olive oil: Effects on plasma lipids and vitamin E in young adults. Am J Clin Nutr 61:1043–1051.
20. Raeini-Sarjaz M, Vanstone CA, Papamandjaris AA, Wykes LJ, Jones PJH. 2001. Comparison of the effect of restriction of dietary fat restriction with that of energy restriction on human lipid metabolism. 73:262–267.
21. Grundy SM, Vega GL. 1986. Plasma cholesterol responsiveness to saturated fatty acids. Am J Clin Nutr 47:822–824.
22. Hayes KC, Khosla P. 1992. Dietary fatty acid thresholds and cholesterolemia. FASEB J 6:2600–2607.
23. Matthan NR, Ausman LM, Lichtenstein AH, Jones PJH. 2000. Hydrogenated fat consumption affects cholesterol synthesis in moderately hypercholesterolemic women. J Lipid Res 41:834–839.
24. Judd JT, Clevidence BA, Muesing RA, Wittes J, Sunkin ME, Podczasy JJ. 1994. Dietary *trans* fatty acids: effects on plasma lipids and lipoproteins of healthy men and women. Amer J Clin Nutr 59:861–868.
25. Katan MB. 1995. Exit trans fatty acids. Lancet 346:1245–1246.
26. Lichtenstein AH, Ausman LM, Jalbert SM, Schaefer EJ. 1999. Effects of different forms of dietary hydrogenated fats on serum lipoprotein cholesterol levels. N Engl J Med 340:1933–1940.
27. Khosla P, Sundram K. 1996. Effects of dietary fatty acid composition on plasma cholesterol. Prog Lipid Res 35:93–132.
28. Abbey M, Nestel PJ. 1994. Plasma cholesteryl ester transfer protein is increased when trans elaidic acid is substituted for cis-oleic acid in the diet. Atherosclerosis 106:99–107.
29. Khosla P, Hajri T, Pronczuk A, Hayes KC.1997. Replacing dietary palmitic acid with elaidic acid (t-C18:1 n9) depresses HDL and increases CETP activity in cebus monkeys. J Nutr 127:531S–536S.

Frontiers in Cardiovascular Health, edited by
N.S. Dhalla, A. Chockalingam,
H.I. Berkowitz & P.K. Singal
Kluwer Academic Publishers, Boston, 2003

Cytoprotection of Cardiac Myocytes by Polyunsaturated Fatty Acids

Alain Grynberg

Summary. Most of the risk factors associated with cardiovascular disease can be controlled by nutrition. Polyunsaturated fatty acids (PUFA) of the ω3 series are known for their beneficial effect on the risk, but can also influence the severity of cardiac disease through their direct action on the myocardium. Introducing ω3 PUFA in the diet results in a marked decrease of the AA/DHA ratio, mainly due to an increase in membrane DHA content. In several experimental models, such structural changes were reported to affect cardiac functions. Among them the membrane ω3 PUFA appear to affect the oxygen cost of energy production by decreasing the fatty acid beta-oxidation in cardiac myocytes, and the improved recovery of mitochondrial function in the post-ischemic heart of rats fed fish oil. On the other hand, the incorporation of DHA in cardiac myocyte membranes induces a large decrease in the biochemical response to catecholamine stimulation. Although the mechanism does not involve a direct modification of the adrenergic receptors, the consequences of DHA intake in vivo reduces heart rate and show some similarity with the cardiac effect of β-blockers. This observation could be correlated with the observations that which occurs during ischemia and reperfusion-induced arrhythmias are largely reduced when cardiac membranes contains 15–20% DHA. In addition, the presence of ω3 PUFAs in the membranes reduces the synthesis of prostaglandines as in other organs. However, they can exert a fine-tuned control of myocardium prostaglandin synthesis in pathological conditions, since during hypoxia and reoxygenation, the effect of ω3 PUFAs becomes more specific to each prostaglandin, with no inhibition of the hypoxia-induced PGE2 synthesis, and a large inhibition of the reoxygenation-induced PGI2 release. The 3 mechanisms reported here may account for the significantly positive effects of dietary ω3 PUFAs reported in epidemiological studies. Each one contributes to cardiac protection in reference to a cardio-active drug (metabolic effectors, β-blockers, or aspirin), largely appreciated in the treatment of cardiac diseases.

***Key words*:** DHA, heart, cytoprotection, adrenergic function, eicosanoids prevention, nutrition, fatty acids.

Lipides Membranaires et Fonctions Cardiovasculaires, INRA UR1154, Faculté de Pharmacie, Université Paris-sud, 5, rue Jean Baptiste Clément, 92290 Châtenay Malabry, France. Tel: 33/146835924, Fax: 33/146835371, E-mail: grynberg@jouy.inra.fr.

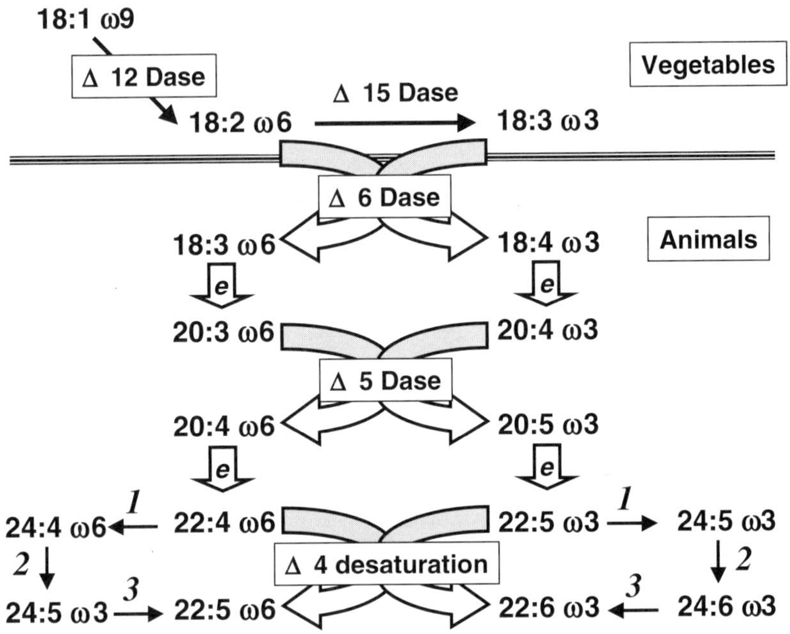

Figure 1. Polyunsaturated fatty acid elongation and desaturation process. (*e*: elongation, Dase: desaturase. The last desaturation requires 3 steps: 1 = elongation step, 2 = desaturation step by Δ6 desaturase, 3 = β-oxidation step).

Food is a key parameter in cardiovascular health as evidenced by the relationship between dietary fat and cardiovascular disease (1,2). A low polyunsaturated fatty acid (PUFA) intake, usually associated to a high saturated fat intake is considered as a major risk factor (3). More than a quantitative reduction of fat intake, the recommendations tend now to more qualitative concerns, including the replacement of saturated fat by unsaturated fat (4), and particularly PUFAs. The main PUFAs are shown on Figure 1. The 18 carbon-long PUFAs (linoleic acid 18:2ω6, and linolenic acid 18:2ω3) are mainly supplied by vegetable oils, whereas longer chains of functional relevance are supplied by either meat (arachidonic acid 20:4ω6, AA) or fish (eicosapentaenoic acid 20:5ω3, EPA, and docosahexaenoic acid 22:6ω3, DHA) (5). On the basis of epidemiological investigations (6–8), the property of PUFAs in cardiovascular disease prevention was attributed to the long chain PUFAs of the ω3 series. These data suggested the correlation between a high EPA and DHA content in plasma and platelets and a low occurrence of coronary disease.

The numerous investigations conducted to determine the mechanism of this prevention demonstrated the pleiotropic effects of the long chain ω3 PUFAs (EPA and DHA). Several authors reported their involvement in the metabolism of eicosanoids affecting platelet function and vascular tone, both involved in atherosclerosis and thrombosis process. The replacement of AA by EPA in platelet and endothelial membranes alters the functional efficiency of the thromboxane/prostacycline balance, favoring vasodilatation and reducing platelet aggregation (9). Leukotriens were also considered to mediate the prevention due to ω3 PUFA, through the replacement of LTB_4 a chemo-attractive agent produced from AA, by LTB_5 produced from EPA with a largely reduced activity (10). The ω3 PUFAs were also reported to increase tissue plasminogen activator (11), to inhibit the synthesis of PAF and fibrinogen (12) and to decrease the endothelial production of platelet derived growth factor, involved in monocyte migration in atherosclerosis plaque (13). Other studies reported the influence of ω3 PUFAs on other atherosclerosis risk factors such as circulating lipids. Their ability to decrease plasma triglycerides was clearly demonstrated (14), but the cholesterol-lowering effect described in animals was not confirmed in humans (15). Moreover, an effect on blood viscosity was reported and attributed to red blood cell shape (16).

The ω3 PUFAs are also considered for their effects on hypertension. In various animal models, fish oil was shown to reduced pressure (17–21), in spite of some controversial reports (22,23). From these data, it can be suggested that ω3 PUFAs may not influence chronic hypertension, but may have a beneficial effect on moderated hypertension, or during the development of hypertension (21). A meta-analysis of the investigations conducted in humans outlined that the large variability of experimental factors (dose, sample size, duration) may account for the discrepancies (24). In spite of the demonstration of the beneficial properties of ω3 PUFAs on the parameters involved in the development of the atherosclerosis process, there is growing evidence that these fatty acids are also involved in the regulation of cardiac function.

The heart is very sensitive to the alterations induced in membrane PUFA composition by any qualitative modification of the PUFA supplied in the diet. The introduction of fish oil in the rat diet (supplying EPA and DHA) thoroughly alters the fatty acid composition of membrane phospholipids (25–26). This diet induces a large increase in DHA (which can represent up to 25% of membrane fatty acids) and a large decrease in AA. These changes, which result in a significant reduction in the AA/DHA ratio, also affect individual membranes such as mitochondria (27). The AA/DHA ratio was shown to decrease progressively during aging. However, in a population of men who died from sudden cardiac death, the AA/DHA ratio in cardiac membranes was markedly higher than expected from the age of the patients (28). These observations supported the hypothesis of a possible interaction between sudden cardiac death and the cardiac membrane fatty acid composition. In the contribution of ω3 PUFAs to the prevention of atherosclerosis or hypertension, the specific recommendation for each dietary fatty acid is poorly documented, since each (EPA and DHA but also α-linolenic acid) was considered as efficient. In the heart, a ω3 PUFAs dietary intake results in a specific DHA increase in membrane phospholipids. This addressed the question of the relationship between dietary ω3 PUFAs and cardiac DHA. The effect of fish oil feeding was investigated by McLennan and co-workers (29,30) who demonstrated the correlation between arrhythmia and ω3 PUFAs. Interestingly, a dietary supply with DHA precursors (Canola oil or Soybean oil) did not show the same efficiency than fish oil. These studies led to the conclusion, that the quantity and nature of PUFA intake was not important, but that the major condition to observe the anti-arrhythmic effect of DHA was a threshold level of DHA (18–20%) in cardiac membranes (31,32). In animal studies, this threshold was achieved only when DHA was supplied in the diet, which addresses the question of a long-term effect of precursor intake. In rats fed fish oil, DHA reaches 20% of phospholipid fatty acids, *vs* 10% only in linseed oil fed rats (rich in α-linolenic acid), and only 4% in sunflower seed oil fed rats. Moreover rat ventricular myocytes in culture do reach 20% of DHA in their membranes, when DHA is present the culture medium. Neither the supply with the sera of linseed oil fed animals (pig or rats), nor the addition of EPA to the medium can bring the cells to a satisfactory DHA level (33). This points out the poor capacity of the cardiac myocyte to achieve the last desaturation step of PUFAs, from the close precursor DPA (22:5ω3) to DHA (22:6ω3) (Figure 1). The occurrence of a Δ4 desaturase was never characterized. The conversion of DPA to DHA requires 3 steps (34) and involves the Δ6 desaturase, and one cycle of β-oxidation on a 24-carbone PUFA, which is probably the inefficient step in the heart.

MEMBRANE PUFAS AND MITOCHONDRIAL FUNCTION

In the ventricular myocyte, the β-oxidation of fatty acids accounts for approximately 60% of oxygen consumption for energy production. The regulation of β-oxidation does not occur at the fatty acid uptake level but at the metabolic level. Acetyl-CoA Carboxylase (ACC) converts the acetyl-CoA produced by β-oxidation to malonyl-CoA, the physiological inhibitor of Carnitine-Palmitoyl-Transferase 1 (CPT1). In case of excessive β-oxidation, the entry of fatty acids in the mitochondria is thus reduced. The activity of ACC is controlled positively by the acetyl-CoA concentration in the cytoplasm (35), and negatively by an AMP activated protein kinase (36). This fine-tuning process is largely hampered in pathological conditions such as ischemia or diabetes. During ischemia, AMP increases in the cytoplasm and activates protein kinase. ACC is inhibited, malonyl-CoA decreases, CPT1 inhibition does not occur and the β-oxidation is stimulated (37). A similar situation can be observed in diabetes, since insulin contributes to the negative regulation of an AMP activated protein kinase. The decrease of insulin efficiency allows the increase in kinase activity, and thus inhibition of ACC, and in turns the decrease in malonyl-CoA, and stimulation of β-oxidation. The mechanism of this effect of insulin remains however to be elucidated (38). The ischemic heart and the diabetic heart display similar abnormalities in fatty acid metabolism, based on an excessive fatty acid contribution (and thus an excessive oxygen cost) to energy production. Any action able to decrease this fatty acid contribution for energy in the heart can thus be considered as cytoprotective, and numerous researches in pharmacy focus on this topic. As shown in isolated perfused rat hearts (39), a decreased MVO_2 and an increased oxygen metabolic efficiency characterize the ω3 PUFA-rich hearts. This observation appears to be independent from cardiac work, since Demaison et al. (40)

reported a reduced production of CO_2 from palmitic acid (and intermediates of the Krebs cycle) in cultured cardiomyocytes enriched with ω3 PUFAs, indicating a lowered β-oxidation. These data were confirmed with isolated mitochondria, showing the reduction of oxygen consumption in mitochondria collected from the heart of ω3 PUFA-fed rats (27). Although these effects of ω3 PUFAs on mitochondria function are of weak amplitude in physiological conditions, they may be much more relevant in pathological conditions. The beneficial effect of ω3 PUFAs on mitochondria appeared clearly after ischemia and reperfusion, with the improvement of metabolic recovery and oxygen consumption (27,40), as well as the systolic ejection volume. These studies showed that in rats fed sunflower seed oil, the recovery of the metabolic function of isolated mitochondria after ischemia and reperfusion was approximately 75% of pre-ischemic value, although in fish oil-fed rats, the recovery was close to 100%. The mechanism of this effect of DHA in mitochondria is largely unknown. Recent indications suggest that DHA could improve in diabetic rat heart myocyte the mitochondrial function through the modification of the Km for ADP, but this needs confirmation.

MEMBRANE PUFAS AND REGULATION OF ADRENERGIC FUNCTION

The influence of the ω6/ω3 PUFA ratio on the activity of functional membrane-bound proteins was also investigated. It was proved to affect the vascular and cardiac noradrenaline sensitivity by alteration of the receptor binding characteristics (41–43). Adenylyl cyclase was often considered as the target of this effect (41,44). Conversely, although the PUFA influence on the functional response of adrenoceptors was also investigated, large differences in methodological approaches led to discordant data. In the cultured cardiomyocyte model, it was shown that the decrease in AA/DHA ratio was associated with a significant decrease in a β-agonist stimulated cAMP synthesis. But very few data were published on the effect of ω3 PUFAs on adrenergic function in pathological conditions. Delerive et al. (45) evaluated the influence of hypoxia and AA/DHA ratio on the ability of cultured rat cardiomyocytes in producing α- and β-adrenergic second messengers. Hypoxia did not affect the basal level of messenger production in un-stimulated cells, but decreased the cAMP production elicited by adrenergic stimulation. Conversely, the decrease in IP production was observed only after long term hypoxia close to irreversible cellular damages. Decreasing the AA/DHA ratio did not alter the basal level of either messenger production in un-stimulated cells. Conversely, the decrease in cAMP production was significantly more pronounced in DHA enriched cardiomyocytes (Table 1), indicating that the presence in the membranes of ω3 PUFAs elicited a decreased biochemical response to β-adrenergic stimulation in these pathological conditions. Moreover, parallel investigations were conducted in the same model on the cell functional response to adrenergic stimulation after hypoxia (46). After post-hypoxic reoxygenation, the chronotropic response to β-adrenergic stimulation (as compared with the control response in normoxia) was significantly enhanced in AA-rich cardiomyocytes but not in DHA-rich cells. Moreover, in response to α-adrenergic stimulation, the chronotropic effect of AA-rich cells but not DHA-rich cells

Table 1. Production of IPs and cAMP after hypoxia and reoxygenation in rat cardiac myocytes in culture, expresses as % of the normoxia value (Mean ± Sem, n = 9). α-adrenergic stimulation was achieved by phenylephrine (10^{-4} M) and β-adrenergic stimulation by isoproterenol (10^{-6} M)

	IPs			cAMP		
	AA rich		DHA rich	AA rich		DHA rich
Normoxia	100		100	100		100
Hypoxia 90 min	97 ± 8	ns	106 ± 9	99 ± 6	ns	98 ± 9
Hypoxia 150 min	100 ± 14	ns	103 ± 10.6	62 ± 20	0.05	38 ± 9.0
Hypoxia 210 min	94 ± 8	ns	99 ± 9	45 ± 18	0.05	29 ± 8.0

appeared significantly enhanced by hypoxia. The enrichment of cardiomyocytes with DHA attenuated the increase in α- and β-adrenergic functional responses observed after hypoxia and reoxygenation. These results suggest that a decrease in phospholipid AA/DHA ratio may partly account for the assumed cardiac protective effect of ω3 PUFAs, through a depressed response to catecholamines (biochemical and functional) in the ischemic myocardium.

As discussed above, the increase in membrane DHA is always associated with a decrease in membrane AA, and the question can be addressed as whether the effect on adrenergic system results from DHA incorporation or from AA decrease. The deficiency of the cardiac myocyte to produce DHA from DPA was used to produce a chimerical model in culture (47). Cardiomyocytes were supplied either with DHA to produce cells high in DHA and poor in AA or with EPA to produce cells high in EPA + DPA but poor in DHA and AA. These 2 groups displayed a similar AA content (10–15%), but the production of cAMP in response to isoproterenol was significantly power in the cells rich in DHA group than in the chimera rich in EPA + DPA and poor in DHA. On the contrary, no difference was observed in phenylephrine stimulated IPs production, although the PUFA composition of phosphatidylinositols was also modified (48). These data confirmed that the PUFA composition of phosphatidylinositols weakly influences their α-adrenoceptor mediated turnover rate (49).

From these data, it appears clearly that the effect of dietary PUFAs on the regulation of cardiac adrenergic function is specifically due to DHA. This specificity was investigated in vivo in a non insulin-dependent rat model. This model is characterized by a moderate increase in blood pressure, in heart rate, and in QT interval length revealed by ECG. The diet of the rats was supplemented with either EPA or DHA. As shown on Table 2, the increase in mean blood pressure was significantly reduced when the rats were fed a ω3 PUFA supplement. This effect on pressure was similar in the EPA and the DHA supplemented groups. Conversely, the ω3 PUFA effect on the cardiac consequences of the pathology was observed only in the DHA-fed group, and not in the EPA-fed group (50). This confirm the reduction by DHA of the cardiac β-adrenergic function, since in addition to the data

Table 2. Mean blood pressure and ECG parameters in insulin-resistant rats (mean ± sem, n = 6). # Statistically different from control ($p < 0.01$)

	Control	EPA	DHA
Mean BP (mm Hg)	143 ± 2	133 ± 2#	134 ± 3#
Heart rate (beat/min)	363 ± 5	363 ± 7	340 ± 6#
QT lenght (ms)	145 ± 3	150 ± 3	129 ± 2#

Control refers to the rats fed the control diet. All the groups presented are insulin-resistant rats.

collected in vitro, the data obtained in vivo evokes the effect of β-blockers on heart function (51).

MEMBRANE PUFAS AND CARDIAC MYOCYTE EICOSANOIDS

The synthesis of eicosanoids in the heart, predominantly prostacyclin (PGI_2) has been described for years. These molecules, known as vasoactive agents and aggregation effectors, were also suspected of direct inotropic and/or chronotropic effects (52). The coronary vessels were considered as the major site of eicosanoid synthesis (53). There is increasing evidence indicating that cardiac myocytes can also produce eicosanoids (54–55), in spite of some uncertainty regarding the metabolites produced by these cells. The cardiac myocyte produces mainly PGI_2 and PGE_2 and a low amount of $PGF_{2\alpha}$ and these compounds are released from the cell. As reported in endothelial cells and platelets, this production is largely dependant on the membrane phospholipid fatty acid composition. However, to our knowledge, the production of 3-series prostaglandins was not reported in the heart. In the cardiac cell, increasing the ω3 PUFA content and decreasing the AA content strongly decreased the synthesis of the 3 compounds. Conversely, increasing the AA content by 30% increased significantly PGE_2 and $PGF_{2\alpha}$, but not PGI_2 (55). Enhanced release of PGI_2 from the heart was reported during post-ischemic reperfusion (56). In cultured cardiomyocytes, ischemia and reperfusion were shown to affect differently the cardiac prostaglandins. The synthesis of PGI_2 was not affected by hypoxia but was strongly stimulated by reoxygenation. Again, increasing the AA content had no effect on these events, but increasing ω3 PUFA and decreasing AA prevented the reoxygenation-induced stimulation (55). On the contrary, the synthesis of $PGF_{2\alpha}$ was stimulated by hypoxia and remained at the same activated level during reoxygenation. The ω3 PUFAs did not influence the hypoxia-induced stimulation but like for PGI_2, prevented the reoxygenation-induced synthesis. The synthesis of PGE_2 was stimulated during hypoxia, and returned to basal level during reoxygenation. Neither the AA increase, nor the ω3 PUFA increase associated with AA decrease could influence the synthesis of PGE_2 during hypoxia and reoxygenation (55). These data suggest that key regulation steps in cardiac prostaglandin synthesis may be related to the specific synthases, downstream the cyclooxygenase step. This view is supported by several observations. Increasing the AA content by 30% does not affect similarly all the prostaglandins, although they all arise from the same cyclooxygenase activity. Decreasing the AA content by 50% (in association with ω3 PUFA increase) also results in individual responses. And both the hypoxia-induced decrease in oxygen and reperfusion-induced oxygen restoration exert a specific influence on the synthesis of each prostaglandin, and also on its sensitivity to the AA/DHA ratio. Additionally, these data suggest that the enhanced release of PGI_2 reported in the heart during post-ischemic reperfusion (56), could be due to myocardial cells rather that endothelial cells, because of the large increase in production, and the mass of the myocardium. Unfortunately, the effect of these prostaglandins is not sufficiently documented. We have to understand why the cardiac cell increases the basal of $PGF_{2\alpha}$ when oxygen decreases and PGI_2 when oxygen is restored. And we have to understand why the AA/DHA ratio affects prostaglandin synthesis in basal conditions and during reoxygenation, but not during hypoxia.

CONCLUSION

In addition to the prevention of atherosclerosis by ω3 PUFAs, DHA exerts specific effects on cardiac function that may account for the prevention of cardiovascular diseases. The results of the Gissi Prevenzione Study demonstrate the beneficial effect of long chain ω3 PUFAs on mortality in post-infarct patients. In addition to the anti-arrhythmic properties of DHA, this paper focused on the 3 properties of DHA that support the comparison with dogmatic drug treatment in cardiac ischemia or diabetes. By reducing cardiac activity, the pharmaceutical treatment tends to lower ATP demand to lower the oxygen cost of cardiac function. DHA reduces the contribution of fatty acids to energy production which results in a decreased oxygen cost of ATP production. β-blockers represent one of the most important treatments in cardiac pathology. DHA also influences the β-adrenergic function of cardiac myocytes. Although the mechanism does not involve a direct modification of the receptor, the consequences of DHA intake show some similarity with the cardiac effect of β-blockers. Finally, like aspirin used for its activity on prostaglandin synthesis, DHA can exert a fine-tuned control on the myocardium prostaglandin synthesis. These conclusions are, however, based of the cardiac cell content in DHA, and more data have to be collected on the nutritional conditions able to fulfil these requirements.

REFERENCES

1. Charnock JS, Abeywardena M, Tan D, McLennan P. 1991. Omega-3 and omega-6 PUFA's have different effects on the phospholipid fatty acid composition of rat myocardial muscle when added to a saturated fatty acid dietary supplement. Nutr Res 11:1013–1024.
2. Horrobin DF. 1993. Omega-6 and omega-3 essential fatty acids in atherosclerosis. Semin Thromb Hemost 19:129–137.
3. Nordoy A. 1999. Dietary fatty acids and coronary heart disease. Lipids 34 Suppl:S19–S22.
4. Dimmitt SB. 1995. Recent insights into dietary fats and cardiovascular disease. Clin Exp Pharmacol Physiol 22:204–208.

5. Carlier H, Bernard A, Caselli C. 1991. Digestion and absorption of polyunsaturated fatty acids. Reprod Nutr Dev 31:475–500.
6. Dyerberg J, Jorgensen KA. 1982. Marine oils and thrombogenesis. Prog Lipid Res 21:255–269.
7. Dyerberg J, Bang HO, Hjorne N. 1975. Fatty acid composition of the plasma lipids in Greenland Eskimos. Am J Clin Nutr 28:958–966.
8. Schmidt EB, Dyerberg J. 1994. Omega-3 fatty acids. Current status in cardiovascular medicine. Drugs 47:405–424.
9. Abeywardena MY, McLennan PL, Charnock JS. 1991. Differences between in vivo and in vitro production of eicosanoids following long-term dietary fish oil supplementation in the rat. Prostaglandins Leukot Essent Fatty Acids 42:159–165.
10. Hirai A, Terano T, Tamura Y, Yoshida S. 1989. Eicosapentaenoic acid and adult diseases in Japan: epidemiological and clinical aspects. J Intern Med 225:69–75.
11. Waeber B, Nussberger J, Brunner H. 1992. Antihypertenseurs. In ≪Pharmacologie—Des concepts fondamentaux aux applications thérapeutiques≫. (Ed Schorderet E et al.) pp. 130–153.
12. Leaf A, Weber PC. 1988. Cardiovascular effects of n-3 fatty acids. N Engl J Med 318:549–557.
13. Sellmayer A, Hrboticky N, Weber PC. 1999. Lipids in vascular function. Lipids 34 Suppl:S13–S18.
14. Horrocks LA, Yeo YK. 1999. Docosahexaenoic acid-enriched foods: production and effects on blood lipids. Lipids 34 Suppl:S313.
15. GISSI group. 1999. Dietary supplementation with n-3 polyunsaturated fatty acids and vitamin E after myocardial infarction: results of the GISSI-Prevenzione trial. Gruppo Italiano per lo Studio della Sopravvivenza nell'Infarto miocardico. Lancet 354:447–455.
16. Knapp HR. 1991. Cardiovascular III: Circulation—Blood Pressure. Hypotensive effects of ω3 fatty acids: mechanistic aspects. In "Health Effects of ω3 Polyunsaturated Fatty Acids in Seafoods" pp. 313–328.
17. Chin JP, Dart AM. 1995. How do fish oils affect vascular function? Clin Exp Pharmacol Physiol 22:71–81.
18. Chen HW, Lii CK, Chen WT, Wang ML, Ou CC. 1996. Blood pressure-lowering effect of fish oil is independent of thromboxane A2 level in spontaneously hypertensive rats. Prostaglandins Leukot Essent Fatty Acids 54:147–154.
19. Rousseau D, Moreau D, Raederstorff D, Sergiel JP, Rupp H, Muggli R, Grynberg A. 1998. Is a dietary n-3 fatty acid supplement able to influence the cardiac effect of the psychological stress. Mol Cell Biochem 178:353–366.
20. Engler MM, Engler MB, Goodfriend TL, Ball DL, Yu Z, Su P, Kroetz DL. 1999. Docosahexaenoic acid is an antihypertensive nutrient that affects aldosterone production in SHR. Proc Soc Exp Biol Med 221:32–38.
21. Rousseau D, Héliès C, Raederstorff D, Moreau D, Grynberg A. 2001. Dietary n-3 polyunsaturated fatty acids affect the development of reno-vascular hypertension in rats. Mol Cell Biochem 225: 109–119.
22. Gray DR, Gozzip CG, Eastham JH, Kashyap ML. 1996. Fish oil as an adjuvant in the treatment of hypertension. Pharmacotherapy 16:295–300.
23. Kenny D, Egan BM. 1994. Is there a role for dietary fish oil in the treatment of hypertension? J Hum Hypertens 8:895–905.
24. Morris MC, Sacks F, Rosner B. 1993. Does fish oil lower blood pressure? A meta-analysis of controlled trials. Circulation 88:523–533.
25. Charnock JS, Abeywardena MY, McLennan PL. 1986. Comparative changes in the fatty acid composition of rat cardiac phospholipids after long term feeding of sunflower seed oil- or tuna fish oil-supplemented diets. Ann Nutr Metab 30:393–406.
26. Hock CE, Holahan MA, Reibel DK. 1987. Effect of dietary fish oil on myocardial phospholipids and myocardial ischemic damage. Am J Physiol 252:H554–H560.
27. Demaison L, Sergiel JP, Moreau D, Grynberg A. 1994. Influence of the Phospholipid n-6/n-3 Polyunsaturated Fatty Acid Ratio on Mitochondrial Oxidative Metabolism Before and After Myocardial Ischemia. Biochim Biophys Acta 1227:53–59.
28. Gudbjarnason S, Hallgrimsson J. 1976. Prostaglandins and polyunsaturated fatty acids in heart muscle. Acta Biol Med Germ 35:1069–1080.
29. McLennan PL, Abeywardena MY, Charnock JS. 1988. Dietary fish oil prevents ventricular fibrillation following coronary artery occlusion and reperfusion. Am Heart J 116:709–717.
30. McLennan PL. 1992. Relative effects of dietary saturated, monounsaturated and polyunsaturated fatty acids on cardiac arrhythmias in the rat. Am J Clin Nutr 57:207–212.

31. McLennan PL, Bridle TM, Abeywardena MY, Charnock JS. 1993. Comparative efficacy of n-3 and n-6 polyunsaturated fatty acids in modulating ventricular fibrillation threshold in the marmoset monkey. Am J Clin Nutr 58:666–669.
32. McLennan PL, Howe PR, Abeywardena MY, Muggli R, Raederstorff D, Mano M, Rayner T, Head RJ. 1996. The cardiovascular protective role of docosahexaenoic acid. Eur J Pharmacol 300:83–89.
33. Liautaud S, Grynberg A, Mourot J, Athias P. 1991. Contribution to the Use of Cultured Cardiomyocytes as a Model in Nutritional Studies: Fatty Acid Composition of the Hearts of Rats Fed Linseed Oil or Sunflower Oil and Cardiomyocytes Grown on their Sera. Cardioscience 2:55–61.
34. Voss A, Reinhart M, Sankarappa S, Sprecher H. 1991. The metabolism of 7,10,13,16,19-docosapentaenoic acid to 4,7,10,13,16,19-docosahexaenoic in rat liver is dependant on an delta-4 desaturase. J Biol Chem 266:19995–20000.
35. Saddik M, Gamble J, Witters LA, Lopaschuk GD. 1993. Acetyl-CoA carboxylase regulation of fatty acid oxidation in the heart. J Biol Chem 268:25836–25845.
36. Kudo N, Barr A, Barr R, Lopaschuk GD. 1995. 5′AMP activated protein kinase inhibition of acetyl CoA carboxylase can explain the high rates of fatty acid oxidation in the reperfused ischemic heart. J Biol Chem 270:17511–17520.
37. Pauly DF, Kirk KA, McMillin JB. 1991. Carnitine palmitoyl transferase in cardiac ischemia. A potential site for altered fatty acid metabolism. Circ Res 68:1085–1094.
38. Gamble J, Lopaschuk GD. 1997. Insulin inhibition of 5′ adenosine monophosphate-activated protein kinase in the heart results in activation of acetyl coenzyme A carboxylase and inhibition of fatty acid oxidation. Metabolism 46:1270–1274.
39. Pepe S, McLennan PL. 1992. Modulation of myocardial oxygen requirements by dietary lipids in the isolated erythrocyte perfused working rat heart. J Mol Cell Cardiol 24:S115.
40. Demaison L, Bouveret P, Grynberg A. 1993. Polyunsaturated Fatty Acid Composition and Lipid Metabolism in Cultured Cardiomyocytes and Isolated Working Rat Heart. Nutr Res 13:1003–1015.
41. Alam SQ, Ren YF, Alam BS. 1988. (^{3}H)Forskolin- and (^{3}H)Dihydroalprenolol-binding sites and adenylate cyclase activity in heart of rats fed diets containing different oils. Lipids 23:207–213.
42. Skuladottir GV, Schioth HB, Gudbjarnason S. 1993. Polyunsaturated Fatty Acids in Heart Muscle and alpha(1)-Adrenoceptor Binding Properties. Biochim Biophys Acta 1178:49–54.
43. Gudmundsdottir E, Benediktsdottir VE, Gudbjarnason S. 1991. Combined effects of age and dietary fat on beta 1-receptors and Ca2+ channels in rat hearts. Am J Physiol 260:H66–H72.
44. McMurchie EJ. 1988. Dietary lipids and the regulation of membrane fluidity and function, in Advances in membrane fluidity, Vol 3, *Physiological Regulation of membrane fluidity. Aloia, Curtain and Gordon Eds*, Alan R Liss Inc., New York. pp. 189–237.
45. Delerive P, Oudot F, Ponsard B, Talpin S, Sergiel JP, Cordelet C, Athias P, Grynberg A. 1999. Hypoxia-Reoxygenation and Polyunsaturated Fatty Acids Modulate Adrenergic Functions in Cultured Cardiomyocytes. J Mol Cell Cardiol 31:377–386.
46. Ponsard B, Durot I, Delerive P, Oudot F, Cordelet C, Grynberg A, Athias P. 1999. Cross influence of membrane PUFA and hypoxia reoxygenation on alpha- and beta-adrenergic function of rat cardiomyocytes. Lipids 34:457–466.
47. Grynberg A, Fournier A, Sergiel JP, Athias P. 1995. Effect of docosahexaenoic acid and eicosapentaenoic acid in the phospholipids of rat heart muscle cells on adrenoceptor responsiveness and mechanism. J Mol Cell Cardiol 27:2507–2520.
48. Grynberg A, Fournier A, Sergiel JP, Athias P. 1996. Membrane DHA versus EPA and the beating function of the Cardiomyocytes through the adrenergic receptors. Lipids 31:S205–S210.
49. Meij JTA, Bordoni A, Dekkers DHW, Lamers JMJ, Guarnieri C. 1990. Alterations in polyunsaturated fatty acid composition of cardiac membrane phospholipids and α1 adrenoceptor mediated phosphatidylinositol turnover. Cardiovasc Res 24:94–101.
50. Rousseau D, Héliès C, Raederstorff D, Moreau D, Grynberg A. 2001. [N-3 polyunsaturated fatty acids in insulin resistance: effect on cardiac rhythm and blood pressure]. Arch Mal Coeur Vaiss 94:369.
51. Extramiana F, Tavernier R, Maison-Blanche P, Neyroud N, Jordaens L, Leenhardt A, Coumel P. 2000. [Ventricular repolarization and Holter monitoring. Effect of sympathetic blockage on the QT/RR ratio]. Arch Mal Coeur Vaiss 93:1277–1283.
52. Karmazyn M, Dhalla NS. 1983. Physiological and pathophysiological aspects of cardiac prostaglandins. Can J Physiol Pharmacol 61:1207–1225.
53. Gerritsen ME, Printz M. 1981. Sites of prostaglandin synthesis in the bovine heart and isolated bovine coronary microvessels. Circ Res 49:1152–1163.
54. Linssen MCJG, Engels W, Lemmens PJMR, Heijnen VV T, Van Bilsen M, Reneman RS, Van Der

Vusse GJ. 1993. Production of arachidonic acid metabolites in adult rat cardiac myocytes, endothelial cells, and fibroblast-like cells. Am J Physiol 264:H973–H982.

55. Oudot F, Grynberg A, Sergiel JP. 1995. Synthesis of Eicosanoids in Cardiomyocytes during Hypoxia and Reoxygenation: Influence of the Polyunsaturated Fatty Acid Composition. Am J Physiol 268:H308–H315.

56. Engels W, Van Bilsen M, De Groot MJM, P Lemmens JMR, Willemsen PHM, Reneman RS, Van Der Vusse GJ. 1990. Ischemia and reperfusion induced formation of eicosanoids in isolated rat hearts. Am J Physiol 258:H1865–H1871.

Frontiers in Cardiovascular Health, edited by
N.S. Dhalla, A. Chockalingam,
H.I. Berkowitz & P.K. Singal
Kluwer Academic Publishers, Boston, 2003

The Effects of Taurine and Astragalus Membranaceus on Ion Currents and Their Expression in Cardiomyocytes After CVB3 Infection

Ying-Zhen Yang, Yan-Gang Su, Wei-Sheng Bao, Gong-Xin Liu, and Haozhu Chen

Shanghai Institute of Cardiovascular Diseases, Zhongshan Hospital of Fudan University, Shanghai 200032, P.R. China

Summary. **Purpose:** To investigate the effects of taurine and astragalus membranaceus (AM) on ion currents in cardiomyocytes and their expression in mouse myocardium after Coxsackie virus B3 (CVB3) infection. **Material and Methods:** Cardiomyocytes from Sprague-Dawley (SD) rats were obtained by retrograde perfusion with collagenase and used for recording current of L-type voltage dependent calcium channel (I_{ca}) and Na^+ current (I_{Na}) by whole cell patch clamp techniques. Cardiomyocytes from neonatal SD rats were prepared by digestion with collagenase and used for recording outward potassium current (*I*out) and inward rectifying potassium current (I_{KI}). To set up the in vitro model of VMC, 1~2 × 10^5 adult and neonatal rat cells were inoculated to the medium with 200 $TCID_{50}$ (50% tissue culture infection dose) and 100 $TCID_{50}$ CVB3 for 2 h, respectively. In vivo model of VMC was caused by intraperitoneal injection of 10 $TCID_{50}$ CVB3 into BALB/c mice. Hearts were removed after 7 days infection and used for examining the expression of L-type voltage dependent Ca^{2+} channel (LVDCC)α1 subunit and voltage-gate potassium channel (Kv) by immunohistochemistry and in situ hybridization, respectively. 1, 8, 16 mmol/L of taurine and 0.2 g/ml of AM were added to the medium of in vitro model. in vivo model, 50 mg/day of taurine was given by mouth and 0.5 ml of AM (2 g/ml) was injected intraperitoneally to the mice per day before sacrificed. **Results:** 1. the I_{ca} and I_{out} were increased while I_{KI} was decreased after inoculation with CVB3 for 2 hours. However, I_{Na} showed no difference

Note: The project was supported by the National Key Projects for the Ninth-five Year Plan of P.R. China (No 969060213).
Author for Correspondence: Ying-Zhen Yang, Shanghai Institute of Cardiovascular Diseases, Zhongshan Hospital of Fudan University, Shanghai 200032, P.R. China. Telephone: 02164041990×2104, Fax: 021-64223006, E-mail: yzyang@zshospital.com.

between normal and infected cells. The positive hybridization signals of LVDCCα1 subunit (antigen) and Kv1.2, Kv2.1, Kv4.2 were much reinforced after CVB3 infection. 2. taurine and AM could thwart the enhancement of *I*ca, *I*out and reduction of I_{KI} after virus infection. Besides, they could lessen the increased expression level of LVDCCα1 subunit as well as Kv mRNA. **Conclusions:** The ion currents and expression of calcium and potassium channels were increased after CVB3 infection. Taurine and AM could exert their beneficial effect on VMC through modulating these changes.

Key words: taurine, astragalus membranaceus, coxsackie virus B, ion channel, mRNA expression.

INTRODUCTION

The pathogenesis and treatment of viral myocarditis (VMC) have received considerable attention recently. The direct damage of virus and virus mediated immunological damage were considered to be related to the pathologenesis of VMC (1).

The effect of virus on ion channels could participate in and/or aggravate cardiomyocytes damage. For example, perforin released from activated cytotoxic T lymphocytes (CTL) and natural killing (NK) cells made a 1390ps non-selective ion channel on myocardial membrane, which leads massive ion motion and forms the basis of cell death (2). Taurine makes up 50% of the total free amino acid pool in mammalian heart and possesses a lot of cell protective actions such as modulating intracellular Ca^{2+} homeostasis, inhibiting lipoperoxide formation, reducing enzyme leakage and maintaining membrane stability (3). Deficiency of taurine was implicated in many heart pathological states and could be reversed by taurine supplement (4). We found that taurine was beneficial to clinical treatment for viral myocarditis (5), cultured rat cardiomyocytes infected with coxsackie virus B3 (CVB3) (6), and the reduction of transmembrane Ca^{2+} inflow was one of the function of taurine's protection to cardiomyocytes (7). Astragalus Membranaceus (AM), one kind of traditional Chinese medicine, has been verified by lots of modern experiments that it possesses good effects on many heart diseases, including VMC (8). Our previous studies showed eutherapeutic effect in treating VMC patients (9). AM could prevent myocardial damage from CVB infection, improve the electric activities of cardiomyocytes in CVB-infected mice, including action potential amplitude, over shoot and maximal upstroke rate of action potential (10), et al. In addition, AM could inhibit the Ca^{2+} influx and CVB3-RNA replication in heart cells (11). However, the transmembrane Ca^{2+} influx involved in a lot of aspects including voltage-dependent Ca^{2+} channel (VDCC), Ca^{2+} leak channel, ATP-dependent Ca^{2+} pump, Na^+/Ca^{2+} exchange, K^+ channel, et al. In this study, we focused on investigating the current of L-type VDCC (I_{ca}), Na^+ current (I_{Na}), outward potassium current (*I*out) and inward rectifying potassium current (I_{KI}) in rat cardiomyocytes by whole cell patch-clamp methods, and, their expression in myocardium of mice infected with CVB3 was studied by in situ hybridization and immunohistochemical techniques. In addition, the effect of taurine and AM on these courses were also investigated. The aim of this study is to further explore the pathogenesis of VMC from the point of ion channel and to provide a basis for the clinical treatment with taurine and AM in VMC.

MATERIALS AND METHODS

1. Models of VMC

In vitro model

1). Isolation of adult rat cardiomyocytes: Cardiomyocytes were isolated from Sprague-Dawley (SD) rats (weighing 200~250 g, clean, from Experimental Animal Center, Shanghai Medical University) as previously described (12). In brief, hearts were quickly moved and mounted on an improved Langendorff apparatus for retrograde perfusion at 37°C, first with Ca^{2+} free Tyrode's solution for 5~7 min, then with the same solution containing 0.05% collagenase(Type 1, Sigma), 40~60 µmol/L $CaCl_2$ and 0.01% BSA for 7~10 min. Afterwards, the hearts were incubated in KB solution for 10~15 min, then minced and dispersed with a pipette for 3~5 min. The suspensions were filtered through a 200 µM mylon mesh, and kept at 15~25°C at least 1 h before transferred to Eagle's minimum essential medium (MEM) including 1~2 mmol/L $CaCl_2$. Cells were used to record I_{ca} and I_{Na}.

2). Isolation of neonatal rat heart cells: Neonatal 5 days rat ventricular myocytes were prepared using the procedure described previously (13). The hearts were removed quickly from SD rats and placed to a culture plate containing Tyrode solution saturated with 100% oxygen. The atrium was removed and ventricle was scissored to 1 $mm^3 \times 1$ mm^3 fragment and digested in Ca^{2+} free Tyrode's solution containing 0.1% collagenase for 50 min at 37°C. The digested tissue then kept in KB solution for 30 min before transferred to Eagle's MEM. Cells were used to record I_{out} and I_{KI}.

3). VMC models in cardiomyocytes: To set up the in vitro VMC models, 1~2 × 10^5 adult rat cells and 1~2 × 10^5 neonatal rat cells were inoculated to the medium with 200 $TCID_{50}$ (50% tissue culture infection dose) and 100 $TCID_{50}$ CVB3 respectively. All cells were incubated for 2 hours at 37°C before use.

In vivo model

Male 4 weeks old BALB/c mice, obtained from the Experimental Animal Department, Shanghai Medical University, were intraperitoneally inoculated with 0.3 ml of 10 $TCID_{50}$ CVB3 served as in vivo VMC model. The hearts were removed after 7 days infection and used for examining the expression of L-type voltage dependent Ca^{2+} channel (LVDCC)α1 subunit and voltage-gate potassium channel (Kv).

2. Groups

There are six groups in the whole experiments. (1). N: normal control group. (2). V: CVB3 infection group. (3). T: taurine control group. (4). AM: AM control group. (5). V + T: group V + taurine. (6). V + AM: group V + AM. In vitro model of taurine therapeutic part, 1, 8 and 16 mmol/L taurine were added to the medium of group T and V + T for 2 h before recording. In vivo model, 50 mg/day of taurine was given to the mice of the groups by mouth with a needle until 7days-post inoculation. In vitro model of AM therapeutic part, final concentration of AM in medium of group AM and V + AM was 0.2 g/ml, while in vivo model, 0.5 ml of AM (2 g/ml) was injected intraperitoneally to the mice of the groups until 7days-post inoculation. The dosage of taurine and AM we used in this study were referred to our prior experiment which showed the dosage had good protective effect in VMC model (6,7,10,11,14).

3. Recording

Whole-cell I_{ca}, I_{Na}, I_{out} and I_{KI} were recorded by Hamill patch-clamp methods (15) using a glass pipette (diameter 1~3 µm). The whole-cell configuration was performed in Tyrode's solution, then the cell was superfused with the external solution. The resting potential was monitored in current clamp mode, compensated the slow capacitance near resting potential. The data were acquired by a Macintosh computer using an EPC-9 amplifier and Pulse + Pulsedfit 8.0 software (German, HEAK). For *I*ca recording, the holding potential (HP) was kept at −50 mV to inactivate Na^+ channel and T-type Ca^{2+} channel, test potential (TP) depolarizing from −40 mV to +60 mV, pulse width 100 ms. For I_{Na} recording, HP was kept at −90 mV, TP was from −80 mV to +60 mV, pulse width 20 ms. For *I*out recording, HP was kept at −60 mV; TP was from −30 mV to +90 mV, pulse width 100 ms. For I_{KI} recording, HP was kept at −40 mV, TP was from −120 mV to +60 mV. For all recording, step was +10 mv, frequency was 0.5 Hz. The mean peak I_{ca}, I_{Na}, I_{out} and I_{KI} were expressed as a function of membrane capacity (Cm), the unit is pA/pF. The data were recorded and calculated by computer automatically.

4. In situ hybridization

The Kv probe was synthesized by Tanka company and labeled by digoxin (the detail method was present on the reagent box, Boringer company). The sequence of three Kv probes as follows: Kv1.2: TGCAAGTGACAAGCTGTCCAAAGATCCCATC CTCCCCTGACCTAA, Kv2.1: GAGAAACACACAGCAATAGGTTCAACTTT GAGGCGGGTGTCCA, Kv4.2: AGAGGCAGCGTGCAAGAACTCAGTACAAT TCAGATCAGATGTGTG. The concentration of the probe is 2 ng/µl. Routine flotation method was used to detect the expression of Kv.

5. Immunohistochemical procedures

Each rat ventricle was taken 2~3 sections for detecting the antigen of LVDCCα1 subunit using routine immunohistochemical ABC methods. The monoclonal antibody of anti- LVDCCα1 subunit of rat was kindly supported by professor J. Ptasienski of Northwestern University.

6. Positive antigen analysis

By means of picture analyzer, five high power fields of each mouse heart section were taken randomly. The positive antigen index was calculated using below formula: positive signal index = area of positive signal × mean positive signal brilliance/total examined area × 100.

7. Solution preparation

(1): Tyrode's solution: NaCl 143, $MgCl_2$ 0.5, $CaCl_2$ 1.8, Glucose 5.5, HEPES 5, pH was adjusted to 7.4 with NaOH. Ca^{2+} free Tyrode's solution is the former solution without $CaCl_2$. (2): KB soultion: K-glutamate 50, KOH 20, KCl 40, taurine 20, $KHPO_4$ 20, $MgCl_2$ 3, Glucose 10, EGTA 1, HEPES 10, pH was adjusted to 7.4 with KOH. (3): External solution for I_{ca}: tetraethylammonium chloride (TEACl) 135, $CaCl_2$ 10, $MgCl_2$ 1, HEPES 10, Glucose 10, pH was adjusted to 7.4 with TEAOH. (4): Internal solution for I_{ca}: CsCl 120, $MgCl_2$ 1, MgATP4, EGTA 10, HEPES 10, pH was adjusted to 7.2 with CsOH. (5): External solution for I_{ca}:TEACl 100, NaCl 40, $MgCl_2$ 1, Glucose 10, HEPES 10, pH was adjusted to 7.4 with TEAOH. (6): Internal solution for I_{Na}: CsCl 120, NaCl 10, $MgCl_2$ 1, MgATP 4, EGTA 10, HEPES 10, pH was adjusted to 7.2 with CsOH. (7): External solution for I_{out}: acetylcholine chloride 126, KCl 5.4, $MgCl_2$ 0.8, NaH_2PO_4 0.33, HEPES 10, Glucose 5.5, TTX 0.02, $BaCl_2$ 2, $CdCl_2$ 0.5, pH was adjusted to 7.4 with Tris. (8): Internal solution for Iout: KCl 135, MgATP 3, EGTA 10, HEPES 10, Glucose 5, pH was adjusted to 7.2 with KOH. (9): External solution for I_{KI}: NaCl 140, KCl 5.4, $CaCl_2$ 1.8, $MgCl_2$ 1.1, Glucose 10, $CdCl_2$ 0.5, HEPES 5, pH was adjusted to 7.4 with NaOH. (10): Internal solution for I_{KI}: KCl 120, Na_2ATP 5, $MgCl_2$ 6, $CaCl_2$ 0.154, EGTA 5, HEPES 10, pH was adjusted to 7.2 with KOH.

8. Drugs

Taurine was purchased from Sigma Chemicals, Co., St. Louis. MO, USA. AM (4g/2ml, No 941207) was purchased from Shanghai Forward Pharamaceutical Co. Ltd. Shanghai.

Statistics: Each value was expressed as mean ± SD. Statistical analysis of data was performed using the Student's paired t test.

RESULTS

1. Alternation of ion currents and their expression after CVB3 infection

(1). Ion currents: Figure 1A and IB showed the waveforms of I_{ca} In normal cardiomyocytes and effect of CVB3 on the I_{ca}, respectively. Figure 2A and 2B showed the waveforms of I_{Na} in normal cardiomyocytes and effect of CVB3 on the I_{Na}, respectively. Figure 3A and 3B showed the waveforms of *I*out in normal cardiomyocytes and effect of CVB3 on the *I*out, respectively. Figure 4A and 4B showed the waveforms of I_{KI} in normal cardiomyocytes and effect of CVB3 on the I_{KI}, respectively. From above figures and data in table 1, we could see that the I_{ca} and I_{out} were increased while I_{KI} was decreased after inoculation with CVB3 for 2 hours. However, I_{Na} showed no difference between normal and infected cells. The voltage depolarizing to peak current (Vp) of I_{ca} in CVB3 infected cardiomyocytes was lower than in normal group although there was no significantly difference.

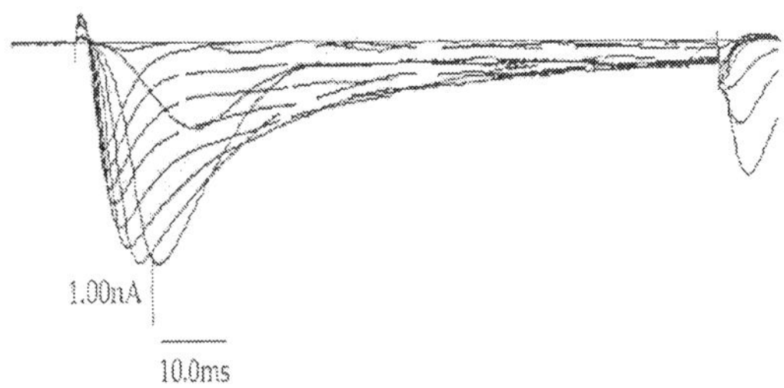

Figure 1A. Waveform of the I_{ca} in normal adult rat ventricular myocytes.

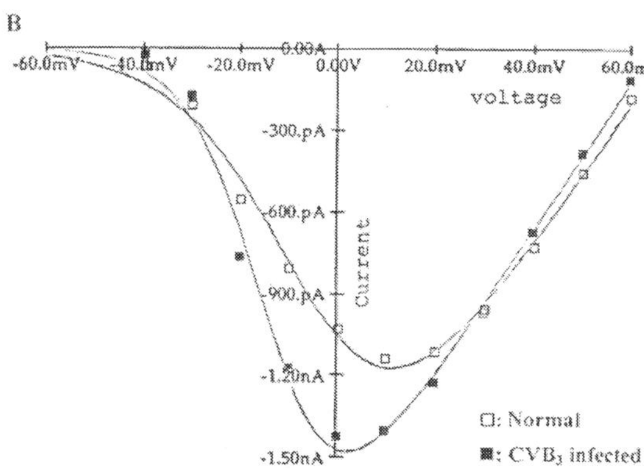

Figure 1B. I-V curve of I_{ca} after CVB3 infection in rat cardiomyocytes.

Figure 1B represent the current-voltage curve (I-V) of I_{ca} which showed that CVB3 not only increased the amplitude of I_{ca}, but also altered its characteristic of voltage-dependent. The curve was deviated to left lower direction after CVB3 infection. It means that I_{ca} trended to reach its peak value at lower membrane potential. Figure 3B and figure 4B which displayed the I-V curve of I_{out} and I_{KI} respectively, showed that current of I_{out} was increased as membrane potential depolarized, while I_{KI} was increased as membrane potential repolarized and some variation were seen post CVB3 infection.

(2). LVDCCα1 subunit and Kv mRNA expression: The results showed in table 2 and Figure 5 and 6. As displayed in Table 2, The positive hybridization signals of LVDCCα1 subunit (antigen) and Kv1.2, Kv2.1, Kv4.2 mRNA in mouse myocardium were much reinforced after CVB3 infection. Tawny LVDCCα1 antigen

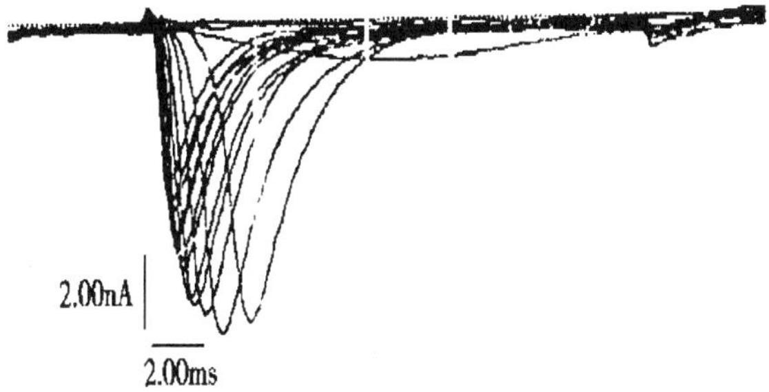

Figure 2A. Waveform of the I_{Na} in normal adult rat ventricular myocytes.

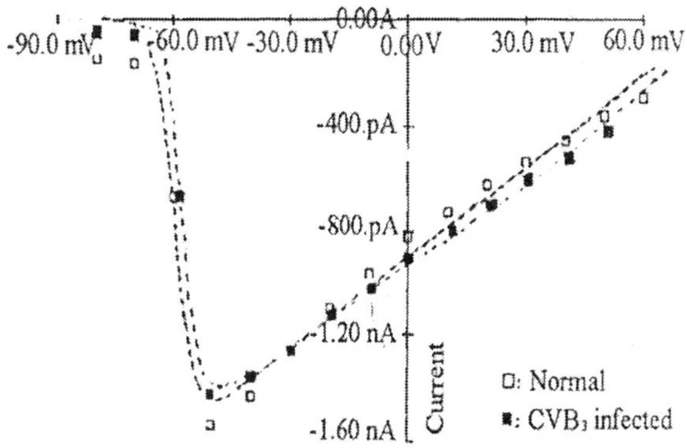

Figure 2B. I-V curve of I_{Na} after CVB3 infection in rat cardiomyocytes.

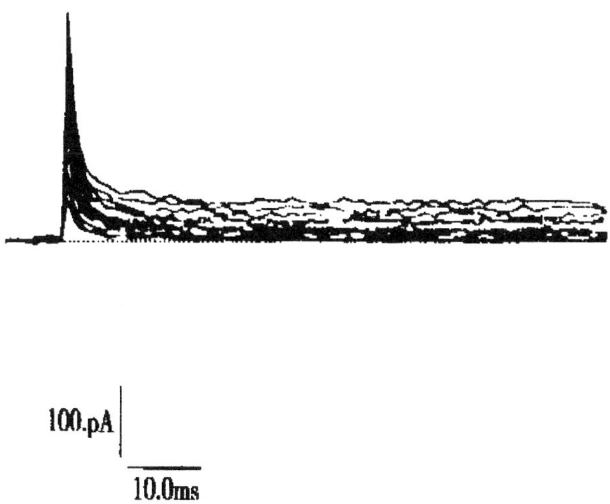

Figure 3A. Waveform of the I_{out} in normal adult rat ventricular myocytes.

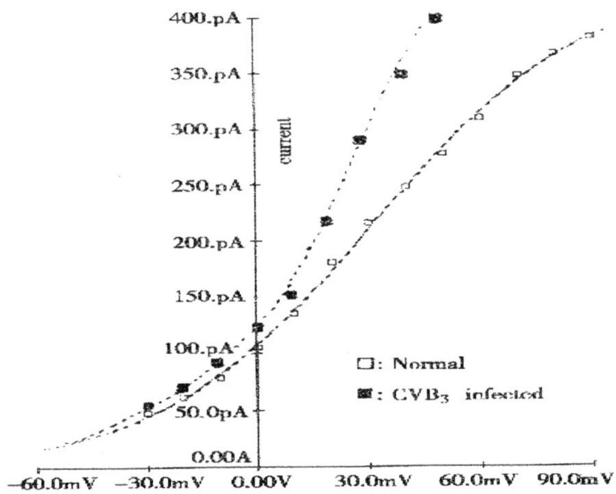

Figure 3B. I-V curve of I_{out} after CVB3 infection in rat cardiomyocytes.

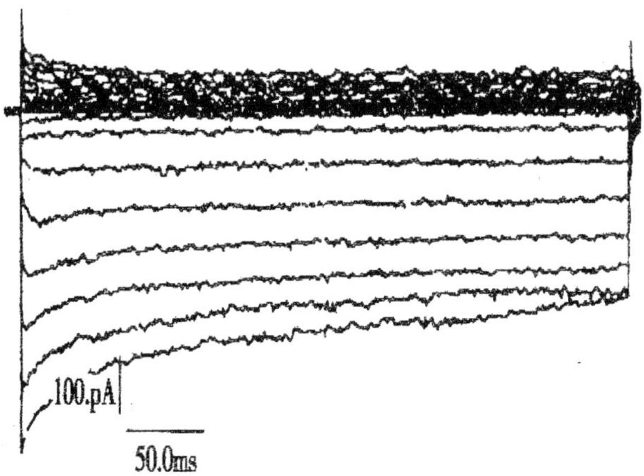

Figure 4A. Waveform of the I_{K1} in normal adult rat ventricular myocytes.

positive signal were seen in the localized ventricle areas in Figure 5. In Figure 6, pale blue or blue granule were the positive hybridization signal of digoxin marked probe of Kv4.2 mRAN (Kv1.2 mRNA and Kv2.1 mRNA were omitted here). Besides, spoiled structure of myocardium fiber by CVB3 infection could be seen in Figures 5 and 6.

Table 1. The effect of taurine and AM on ion currents after CVB3 infection

Groups	I_{ca} (pA/pF)	Vp (mV)	I_{Na} (pA/pF)	I_{out} (pA/pF)	I_{KI} (pA/pF)
N	4.1 ± 0.8 (Cm = 263 ± 64PF) (n = 23)	8.3 ± 7.8 (n = 23)	10.0 ± 2.7 (Cm = 196 ± 44PF) (n = 16)	15.4 ± 1.2 (Cm = 24.6 ± 1.2PF) (n = 10)	15.8 ± 1.4 (Cm = 24.8 ± 1.6PF) (n = 10)
T1	3.9 ± 0.4 (Cm = 262 ± 58PF) (n = 10)	7.0 ± 6.8 (n = 10)		15.0 ± 1.1 (Cm = 26.0 ± 2.1PF) (n = 10)	15.7 ± 1.6 (Cm = 26.2 ± 1.9PF) (n = 10)
T8	3.7 ± 0.6 (Cm = 231 ± 38PF) (n = 10)	11.0 ± 3.1 (n = 10)		14.9 ± 0.8 (Cm = 25.9 ± 1.9PF) (n = 10)	15.6 ± 1.7 (Cm = 25.9 ± 1.7PF) (n = 10)
T16	3.5 ± 0.5* (Cm = 284 ± 53PF) (n = 10)	8.8 ± 5.0 (n = 10)		14.6 ± 0.9 (Cm = 26.2 ± 1.7PF) (n = 10)	15.9 ± 1.3 (Cm = 26.3 ± 1.8PF) (n = 10)
AM	4.0 ± 0.7 (Cm = 290 ± 74PF) (n = 14)	11.0 ± 3.6 (n = 14)		15.2 ± 0.9 (Cm = 25.7 ± 1.4PF) (n = 10)	15.6 ± 1.5 (Cm = 26.2 ± 1.6PF) (n = 10)
V	4.9 ± 1.4** (Cm = 260 ± 44PF) (n = 14)	4.9 ± 3.4 (n = 14)	10.0 ± 2.6† (Cm = 196 ± 44PF) (n = 12)	25.1 ± 2.2*** (Cm = 25.1 ± 2.3PF) (n = 10)	12.2 ± 0.8*** (Cm = 26.4 ± 1.7PF) (n = 10)
V + T16	3.8 ± 0.8# (Cm = 289 ± 81PF) (n = 10)	7.9 ± 4.3# (n = 10)		22.8 ± 1.9# (Cm = 25.2 ± 3.3PF) (n = 10)	13.4 ± 1.5# (Cm = 26.0 ± 1.5PF) (n = 10)
V + AM	4.3 ± 0.9# (Cm = 306 ± 78PF) (n = 12)	11.7 ± 7.1# (n = 12)		23.2 ± 1.6# (Cm = 26.2 ± 3.0PF) (n = 10)	13.3 ± 1.2# (Cm = 25.8 ± 1.9PF) (n = 10)

Note: N: control group, V:CVB3 infection group, V + T: CVB3 infection + taurine group, V + AM: CVB3 infection + AM group. T1: 1 mmol/L taurine, T8: 8 mmol/L taurine, T16: 16 mmol/L taurine. *$P < 0.05$, **$P < 0.01$, ***$P < 0.001$ vs group N, †$P > 0.05$ vs group N, #$P < 0.05$ vs group V.

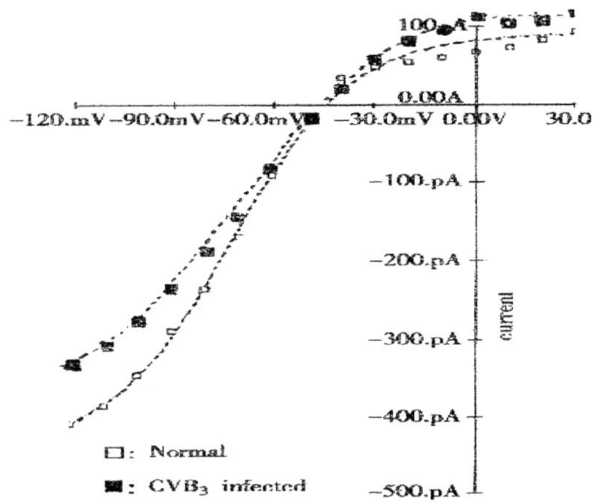

Figure 4B. I-V curve of I_{KI} after CVB3 infection in rat cardiomyocytes.

Table 2. The effect of taurine and AM on the expression of ion channel after CVB3 infection

Groups	n	Kv1.2mRNA	Kv2.1mRNA	Kv4.2mRNA	LVDCCα 1 Subunit
N	10	40.3 ± 6.8	42.3 ± 7.5	53.6 ± 7.9	36.1 ± 5.2
V	10	49.6 ± 7.2★★	52.5 ± 8.2★★	64.4 ± 8.7★★	67.3 ± 7.8★★★
V + T16	10	43.2 ± 6.0#	45.7 ± 6.1#	56.9 ± 6.4#	59.9 ± 6.8#
V + AM	10	42.9 ± 6.3#	45.1 ± 6.6#	56.6 ± 7.0#	60.3 ± 7.0#

Note: N: control group, V:CVB3 infection group, V + T16: CVB3 infection + 16 mmol/L taurine group, V + AM: CVB3 infection + AM group. ★★P < 0.01, ★★★P < 0.001 vs group N, #P < 0.05 vs group V.

2. Effect of taurine and AM on ion currents and their expression after CVB3 infection

(1). Ion currents: As showed in table 2, although taurine 1, 8 and 16 mmol/L decreased I_{ca} in a concentration-dependent manner, only taurine 16 mmol/L caused substantial effects on the basal I_{ca} at high extracellular calcium concentration (10 mmol/L) compared with normal group ($P < 0.05$). Taurine had no effect on Vp in normal cardiomyocytes. With CVB3 infection, the I_{ca} increased and Vp was little lower than in normal group while taurine 16 mmol/L counteracted the effects of CVB3 on I_{ca} and normalized the decreased Vp. AM had no effect on the I_{ca}. However, AM could significantly inhibit attenuation of I_{ca} along with time. I_{ca} was weaken to 51 ± 12% at 10 minutes in group N, while in the same time it was 75 ± 8% in the group AM ($P < 0.05$). AM could attenuate the increased I_{ca} after CVB3 infection and made the Vp restored to the normal. Besides, taurine and AM could thwart the enhancement of Iout and reduction of I_{KI} after virus infection even though taurine and AM have no effect on Iout and I_{KI} in normal rat cardiomyocytes.

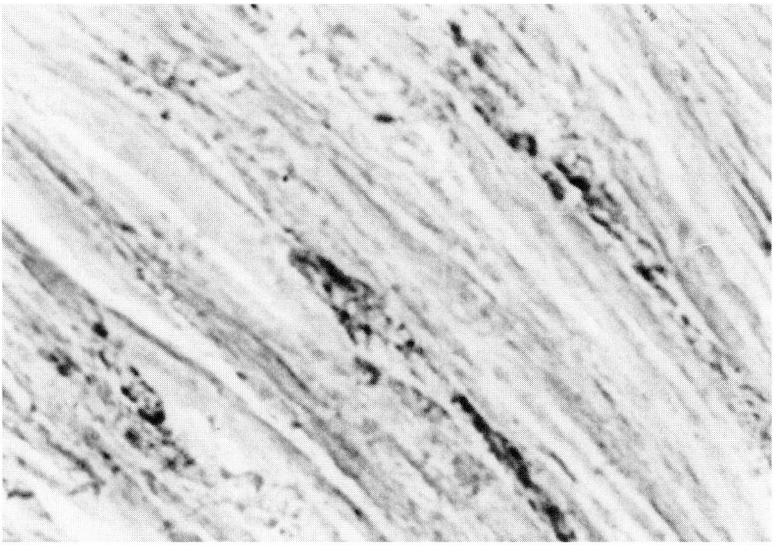

Figure 5A. LVDCCα1 antigen in myocardium of normal mice.

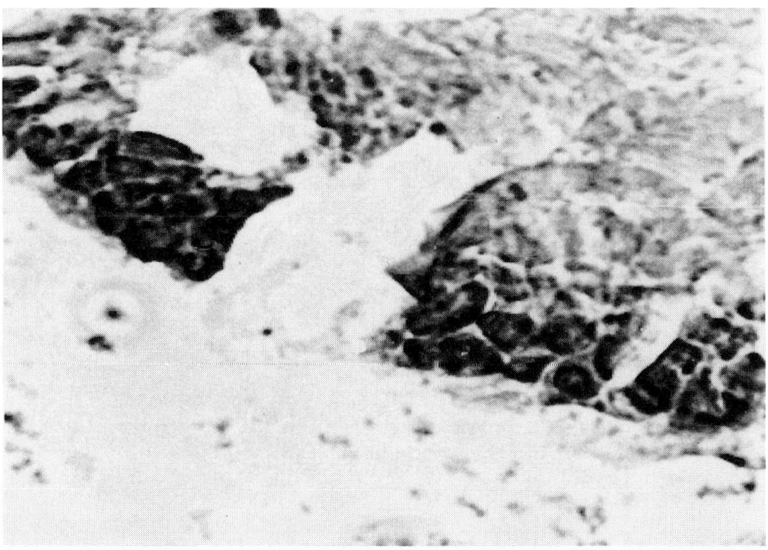

Figure 5B. LVDCCα1 antigen in myocardium infected with CVB3.

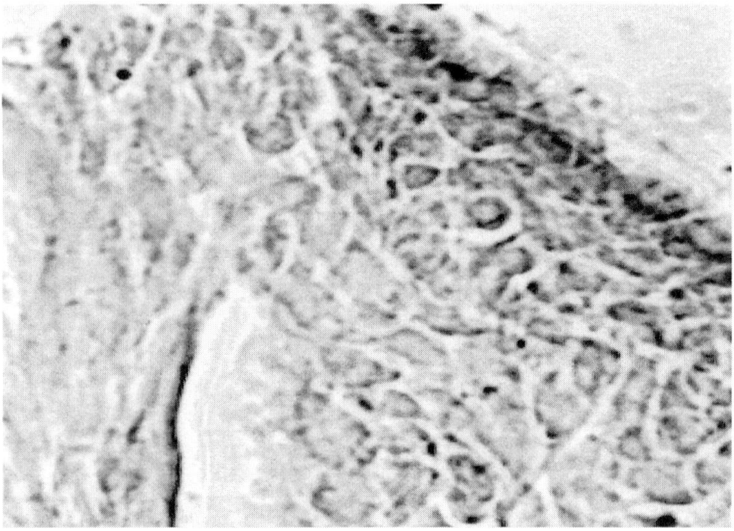

Figure 5C. Taurine on LVDCCα1 antigen in myocardium of VMC mice.

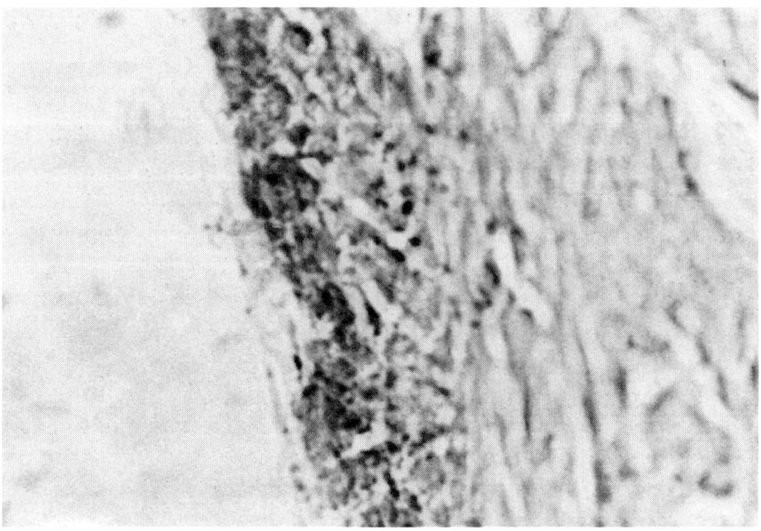

Figure 5D. AM on LVDCCα1 antigen in myocardium of VMC mice.

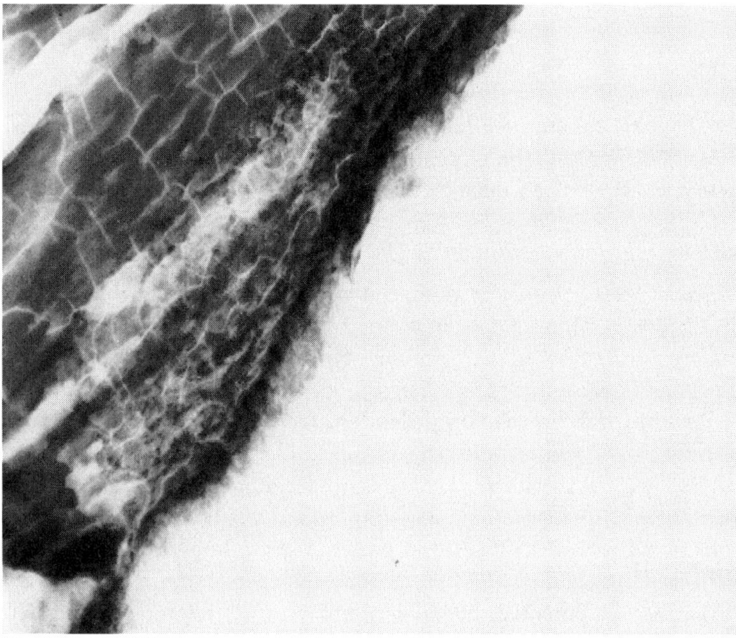

Figure 6A. Kv4.2 MRNA expression in myocardium of normal BALB/c mice (in situ hybridization ×200).

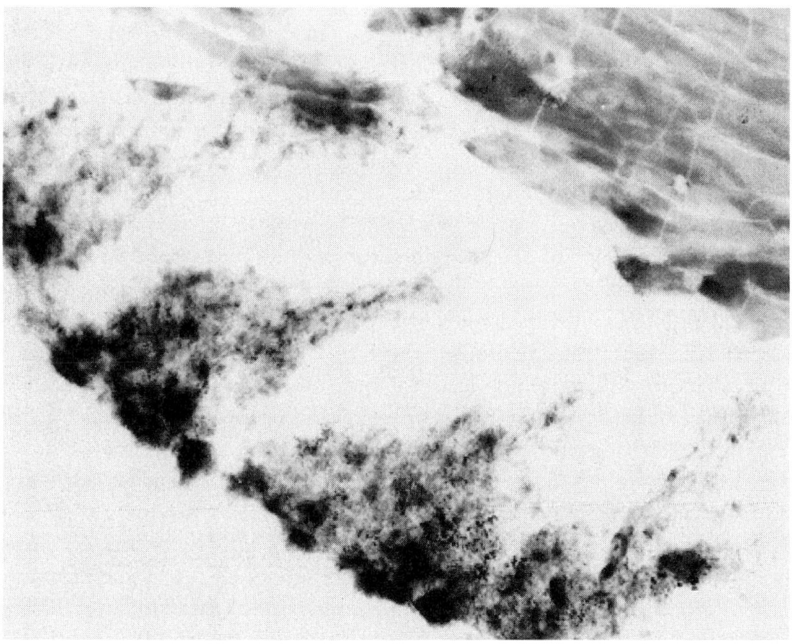

Figure 6B. Kv4.2 mRNA expression in myocardium of mice infected with CVB3 (in situ hybridization ×200).

(2). LVDCCα1 subunit and Kv mRNA expression: Taurine and AM could lessen the increased expression level of positive hybridization signals of LVDCCα1 subunit as well as Kv mRNA (see Table 2, Figure 5C and D).

DISCUSSION

Mechanism of VMC is unclear though it maybe due to destroying the heart cells by virus directly or through immunologic injury (1). Ion channel should take part in the course of destroying the cardiomyocytes in VMC since lots of pathophysiological process is related to this changes and we already found increased calcium influx after virus infection (11). Voltage-dependent calcium channels in myocardial cells consists of T type and L type channel. L-type voltage dependent calcium channel (LVDCC) is the main pathway for determining calcium influx. LVDCC is a peptide complex composed by α1, α2, δ, β and γ subunits, in which α1 subunit is the functional part of LVDCC and possesses diphydropyridine (DHP) receptors. Calcium entered through LVDCC not only increases intracellular Ca^{2+} accumulation during action potential, but also promotes Ca^{2+} releasing from sarcolemmal reticulum. Some pathological situation, e.g. ischemia and heart failurecan change the electrophysiologic characteristics of LVDCC (16,17). Our study demonstrated that CVB3 infection increased *I*ca and trended to decrease the Vp. In other words, the LVDCC could be activated at lower membrane potential after CVB3 infection. The extra calcium influx and the shifted Vp resulted in intracellular calcium overload and abnormal electric activities, thus, caused cell damage in viral infection.

Other than calcium, CVB3 infection has no influence on Na^+ channel. One of the reasons for calcium overload was contributed to activating Na^+/Ca^{2+} exchange by enhanced intracellular sodium. Our results indicated that the increased intracellular sodium might be due to leakage of destroyed membrane by virus other than alternation of sodium channel.

Potassium channel plays an important role in maintaining rest potential, controlling excitability and plateau of action potential in cardiomyocytes. Our study showed that *I*out was increased and I_{KI} was decreased after CVB3 infection. Descent of intracellular potassium lowered the rest potential and evoked arrhythmia. Besides, enhanced potassium efflux reinforced the K^+/Ca^{2+} exchange and aggravated intracellular calcium overload, which leads to myocardial damage.

Alternation of spatial configuration or expression of ion channel, which happened during virus adhering and penetrating to cell membrane, may contribute to the above changes of ion channel. In this study, we tried to elucidate whether virus could effect the ion channel expression. As we know, there are more than 17 types of Kv. Because of the high expression level of Kv1.2, Kv2.1 and Kv4.2 in rat myocardium (18), we selected these 3 kinds of probes to detect the voltage-gated potassium channel mRNA expression. It is generally thought that Kv4.2 is the main part of transient outward potassium current (I_{to}). Kv2.1 is the main part of postponement rectified postassium currents (I_K). The action of Kv1.2 has not been known yet. Maybe it relates to the construct of slow inactivated potassium currents (I_{Kslow}) (19). We found that the LVDCCα1 subunit was much reinforced and positive hybridization signals of Kv1.2, Kv2.1 and Kv4.2 mRNA were increased after CVB3 infection. It means CVB3 infection not only changed the current characteristic through the ion channel, but also affected its expression which leads to further increasing intracellular calcium overload and potassium efflux.

Former study revealed that taurine affected the intracellular calcium by a dual effect that depended on calcium concentration (20). In this study, the result showed that taurine plays a role of decreasing Ca^{2+} entry with Ca^{2+} 10 mmol/L in external solution. In addition of the good effects of taurine and AM on experimental CVB myocarditis and patients with VMC, we also have found that combination therapy of taurine and AM were more beneficial to patients and VMC mice (21,22). In the cultured rat cardiomyocytes infected with CVB3, taurine and AM could improve the percentage of active and beating cells as well as inhibit the calcium influx postinfected with CVB3 (7,11). Above results indicated that one of the protective effect of taurine and AM on myocardium would be their beneficial action on ion channels. Our results exhibited that taurine and AM could reverse the influence by CVB3 infection on ion channel (I_{ca}, Vp, *I*out and I_{KI}). In addition, enhanced expression of LVDCCα1 subunit and Kv mRNA postinfection were also lessened by taurine and AM. Probably, their beneficial action on ion channel would be one of the protective effect on infected myocardium.

CONCLUSION

Taurine and AM could exert beneficial action on VMC through modulating current and expression of ion channel after CVB3 infection.

REFERENCES

1. Kearney MT, Cotton JM, Richardson PJ, Shah AM. 2001. Viral myocarditis and dilated cardiomyopathy: mechanism, manifestition and management. Postgrad Med J 77:4–10.
2. Binah O, Kline R, Beake G, Hoffman B. 1993. Mechanisms whereby lytic granules from cytotoxic T lymphocytes damage guinea pig ventricular myocytes. Scand J Immunol 37:53–59.
3. Takahashi K, Ohyabu Y, Schaffer SW, Azuma J. 2000. Taurine prevents ischemia damage in cultured neonatal rat cardiomyocytes. Adv Exp Med Biol 486:109–116.
4. Schaffer S, Solodushro V, Azuma J. 2000. Taurine-deficient cardiomyopathy: role of phospholipids, calcium and osmotic stress. Adv Exp Med Biol 483:57–69.
5. Chen RZ, Yang YZ, Ye YC, Chen HZ. 1998. Effects of taurine plus ubidecarenone on viral myocarditis. Chin J New Drugs Clin Remedies 17:83–85.
6. Su YG, Yang YZ, Guo Q, Chen HZ, Gu QB, Zhao JX. 1997. Effect of taurine on cultured rat cardiomyocytes infected with coxsackie Be virus. Chin Pharmacological Bulletin 13:56–60.
7. Su YG, Yang YZ, Gu Q, Guo Q, Zhao JX, Chen HZ. 1996. Effect of taurine on calcium influx in rat cultured cardiomyocytes after coxsackie virus B3 infection. J Shanghai Med Univ 23:339–342.
8. Miller AL. 1998. Botanical influences on cardiovascular diseases. Altern Med Rev 3:422–431.
9. Li L, Yang YZ, Ye YC, Jin PY, Wu WZ, Shan YF. 1992. An oral solution of Radix Astragali for therapy of viral myocarditis in 50 patients. New Drugs and Clinical Remedies 11:12–14.
10. Rui T, Yang YZ, Zhou TS, Yang XY, Chen HZ. 1993. Effect of Astragalus membranaceus on electrophysiological activities of acute experimental coxsackie B3 viral myocarditis in mice. Chin Med Sci J 8:203–206.
11. Guo Q, Peng TQ, Yang YZ, Gu QB, Zhao JX, Chen HZ. 1996. Effect of Astragalus membranaceus on Ca^{2+} influx and CVB3 RNA replication in cultured neonatal rat heart cells infected with CVB3. CJIM, 2:64–67.

12. Liu GX, Gu QB, Guo Q, Yang YZ. 1997. A simple, rapid method to isolate cardiac myocytes from rat and guinea pig. Chin J Appl Physiol 13:361–362.
13. Yang YZ, Dyke JW. 1985. Coxsackie B-2 virus infection in rat beating heart cell culture. JVM 12:217–224.
14. Su YG, Xiong DD, Yang YZ, Guo Q, Gu QB, Chen HZ. 1997. Effects of taurine on coxsackie virus B3 murine myocarditis. Chin J Cardiolva 2:69–72.
15. Hamill O, Marty A, Neher Z, Sakmann B, Sigworth FJ. 1981. Improved patch-clamp techniques for high resolution current recording from cells and cell free membrane paths. Pfluger Arch 391:85–100.
16. Gidh-Jain M, Huang B, Jain P, Battula V, el-Sherif N. 1995. Reemergence of the fetal pattern of L-type calcium channel gene expression in non infarcted myocardium during left ventricular remodeling. Biochem Biophys Res Commun 216:892–897.
17. Uechi M, Asai K, Sato N, Vatner SF. 1998. Voltage-dependent calcium channel promotor restores broreflex sensitivity in conscious dogs with heart failure. Circulation 98:1342–1347.
18. Dixon JE, Mckinnon D. 1994. Quantitative analysis of potassium channel mRNA expression in atrial and ventricular muscle of rats. Circ Res 75:252–260.
19. Barry DM, Trimmer JS, Merlie JP, Nerbonne JM. 1995. Differential expression of voltage-gated K+ channel subunits in adult rat heart. Circ Res 77:361–369.
20. Satoh H. 1998. Cardiac actions of taurine as a modulator of the ion channel. Adv Exp Med Biol 44:21–28.
21. Collaborative group of "Key national medical projects for the Ninth-Five year plan research". 1999. Study of drug therapy in acute viral myocarditis. Chin J Cardiol 27:413–415.
22. Xiong DD, Yang YZ, Su YG, Hu Y, Chen HZ. 1998. Experimental study on treatment of viral myocarditis in mice by integrated traditional Chinese and Western medicine. Chin J Intergr Med 18:480–482.

Frontiers in Cardiovascular Health, edited by
N.S. Dhalla, A. Chockalingam,
H.I. Berkowitz & P.K. Singal
Kluwer Academic Publishers, Boston, 2003

CoQ10 in the Treatment of Heart and Vascular Disease

Ram B. Singh,[1] Kumar Kartikey,[2] Mahmood Moshiri,[3] Narankar S. Neki,[4] Daniel Pella,[5] Shanti S. Rastogi,[6] Shiv S. L. Srivastav[7], and Atul Krishna[7]

Medical Hospital and Research Centre, Subharti Medical College, Meerut(UP)[1,2,4,6,7], *Cardiovascular Research Centre, Tehran*[3], *Safaric University, Kosice, Slovakia*[5]

Summary. CoQ10 (CoQ10) deficiency has been reported in apparently healthy subjects as well as in patients with congestive heart failure, angina pectoris, coronary artery disease, cardiomyopathy, hypertension, mitral valve prolapse, diabetes mellitus and after coronary revascularization. Since CoQ10 bolsters the synthesis of ATP and inhibits free radical damage, its administration may be useful in cellular energy production as well as preventing cellular damage during ischaemia-reperfusion injury. Clinical benefits of CoQ10 are mainly due to its ability to improve energy production, antioxidant activity, and membrane stabilizing properties. Several small scale studies indicate that CoQ10 could be useful in patients with congestive heart failure, angina pectoris, cardiomyopathy, coronary artery disease, acute myocardial infarction, diabetes, and in the preservation of myocardium. It may also decrease plasma lipoproteins, insulin and angiotensin converting enzyme. CoQ10 is normally present in the low density lipoprotein cholesterol fraction and inhibits its oxidation, indicating that it can inhibit atherosclerosis. CoQ10 also regenerates vitamin E. These actions of CoQ10 indicate that it can inhibit the development of atherosclerosis and prevent the instability and disruption of plaques. The adverse effects of CoQ10 are minor gastrointestinal discomfort and elevation in SGOT and LDH.

***Key words*:** Antioxidant, free radical stress, ubiquinone, coronary artery disease, hypertension, heart failure, cardiomyopathy, myocardial infarction, atherosclerosis.

Corresponding Author: Dr. R.B. Singh, MD, Professor of Medicine, Subharti Medical College, Civil Lines, Moradabad-10 (UP) 244001, India. E-mail: icn@mickyonline.com.

INTRODUCTION

Plant and animal cells (1–3) contain CoQ10 (CoQ10). It is naturally present in foods and synthesized in all body tissues. The biosynthesis of CoQ10 from the amino acid tyrosine is a multi-stage process requiring at least eight vitamins and several trace elements (1–4). Therefore, deficiency of any of these micronutrients can cause CoQ10 deficiency. CoQ10 was first identified by Moor et al. in 1940. In 1957, Crane et al. demonstrated that it has an important role as a redox carrier in the mammalian respiratory transport chain (1). Professor Morton of UK introduced the name ubiquinone and Folkers determined the chemical formula of CoQ10. However, Yamamura and his group were the first to use CoQ10 for the treatment of cardiovascular disease (CVD) in the 1960's. In 1972, Littarru, of Italy and the late Prof. Folkers from Texas, documented a deficiency of CoQ10 in human heart disease particularly among patients subjected to bypass surgery in Houston, USA. Stocker and coworkers as well as Singh et al. demonstrated for the first time that CoQ10 can inhibit atherosclerosis and modulate the quality and chemical composition of atheroma (1–4).

MECHANISM OF ACTIONS

CoQ10 has a strong influence on at least three mitochondrial enzymes (complexes I, II and III) as well as enzymes in other parts of the cell (2). These enzymes are concerned with oxidative phosphorylation pathway and thus, are essential for the synthesis of ATP which is required for cell function (2,3). It may be useful in preventing cellular damage during myocardial ischaemia and reperfusion. CoQ10 may prevent the oxidation of LDL cholesterol and inhibit atherosclerosis and disruption of plaque. Its clinical benefits are mainly due to its ability to improve ATP production, antioxidant activity and membrane stabilizing properties (1–4). These effects are beneficial in the prevention and treatment of heart disease. The antioxidant activity confers protection against lipid peroxidation and works together with vitamin E in prevention of damage to lipid membranes and plasma lipids (5). Treatment with CoQ10 may offer significant protection against atherosclerosis by activating smooth muscle cells in which it is rich, and by preventing lipid peroxide formation and oxidation of low density lipoprotein cholesterol (6–8). It might have some ability to maintain the integrity of myocardial calcium ion channels, sodium channels and potassium channels during ischemic insults. CoQ10 might therefore activate potassium channels similar to nicrondil and modulate calcium channels resulting into decreased cellular calcium and improved cardiac integrity during ischemia (9–11). Reduction in cytoplasmic calcium may be associated with hyperpolarization of cell membrane which may mediate vasorelaxation and decrease in cell damage. There is evidence that free radicals play an important role in cardiac damage that occurs during myocardial ischaemia and reperfusion (12,13). Free radicals are molecules containing an unpaired electron in the outer orbit rendering it chemically active. If a free radical reacts with a nonradical species, another free radical is produced. This property of self-perpetuation enables free radicals to initiate and per-

Table 1. Possible mechanisms of action of CoQ10

1.	Repletion of CoQ10 deficiency.
2.	Antioxidant activity.
3.	Spares Vitamin E.
4.	Direct free radical scavenger via semiquinone species.
5.	Membrane stabilizing effect due to phospholipid protein inter-action.
6.	Preservation of myocardial Na-K-ATPase activity and ATP manufacturing.
7.	Correction of mitochondrial "leak" of electrons during oxidative respiration.
8.	Induction of DT diaphorase which is an inhibitor of free radicals.
9.	Beneficial effect on prostaglandin metabolism.
10.	Inhibition of intracellular phospholipases.
11.	Stabilization of integrity of calcium ion dependent slow channels and possibly potassium channels.
12.	Spares vitamin C, A and beta carotene by decreasing their cell consumption.

petuate chain reactions. Superoxide anion (O2), hydroxyl radical, hydrogen peroxide and nitric oxide are major species of free radicals which are produced during ischaemia (10,11), (Table 1).

Oxygen is the major source of free radicals during myocardial ischaemia. ATP is catabolized to adenosine, inosine and hypoxanthine, which are oxidants. In addition, xanthine dehydrogenase is selectively converted into xanthine oxidase via limited protolysis or by oxidation of the thiol groups. Oxygen combines with hypoxanthine, in the presence of xanthine oxidase reperfusion, which generates superoxide anion and other free radicals. Neutrophil is another potential source of free radicals due to the activation of NADPH oxidase (2). This enzyme system produces superoxide radicals while mitochondria is the third source of free radicals during myocardial ischaemia.

Electrons may leak out of the mitochondrion via pathways involving NADH dehydrogenase and ubisemiquionoe to produce superoxide radical. Lipid peroxidase and hydroperoxidase, present in the cell membrane lipids, are activated during ischaemia which release arachidonic acid. Arachinonate in turn, accelerates the production and perpetuation of free radicals due to actions of cycloxygenase and lipooxygenase. Release of free iron and copper during ischaemia also cause the production of hydroxyl radicals (1,4). These multiple mechanisms involved in the production of free radicals can result in damage to the cell membrane. As a result, there may occur a handling of calcium gradients, activation of calcium dependent phospholipases, protein kinases, contractile elements and accumulation of mitochondrial calcium leading to further cellular damage and necrosis. There is evidence that treatment with endogenous free radical scavengers such as superoxide dismutase and catalase can enhance cardiac function during ischaemia (1,2). CoQ10 protects ischemic tissue from reperfusion damage by its antioxidant membrane stabilizing property and free radical scavenging activity. Furthermore, ubiquinone provides protection to myocardium by preventing oxidation of low density lipoprotein cholesterol. These actions provide the rationale for the experimental and clinical use of coenzyme Q in cardiovascular disease (1–3). These actions are similar to

ACE-inhibitors and potassium channel activators. It is possible that there is "in vivo" reduction of CoQ4 to its reduced Quinol form. This short, side chain Quinol might act as a radical scavenging antioxidant by donating phenolic hydrogen to peroxyl radicals (1,2). The other possible antioxidant action may be in the capacity of ubiquinols to reduce the alphatocopheryl radical, thus allowing regeneration of the active form of vitamin E.

ABSORPTION AND EXCRETION

CoQ10 is slowly absorbed from the gastrointestinal tract because of its solubility in lipids. The mean plasma level after a single 100 mg oral dose of CoQ10 in human subjects is 1.004 + 0.37 ug/ml (1,2). The mean steady state level after three daily administrations of 100 mg has been estimated to be 5.4 ug/ml. A softsule developed by Tishcon Corporation (USA) may provide better serum levels. It has a relative long plasma half life of 33.9 + 5.32 hours, indicating a low clearance rate from the plasma. The major portion of an exogenous dose of CoQ10 is deposited in the liver and packaged into very low density lipoprotein. The excretion is via the biliary tract and approximately 62.5% of the drug may be recovered in the stools. During chronic administration, the drug is concentrated in adrenal, spleen, lung, kidney, liver, brain and myocardial tissue, which poses the possibility that it may have beneficial effects on these organs.

DEFICIENCY OF CoQ10

CoQ10 deficiency (1–6) may be due to insufficient dietary intake, impairment in CoQ10 biosynthesis, excessive utilization by the body or a combination of any three (1–4). There is an increased requirement of CoQ10 by body tissues due to their consumption by the cells in several diseases such as angina pectoris, congestive heart failure, mitral valve prolapse, etc. (Table 2). It is possible that poor body stores or low dietary intake can predispose several of the diseases mentioned in the Table 2 and CoQ10 supplementation may be protective. Environmental oxidants such as pollutants, pesticides, heavy metals, industrial fumes, radiation and increased consumption of linoleic acid may enhance oxidative stress in the tissues and may enhance the requirement of CoQ10. Decreased synthesis and poor supply may cause CoQ10 deficiency. All animal and plant cells contain CoQ10. Fruits, vegetables, legumes and nuts, as well as animal organ meat, soy oil, peanuts, sweet potato, sardines, mackerel, etc. are important sources of CoQ10. However, the amount from dietary sources is probably insufficient to produce the clinical effects observed with therapeutic doses of the nutrient (1–4). The plasma level of CoQ10 is approximately two-fold higher among vegetarians than in omnivores, indicating that a high intake foods may also provide high CoQ10 levels (0.86 vs. 0.44 ug/ml) (1–4).

CLINICAL USES OF CoQ10

The deficiency of CoQ10 and experimental observation of myocardial protection during ischaemia (13) by CoQ10 reasonably constitutes one of the sound reasons for the therapeutic use of CoQ10 in human heart disease. Indications for CoQ10

Table 2. Diseases associated with CoQ10 deficiency

Noncardiovascular Conditions	Cardiovascular Diseases
1. Persistent nausea, vomiting and diarrhoea	1. Angina pectoris
2. Cachexia	2. Coronary artery disease
3. Chronic malnutrition	3. Congestive heart failure
4. Suboptimal dietary intake of CoQ10	4. Hypertension
5. Aging	5. Cardiomyopathy
6. Obesity	6. Mitral valve prolapse
7. Acute shock states	7. Revascularization
8. Diabetes mellitus	
9. Cancer	
10. Immune deficiency	
11. Peridontal disease	
12. Muscular dystrophy	
13. Drug therapy eg. statins, adriamycin, diuretics (possible)	
14. Excessive exertion	
15. Hypermetabolism	

Table 3. Clinical controlled studies on CoQ10 in chronic stable angina

Author	n	CoQ10, Daily Dose	Significant Findings
Hiasa (1984)	18	1.5 mg/kg 1.V.	Increased exercise tolerance, less angina
Kamikawa (1985)	12	150 mg, oral	Improved exercise tolerance, longer time to ST depression
Schardt (1986)	15	600 mg, oral	Less ST depression
Wilson (1991)	58	300 mg, oral	Improved exercise tolerance, longer time to angina
Serra (1991)	20	60 mg, oral	Improved cardiac output, less angina, less nitrate use

administration are growing gradually. The majority of patients with heart disease have CoQ10 deficiency. Treatment with CoQ10 has been shown to improve clinical manifestations such as dyspnea, angina, improvement in ejection fraction, work capacity decrease in catecholamines and angiotensin converting enzyme.

CORONARY ARTERY DISEASE

Hiasa (15) performed thc first controlled trial with CoQ10, specifically in patients with angina. CoQ10 group showed a prolongation in exercise time with 8 to 12 patients. This showed an increase of 1 stage or more on a modified Bruce protocol and no increase in exercise duration in the placebo group. Treatment with CoQ10 decreased ST segment depression without any influence on heart rate, blood pressure or double product. It is noteworthy that five controlled trials from 1984–1991 showed rapid and marked improvement in the symptoms of angina as well as a reduction in the degree of ischemic ST segment depression with exercise stress testing with no change in hemodynamics (Table 3).

Kamikawa et al. (17) gave oral CoQ10 (150 mg/day) or placebo for 4 weeks in 12 patients with chronic stable angina. This was followed by a crossover to the opposing treatment regimen for another 4 weeks. Exercise time and time to 1 mm electrocardiographic ST-depression were significantly increased in the CoQ10 group compared to placebo group. Schardt et al. (18) compared the effect of 600 mg/day of oral CoQ10 with placebo and the combination of pindolol (7.5 mg/day) and isosobidedinitrate (30 mg/day) in 15 patients with chronic stable angina. Treatment with CoQ10 was associated with a significant reduction in cumulative exercise induced ST-segment depression compared to placebo. CoQ10 in doses of 150 or 300 mg/day was compared with placebo in 37 patients on exercise duration in stable angina at 10 different centres. CoQ10 monotherapy caused an increase in exercise duration to onset of angina of 70 seconds in the 300 mg group and 65 in the 150 mg group at end of first week; 140 and 127 seconds respectively by week 4.

There was a 60% decrease in the frequency of anginal attacks in the 150 mg group. In post infarction patients, 19 treatments with CoQ10 caused a significant beneficial effect on work capacity and significantly lower level of malondialdehyde in the treatment group compared to placebo. In one 58 year old patient with diabetes mellitus and refractory unstable angina, the addition of CoQ10 (60 mg/day) to treatment with nitrates and calcium blockers was associated with exercise tolerance and relief in angina within 2 weeks; no response was observed during the last 4 weeks with conventional drugs (3–5).

CONGESTIVE HEART FAILURE

Heart failure is the main indication for treatment with CoQ10 among all other symptoms (Table 4) (22–38). Most clinical trials with CoQ10 focus on heart disease due to the known high CoQ10 content of the myocardium and to the high amount of energy required for normal heart function. After the publication of pioneering Japanese studies in the late 1960's and early 1970's, there have been 15 randomized controlled trials involving 1366 patients with various causes of heart failure. Our randomized controlled trial in 42 patients increased this number to 1408 subjects in which CoQ10 was administered for the treatment of heart failure. In Japan, about 48 controlled and open trials have been conducted to study the role of CoQ10 in heart failure (33). In the early trials, beneficial effects in the manifestations of heart failure was observed with smaller doses of 30 mg CoQ10 per day. However, rapid recovery in heart failure was noted using up to 200 mg/day of CoQ10 in later studies when more attention was paid to the therapeutic levels of the drug.

Serum level of CoQ10 > 1.0 ug/ml is usually associated with optimal improvement in heart function and this level is considered as normal. CoQ10 deficiency is considered when the level is <0.5 ug/ml and the therapeutic level, when it is >2.0 ug/ml. The requirement for a supraphysiologic level of CoQ10 is not clear but high blood CoQ10 level may be required to attain adequate tissue levels. It is possible that more data on blood and myocardial tissue levels of CoQ10 would be necessary to explain this question.

Table 4. Controlled trials of CoQ10 in heart failure

Author	No. of Patients	Diagnosis	CoQ10 Daily Oral Dose	Significant Findings
Hashiba (1972)	197	CHF	30 mg	Imp. NYHA class
Iwabuchi (1972)	38	CHF	30 mg	Imp. NYHA class
Langsjoen (1985)	19	CHF	100 mg	Increased EF
Vanfrachem (1986)	15	CHF	100 mg	Imp. Co. EF. SV Areobic capacity
Judy (1986)	14	CHF	100 mg	Imp. Co. & EF
Schneeberger (1986)	12	CHF	100 mg	Imp. Co. & EF
Oda (1990)	40	MVP with DD	3 mg/kg	Imp. DF
Rossi (1991)	20	ICM	200 mg	Imp. Exercise tol.
Poggesi (1991)	20	ICM & IDCM	100 mg	Imp. EF
Judy (1991)	180	CHF	100 mg	Imp. 8 yr. survival
Permanetter (1992)	25	IDCM	100 mg	No benefits
Rengo (1993)	60	CHF	100 mg	Imp. EF Imp. NYHA class
Morisco (1993)	641	CHF	2 mg/kg	Less hosp. for CHF at 1 yr
Morisco (1994)	6	CHF	150 mg	Imp. EF SV Co. by MUGA scan
Hofman-bang (1995)	79	CHF	100 mg	Imp. Vol. load EF
Watson et al (1999)		CHF	200 mg	No effect
Khatta et al (2000)	55	CHF	200 mg	EF, no effect
Singh RB (unpublished)	42	CHF	120 mg	Imp. NYHA class, EF

Abbreviations: Imp., improved; LV, left ventricular; EF, ejection fraction; CO, cardiac output; SV, stroke volume; CHF, congestive heart failure unspecified aetiology; MVP, mitral valve prolapse; DD, diastolic dysfunction; ICMN ischemic cardiomyopathy; IDCM, idiopathic dilated cardiomyopathy; hosps., hospitalizations; vol., volume.

Mortenson and Folkers (25) reported that patients in NYHA classes III and IV showed diminished contents of cardiac CoQ10 when compared to patients in class 1 and 2. It is possible that there may be an impairment in CoQ10 biosynthesis, accelerated catabolism, or a combination of both which caused a deficiency. Increased antioxidant commitment of CoQ10 may somehow lead to accelerated consumption leading to deficiency. It is possible that exogenous CoQ10 administration may increase the velocity of electron transfer, especially when endogenous pool is diminished as in cases of higher levels of lipid peroxidation. In one study (23) involving 79 patients of heart failure in a double blind crossover trial, the intervention group showed improvement in physical performance and exercise capacity consistent with captopril-digoxin multicentre research trial. In another double blind trial (24) involving 33 centres and comprising of 641 patients, 319 were administered CoQ10 and 322 placebo for 12 months. Although deaths (16 vs 21) were not significantly less, incidence of acute pulmonary oedema, arrhythmias, hospitalizations and incidence of class III and IV heart failure were significantly lower in the CoQ10 group. Clinical benefit score 1.4 was much higher in the treatment group. In another double blind and controlled study (22) Ursini et al. (Paciarioni group), treatment with CoQ10 was associated with significant reduction in catecholamines.

There was also clinical improvement in the intervention group compared to control group in a group of elderly heart failure patients. However, a German double blind study (26), showed no benefit of CoQ10 in patients with well-preserved cardiac function. In a long-term randomized survival study among 90 class IV congestive heart failure patients by Judy et al. (27), treatment with 100 mg/day of CoQ10 showed significant benefit compared to control group during a follow-up of 8 years.

In congestive heart failure due to CAD, there may be an ischaemia-reperfusion induced free radical stress in conjunction with higher serum catecholamines (34), insulin and angiotensin converting enzyme. Higher sympathetic activity and catecholamines, as well as angiotensin II in heart failure, may be associated with a deficiency of endogenous antioxidants such as catalase and super-oxidedismutase, glutathione as well as antioxidant vitamins A, E and C and betacarotene and CoQ10 which further enhance the oxidative stress. These biochemical abnormalities may cause worsening of heart failure. In experimental animals, an improved myocardial redox state with long-term antioxidant therapy has been shown to modulate the development and progression of heart failure (34). This study provides further proof to the rationale regarding the use of antioxidants in heart failure. Carvedilol, an antioxidant and betablocker, has also been found to retard heart failure indicating that a decrease in oxidative stress and sympathetic activity may be of benefit in heart failure (34). CoQ10 has also been successfully used in patients with refractory heart failure (35). In one metaanalysis of randomized trials (36), published between 1984–1994, only 8 out of 14 studies met the inclusion criteria. These studies comprised a total of 356 patients. Treatment with CoQ10 was consistent with improvement in stroke volume, ijection fraction, cardiac output, cardiac index and end diasobolic volume index compared to control group. However, a few studies (37,38) showed no benefit of CoQ10 in congestive heart failure, mainly due to lack of sufficient rise in plasma CoQ levels.

CARDIOMYOPATHY

There is no scientific proof that CoQ10 deficiency is the cause or effect of cardiomyopathy (19,20). In one study, tissue levels of CoQ10 were significantly lower among NYHA class IV subjects of cardiomyopathy compared to class 1 and 2 subjects (4). The greater the deficiency of CoQ10, the better the response to treatment with CoQ10, indicating cardiomyopathy. Significant improvement was noted in patients with dilated cardiomyopathy with class III and IV heart failure in a randomized double blind study when they were administered CoQ10 (14). In other studies of patients with cardiomyopathy, coenzyme Q treatment showed adequate benefits (22–25).

MYOCARDIAL PRESERVATION AND INTERVENTION

There is evidence that prior CoQ10 therapy provides protection against ischemic reperfusion (1–4) (Table 5). In a rabbit heart model of ischaemia and reperfusion, a role of CoQ10 in preserving ischemic myocardium was observed. Myocardium,

Table 5. Controlled trials of CoQ10 in cariac surgery

Author	No. of Patients	CoQ10 Daily Dose	Significant Postoperative Findings
Tanaka (1982)	50	30–60 mg p.o. 6 days preop	Imp. Co
Sunamori (1991)	78	5 mg/kg, i.e. 2 hrs preop 14 days preop	Imp. LV stroke work index, decreased CPK—MB Imp. LV ejection fraction, shortened recovery time
Judy (1993)	20	100 mg, 14 day, preop	EF improv, recovery time less
Chello (1994)	40	150 mg p.o.	Decreased markers of oxidative damage
		7 days preop.	Less arrhythmia, less need for inotropes
Chen (1994)	22	150–200 kg, p.o. 5–7 days preop.	Increased pulse pressure Imp. LV ultrastructure
Taggart (1994)	20	600 mg p.o. 12 hrs, preop.	No benefit

Abbreviations: No. = number of; p.o. = per os; ejection fraction; CO = cardiac output; Imp. = improved; preop. = preoperatively; LV = left ventricular.

pretreated with CoQ10, was relatively protected against both structural and functional changes induced by ischaemia and reperfusion. The animals pretreated with CoQ10 were able to maintain oxidative phosphorylation and cellular ATP generating capacity and showed that cellular and mitochondrial calcium overload was prevented by pretreatment with CoQ10. The clinical and metabolic beneficial effects were similar in magnitude to those seen with propranolol and verapamil (1). CoQ10 has been demonstrated to protect both Ca dependent and Na-K dependent ATPase activity. The effectiveness of CoQ10 in preventing low cardiac output states following cardiac surgery was compared in a randomized study in humans. Judy et al. (37) demonstrated myocardial preservation by prior treatment with CoQ10 for 15 days before heart surgery and compared with 30 days treatment after the surgery. The CoQ10 group showed optimal blood and tissue CoQ10 and tissue ATP levels, improvement in cardiac pumping and ijection fraction, as well as an uncomplicated and short recovery period compared to placebo group.

CARDIAC ARRHYTHMIAS

In experimental coronary artery ischaemia, pretreatment with CoQ10 increased the ventricular fibrillation threshold while minimizing the impairment in contractility and myocardial stunning (39). The antiarrhythmic effect of CoQ10 has been studied in several experiments. Treatment with CoQ10 was associated with prolongation of action potential duration in right ventricular papillary muscles. Clinical studies on the role of CoQ10 in patients with ventricular ectopic activity indicate that 20–25% of patients respond to treatment with this agent (1,2). These studies also showed a consistent effect of CoQ in shortening the QT interval, including QTc. CoQ10 may have similar effect on QT interval in patients receiving psychotropic agents. It seems that CoQ10 prevents the stimulation of excitable tissues in the heart as well as in the brain. Therefore treatment with CoQ10, similar to n-3 fatty acids might modulate the acute precipitating trigger that lies in the excitable tissue of brain and the chronic electrical instability of the myocardium, contributing to prevention of sudden cardiac death.

HYPERTENSION

There are not very many studies on the role of CoQ10 in hypertension (40–42). In earlier studies, Yamagami et al. used CoQ10 in 29 patients of hypertension with some success. In a randomized double blind trial in 59 patients receiving antihypertensive drugs, the effects of oral treatment with CoQ10 (60 mg twice daily) were compared for 8 weeks in 30 intervention group and 29 control group patients known to have hypertension and presenting with acute CAD (42). After 8 weeks of follow-up, the following indices were reduced in the CoQ10 group: systolic and diastolic blood pressure, fasting and 2-h plasma insulin, glucose, triglycerides, lipid peroxides, malondialdehyde and diene conjugates. The following indices were increased; HDL cholesterol, vitamins A, C, E and beta-carotene ($P < 0.05$). These findings indicate that treatment with CoQ10 decreases blood pressure possibly by decreasing oxidative stress and insulin response in patients with known hypertension receiving conventional antihypertensive drugs. Digiesi et al. (40) also studied the role of CoQ10 in hypertension and reported a decrease in total peripheral resistance which may be due to improvement in arterial smooth muscle cell metabolism. In a recent study by Langsjoen et al. (41) in 109 patients with known essential hypertension, CoQ10 (225 mg/day average) was administered to achieve serum level of 2 ug/ml, in conjunction with anti-hypertensive drugs. There was a need to withdraw one to three drugs in 51% of patients. The decrease in systolic blood pressure was from 159 to 147 mmHg, mean and in diastolic blood pressure from 94 to 85 mmHg. A further study (22), showed that CoQ10 causes a significant decrease in serum catecholamines and possibly reduces peripheral vascular resistance. The available data indicate that a double blind randomized study should be conducted with higher doses (100–200 mg/day) of CoQ10 with a long-term follow up.

ADRIAMYCIN MYOCARDIAL TOXICITY

Adriamycin, an anthracycline and mixed quinoid and hydroquinoid compound may have inhibition effects on CoQ10 enzyme systems (1). Repletion with CoQ10 can prevent the inhibition of CoQ10 enzymes in mitochondrial preparations. In several other experimental studies, the role of exogenous CoQ10 in preventing adriamycin toxicity was corroborated (1). Clinical studies also showed beneficial effects on systolic time intervals of pretreatment with CoQ10 (a manifestation of adriamycin toxicity) in cancer patients. In a randomized (36) and controlled study in 20 patients with cancer, 10 were supplemented with 200 mg/day of CoQ10 for the duration of treatment with anthracyclins (43). Echocardiographic monitoring showed protective effects on the left ventricular contractile function in the form of less decrease in ijection fraction and of shortening fraction in the CoQ10 group compared to control subjects. It is possible that CoQ10 therapy causes repletion of a CoQ10 deficiency induced by adriamycin and inhibits adriamycin induced lipid peroxidation and free radical generation.

PLASMA LIPOPROTEINS

In one in vitro experiment (6), it has been demonstrated that following exposure to free radical source (Azo componds), low density lipoproteins (LDL) deployed their antioxidant reserve which were consumed while inhibiting the oxidative attack. When LDL, depleted of abscorbic acid, was exposed to free radical source, peroxidation remained under control as long as some uniquinol was present. The findings suggested that ubiquinol as an antioxidant may be more efficient than tocopherol and carotenoids in preventing the oxidation of LDL.

A double blind controlled study (6), in patients with hypercholesterolemia showed that treatment with HMGCOA reductase-I (lovastatin) was associated with significantly lower plasma level of CoQ10 compared to placebo (44). The decrease in CoQ10 appears to be due to the fact that cholesterol and CoQ10 share the same biosynthetic pathway. These findings were confirmed in a crossover trial with CoQ10 and HMGCOA inhibitors (45). This study showed a decrease in CoQ10 in plasma, as well as in platelets which was prevented by concomitant administration of CoQ10. In one experimental study, Singh et al. (46) demonstrated that lovastain has a modest antioxidant activity which may be similar to fluvastatin. Despite a reduction in CoQ10, induced by statins, oxidation of LDL is inhibited by the statins with no serious adverse effect of CoQ10 deficiency. However, treatment of hypercholesterolemia with HMGCOA reductase inhibitors in conjunction with CoQ10 may provide greater benefit in the regression of coronary atherosclerosis and prevention of cardiac events. We also observed in a sub study that CoQ10 treatment may be associated with significant reduction in lipoprotein level and plasma insulin levels in patients with acute coronary syndromes (42,47). In a randomized, double blind, placebo controlled trial (51) in 47 patients with acute CAD and moderately raised lipoprotein(a) {Lp(a)}, treatment with CoQ10 (60 mg twice daily) in 25 interventions and 22 control group patients were given. After 28 days, serum Lp(a) level showed significant reduction in CoQ10 group compared with the placebo group (31.0 vs 8.2%, $P < 0.001$) with a net reduction of 22.6% attributed to CoQ10. HDL cholesterol showed a significant increase in the intervention group. CoQ10 treatment was also associated with significant reductions in thiobarbituric acid reactive substances, malondialdehyde and dien conjugates indicating an overall decrease in oxidative stress.

The effects of the administration of CoQ10 (5 mg/kg/day) (group A, $n = 10$) and placebo (group B, $n = 10$) were compared over 24 weeks in a randomized, single blind controlled trial (52). There were two groups of rabbits receiving a trans fatty acid rich diet (5–8 g/day) for 36 weeks. Oxidized rabbits chow with vitamin C plus ferric chloride was administered for 4 weeks in all rabbits. Intervention with CoQ10 after feeding of TFA rich diet was associated with a significant decline in thiobarbituric acid reactive substances (TBARS), diene conjugates and malondialdehyde, as well as an increase in plasma levels of vitamin E in the CoQ10 group compared to placebo group. The aortic and coronary artery plaque quality also showed beneficial effects which would be discussed later (48).

ACUTE MYOCARDIAL INFARCTION

A recent study has shown that CoQ10 can inhibit human vitronectin receptor expression indicating that it might inhibit thrombosis (49). In one study by Kuklinski et al. (50), in patients with AMI, treatment with CoQ10 + selenium for 6 months was associated with significant less patients with prolonged QT interval compared to control group. There were no deaths in the treatment group (0 vs 6) during a follow up of 6 months. Singh et al. (51), conducted a randomized, double blind, controlled trial in 144 patients with AMI. Treatment with CoQ10 (60 mg twice a day) was associated with significant decrease in arrhythmias, angina and cardiac enlargement in the intervention group compared to control group during the follow up of 4 weeks. Nonfatal infarction and cardiac deaths were significantly less in the CoQ10 group than control group (15 vs 31%, $P < 0.02$).

ATHEROSCLEROSIS AND UNSTABILITY OF ATHEROMA

CoQ10 and vitamin E can have synergestic effects and CoQ deficiency may decrease the beneficial effect of vitamin B6 (52). Littarru and coworkers (53,56) demonstrated a deficiency of CoQ in cardiac muscle and possibly in the arterial smooth muscle which are important in the pathogenesis of left ventricular hypertrophy (LVH) and atherosclerosis respectively (55–59). LVH and atherosclerosis are risk factors of acute myocardial infarction (AMI) and sudden cardiac death (SCD). It is now widely accepted that unstable atheroma and subsequent plaque rupture is a major cause of myocardial infarction and stroke (59–62). Clinical trials with statins (46,63,64) only showed minor effects on the size of existing lesions but major reduction in clinical events, despite the fact that these agents decrease CoQ as a side effect of drugs. These results indicate that despite statin induced CoQ deficiency, there is a beneficial effect on stability and chemical composition of atherosclerotic plaque (63). There is a need to know how active the plaques are rather than just the severity of stenosis that is routinely assessed by angiography. Antioxidants such as vitamin E, C, beta carotene, minerals, selenium, zinc, copper, magnesium and calcium and lycopene, CoQ10, n-3 fatty acids, amino acids in conjuction with lipids, appear to be important determinants of the chemical composition and quality of atherosclerotic plaque (65). While regular physical activity stabilizes the atheroma, tobacco consumption, sedentary behaviour, hyperinsulinemia, hyperglycemia, hypertriglyceridemia and low high density lipoprotein (HDL) may increase the vulnerability of the plaque. Thrombosis is also the major initiating factor in unstable angina particularly when chest pain is recent and increasing in severity. However, the thrombosis in unstable angina is mainly due to white platelets which do not respond to fibrinolytic streptokinase.

THE ATHEROSCLEROTIC PLAQUE

The fully developed human fibrolipid, atherosclerotic plaque as defined by American Heart Association (Type IV or Type V) has a core of lipid surrounded by a capsule of connective tissue (60–62). It begins as a subendothelial accumulation of lipid-laden monocyte derived foam cells and associated T-cells which form a non-stenotic fatty streak. Progression of fatty streak results into plaque having extracellular lipid cholesterol and its esters bounded by an endothelized fibrous cap containing vascular smooth muscle cell (SMC) and inflammatory cells. It predominantly macrophages with some T-cells and mast cells which tend to accumulate at the shoulder regions of the plaque (60,61). In the advanced lesions, new blood vessels and deposits of calcium may be present. The macrophages may be laiden with cholesterol or lipids which are called foam cells. These macrophages are derived from monocytes which crossed the endothelium from the arterial lumen. These macrophages are highly activated producing procoagulant tissue factor and a host of inflammatory cell mediators such as tumor necrosis factor, interleukins and metaloproteinases. The connective tissue capsule which surrounds above inflammatory mass is collagen synthesized by the SMCs. This portion of the capsule separating the core from the arterial lumen itself is the plaque cap which is fibrous and determines the stability of the plaque. Although recruitment of inflammatory cells is important for plaque development, they do not accumulate in the intima in the absence of lipids. Therefore lipid accumulation is the initiating event and that inflammatory cells play a permissive role in lesion progression.

OXIDIZED LOW DENSITY LIPOPROTEIN CHOLESTEROL

Oxidized LDL exhibits a variety of pro-atherogenic actions including inflammation, endothelial dysfunction, the attraction and retention of blood monocytes in the intimal space and the promotion of foam cells as well as cytotoxicity and SMC proliferation. Myeloperoxidase-derived oxidants, reactive nitrogen intermediates, oxygen centered radicals and also possibly 15 lipoxygenase, transition metal ions are important in oxidising LDL. However, the exact oxidants involved and the extent of molecular mechanisms of LDL oxidation in human body are yet to be studied. Therefore, apart from hypolipidemic agents, LDL antioxidants appear to be potential anti-atherosclerotic agents in the management of atherosclerosis. There is some evidence (65–67) which indicates that to be anti-atherogenic, an antioxidant needs to be associated with LDL in adequate concentrations. Human LDL contains a number of endogenous antioxidants such as alphatocopherol, which is higher than ubiquinol-l0, gama tocopherol, lycopene and carotenoids. There is also evidence that higher doses of alpha tocopherol can decrease the availability of CoQ as well as gama-tocopherol which may have adverse effects including enhanced proinflammatory responses in the atherosclerotic plaque. CoQ10H2 is the first antioxidant consumed in LDL exposed to various oxidants and it inhibits LDL lipid peroxidation by reducing the chain carrying alpha-tocopheroxyl radical and exporting the radical from the lipoprotein particle. Enrichment of LDL with CoQ10H2 by dietary supplementation with CoQ10 inhibits exvivo LDL oxidation.

OXIDATION OF LDL AND CoQ10

Experimental studies indicate that when LDL is exposed to oxidants, reduced CoQ10 is the first antioxidant to be consumed (8,66–68). Formation of oxidized lipids is markedly suppressed while reduced CoQ is present in the LDL. Fresh and rapidly isolated LDL contains comparatively smaller amount of reduced CoQ than vitamin E. Only second LDL particle contains on average, one molecule of reduced CoQ10 in unsupplemented human subjects. However, dietary supplementation with CoQ (100–300 mg/day) may cause greater concentrations of reduced CoQ in plasma and all of its lipoproteins (68). A maximal concentration is achieved in LDL after 4–5 days of daily CoQ administration (from 0.5–0.8 normal to 2.0–3.0 CoQ10 reduced molecules per LDL). Increased concentration of reduced CoQ10 also overcomes and fully prevents the pro-oxident effect seen with alpha-tocopherol supplementation (68,69). It is not clear how such small levels of reduced CoQ provide significant antioxidant protection against low fluxes of a variety of different oxidants. It seems that reduced CoQ exhibits antioxidant activity for LDL lipids by inhibiting the chain transfer activity of alpha-tocopheroxyl radicals (68,69).

Experimental studies (8) reveal that scavenging of alpha-tocopheroxyl by reduced CoQ can explain that co-supplementation with reduced CoQ10 inhibits the proxidant effect of supplementation with alphatocopherol alone. In other words, alphatocopherol requires co-antioxidants for efficient antioxidation of LDL lipids. Increased number of reduced CoQ10 molecules per LDL particle from <1 to >1 is likely to substantially increase the resistance of the lipoprotein towards lipid peroxidation and may be crucial with respect to effecting antioxidant protection of LDL.

INFLAMMATION

The lipid laden monocytes accumulate in the subendothelial space and exacerbate the local inflammatory reaction which becomes more severe if the lipids are oxidized (59–62). Subendothelial lipids also maintain activation of the overlying endothelium resulting into continued expression of selectin and adhesion molecules and also expression of chemokines in particularly monocyte chemoattractant proteins-l (MCP-l). Chemokines are proinflammatory cytokines that function in leucocyte chemoattraction and activation. The inflammatory cells once captured, migrate into the subendothelial space where they are activated by local chemokines. Activated macrophages and T cells also express a variety of proinflammatory cytokines and growth factors that contribute to the evolution of the plaque. It is possible that a subendothelial inflammatory stimuli and the local adaptive wound healing response of vascular smooth cells interact to form atherosclerotic plaque (61,62). CoQ can inhibit atheroma development by inhibiting pro-inflammatory agents as well as by SMC activation due to energy production in the cells.

ARTERIAL SMOOTH MUSCLE CELLS

Smooth muscle cells (SMC) gene expression of the intima in atherosclerosis and SMCs in the early developing blood vessel have many similarities indicating that intimal SMCs are likely to be performing a reparative rather than a permissive role in atherosclerosis (14). In adopting a repair phenotype, SMCs express the proteinases that break down the basement membrane to facilitate their migration to the site of injury (69,70). SMCs produce growth factors which help in their proliferation at the site of injury and they also produce collagen and elastin to repair the artery (67,68). Expression of this repertoire of genes is essential for the formation of a fibrous cap over the lipid core of a plaque. It is clear that SMC is the only capable cell which synthesizes the cap and plays a pivotal role in maintaining plaque stability (63). The fibrous cap separates the highly thrombogenic lipid-rich core from circulating platelets and proteins of coagulation cascade and confers structural stability to a lesion (63). Since CoQ deficiency is an important factor in predisposing atherosclerosis, it is possible that SMC deficiency of CoQ might decrease energy production in the cells and alter their capability of forming a strong fibrous cap. It is also possible that CoQ supplementation would enhance the capability of SMC to form a stronger fibrous cap, as well as attenuate their proliferation to prevent atherogenesis and unstability of atheroma (61,69,70).

INTERACTIONS OF CELLS AND PLAOUE RUPTURE

There is an accumulation of platelets leading to intravascular thrombosis if the atherosclerotic plaque ruptures or erodes resulting into acute coronary syndromes of unstable angina, and myocardial infarction (61). The most important determinant of plaque rupture such as large lipid pool, thin fibrous cap of atheroma and proponderance of inflammatory cells produce metaloproteases and metaloproteinases, (which degrade matrix proteins and weaken the cap of plaque) and proinflammatory cytokines in particular interfer on gamma which inhibits SMC proliferation and collagen synthesis (62). They also secrete inflammatory cytokines, in particular interleukin 1 beta, tumour necrosis factor-alpha and interferon gamma that are synergistically cytotoxic for SMCs. Activated macrophages can also induce SMC apoptosis by direct cell to cell contact which possibly becomes worse if there is a CoQ deficiency in the cells. These mechanisms are compounded by the phenotype of the SMCs within the fibrous cap of a mature plaque which has a reduced ability to proliferate and an enhanced susceptibility to apoptosis (61,62). It is clear that inflammatory cells can destroy the fibric of the fibrous cap which becomes greater due to the paucity of SMC and their lack of compensatory capability (59–61).

These characteristics are often present in small, non-significant atherosclerotic plaques that are clinically silent and angiographically invisible. Therefore, it seems that plaque quality and possibly chemical composition are far more important than plaque size in determining outcome. A rupture or erosion of the fibrous cap exposes the highly thrombogenic collagenous matrix and lipid core to the circulation causing platelet accumulation and activation. In turn, this leads to fibrin deposition, thrombus formation and finally arterial occlusion which is not inevitable. In one study, up to 70% of plaques causing high-grade stenosis had evidence of previous plaque rupture and repair in the absence of vessel occlusion or a clinical event (59–61). It is possible that these episodes of non-occlusive plaque rupture induce recruitment of new SMCs under the influence of mitogens, in particular platelet derived growth factor and thrombin possibly due to CoQ deficient SMCs. Thrombus also contains large quantities of transforming growth factor beta which is a potent stimulator of SMC matrix synthesis. These factors enhance formation of new fibrous cap over the thrombus resulting into increased size of the lesion continue increasing by rupture and repair. When the rupture and repair process is rapid, it results into occlusive CAD. It is clear that inhibition of silent plaque rupture and anti-platelet agents are therefore important in reducing progression of atherosclerosis.

INTERACTIONS OF ANTIOXIDANTS AND CHEMICAL COMPOSITION OF PLAQUE

There is evidence that oxidative modification of LDL may be associated with depletion of antioxidants indicating that the levels of alpha-tocopherol and reduced CoQ in the blood of the patients with atherosclerosis may be lowered. Since reduced CoQ10 is consumed before alpha-tocopherol and is associated with LDL with a decrease in its redox status (higher level of CoQ10), it could be a useful diagnostic indicator for in vivo lipoprotein oxidation. In one study (70–72), reduced plasma CoQ10 and CoQ10 redox status were slightly lower while levels of alpha-tocopherol were slightly higher in patients exhibiting clinical indices of CAD compared to controls. The levels of antioxidants in isolated LDL hydroperoxides of cholesteryl esters from patients and controls were undetectable, indicating that plasma and LDL levels of lipophilic antioxidants including reduced CoQ are only partially oxidized.

Recent studies (72,73) indicate that homogenates of advanced atherosclerotic lesions and lesion lipoprotein fractions derived from them contain substantial levels of both oxidized lipids and alpha tocopherol. This indicates that the vitamin remains present in normal levels or that it may be slightly lower in the majority of lipoprotein isolated from the lesions. Diseased and normal arteries contained similar levels of total CoQ10 and did not contain detectable reduced CoQ10. The absence of reduced CoQ in these arteries may, however, be due to autooxidation during the homogenization procedure carried out during sample preparation (72–74). If CoQ is presently predominant as CoQ10 in the arterial wall, it would increase the susceptibility of lipoproteins towards oxidation. Therefore reduced CoQ10 should be present in adequate amounts in the atherosclerotic plaque to stabilise the plaque.

Above studies suggest that the reduced CoQ10 is a candidate for an in vivo antioxidant activity for a number of reasons for inhibition of lipid peroxidation. Unlike the aqueous co-antioxidants, ascorbate and 3-hydroxyanthronilic acid, reduced CoQ10 is incorporated in lipoproteins and thereby can exhibit site specific co-antioxidation. Reduced CoQ10 inhibits LDL lipid peroxidation induced by both strong and mild oxidising conditions. Reduced CoQ10 is a first line of lipophilic antioxidant defense in lipoproteins and plasma against many oxidants including those of potential physiological function such as hypochlorite, 15-lipoxygenase, transition metals and peroxynitrite. CoQ supplementation increases the lipoproteins content of reduced CoQ10 from <1 to >1 molecule per particle which enhances the

Table 6. Effect of coenzyme Q on chemical composition of atheroma

	Coenzyme Q Group A	Placebo Group B
Aortic cholesterol (mg/g wet wt)	1.88 ± 0.6*	4.26 ± 1.4
Aortic triglycerides (mg/g wet wt)	3.85 ± 1.8*	6.92 ± 4.2
Coronary cholesterol (mg/g wet wt)	2.01 ± 0.5*	6.41 ± 3.2
Coronary triglycerides (mg/g wet wt)	4.01 ± 1.9*	7.21 ± 4.5
Aortic insulin (mU/L)	0.05 ± 0.01*	0.22 ± 0.05
Aortic angiotensin converting enzyme (10)	25.5 ± 5.5*	42.6 ± 7.6
Aortic vitamin E (umol/L)	3.2 ± 4.5*	0.45 ± 0.11
Diene conjugates (OD units)	22.8 ± 4.5*	32.6 ± 6.2
Malondialdehyde (pmol/L)	1.1 ± 0.21*	4.5 ± 0.9
TBARS (pmol/L)	0.68 ± 0.6*	3.1 ± 0.6

resistance to oxidation. CoQ is a safe dietary supplement without known adverse effects, even in a dosage of 120 mg/day.

In one randomized controlled intervention trial (48), in an experimental study of atherosclerosis in rabbits, TBARS, diene conjugates, insulin and angiotensin activity, malondialdehyde, aortic and coronary triglycerides, and cholesterol showed a marked decline in plasma as well as in atherosclerotic plaque in the CoQ10 group compared to control group (Table 6). However, vitamin E both in plasma and plaque, showed significant increase in the CoQ group than control group. Increased availability of Vitamin E in the plasma and atheroma indicates that recycling of vitamin E by ubiquinol results in a 600% greater availability and is an important mechanism of antioxidant activity in this study (65). It is possible that antioxidant activity of CoQ is mainly exerted by being fully reduced from CoQH2. This is useful as it may react with different types of oxygen radicals. CoQH2 is present in relatively higher amount in the mitochondrial pool and can be readily recycled by electron transport. Reduction in plasma insulin and angiotensin converting enzyme by CoQ in our study indicates that it may have also repaired coexistent CoQ deficiency of beta-cells of pancrease and justaglomemlar cells of kidneys respectively by inhibiting renin-angiotensin aldosterone-system. Insulin and angiotensin II and III are damaging to arterial intima and help in the proliferation of smooth muscle cells and activate the pro inflammatory macrophages indicating that both the agents may be responsible for instability of atheroma (74). One recent study (74), reported adequate levels of alpha-tocopherol in the atheroma, whereas another one found decreased level in the control group including a significant increase in the lovastatin + vitamin E treatment group (46).

COENZYME Q10, THE DYNAMIC BALANCE OF ATHEROSCLEROSIS AND ARTERIAL REMODELING

Plaque growth does not always lead to the coronary artery stenosis. The atherosclerotic artery can adapt and remodel to accommodate the expanding plaque while still maintaining a near normal luman diameter, making a large lesion still silent.

Table 7. Effect of CoQ10 on atherosclerosis

	CoQ10 Mean + SD	Control
Aortic sudanophilia (% score)	7.5 + 1.2*	17.5 + 3.3
Aortic plaque height (um)	97.5 + 7.5**	345 + 18.8
Coronary plaque height (um)	42.6 + 4.8*	87.6 + 8.6
Coronary atherosclerosis index	3.6 + 1.2*	16.6 + 3.2
Aortic atherosclerosis score	5.7 + 1.4*	14.3 + 3.1
Coronary atherosclerosis score	1.2 + 0.3*	5.6 + 0.8

* = $P < 0.05$, ** $P < 0.01$ by analysis of variance.

Arterial remodeling is a beneficial adaptive mechanism which is associated by thickening of the artery due to atherosclerosis without narrowing of the arterial lumen. It is possible that the biochemical changes associated with the CoQ treatment may facilitate coronary arterial remodeling in the initial phases of atherosclerosis. CoQ induced biochemical changes may inhibit and prevent the unstability of atherosclerotic plaque.

In one study (74) by Stockers group, dietary supplementation with CoQ (0.5 or 10%) and vitamin E (0.2%) either alone or together, resulted in an increase in both plasma and aortic content of both the agents; heart, brain and muscle content of CoQ remain unchanged. In co-supplemented mice the tissue concentration of lipid hydroperoxides was decreased, whereas the contents of the secondary lipids oxidation products were unaffected. CoQ10 (10%) and CoQ10 (0.5%) plus vitamin E significantly decreased the extent of atherosclerosis at all the sites examined. CoQ10 alone significantly decreased atherosclerosis at the aortic arch but not the descending thoracic aorta whereas vitamin E alone was anti-atherogenic at the aortic root only. These workers are also studying the effect of CoQ on atherosclerosis in rabbits.

QUALITY OF ATHEROMA AND CoQ10

In our experimental study in rabbits (48) the mean aortic and coronary artery plaque heights, as revealed by micrometer, were significantly smaller in the CoQ group compared to control group (Table 6). Coronary atherosclerosis index, aortic atherosclerosis score and coronary atherosclerosis score were significantly lower in CoQ group than control group. We also observed a variable degree of intimal thickening which was observed in both groups of rabbits as revealed by paraffin sections of aortic and coronary arteries. Fatty streaks, atheromatous plaques and fibrous plaques were noted in all the rabbits in the control group, whereas these changes occurred significantly less in the CoQ group (Table 7). Control group rabbits also showed significantly more ulceration, hemorrhages and thrombosis, indicating complicated lesions in the coronary arteries which were rarely observed in the CoQ group rabbits (Table 8). General assessment by appearance and manipulation with a pointer revealed that in the CoQ group, the plaques were more flat, strong, fibrous and less fragile without any cracks and fissures. In comparison with the control

Table 8. Effect of CoQ10 on qualities of lesions

Frequencies (%)	CoQ10	Control Group
Aortic plaque frequency	28.6*	51.3
Coronary plaque frequency	12.8*	26.8
Aortic plaque ulceration	2.3*	18.2
Coronary plaque ulceration	1.8*	16.6
Aortic plaque thrombosis and hemorrhage	1.6*	12.6
Coronary plaque thrombosis and hemorrhage	1.8*	14.5
Aortic plaque cracks and fissures	3.1*	17.2
Coronary plaque cracks and fissures	3.4*	16.4

* = P < 0.02 by X2 test.

Table 9. Cardiac events in the intervention and control groups after 1 year

Cardiac Events (95%)	CoQ10 (n = 73)	B Vitamins (n = 71)	Relative Risk
Sudden cardiac death (1 hr.)	3 (4.1)	5 (7.0)	0.58
Fatal myocardial infarction	5 (6.8)	9 (12.7)	0.53
Nonfatal myocardial infarction	10 (13.7)*	18 (25.3)	0.54
Total cardiac deaths	8 (10.9)	14 (19.7)	0.55
Stroke	1 (1.4)	3 (3.1)	0.45
Angioplasty or CABG	—	2 (2.8)	0.46
Total cardiac events	18 (24.6)**	32 (45.0)	0.54
Total cardiovascular events	18 (24.6)**	34 (47.8)	0.51
Total cardiac endpoints	19 (25.9)**	37 (52.0)	0.49

CABG—Coronary artery bypass grafting * = P < 0.05, ** = P < 0.02 P value was obtained by comparison of intervention and control group by Z score test of proportions.

group, the plaques were more atheromatous and fragile and revealed cracks and fissures and were more lipid in the body of the lesions (Table 9). These qualities of atheroma are predisposing factors for unstability of plaque. The findings indicated for the first time that treatment with CoQ may modulate the chemical composition and biology of atherosclerotic plaque.

CoQ10 AND RISK OF ATHEROSCLEROSIS IN HUMANS

The clinical diagnosis of coronary disease is made by coronary angiogram. However, coronary angiography is able to detect those lesions which impinge significantly on the lumen, without providing any information on the composition of stenotic lesion. Since it is the composition, rather than the size that determines the likelihood of plaque rupture, it seems that angiography may be a poor predictor of clinical events. Falk et al. (75) showed that most of the lesions that cause AMI produce less than a 50% stenosis. Therefore, AMI occurs more commonly in patients who have experienced no previous symptoms and emphasizes the reason better diagnostic tools are required. Despite pivotal role in evaluation and management of symptomatic coronary disease, angiography has a minor role in risk prediction or therapeutic monitoring in the asymptomatic population. However, in AMI, angiography may be important even in the asyptomatic patients.

Intravascular ultrasound, even though it provides much more information than angiography, on the extent and composition of targeted, proximal pressures components. However, image resolution and movement artifact remain substantial obstacles to the use of MRI to monitor coronary disease. While MRI may provide fine anatomical details, it is unlikely to provide details of inflammatory activity within plaques. Arterial thermography, which measures the temperature of the plaque, is an additional method to find inflammatory activity in the plaque. Serial MRI and thermography may also reveal how plaques respond to treatment with statins and CoQ10 and other antiatherosclerotic measures. MRI spectroscopy provides anatomical information and Positron Emission Tomography offers the potential to measure and monitor plaque inflammatory cell content and activity. Early animal studies to measure plaque metabolic activity have been encouraging and resolution is a measure in studies in humans.

Biochemical markers of inflammation in the atherosclerotic plaque such as non-specific serum amyloid, c-reactive protein (CRP), TNF-alpha and other specific markers for vascular inflammation such as ICAM 1 and VCAN 1 are important factors for evaluation of risk factors of atherosclerosis. In one randomized controlled intervention trial in 144 patients with AMI, CoQ was administered for one year (51). There was a significant decrease in c-reactive protein in the intervention group compared to a subgroup of patients in which c-reactive protein was done. After one year, total cardiac events including nonfatal MI and cardiac death showed significant decline in the CoQ group compared to control group (Table 9). These beneficial effects of CoQ may be due to its effects on thrombosis, atherosclerosis, endothelial function and heart failure (78–80).

In brief, it is possible to suggest that energy deficiency in the arterial SMC and myocardial cell, in association with CoQ10 deficiency appear to be important predictors of atherosclerotic plaque inflammation and unstability of atheroma. Treatment with CoQ may inhibit inflammation by decreasing oxidative damage and increasing ATP generation and repair process in the SMC resulting into decrease in the extent of atherosclerosis as well as improvement in the chemical composition and biology of atheroma. CoQ administration in humans may decrease the risk of atherosclerosis resulting into a significant reduction in total cardiac events in patients of recent AMI. It is possible that a better understanding of the molecular regulators of SMC behaviour in relation to intracellular CoQ concentration may provide better treatment aimed at enhancing fibrous cap formation.

CONTROLLED TRIALS IN CARDIAC SURGERY

It has been shown for the first time that administration of CoQ10 before open heart surgery showed a significant reduction in the incidence of low cardiac output during recovery (1–4). There have been 6 controlled trials in patients with open

Table 10. Age related changes in ubiquinone content in human organs

Organ	1–3 Days	0.7—Years	19–21 Years	39–41 Years	77–81 Years
Heart	36.7	78.5	110	75	47
Kidney	17.4	53.4	98	71	64
Liver	13	45	61	58	51
Pancreas	9	38	21	19	6.5
Spleen	21	80	33	29	13
Adrenal	17.5	58	16	12	8.5
Lung	2.2	6.4	6	6.5	3

heart surgery, 5 of which showed significant benefit in post operative measurements of cardiac function after pretreatment (Table 5) (81–84). There was a decline in the incidence of postoperative low cardiac output state in post operative arrhythrrias including a shorter recovery time with a significant reduction in the need for inotropic support (81). In one study, 600 mg of oral CoQ10 was administered 12 hours before surgery; no benefit was noted (84). Only one study (82), used an intravenous form of CoQ10 and showed benefits even though CoQ10 was given just 2 hours before surgery. In cardiac surgery, as in CHF and myocardial ischaemia, CoQ10 appears to be safe, simple and a cost effective means of patient support. It promises to decrease the morbidity and mortality of open heart surgery, particularly in the elderly or in patients with compromised myocardial function. The results of ongoing surgical trials in Australia with CoQ10 are eagerly awaited as the results will have important implications.

MISCELLANEOUS

In diabetes, stroke, immunodeficiency, muscular dystrophy, polymyositis, renal failure, myopathy, and tuberculosis, treatment with CoQ10 may be beneficial (1,4). However, in a recent 12 week randomized controlled trial, treatment with CoQ10 in 40 patients with type two diabetes showed no benefit. We have administered CoQ10 in refractory heart failure (n = 2), cardiogenic shock (n = l), refractory angina (n = l) and ectopics (n = l) showing beneficial effects in all the 5 cases (4). All patients who also had associated diabetes (n = 3) showed improvement in glucose levels. Higher tissue levels of CoQ10 may be seen during thyroid hormone treatment, cold adaptation and exercise due to increased biosynthesis as an adaptive response to oxidative stress. Age related changes in CoQ10 levels have also been reported (Table 10). Mitral valve prolapse may also be associated with CoQ10 deficiency (1). Clinical studies suggest that CoQ10 may improve cardiac performance under exercise conditions in patients with mitral valve prolapse.

DOSAGE

Evidence indicates that in various conditions, the dosage varies between 30–300 mg/day in two to three divided doses. The optimal doses in heart disease appear to be 50 to 200 mg/day or 2–6 mg/kg body weight. Longterm, followup studies in

Table 11. Possible therapeutic uses of coq10

Cardiovascular Diseases	Non-Cardiovascular Diseases
1. Congestive heart failure	1. Muscular dystrophy
2. Angina pectoris and AMI	2. Peridontal disease
3. Coronary artery disease	3. Aging
4. Toxin induced cardiomyopathy	4. Cancer
5. Myocardial preserving agent	5. Diabetes mellitus
6. Hypertension	6. Immune deficiency
7. Arrhythmias	7. Cerebral ischaemia
8. Cardiomyopathy	8. Physical performance
9. Mitral valve prolapse	9. Polymyositis
10. Potential imaging agent	10. Nephrophathy and renal failure
	11. Liver damage

a large number of subjects would be necessary to demonstrate the exact therapeutic dosage of CoQ10 in heart disease.

ADVERSE MANIFESTATIONS

Major adverse effects (11-3) of CoQ10 administration in pharmacological dosages of 30–300 mg/day have not been observed. These side effects attributed to CoQ10 therapy may be mainly gastrointestinal such as decreased appetite, epigastric discomfort, and loose stools. Asymtomatic elevations of lactic dehydonogenase (LDH) and serum glutamicoxaltransferase (SGOT) can occur with higher doses above 300 mg/day of CoQ10. Oral hypoglycemic agents and HMGCoA reductase inhibitors (44) and also possibly diuretics may enhance the requirement of CoQ10 and need supplementation. Further studies using higher doses of CoQ10 in the treatment and longterm administration would be necessary to find out the safety of this drug.

CoQ10 is still in the investigational stages and the list of possible indications appears to be quite large (Table 11). It is sold as a health product in United States (Tishcon Corporation, USA) and its therapeutic uses cannot be patented, hence drug industry is not interested in research on CoQ10. The most intriguing property of CoQ10 is its potential ability to protect and preserve ischemic myocardium. However, no randomized controlled intervention trial exists on its use in decreasing myocardial infarction size. CoQ10 has been used in the prevention of complications in patients with acute myocardial infarction in only two studies (50,51). In acute myocardial infarction, ischemic reperfusion injury is an important determinant of complications. Therefore, CoQ10 should be administered immediately upon suspicion of infarction, preferably intravenously and before the thrombolytic agents, to achieve maximum protection. Since this drug has no side effects, and thus may not require ethical approval for conducting trials with CoQ10.

ACKNOWLEDGEMENTS

Acknowledgements are due to Mr. Raj Chopra, Tishcon Corporation, NY, USA for a grant for completion of this work.

REFERENCES

1. Greenberg S, Frishman WH. 1990. CoQ10. A new drug for cardiovascular disease. J Clin Pharmacol 30:596–608.
2. Ernster L, Dallner G. 1995. Biochemical, physiological and medical aspects of ubiquinone function. Biochemica Biophys Acta 1271:195–204.
3. Langajoen PH, Langajoen AM. 1998. CoQ10 in cardiovascular disease with emphasis on heart failure and myocardial ischemia. Asia Pac Heart J 7:160–168.
4. Singh RB, Niaz MA, Rastogi V, Rastogi SS. 1998. Coenzyme Q in cardiovascular disease. JAPI 46:299–306.
5. Kagan V, Packer L. 1993. Electron transport regenerates vitamin E in mitochondria and microsomes via ubiquione: an antioxidant duet. In: Free radicals and antioxidants and nutrition. Ed. F Corongni, S Banni, MA Desai and C Rice Evans, 27–36. London: Richelieu Press.
6. Stocker R, Bowry WE, Frei B. 1991. Ubiquionol-10 protects human low density lipoprotein more efficiently against lipid peroxidation than does alpha-tocopherol. Proc Natl Acad Sci USA 88:1646–1650.
7. Merati G, Pasquali P, Vergani C, Landi L. 1992. Antioxidant activity of ubiquinone-3 in human low density lipoprotein. Free Rad Res Common 16:11–17.
8. Mohr D, Bowry VW, Stocker R. 1992. Dietary supplementation with CoQ10 results in increased levels of ubiquionol-10 within circulating lipoproteins and increased resistance of human low density lipoprotein to the initiation of lipid peroxidation. Biochim Biophys Acta 1126:247–254.
9. Esconde D, Cavero I. 1992. Potassium channel openers: moving towards cardioprotection via strengthening of a natural mechanism. Trends Pharmacol Sci 13:269–272.
10. Singh RB, Rastogi SS, Moshiri M. 1999. CoQ10 and its role in heart disease. J Clin Biochem Nutr 26:109–118.
11. Singh RB, Niaz MA. 1996. Antioxidants, oxidants and free radical stress in cardiovascular disease. J Asso Phys India 44:43–48.
12. Sundarroa M, Quinn P. 1986. Proton magnetic resonance spectroscopic studies of the interaction of ubiquinone-l0 with phospholipid membranes. Int J Biochem 155:353–358.
13. Niki E. 1993. Chemistry and biochemistry of vitamin E and coenzyme Q as antioxidants. In: Free radicals and antioxidants in nutrition. Ed. F Corogin, S Banni, MA Desai and C Rice-Evans, 13–25. London: Richelieu Press.
14. Langsjoen PH, Vadhanavikit S, Folkers K. 1994. Effective treatment with CoQ10 of patients with myocardial disease class III and IV. In: Biomedical Clinical aspects of coenzyme Q, Vol. 4. Ed. K Folkers and Y Yamamura, 325–339. Amsterdam: Elsevier.
15. Hiasa Y, Ishida T, Maeda T, Iwanc K, Aihara T, Mori H. 1984. Effects of CoQ10 on exercise tolerance in patients with stable angina. In: Biomedical and Clinical Aspects of CoQ10. Ed. K Folker, T Yamagami and GP Littarru, 291–301. Amsterdam: Elsevier.
16. Serra G, Lissoni F, Piemonti C, Mazzda C. 1991. Evaluation of CoQ10 in patients with moderate heart failure and chronic stable angina. In: Biomedical and Clinical Aspects of CoQ10. Ed. K Folker, T Yamagami and GP Littarru. Amsterdam: Elsevier.
17. Kamikawa T, Kobayashi A, Yamashita T, Hayashi H, Yamasaki N. 1985. Effects of CoQ10 on exercise tolerance in chronic stable angina pectoris. Am J Cardiol 56:247–251.
18. Schardr F, Welzel D, Schess W, Toda K. 1986. Effect of CoQ10 on ischaemia induced ST-segment depression: a double blind placebo controlled crossover study. In: Biomedical and Clinical Aspects of CoQ10, Vol. 5. Ed. K Folkers and Y Yamamura, 385–394. Amsterdam: Elsevier.
19. Rossi E, Lombardo A, Testa M, Lippa S, Oradei A, Littarru GP, Lucente M, Coppola E, Manzoli U. 1991. CoQ10 in ischemic cardiopathy. In: Biomedical and clinical aspects of coenzyme Q, Vol. 6. Ed. K Folkers, GP Littarru and T Yamagami, 321–326. Amsterdam: Elsevier.
20. Wilson MF, Frishman WH, Giles T, Sethi G, Greenberg SM, Brackett DJ. 1991. CoQ10 therapy and exercise duration in stable angina. In: Biomedical and clinical aspects of coenzyme Q. Vol. 6. Ed. K Folkers, GP Littarru and T Yamagami, 339–348. Amsterdam, Elsevier.
21. Mazzola C, Guffanti EE, Vaccarella A, Meregalli M, Colmago R, Ferrario N, Cantoni V, Marcherri G. 1987. Noninvasive assessment of CoQ10 in patients with chronic stable effort angina and moderate heart failure. Curr Ther Res 41:923–930.
22. Ursini F, Gambini C, Paciaroni E, Littarru GP. CoQ10 treatment of heart failure in elderly. preliminary results. In: Biomedical and clinical aspects of coenzyme Q, Vol 6. Eds. K Folkers, GP Littaru and T Yamagami, 473–480. Amsterdam, Elsevier.
23. Hofman-Bang C, Rehnqvist N, Swedberg K, Astrom H. 1992. CoQ10 as an adjunctive in treatment of congestive heart failure. J Am Coll Cardiol 19(Suppl):774–776.

24. Morisco C, Trimarco B, Condorelli M. 1993. Effect of CoQ10 therapy in patients with congestive heart failure: a long term multicentre randomized study. Clin Invest 71(Suppl):134–136.
25. Mortensen SA, Vadhanavikit S, Folkers K. 1984. Apparent effectiveness of CoQ10 (CoQ) to treat patients with cardiomyopathy and CoQ levels in blood and endomyocardial biopsies. In: Biomedical and clinical aspects of coenzyme Q, Vol 6. Ed. K Folkers and T Yamagami, 391–402. Amsterdam, Elsevier.
26. Permanetter B, Rossy W, Weingartner F, Baner R, Seidi KF, Klein G, Fehende Wirksamkeit von. 1989. CoQ10 (Ubiquinone) bei der Iangzeitbehandlung der dilatativen Kardiomyopathie. Z. Kardiol 78:360–365.
27. Judy WV, Folkers K, Hall JH. 1991. Improved long-term survival in CoQ10 treated congestive heart failure patients compared to conventionally treated patients. In: Biomedical and clinical aspects of coenzyme Q, Vol 6. Ed. K Folkers, GP Littarru and T Yamagami, 291–298. Amsterdam, Elsevier.
28. Longsjoen PH, Vadhanavikit S, Folkers K. 1985. Response of patients in class III and IV of cardiomyopathy to therapy in a blind and crossover trial with CoQ10. Proc Natl Acad Sci USA 82:4240–4244.
29. Vanfraechem JPH, Pikalausa C, Folkers K. 1986. Effects of CoQ10 on physical performance and recovery in myocardial failure. In: Biomedical and clinical aspects of CoQ10. Ed. K Folkers and Y Yamamura, 5:371–377. Amsterdam, Elsevier.
30. Judy Wr, Hall JH, Toth PD, Folkers K, Yamamura Y. 1986. Double blind, crossover study of coenzyme Q10 in heart failure. In: Biomedical and Clinical Aspects of CoQ10, 5:315–323. Amsterdam: Elsevier.
31. Oda T. 1990. Effect of CoQ10 on load-induced cardiac dysfunction: double blind study and investigation of dose response relationship. In: Highlights in buiquinone research. Ed. G Lenaz, Q Bamabei, A Rabbi, and M Battino, 232–237. London: Taylor and Francis.
32. Poggesi L, Galanti G, Comeglio M, Toncelli L, Vinci M. 1991. Effect of CoQ10 on left ventricular function in patients with dialated cardiomyopathy. A medium term randomized double blind study versus placebo. Curr Ther Res, 49: 878–886.
33. Yamamura Y. 1985. A survey of therapeutic uses of CoQ10. In: Biochemistry, Bioenergetics, and Clinical Applications of Ubiquinone. Ed. G Lenaz, 479–505. Chickester: Lok Wiley L Sons.
34. Dhalla AK, Hill MF, Singal PK. 1996. Role of oxidative stress in transition of hypertrophy to heart failure. J Am Coll Cardiol, 28:506–514.
35. Sinatra ST. 1997. Treatment of congestive heart failure with CoQ10 illuminated by metaanalysis of clinical trials. Molec Aspects Med 18:299–305.
36. Soja AM, Mortensen SA. 1997. Treatment of congestive heart failure with CoQ10 illuminated by metannalysis of clinical trials. Molec Aspects Med. 18:159–168.
37. Watson PS, Scalia GM, Galbraith A, Burstow DJ, Bett N, Aroney CN. 1999. Lack of effect of coenzyme Q on left ventricular function in patients with congestive heart failure. J Am Coll Cardiol 33:1549–1552.
38. Khatta M, Alexandewr BS, Krichten CM, Fisher ML, Frendanberger R, Rovinson SW, Gottleit SS. 2000. The effect of CoQ10 in patients with congestive heart failure. Ann Intern Med 132:636–640.
39. Takasawa K, Fuse K, Konishi T, Watanabe Y. 1991. Prevention of premature ventricular contractions with CoQ10 after coronary artery bypass grafting. In: Biomedical and Clinical Aspects of coenzyme Q, Vol. 6. Ed. K Folkers, CP Littarru and T Yamagami, 357–359. Amsterdam: Elsevier.
40. Fihirdi B, Vsnyini G, Oradei A, Biusi G, Guarino GC, Brocchi A, Bellandi F, Mancini M, Littarru GP. 1994. CoQ10 in essential hypertension. Mol Aspects Med 15(Suppl):275–283.
41. Langsjoen P, Wills R, Folkers K. 1994. Treatment of essential hypertension with CoQ10. Mol Aspects Med 15(Suppl):265–272.
42. Singh RB, Niaz MA, Rastogi SS, Shukla PK, Thakur AS. 1999. Effect of hydrosoluble CoQ10 on blood pressures and insulin resistance in hypertensive patients with coronary artery disease. J Human Hyper 13:203–208.
43. Iarussi D, Auricchi U, Murano A, Giuliano M, DI Tullio MT, Iacono A. 1994. Protective effect of coenzyme Q on anthracyclines cardiotoxicity: control study in children with acute hymphoblastic leukemia or non-Hodgkin lymphoma. Mol Aspects Med 15(Suppl):207–212.
44. Ghirlanda G, Oradei A, Manto A, Lippa S, Uccioli L, Caputa S, Greco AV, Littaru GP. 1993. Evidence of plasma CoQ10 lowering effect by HMGCOA reductase inhibitors, a double blind placebo controlled trial. J Clin Pharmacol 33:226–229.
45. Bargossi AM, Battino M, Gaddi A, Fiorella PL, Grossi G, Barozzi G, Di Giulio R, Descovich G, Sassi S, Genova ML, Lenaz G. 1994. Exogenous CoQ10 preserves plasma ubiquinone levels in patients

treated with 3-hydroxy-3-methylglutaryl coenzyme A reductase inhibitors. Int J Clin Lab Res 24:171–176.
46. Singh RB, Singh NK, Rastogi SS, Wander GS, Aslam M, Onouchi Z, Kummerow FA. 1997. Antioxidant effects of lovastatin and vitamin E on experimental atherosclerosis in rabbits. Cardiovas Drug Ther 11:575–580.
47. Singh RB, Chopra RK, Niaz MA, Kapoor R. 1999. Serum concentration of lipoprotein (a) decreases on treatment with hydro soluble CoQ10 in patients with acute coronary artery disease. Discovery of a new role. Int J Cardiol 68:23–29.
48. Singh RB, Shinde SN, Chopra RK, Niaz MA, Thakur AS, Onouchi Z. 2000. Effect of CoQ10 on experimental atherosclerosis and chemical composition and quality of atheroma. Atherosclerosis 148:275–282.
49. Serebruany VL, Ordonez JV, Herzog WR, Rohde M, Mortensen SA, Folkers K, Gurbel PA. 1997. Dietary CoQ10 supplementation alters platelet size and inhibits human vitronectin (CD 51/CD61) receptro expression. J Cardiovasc Pharmacol 29:16–22.
50. Kuklinski B, Weissenbacker E, Fahnrich A. 1994. CoQ10 and antioxidants in acute myocardial infarction. Mol Aspects Med 15(Suppl):143–147.
51. Singh RB, Wander GS, Rastogi A, Shukla PK, Mittal A, Sharma JP. 1998. Randomized, double blind, placebo controlled trial of CoQ10 in patients with acute myocardial infarction. Cardiovasc Drug Ther 12:347–353.
52. Quinn PJ, Fabisiak JP, Kagan VE. 1999. Expansion of antioxidant function of vitamin E by coenzyme Q. Bio Factors 4:149–154.
53. Littarru GP, Ho L, Folkers K. 1972. Deficiency of CoQ10 in human heart disease II. Int J Vit Nutur Res 42:413–415.
54. Littarru GP, Ho L, Folkers K. 1972. Deficiency of CoQ10 in human heart disease. Int J Vit Nutur Res 42:291–295.
55. Thomas SR, Neuzil J, Stocker R. 1996. Co-supplementation with coenzyme Q prevents the prooxidant effect of alpha-tocopherol and increases the resistance of LDL to transition metal-dependent oxidation initiation. Arterio Thromb Vas. Biol 16:687–696.
56. Aejmelaeus R, Metsa-Ketela, T, Laippala P, Alho H, Solakvi T. 1997. Ubiquinol-10 and total peroxyl radical trapping capacity of LDL lipoproteins during aging the effect of Q10 supplementation. Mol Aspects Med 18(Supple):113–120.
57. Alleva R, Tomasetti M, Battino M, Curatola G, Littarru GP, Folkers K. 1995. The role of CoQ10 and vitamin E on peroxidation of human low density subfractions. Proc Natl Acad Sci USA 92: 9388–93.
58. Rudney H, Nambudiri AMD, Ranganathan S. 1981. The regulation of the synthesis of coenzyme Q in fibroblasts and in heart muscle. In: Biomedical and Clinical Aspects of coenzyme Q. Ed. K Folkers and Y Yamamura, 279–290. Amsterdam: Elsevier North Holland Press.
59. Davies M. 1996. Stability and unstabi1ity: two faces of coronary atherosclerosis. Circulation 94: 2013–2020.
60. Davies MJ. 2000. Pathophysiology of acute coronary syndromes. Heart 83:361–366.
61. Libby P, Aikawa M. 1998. New insights in plague stabilization by lipid lowering. Drugs (Suppl):9–13.
62. Wesissberg PL. 2000. Atherogenesis: current understanding of the causes of atheroma. Heart 83:247–252.
63. MAAS Investigators. 1994. Effect of simvastatin on coronary atheroma. The multicentre Anti Atheroma Study (MAAS) Lancet 334:633–638.
64. LIPID Study Group. 1998. Prevention of cardiovascular events and death with pravastatin in patients with coronary heart disease and a broad range of initial cholesterol levels. The Long term Intervention with Pravastatin in Ischemic. Disease (LIPID) Study. N Engl J Med 339:1349–1357.
65. Thomas SR, Witting PK, Stocker R. 1999. A role of reduced coenzyme Q in atherosclerosis. Bio Factors 9:207–224.
66. Tomasetti M, Alleva R, Solenghi MD, Littarru GP. 1999. Distribution of antioxidants among blood components and lipoproteins. Significance of lipids/CoQ10 ratio as a possible marker of increased risk of atherosclerosis. Bio Factors 9:225–230.
67. Thomas SR, Neuzil J, Mohr D, Stocker R. 1995. Co-antioxidants made alphatocopherol an efficient antioxidant for LDL. Am J Clin Nutr 62:13575–13645.
68. Thomas SR, Neuzil J, Stocker R. 1996. Co-supplementation with coenzyme Q prevents the proxidant effect of alpha-tocopherol and increase the resistance of low density lipoprotein towards transition metal-dependent oxidation initiation. Arterioscler Thromb Vase Biol 16:687–696.

69. Shanalan C, Weissberg P. 1998. Smooth muscle cell heterogeneity: Patterns of gene expression in vascular smooth muscle cells in vitro and in vivo. Arterioscler Thromb Vase Biol 18:333–338.
70. Cleary J, Mohr D, Adams MR, Celermager DS, Stocker R. 1997. Plasma LDL levels of major lipophilic antioxidants are similar in patients with advanced atherosclerosis and healthy controls. Free Radic Res 26:175–182.
71. Lagendijk J, Ubbink JB, Delport R, Vermaak WJ, Human JA. 1997. Ubiquinol/ubiquinone ratio as marker of oxidative stress in coronary artery disease. Res Commu Mol Pathol Pharmacol 95:11–20.
72. Surana C, Dean RT, May J, Stocker R. 1995. Human atherosclerotic plaque contains both oxidized lipids and relatively large amounts of alpha-tocopherol and ascorate. Arterioscler Thromb Vasc Biol 15:1616–1624.
73. Niu E, Zammit V, Upston JM, Dean RT, Stocker R. 1999. Co-existence of oxidized lipids and alpha-tocopherol in lipoprotein fractions isolated from advanced human atherosclerotic plaques. Arterioscler Thromb Vasc Biol (in press).
74. Leichtweis S, Lau A, Thomas S, Witting P, Kap Choy, Patterson K, Croft K, Mori T, Brown A, Stocker R. 2000. Inhibition of in vivo lipoprotein lipid peroxidation and atherosclerosis by CoQ10 in two animal models. 2nd conference of CoQ10 Association, Abstract 10:60–62.
75. Falk E, Shah P, Fuster V. 1995. Coronary plaque disruption. Circulation 92:657–671.
76. Langsjoen PH, Langsjoen AM. 1999. Overview of the use of CoQ10 in cardiovascular disease, Bio Factors 9:273–284.
77. Nibori K, Wroblewski KP, Yokoyama H, Juan A, Crestanello JA, Whitman GJR. 1999. Bioenergetic effect of liposomal CoQ10 on myocardial ischaemia reperfusion injury. Bio Factors 9:307–313.
78. Herzog WR, Schlossberg ML, Mortensen SA, Serebruany VL. 1995. Dietary supplementation with CoQ10 reduces platelet aggregability in swine. coenzyme Q. Res Biol Med 3:5–8.
79. Kontush A, Reich A, Baum K, Spranger T, Finckh B, Kohlschutter A, Beisiegel U. 1997. Plasma ubiquinol is decreased in patients with hyperlipidemia. Atherosclerosis 129:119–126.
80. Baggio G, Gandini R, Planchar AC, Passeri M, Carmosion G. 1994. Italian multicentre study on the safety and efficacy of CoQ10 as adjunctive therapy in heart failure. Mol Aspects Med 15(Suppl.): 287–294.
81. Sunamori M, Suzuki A. 1998. Improved efficacy of intra aortic balloon pumping by pharmacological myocardial protection of postoperative pump failure after coronary revascularization. Jpn J Surg 18:61–67.
82. Judy WV, Stogsdill WW, Folkers K. 1993. Myocardial preservation by therapy with CoQ10 during heart surgery. The Clin Invest 71(Suppl 8):155–161.
83. Chen YF, Lin TY, Wu SC. 1994. Effectiveness of CoQ10 on myocardial preservation during hypothermic cardioplegic arrest. J Thor Cardiovasc Surg 107:242–247.
84. Taggart DP, Jenkins M, Hooper J, Handjinikolas L, Kemp M, Hue D, Dennett G. 1996. Effects of short term supplementation with CoQ10 on myocardial protection during cardiac operations. Ann Thorac Surg 61:829–833.

III. Lifestyle and Global Cardiovascular Burden

Frontiers in Cardiovascular Health, edited by
N.S. Dhalla, A. Chockalingam,
H.I. Berkowitz & P.K. Singal
Kluwer Academic Publishers, Boston, 2003

Global Burden of Cardiovascular Disease: Impending Pandemic in Developing Countries and Economies in Transition

Arun Chockalingam[1] and Mario F. de Camargo Maranhao[2]

[1] *Assistant Director, Institute of Circulatory and Respiratory Health, Canadian Institutes of Health Research, & Clinical Professor of Health Care and Epidemiology, University of British Columbia, Vancouver, B.C., Canada*
[2] *President, World Heart Federation, Geneva, Switzerland & Professor of Cardiology, Evangelical School of Medicine and Hospital, Curitiba, Brazil*

Summary. As the second millennium ended, Cardiovascular disease (CVD) (heart disease and stroke) accounted for over 15 million death world-wide. Much of these deaths due to CVD occurred in the developing countries (DC) and economies in transition (ET) (former Soviet Union countries). The projections for the next two decades are even more alarming for DC and ET, as the CVD would become the number one cause of death. Many of the international organizations including World Health Organization (WHO), World Heart Federation (WHF), World Bank (WB), and others are concerned about this growing epidemic. As the non-communicable diseases are rising in the DC and ET, in contrast to the decline in developed countries, they face a double jeopardy of both communicable and non-communicable disease burden.

In an attempt to combat the pandemic of CVD in DC and ET, the WHF assessed the global situation to take stock of (i) available resources—both human and fiscal; (ii) base-line data on which to embark on programs; (iii) prevention programs and legislations. The outcome of this effort was a resource document entitled "*Global Pandemic of Cardiovascular Disease: Opportunities for prevention and control of cardiovascular disease in developing countries and economies in transition*", often referred to as the **WHF White Book**.

This paper describes the magnitude of the problem of CVD, burden of disease, lack of baseline data, prevention programs and absence of legislation against tobacco. Based on the White Book, it is clear that the DC and ET can not afford to follow the western medical strategy to solve the CVD epidemic, since the available resources in many of these countries is $25, or less, per person per year for the entire health care. It is essential to approach this

Correspondence to: Dr. Arun Chockalingam, ICRH/CIHR, 1081 Burrard Street, Suite 553, Vancouver, B.C., Canada V6Z 1Y6. Tel: 604-806-8932, E-mail: achockalingam@mrl.ubc.ca.

issue largely through health promotion, and primordial and primary prevention. At the same time, clinical care should be provided to those who have been manifested with the disease. Available resources must be equitably expended with careful planning. There is a role for health professionals and voluntary agencies to partner with international agencies, the public and governments in addressing the CVD pandemic. The lessons learnt from the west could be adopted in the DC and ET with appropriate cultural sensitivities. This is a global problem and the solutions must be global too.

Key words: Cardiovascular disease, prevention, developing countries, health promotion, partnership.

INTRODUCTION

"No era in human history has been distinguished by so much scientific and cultural advance, at the same time burdened with so much abysmal barbarism. We physicians have a role in preventing the new millennium from becoming overwhelmed by tribalism, nuclearism and savagery. To fulfill this role requires expanding the outreach of our health professionalism.

We are witnessing the emergence of an all encompassing globalism. This has not slowed the growing divide between the industrialized nations living amidst prodigious wealth and the developing countries subsisting in profound poverty. Such a world order is an augury for mounting tensions and endless wars. In an age bristling with nuclear as well as other pernicious weapons of mass destruction, threatened is unprecedented misery and a further despoiling of an already frayed global environment.

A hopeful fact though is that healthy people have deeper social stakes in their communities and are less likely to resort to desperate means. Good health is a major factor favoring social cohesion and stability."

Bernard Lown, Nobel Laureate (1)

The world we live in faces a dramatic change in the pattern of health and disease as we move into the new millennium. As highlighted in reports from the World Health Organization (WHO) (2), Victoria Declaration (3) the World Bank (4) and Murray and Lopez (5), the burden of disease in developing countries will become more closely aligned with the one that currently afflicts developed countries. As documented in the 1997 World Health Report (2), cardiovascular diseases (CVD) represent more than 30% of all deaths worldwide today or close to 15 million each year, with about 9 million of those in developing countries and 2 million in economies in transition (formerly socialist countries of central and eastern Europe), as shown in Table 1. The two most frequent causes of cardiovascular disease are coronary heart disease (CHD) and cerebrovascular disease or stroke. By 1990, the single biggest cause of death worldwide was CHD. In fact, CHD accounted for over 6 million deaths, with 1.7 million in the established market economies, 1 million in economies in transition and 3.6 million in developing countries. Cerebrovascular diseases, especially stroke, accounted for more than 4 million deaths, and of these the vast majority, 3 million, were in developing countries (4). Rheumatic fever and rheumatic heart disease (RF/RHD) and inflammatory heart disease accounted for close to half a million deaths each in 1990 (5) (see Table 2). RF/RHD are among the most, if not *the* most, preventable of cardiovascular diseases.

Table 1. Total and cardiovascular mortality[5] (in thousands) in 1990 and 2020 (baseline scenario)

		Total Mortality			Cardiovascular Mortality		
Year	Population	Numbers	Rate per 100,000	% Difference	Numbers	Rate per 100,000	% Difference
WORLD							
1990	5,267,000	50,467	958	−9.1	14,326	272	+16.2
2020	7,844,000	68,337	871		81,324	316	
ESTABLISHED MARKET ECONOMIES							
1990	798,000	7,121	892	+7.4	3,175	398	+1.8
2020	905,000	8,651	958		3,663	405	
ECONOMIES IN TRANSITION							
1990	346,000	3,791	1,095	+21.5	2,071	599	+19.4
2020	365,000	4,854	1,330		2,608	715	
DEVELOPING COUNTRIES							
1990	4,123,000	39,554	959	−13.0	9,081	220	+28.2
2020	6,574,000	54,832	834		18,542		282

Some totals may not be the same as the one shown for WORLD since the numbers have been rounded off.

Table 2. Estimates of cardiovascular deaths in 1990[5]

	Populations (millions)	Deaths (thousands)						
		All	CVD	CHD	Stroke	RHD	InHD	Other HD
MEN								
World	2,654	26,962	6,942	3,126	2,022	141	247	1,407
Established market economies	390	3,659	1,491	829	322	6	33	301
Economies in transition	165	1,908	885	468	239	10	19	148
India	439	4,875	1,165	619	227	29	41	249
China	585	4,829	1,322	386	672	69	33	163
Other Asia & Islands	343	3,044	681	233	190	5	43	210
Sub-sahara Africa	344	4,324	344	92	152	9	28	63
Latin America & Caribbean	222	1,654	395	179	121	3	12	80
Middle Eastern Crescent	256	2,399	658	319	99	10	37	194
WOMEN								
World	2,614	23,775	7,385	3,134	2,359	199	249	1,444
Established market economies	407	3,462	1,684	838	467	14	32	332
Economies in transition	181	1,883	1,186	559	400	15	20	193
India	410	2,356	1,100	556	220	41	42	241
China	548	4,056	1,246	377	601	94	33	142
Other Asia & Islands	340	2,490	667	227	200	6	39	196
Sub-sahara Africa	258	3,878	471	117	231	11	35	77
Latin America & Caribbean	223	1,355	394	169	127	6	12	80
Middle Eastern Crescent	247	2,154	637	291	113	14	35	184

CVD = cardiovascular, CHD = coronary heart disease, RHD = rheumatic heart disease, InHD = inflammatory heart disease.

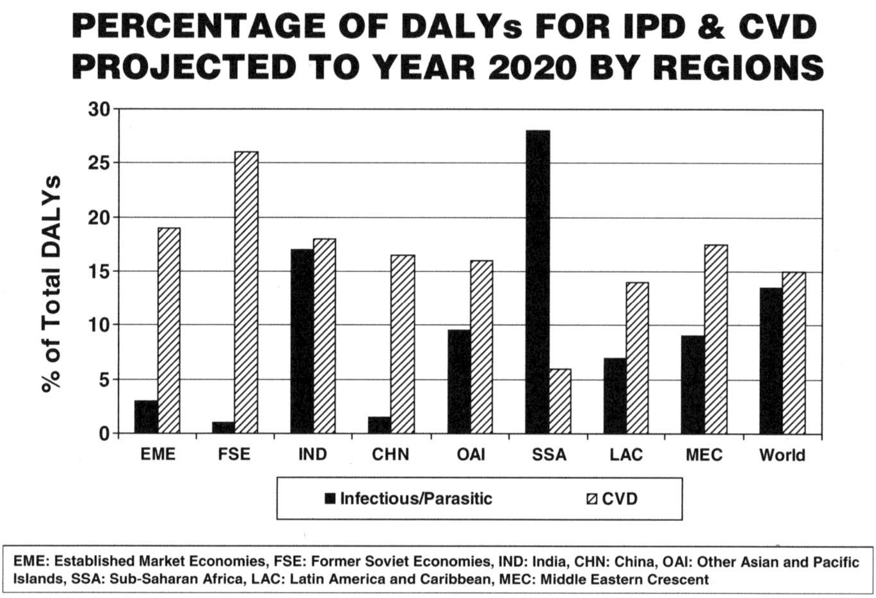

Figure 1. Percentage of Dalys for IPD & CVD Projected to Year 2020 by Regions.

By the year 2020, cardiovascular diseases (CVD) will be added to infectious diseases as the leading causes of death and disability. Such a burden of disease expressed in terms of disability adjusted life years (DALYs) for infectious/parsitic diseases (IPD) and CVD projected to year 2020 is shown in Figure 1 (5). In addition, in countries with economies in transition the CVD burden is much higher than that observed in developed countries, and with some exceptions there is no decline in mortality rates.

Why are we observing such changes in the pattern of diseases and the massive increase in heart disease in the developing world? The dynamics of this transition have been extensively analysed in two significant reports (6,7) and the major determinants identified:

1. the growing life expectancy;
2. the falling infant mortality rate;
3. the decline in infectious disease rates;
4. the increase in gross national product and in per capita income enabling the populations of these nations to adopt the "unhealthy" lifestyles and behaviours of the more developed countries; and
5. the genetic and environmental interaction.

ISSUES AND TASKS

There are three main issues.

- First, there is great variation in the prevalence and trends in CVD between developing countries, economies in transition and developed countries, as seen in rates of RF/RHD, risk factors, Coronary Artery Disease (CAD) and stroke. Corresponding tasks are to define the gaps in our knowledge, and to bring together data on the extent of the growing cardiovascular burden in each country or region. Note that many countries do not have base-line data on the prevalence and incidence of CAD and stroke.
- Second, there are huge disparities in the health care resources available in each country, whether this is money, skilled personnel or the infrastructure needed to mount effective campaigns at the population or the clinical level. The corresponding task is to determine the current levels of available resources in each of the developing countries and economies in transition to fight heart disease in the same region.
- Third, there is a need to coordinate global, regional and local programmes with a clear differentiation of the programme in each region or country to match the available resources. Corrseponding task is to put forward a comprehensive strategic framework for international action to minimize this "second epidemic wave" of cardiovascular disease.

METHODS

To address these issues the World Heart Federation commissioned an international expert committee to gather the data and provide possible solutions. The committee published its findings as a reference book, popularly known as the *White Book* (1). The problems caused by the second epidemic wave catching up with the first wave, are the focus of this book and of the programme of action of the WHF in the years ahead.

Apart from the references to published data, the chief source of information for the White Book has come from two detailed questionnaires, one on public health and the other on clinical resources, sent to 106 countries (54 WHF members and 52 non-members).

The **public health information questionnaire**, assessing the importance of CVD prevention, elicited information on the current status of CVD policies and programmes in all these countries, i.e. on the availability of epidemiologic data, national/regional surveys, CV risk factors, the existence of guidelines for individual risk factors, availability of drugs, sources of funding for prevention, evaluation of different resources, and government's priority for CVD. This questionnaire was circulated in the month of June 1998 and responses were collected until February 1999.

The **clinical resources questionnaire** evaluated the resources available by eliciting information on the current status of clinical care capacity and infrastructures in order to meet the need for CVD prevention and treatment. This questionnaire on clinicians, hospitals and beds, CVD procedures and schools of cardiology was sent out to national societies of cardiology, national heart foundations and some government agencies and returns were collected between September 1997 and September 1998.

In analysing the data on the activities, resources and infrastructures existing in the different nations, it seemed reasonable to divide all countries into three separate regions. Although it is recognized that the availability of resources varies considerably among countries of the same region and among regions, this grouping allows an overall view of the issues concerned. At the same time it is possible to identify common areas in which the same strategies and actions could improve health and prevent CVD.

1. The first region is economies in transition (Eastern and Central Europe [ECE]), in which resources, CVD infrastructures and procedures are available and some sort of CVD prevention programmes are undertaken. These countries need implementation and guidelines to carry on and develop what already exists.
2. The second region is Latin America and Caribbean (LAC) and the Middle Eastern Crescent (MEC). Even though they are geographically apart, all these countries have a similar background. They lack infrastructures, despite the proportion of human resources available. These countries seem to need encouragement and sensitization to increase effective policies and programmes to improve health.
3. The third region is Asian and African (AF&AS) countries. In this particular situation, in order to cope with the complete deficiency of all resources, it is necessary to start from the basics to ensure improvements in protecting and promoting health.

RESULTS

Mortality

Out of the estimated 52 million deaths worldwide in 1996, about 40 million occurred in the developing world and 12 million in developed countries. Of the latter, 4.4 million deaths occurred in economies in transition. Overall, CVD accounted for nearly 30% of total mortality. Of the 15.3 million CVD deaths per year, 5.5 million deaths occurred in developed countries (45%), including economies in transition, and 10 million deaths occurred in developing countries (25%). Infectious and parasitic diseases are still a frequent cause of death in developing countries, particularly perinatal and neonatal deaths (2) (Table 3).

Morbidity

Data on **morbidity** attributed to CVD are very scarce and come mainly from the WHO MONICA Project (8), which registered acute events in small geographic areas in developed countries, economies in transition and developing countries, such as the People's Republic of China.

The rising CVD rates of mortality and morbidity in developing countries and the already high rates in economies in transition raise concerns about the quality

Table 3. Worldwide estimates of causes of death in 1996[2]

Yearly Deaths, in thousands, (percentage of total)	Entire World	Developed World*	Developing World
All causes	52,037	12,116	39,921
Circulatory system	15,300 (29.0%)	5,522 (45.6%)	9,778 (24.5%)
Cancer	6,346 (12.0%)	2,544 (21.0%)	3,802 (9.5%)
Respiratory system	2,888 (6.0%)	979 (8.0%)	1,909 (4.8%)
Infectious & parasitic disease	17,312 (33.0%)	151 (1.2%)	17,161 (43.0%)
Peri & neonatal disease	3,745 (7.0%)	119 (1.0%)	6,626 (9.1%)
Maternal causes	585 (1.0%)	3 (0.0%)	582 (1.0%)
Other & unknown	5,861 (12.0%)	2,798 (23.1%)	3,063 (7.0%)

*Including the economies in transition of Europe.

of clinical care available to people with manifest CVD in these regions and about the quality of life of those with CVD. Information on case-fatality rates, clinical practice patterns (selected for both disease and risk factor management) and quality of life measures is required for such an appraisal. However, such data are very scarce in both developing countries and economies in transition.

Gross national product (GNP)

Great variation was observed in the GNP and in its percentage allocated to health care resources. The national health system provides coverage of the entire population in economies in transition (Eastern and Central Europe) and in only a few countries in the developing world. In many countries it covers only a small percentage of the population. Also, private insurance companies play a role only in a few developing countries. The financial resources available for the whole population are still very limited if we compare the GNP and the number of inhabitants. On average, many developing countries have a health care budget of less than $25 US per person per year. In the world's most populous countries, such as India and China, the per capita health care budget is $17 and $31 respectively (9).

Public health issues

Only 47 out of 105 countries responded. To the question "whether representative data from CVD and risk factor surveys were carried out in the past five years" only 32 (13 reported having representative data at the national level, 17 countries at the regional level and 14 countries in selected communities) responded positively.

With respect to practice guidelines, of the 11 items assessed, the maximum positive response was for hypertension (58%), followed by lipids (43%), rheumatic heart disease (40%), acute myocardial infarction (36%), congestive heart failure (34%), tobacco control (28%), dietary recommendations (26%), stroke (23%), diabetes mellitus (21%) and physical activity (21%). The lowest positive response, of 9%, was reported for obesity guidelines.

When the question was asked whether the guidelines were developed by national expert bodies, a positive response was given less than 50% of the time for all guideline areas: hypertension (40%), followed by diabetes mellitus (36%), lipids (32%), rheumatic heart disease (28%), acute myocardial infarction (28%), congestive heart failure (23%), dietary recommendations (23%), tobacco control (19%), stroke (13%), physical activity (13%) and obesity (9%).

When countries were asked whether international guidelines had been adopted, positive responses were even less common. Strikingly, the maximum response, based on regional analysis, came from ECE countries. This could perhaps be attributable to three factors: 1. the active CINDI (Country-wide Integrated Non-communicable Disease Intervention) programmes in these countries; 2. the implementation of many prevention programmes during the socialist period, developed as a result of their expressed needs and cooperation with WHO; and 3. the commitment of the cardiological societies of these countries to implement the recommendations of the Task Force of the European Society of Cardiology, European Atherosclerosis Society and European Society of Hypertension on prevention of coronary heart disease in clinical practice (10,11).

In terms of implementation of these guidelines at the practitioner level, the responses were dismal. They ranged from 19% for conditions such as hypertension and tobacco control down to 2% for dietary recommendations and further down, to 0%, for obesity. Because the numbers are small, regional analysis is not possible.

Only a third of the respondent countries reported having national programmes on the prevention of (a) CVD, including stroke, (b) hypertension, (c) tobacco consumption, (d) rheumatic heart disease and (e) diabetes.

A mere 49% of the countries (note: response rate was 47/105) reported a positive response for programmes targeted towards children, followed by women (34%), elderly people (23%) and those at the work site (19%).

Nearly two-thirds of respondent countries reported that essential cardiovascular and metabolic drugs are easily available. However, only half of them reported that these drugs are affordable by the majority of the population.

A very low response rate was registered for the question of national legislation related to tobacco sale, tobacco advertising, public smoking, food labelling and drug pricing. Legislation varies among countries and among regions of the world. For many of the issues, the responses are far from optimal. The low response for "tobacco sale" indicates the influence of multinational tobacco companies on national governments.

Finally, with respect to the question: "Does your government consider CVD prevention a national reality?", a positive response was given by four countries in Africa (Benin, Seychelles, Tunisia and Zimbabwe), three in Asia (China, Sri Lanka and Thailand), none from Latin America and the Carribean, three from the Middle Eastern Crescent (Egypt, Iran and Syria), and nine countries from Eastern and Central Europe (Bulgaria, Croatia, Georgia Republic, Hungary, Latvia, Lithuania, Macedonia, Russian Federation, and Ukraine). Thus 19 out of 47 (40%) respondent countries said "Yes" to this question, which is a surprisingly high rate. In reality, it

Table 4. Human resources per million population (cardiovascular only)

Region	Cardiologist	Cardiac surgeons	Cardiology trainees	Cardiovascular nurses
Spain (Reference)	50.21	6.41	7.55	12.53
AF&AS	2.12	0.93	0.46	1.67
LAC&MEC	65.04	5.04	6.99	5.06
ECE	41.91	6.04	7.84	102.5

could be the wishful thinking of the people who filled in the questionnaire, since there is no information to corroborate government policies towards CVD prevention in many of these countries. This situation needs to be carefully examined further.

Resources

To compare the resources between developing and developed countries, Spain was chosen to represent developed countries.

a) Human

There is a lack of adequately trained personnel throughout Asia and Africa, which have fewer than three cardiology specialists per million inhabitants (Table 4). Other developing countries and economies in transition have between 10 and 150 cardiologists per million, while more than 100 per million were reported in Georgia, Argentina and Uruguay. A relation was observed between the number of cardiologists in each country and the number of general physicians (GPs). No adequate information was available from China and India.

b) Cardiovascular infrastructures

- Departments of cardiology are less than 1 per million inhabitants in nearly all the developing countries, with the lowest points reached in Asia and sub-Saharan Africa (less than 0.2). Economies in transition (Central and Eastern Europe) have between 1 and 11 departments of cardiology per million, except for Albania (0.3).
- Only Uruguay and Lebanon have more than one department of cardiac surgery per million. Asian and sub-Saharan countries have less than 0.2 per million and some African countries have none at all.
- Intensive care units, cardiovascular rehabilitation centres, exercise testing facilities, Holter electrocardiography and echocardiography facilities are more common, but still scarce, in economies in transition and in Uruguay and Syria. The African nations have very low rates of these facilities per million inhabitants.
- The countries that reported having at least one nuclear medicine facility or a catheter laboratory per million were Croatia, Slovakia, Slovenia, Uruguay, Latvia, Lithuania, Lebanon and Syria.

c) Diagnostic and therapeutic cardiovascular procedures

Facilities for invasive procedures per million populations are lacking in sub-Saharan Africa and are limited in many countries in Asia. Even though a large number of procedures are carried out in countries like China and India, the volume appears to be low relative to the perceived needs of the population. Compared with Germany, AS&AF perform only 2.8%, LAC&MEC 12.5% and ECE 22.5%. This shows a clear disparity between the rich and poor countries.

DISCUSSION

The second half of the 20th century has witnessed the emergence of the CVD epidemic as the major public health challenge of our times. The fact that the epidemic of CVD has now become a global problem requiring urgent attention and action is clear from both the present magnitude of the problem in developing countries and economies in transition, and the menacing proportions of its projected extent over the next two decades. Most of the countries of Latin and Central America, Asia and Africa will experience rising burdens even though the absolute burdens may vary according to the stage of epidemic transition. Even in countries that are experiencing a recent decline in CVD mortality, the absolute burden will remain high and disproportionate to the available health care resources, mainly because of the increase in people attaining the age at which CVD are more frequent. The economies in transition of Eastern Europe present a picture of mounting burdens in most countries and recent reductions in a few. The direction of the epidemic in this region will depend on the dynamics of development over the next two decades. Whatever the trends may be, the alarmingly high current burdens constitute a public health emergency. The future burdens, too, are likely to be very high.

Fortunately, there is a wealth of global scientific knowledge that can assist the development of preventive and clinical care strategies in developing countries and economies in transition. The experience of developed countries has demonstrated that cardiovascular diseases (including cerebrovascular, renovascular, peripheral vascular, rheumatic fever, rheumatic heart disease and Chagas' diseases) are preventable (3). Extensive knowledge about risk behaviours and risk factors as well as knowledge about effective interventions that reduce risk in individuals and populations has accrued from observational and experimental research in the industrialized countries. Much of this is generalizable to the countries now experiencing the advancing epidemic. It is imperative that this knowledge and expertise be transferred to developing countries and economies in transition, which are already beginning to face this modern epidemic. Although the scientific content of this knowledge may need to be adapted to the specific context of the populations in which it is to be applied, the availability of such knowledge greatly empowers the global community to initiate early responses in order to contain the epidemic.

It is essential that a partnership be forged between developed and developing countries and that the two groups should be on an equal footing at all stages of any cardiovascular programme, from its formulation (to identify the needs of developing countries) to ultimate implementation. Global partnerships, exemplified by the World Heart Federation, can catalyze these responses through shared expertise and experience.

Overall, there is clear evidence that CVD are a global public health problem, and appear to be a growing problem. It is estimated that by the year 2020 these diseases will be responsible for up to 24.8 million of all deaths in the world, of which 18.6 million (74.73%) will occur in developing countries. Coronary heart disease will top the list of major public health problems, and stroke will rank third.

As the population's longevity has increased in all regions of the world in response to better control of communicable diseases, the people of developing countries and economies in transition are now exposed to chronic non-communicable diseases. The problem is compounded by the urban lifestyle—lack of physical activity, increased pollution, and high-calorie fast food. Furthermore, lack of awareness of risk factors is a major impediment.

The capacity of the public health system can be viewed from two perspectives: ability to meet the demands of a growing CVD epidemic from a public health point of view (primordial and primary prevention and health promotion) and ability to provide adequate clinical care to those already at risk or afflicted.

Overall, most of the developing countries and economies in transition are not geared toward prevention. This is reflected in their lack of capacity for data collection, preparation of national guidelines for many of the risk factors, planning and execution of prevention programmes and financial support for prevention programmes. These issues have to be addressed and corrected if we wish to control the impending CVD epidemic.

The White Book survey data indicates that neither developing countries nor economies in transition have the necessary infrastructure and manpower required to meet this challenge. The question arises whether developing countries and economies in transition should follow the course charted by Western countries, namely curative and high-tech medicine.

Although many of the developing countries and economies in transition are facing a multitude of problems besides health conditions, let alone non-communicable disease or CVD, their budget allocation for the entire health services is about 5% GNP or less. When the percentage of GNP is translated into actual dollar figures, the anticipated budget allocation for health care per person per year varies anywhere between US $4 (Mozambique) and about $870 (United Arab Emirates), and the median figure is somewhere around US $100. This median amount is a hypothetical figure based on 5% GNP invested in health care. In reality, most developing countries spend 3% or less. In many of the sub-Saharan African countries the amount of health care dollars allocated per capita is somewhere between US$4 in Mozambique to $91 in Tunisia, with an average of $27. This amount is far below that of any of the developed countries. It is also clear from the experience of the Western countries that their own per capita health care funding (ranging any where from $2500 to $16,000) is inadequate.

Most Western countries are now turning towards population health and prevention of the onset of diseases, particularly CVD. This might reflect the failure of high technology medicine to cater to the needs of the population even in developed countries. They are taking the preventive approaches seriously and encouraging their populations to follow better lifestyles and modify their behaviours. The solution for developing countries and economies in transition is, therefore, to focus on health promotion and disease prevention. However, those who have been afflicted by CVD need to be treated. The meagre health care dollars available should be put into best practice for favourable overall health outcomes.

The lack of a solid economic base in most developing countries puts a heavy premium on prevention at the population level, and such prevention efforts should cover the entire life span, from childhood to old age. For many of these countries, highly technical interventional cardiology may not be the appropriate solution. Furthermore, the views of clinical cardiologists and those of public health workers will often differ, and it will be important to maintain a balance between primary health care and preventive strategies on the one hand, and effective clinical strategies on the other. Cost-benefit considerations will be paramount in developing countries, and cultural sensitivities must be respected.

CONCLUSIONS

Strategies for prevention and control of CVD

The emerging epidemic of CVD in developing counties as well as the established epidemics in economies in transition call for early identification and effective implementation of interventions, which encompass the following:

Population-based risk modification strategies to

- prevent the acquisition or augmentation of risk factors in communities that at present have a low-risk profile for CVD (primordial prevention). Rural communities in most developing countries and children of all nations would be the prime beneficiaries.
- reduce the mean level of risk factors in populations where they are already high, i.e., shift the distribution of those risk factors to the lower end of the scale so that all members of the community will benefit from even modest reductions in risk (primary prevention). Urban communities in most developing countries and the populations of economies in transition would be the appropriate targets for such interventions.
- **Strategies for identifying and protecting individuals** whose risk factor profile places them at a high relative risk of manifesting CVD. Such individuals exist in virtually all communities, and their number would increase proportionally with an increase in the mean population levels of CVD risk factors. Although population-based risk modification would reduce their numbers over time, it is necessary to identify individuals who are currently vulnerable and actively reduce their risk of CVD (primary prevention).

- **Strategies for early case detection and cost-effective clinical care of clinically manifest CVD**, at all levels of health care. Even as primordial and primary prevention strategies are vigorously pursued to reduce the risk of CVD, individuals who have already advanced to the stage of clinical disease need to be identified and provided with cost-effective health care that can improve survival and avoid or reduce disability at costs affordable by those individuals as well as by society.

All these strategies are not mutually exclusive but are synergistically complementary. The population-based strategy not only provides for risk reduction across the wide spectrum of risk in the community, with large cumulative societal benefits, but also ensures a supportive environment for individuals at high risk who wish to alter their lifestyles so as to radically reduce risk. The "high risk" prevention strategy, in return, provides clear and convincing demonstration of the benefits of modifying risk factors so that the population strategy finds incentives and gains impetus. The clinical care of a person affected by CVD is not merely a commitment of compassion but is also a required service essential for establishing the credibility of CVD control programmes in the community by saving valuable lives and alleviating suffering. Thus the continuity of health care programmes for CVD control must span the entire spectrum in the natural history of CVD, starting with the determinants of health behaviour in the community and culminating in the critical care of individuals with debilitating disease.

Specific population-based risk factor control programmes

a. Tobacco control

Effective strategies for tobacco control will need to combine a "top down approach" of regulation and legislation and a "bottom up approach" of community education and mobilization. Since the determinants are both global and local, the responses, too, need to emanate from both levels. Local responses would involve health education (to promote abstinence among persons at risk of acquiring the habit and abandonment by those already addicted), regulatory restraint of advertising and sale to minors, statutory warnings effectively displayed, legislation to ban smoking in public places and transport utilities, taxation-linked disincentives and agro-industrial policies favouring tobacco substitution with other crops and commodities. International cooperation can greatly facilitate these efforts both through shared experience and expertise for strengthening local action and by forging a global coalition for advocacy of effective tobacco control measures.

b. Nutrition

Dietary practices conducive to health promotion and CVD prevention must be advocated and made feasible for adoption by the community. Healthy food choices must become widely available, affordable and acceptable and must provide appropriate nutrition to protect against CVD. Though the specific dietary recommendations will depend on the cultural and economic context of each country, the following dietary practices must be promoted in all populations:

- increased consumption of fresh fruit and vegetables
- reduced consumption of saturated fat and cholesterol
- reduced consumption of salt
- reduced consumption of simple sugars
- calorie intake appropriate to age and activity, in order to attain and maintain ideal body weight for height and avoid both general and central obesity

Dietary behaviour and nutritional trends are influenced by both local and global factors. National policies on agricultural production and food processing interlink with international factors that influence world food prices and transnational marketing of raw, unprocessed foods. Cultural factors influencing local food preferences compete with the global market, which promotes certain foods as part of a "common culture". We cannot be indifferent to the global expansion of fast food hamburger outlets (for example MacDonalds) and must set the same standards in the international developing world market as those in the home countries in terms of fat consumption and food composition.

c. Physical activity

Nutrition has to be appropriately matched to physical activity. Regular leisure time exercise and increase in daily physical activity levels need to be promoted through community education, work-site and school-based programmes, enhancement of community-centre recreational facilities and exercise-friendly urban transport systems such as protected cycle lanes.

d. Stress management

Stress is a widely implicated but inadequately studied risk factor for CVD. Prevention strategies need to promote stress management techniques that are appropriate to the context of each country. These may involve community dynamics or individual practice. Traditional stress management systems, such as yoga and meditation, which are accepted and available in the developing countries may be preserved and promoted.

Strategies for risk reduction in persons at high risk of CVD

Even though population-based risk modification strategies will modify the risk of most persons in the community and eventually reduce the number of those at high risk, efforts are also needed to identify individuals who are currently at high relative risk of developing CVD, those who have marked elevation of a single risk factor, or those with a confluence of multiple, moderately elevated risk factors.

Mass screening of populations to identify such high-risk individuals is neither feasible nor cost-effective in most countries. Economic costs are clearly prohibitive, and the biologic and psychological costs of "false labelling" consequent to the reduced positive predictive value of diagnostic tests in populations with a low prevalence of CVD may be unacceptable. Further, periodic screening at frequent intervals would be needed to identify new entrants to the high-risk group. The limited human and financial resources available for health care are unlikely to permit such recurrent screening for CVD risk factors.

In order to make these screening strategies effective, it is necessary to promote public and provider education emphasizing the need as well as benefits of such programmes. The community would then be prepared to ask for such evaluation or accept it when advised. Health care providers, too, would be better prepared to apply these screening techniques as a part of routine health care rather than viewing it as a sporadic activity to be performed in special "heart camps".

The activities of the opportunistic and targeted screening would be included in the ordinary work of the primary care teams, in a form that would be appropriate to the resources and manpower available.

Political will

Political will is lacking in most developing countries, and international organizations should endeavour to inform the politicians and policy makers of these countries about the impending epidemic of CVD and persuade them of its importance (12). Ministries of health in these countries should be encouraged to work closely with non-governmental organizations (NGOs), such as cardiac societies and heart foundations, towards the prevention of CVD. Well-directed lobbying by the NGOs in their own countries could be very effective in articulating the voice of the people. Intersectoral collaboration between ministries of health, agriculture, industry and finance is equally crucial in our efforts to prevent CVD, and international trade laws (in particular tobacco control) and control of food safety are serious issues in global CVD prevention (13).

Political will should be based on the interests of the population and its right to self-determination rather than on religious values and external charity. For programmes to be sustainable, the local population should be encouraged to accept responsibility. Otherwise, when the external funding from outside donors runs out, the programmes will fall apart. Clearly, a peaceful global order will be threatened if there is not greater parity and equality in the world.

ACKNOWLEDGEMENT

This report is based on the World Heart Federation's White Book (1).

REFERENCES

1. Chockalingam A, Balaguer-Vintro. 1999. Impending Pandemic of cardiovascular diseases: Challenges and opportunities for prevention and control of cardiovascular diseases in developing countries and economies in transition. Prous Science, Barcelona.
2. The World Health Report. 1997. Conquering, suffering, enriching humanity. Geneva, World Health Organization.
3. International Advisory Board. 1992. Victoria declaration on heart health. Victoria, Canada, Health and Welfare Canada.

4. World Bank. 1997. Human development and network strategy. Health, Nutrition and Population Division, World Bank, Washington, DC.
5. Murray ChJL, Lopez AD. 1997. Mortality by cause for eight regions of the world: Global Burden of Disease Study. Lancet 349:1269–1276.
6. World Bank. 1993. World Development Report, Investing in Health. New York, Oxford University Press.
7. Report of the Ad Hoc Committee on Health Research Relating to Future Intervention Options: investing in health research and development. World Health Organization, Geneva, 1996.
8. The WHO MONICA Project. 1989. A worldwide monitoring system for cardiovascular diseases. World Health Statistics Annual, WHO, Geneva, pp. 27–149.
9. The World Bank. 1997. World development report—1997. Washington, DC., 214–214.
10. Pyorala K, De Backer G, Graham I, Poole-Wilson P, Wood D, on behalf of the Task Force. 1994. Prevention of coronary heart disease in clinical practice: Recommendations of the Task Force of the European Society of Cardiology, European Atherosclerosis Society and European Society of Hypertension. Eur Heart J 15:1300–1331.
11. Wood D, De Backer G, Faergeman O, Graham I, Mancia G, Pyorala K. 1998. Prevention of coronary heart disease in clinical practice: Recommendations of the Second Task Force of the European and Other Societies on Coronary Prevention. Eur Heart J 19:1434–1503.
12. Singapore Declaration, Forging the will for heart health in the next millennium. 1998. Singapore National Heart Association.
13. Chockalingam A, Chalmers J, Liu L, Labarthe D, MacMahon S, Martin I, Whitworth J. (On behalf of discussants and contributors at the WHO-ISH Meeting on Prevention of Hypertension and Associated Cardiovascular Diseases, Beijing, China, October 6–9, 1999). 2000. Prevention of Cardiovascular Diseases in Developing Countries: Agenda for Action. Statement from a WHO-ISH Meeting in Beijing—October 1999. Simultaneous publication in CVD Prev. 3(3):255–258 and J Hypertens 18(12):1705–1708.

Frontiers in Cardiovascular Health, edited by
N.S. Dhalla, A. Chockalingam,
H.I. Berkowitz & P.K. Singal
Kluwer Academic Publishers, Boston, 2003

Cardiovascular Risk Factors in Women

Geetha Bhat

University of Louisville Division of Cardiology 550 South Jackson Street ACB Bldg, 3rd Floor

Louisville, KY 40292 USA

Summary. Cardiovascular disease (CVD) is the leading cause of death and disability for women in the United States. Most of the risk factors for CVD and benefits of risk reduction are similar in women and men with some risk factors varying in magnitude and other risk factors unique in women. Even though heart disease remains the leading cause of mortality in women, healthy life style changes in addition to modification of traditional risk factors for CVD can impact positively on the incidence of CVD. Inspite of known benefits, CVD risk reduction strategies are underused. Prevention and treatment strategies in women need to be more aggressive. The CVD risk factors in women and benefits of risk factor modification are reviewed here.

Key words: Cardiovascular Disease, Women, Risk Factors, Prevention.

INTRODUCTION

Cardiovascular disease (CVD) is the leading cause of death among both women and men in the United States. Nearly twice as many women die of heart disease as from all forms of cancer, including breast cancer (1). For African-American and Hispanic women the risk of CVD is even higher (2). There is widespread awareness among women about breast cancer and osteoporosis being serious challenges to their health with less knowledge about their risk factors for heart disease. Early recognition of risk factors and strategies to prevent heart disease should be instituted in younger women. Unfortunately, a recent survey indicates that four in five women and one in three primary care physicians appear to be unaware that CVD is the major cause

Geetha Bhat, Ph.D., M.D., University of Louisville, Division of Cardiology, 550 South Jackson Street, ACB Bldg, 3rd Floor, Louisville, KY 40292. Telephone: 502-587-2883, Fax: 502-587-4846, E-mail: g0bhat01@gwise.louisville.edu.

of death in women (3). Most of the risk factors for coronary heart disease (CHD) and the benefits of risk factor modification among men are also important in women (4). All the risk factors that promote atherosclerosis in men also affect women, including hypertension, diabetes mellitus, dyslipidemia, smoking and obesity. The magnitude of the risk factors may be different and some of the risk factors are unique to women. Aging and family history are nonmodifiable risk factors in women and men. Women develop CVD about a decade later than men. Their outcome may be worse than men when heart disease develops because of more concomitant diseases. CHD risk increases with age, and this risk is more dramatic in women (5). Although most risk factors are more favorable in females, the gender effect decreases with increasing age.

Incidence of CVD is lower in premenopausal women compared with men. Menopause plays an important role in the development of CVD and the risk of mortality from CVD increases in postmenopausal women (6). Although most CVD risk factors in women and men are similar there are unique challenges in addressing risk factors in women. The diagnosis of CVD poses greater challenge in women as symptoms may be atypical. Treadmill exercise testing has lower predictive value for women. It has been suggested that female patients be stratified based on low, intermediate and high likelihood of CHD for better diagnosis (7). Risk factors play an important role in the accurate diagnosis of CVD in women. The CVD risk factors in women and benefits of risk factor modification are reviewed in this article.

HYPERTENSION

Number of prospective studies have shown strong association between hypertension and CHD in both men and women (4). More than twice as many women as men develop hypertension after age 50. About 60 percent of all women ages 65 to 74 have elevated blood pressure (5). Isolated systolic hypertension is more prevalent in elderly females than males affecting about 30 percent of women over 65 years old (8).

Benefits of treating hypertension apply both to men and women. Systolic hypertension in the Elderly Program, which had 57 percent women in the study population showed that antihypertensive therapy resulted in 36 percent reduction in the incidence of stroke and 25 percent reduction in CHD (9).

DIABETES MELLITUS

Diabetes mellitus is a more important risk factor in women than men. Diabetes eliminates the protective effect of female gender. Postmenopausal women with diabetes have approximately the same risk as diabetic men of the same age. Diabetes increased the risk of CVD events more than twofold in men and almost fourfold in women, virtually eliminating women's advantage over men (6). After a myocardial infarction, diabetic women have a higher mortality rate compared with nondiabetic persons (10). One third of women with gestational diabetes subsequently develop noninsulin dependent diabetes compared with only 5 percent of those with normal pregnancies (4). Efforts should be made to identify and control diabetes in women, including modification of concomitant risk factors such as dyslipidemia or hypertension (6).

DYSLIPIDEMIA

In women over age of 55, over half have cholesterol levels of 240 mg/dl, or higher. Women's cholesterol is higher than men's from age 55 on. Similar to men, low HDL cholesterol and high triglycerides are important risk factors in women. Low levels of HDL cholesterol appear to be a stronger risk factor for women than for men (11). High triglycerides may increase the risk for women more than for men. In the Scandinavian Simvastatin Survival Study, major coronary events were reduced by 35 percent in women similar to men. Cholesterol and Recurrent Events (CARE) trial showed that risk of coronary events in women decreased twice that in men (12).

SMOKING

Cigarette smoking is the leading preventable cause of CHD. Smoking is a potent CHD risk factor in women, as in men. Approximately one in four women smoke cigarettes in the United States. First myocardial infarctions occur 7 years earlier in male smokers compared to nonsmokers; whereas first myocardial infarctions in female smokers precede nonsmokers by 19 years (12).

The Nurses' Health Study demonstrated that excess risk for CHD due to smoking was eliminated within 2 years after smoking cessation. Nurses Health Study of 84,129 registered nurses during 14-year follow-up for primary prevention of CHD showed that smoking is the most important CHD risk factor (13). The risk of CHD in both men and women begins to decline within months and falls to the level of risk of nonsmokers within three to five years after cessation (4).

OBESITY

About one third of adult women in the United States can be classified as obese. Excess weight is positively associated with increased CHD risk in both men and women (14). In the Nurses' Health Study, the risk of CHD was over three times higher among women with a body-mass index (BMI) of 29 or higher than among lean women (BMI < 21). Women who had life styles with good diet, moderate exercise, BMI < 25, no smoking and moderate alcohol consumption had low risk for CHD (13). In addition to BMI, central obesity is an important predictor of CHD in women (12).

PHYSICAL ACTIVITY

Observational studies have shown 60 to 75 percent lower risk of CHD in physically active women than in sedentary women (4). Even light-to-moderate activity is associated with low CHD rates in women (15). Women are less likely to exercise than men, and elderly females tend to be less active. An eight-year prospective study of 3120 healthy women demonstrated association between physical fitness and decreased rates of mortality from CVD (16).

HORMONE REPLACEMENT THERAPY

Observational data and meta-analysis have suggested that hormone replacement therapy (HRT) is cardioprotective and can reduce CHD risk by as much as 35 percent to 50 percent (17). HRT has beneficial effects on dyslipidemia. The Nurses' Health Study reported a 61 percent lower risk of CHD in those on combined estrogen-progestin therapy as compared with a 40 percent risk reduction in those on estrogen alone (18). Despite this, HERS (Heart and Estrogen/progestin Replacement Study) a large, randomized double-blind, placebo-controlled secondary prevention trial found that while hormone replacement therapy decreased LDL-C levels and increased HDL-C and triglyceride levels, it was not associated with any change in the combined endpoints of nonfatal MI and CHD death (17).

The Women's Health Initiative (WHI) is an ongoing large clinical trial evaluating HRT for primary prevention of CHD in postmenopausal women (19). Hopefully, WHI will clarify benefits of HRT in postmenopausal females. Previously oral contraceptive use had been associated with risk of myocardial infarction. It has now been shown that CVD among oral contraceptive users occurs predominantly in smokers and women with risk factors (20). The Raloxifene Use for the Heart (RUTH) trial is currently evaluating a selective estrogen receptor modulator in postmenopausal women at risk for CHD.

NEW RISK FACTORS FOR CHD

In both men and women investigations are underway to evaluate the effectiveness of controlling novel risk factors such as homocysteine (21), Lipoprotein (a) (22), C-reactive protein (23), insulin resistance, and hemostatic factors (12). Diet and lifestyle factors have become additional important determinants of risk for CVD (24).

CONCLUSION

CVD is the single leading cause of death among women in the United States. A new American Heart Association survey reveals that 62 percent of women still believe that cancer is the greatest health threat for women (25). Prevention and treatment strategies are still less aggressive for women than men. Early risk factor assessment, modification of risk factors, and healthy life style choices can help women as much or more than men to reduce the incidence of CVD and avoid the devastating outcomes of CVD.

REFERENCES

1. American Heart Association. 2001. Heart and Stroke Statistical Update. Dallas, Texas: American Heart Association, 2000.
2. Winkleby MA, Kraemer HC, Ahn DK, Varady AN. 1998. Ethnic and socioeconomic differences in carediovascular disease risk factors. JAMA 280:356–362.

3. Wenger NK. 1998. Preventive coronary care in women: The challenge to institute coronary risk reduction. Prev Cardiol 1:25.
4. Rich-Edwards JW, Manson JE, Hennekens CH, Buring JE. 1995. The primary prevention of coronary heart disease in women. N Engl J Med 332:1758–1766.
5. Mosca L, Manson JE, Sutherland SE, Langer RD, Manolio T, Barrett-Connor E. 1997. Cardiovascular disease in women: A statement for healthcare professionals from the American Heart Association writing group. Circulation 97:2468–2482.
6. Mosca L, Grundy SM, Judelson D, King K, Limacher M, Oparil S, Pasternak R, Pearson TA, Redberg RF, Smith SC, Winston M, Zinberg S. 1999. Guide to preventive cardiology for women. Circulation 99:2480–2484.
7. Douglas PS, Ginburg GS. 1996. The evaluation of chest pain in women. N Engl J Med 344: 1311–1315.
8. National high blood pressure education program working group: National high blood pressure working group report on high blood pressure in the elderly. 1994. Hypertension 23:275–285.
9. SHEP Cooperative Research Group. 1991. Prevention of stroke by antihypertensive drug treatment in older persons with isolated systolic hypertension: final results of the Systolic Hypertension in the Elderly Program (SHEP). JAMA 265:3255–3264.
10. Zuanette G, Lantini R, Maggioni AP, Santoro L, Franzosi MG. 1993. Influence of diabetes on mortality in acute myocardial infarction: data from the GISSI-2 Study. J Am Coll Cardiol 22:1788–1794.
11. Welty FK. 2001. Cardiovascular disease and dyslipidemia in women. Arch Intern Med 161:514–522.
12. Tsang TSM, Barnes ME, Gersh BJ, Hayes SN. 2000. Risk of coronary heart disease in women: Current understanding and evolving concepts. Mayo Clin Proc 75:1289–1303.
13. Stampfer MJ, Hu FB, Manson JE, Rimm EB, Willett WC. 2000. Primary prevention of coronary heart disease in women through diet and lifestyle. N Engl J Med 343:16–22.
14. Jousilahti P, Tuomilehto J, Vartiainen E, Pekkanen J, Puskha P. 1996. Body weight, cardiovascular risk factors, and coronary mortality: 15-year follow-up of middle aged men and women in eastern Finland. Circulation 93:1372–1379.
15. Lee IM, Rexrode KM, Cook NR, Manson JE, Buring JE. 2001. Physical activity and coronary heart disease in women. JAMA 285:1447–1454.
16. Blair SN, Kohl HW, Paffenbarger RS. 1989. Physical fitness and all-cause mortality: a prospective study of healthy men and women. JAMA 262:2395–2401.
17. Blakely JA. 2000. The heart and estrogen/progestin replacement study revisited. Arch Intern Med 160:2897–2900.
18. Goldstein F, Stampfer MJ, Manson JE, Colditz GA, Willett WC, Rosner B, Speizer FE, Hennekens CH. 1996. Postmenopausal estrogen and progestin use and the risk of cardiovascular disease. N Engl J Med 335:453–461.
19. The Women's Health Initiative Study Group: Design of the Women's Health Initiative Clinical Trial and Observational Study. 1998. Control Clin Trials 19:61–109.
20. Chasan-Taber L, Stampfer MJ. 1998. Epidemiology of oral contraceptives and cardiovascular disease. Ann Intern Med 128:467–477.
21. Pearson TA. 2002. New tools for coronary risk assessment. Circulation 105:886–892.
22. Orth-Gomer E, Mittleman MA, Schenck-Gustafsson K, Wamala SP, Eriksson M, Belkic K, Kirkeeide R, Svane B, Ryden L. 1997. Lipoprotein(a) as a determinant of coronary heart disease in young women. Circulation 95:329–334.
23. Ridker PM, Buring JE, Shih J, Matias M, Hennekens CH. 1998. Prospective study of C-Reactive protein and the risk of future cardiovascular events among apparently healthy women. Circulation 98:731–733.
24. Kromhout D, Menotti A, Kesteloot H, Sans S. 2002. Prevention of coronary heart disease by diet and lifestyle. Circulation 105:893–898.
25. Robertson RM. 2001. Women and cardiovascular disease. The risk of misperception and the need for action. Circulation 103:2318–2320.

Frontiers in Cardiovascular Health, edited by
N.S. Dhalla, A. Chockalingam,
H.I. Berkowitz & P.K. Singal
Kluwer Academic Publishers, Boston, 2003

Cardiovascular Disease in Women in the Middle East

Wafia B. Eteiba

Professor and Head of Cardiology Department, Al-Azhar University (Girls)
Cairo, Egypt

***Summary*:** Each country seems to have a range of heart disease incidence, morbidity and mortality that characterizes its population. Some cardiovascular disease (CVD) entities characterize the health profile and disease trends in women in the Middle East. These disease entity characteristics are linked to the women age group. In the childbearing age group, rheumatic heart disease and its related problems are the most common, and in the postmenopausal age group, IHD and hypertension are the most common CVD entities in many Middle east countries. This article highlights the results of some studies dealing with CVD in women with special emphasis on prevalence and risk factor profile in some Middle East countries including Egypt.

***Key words*:** Women's health, Middle East, Prevalence, Risk profile, Cross-sectional studies.

Most of knowledge of cardiovascular disease (CVD) comes from studies involving men. New emphasis on women's health in general and in cardiovascular health in particular, has led to increasing evidence that sex differences do exist in the incidence of CVD, in risk factors and in the modification of cardiovascular risk among women.

CVD is the leading cause of morbidity and mortality among women and most deaths occur in the postmenopausal years.

Each country seems to have a range for heart disease incidence, morbidity and mortality that characterizes its population. Some cardiovascular disease entities characterize the health profile and disease trends in women in the Middle East. These disease entities are related to the women's age group.

In the childbearing age group, rheumatic heart disease and its related problems as atrial fibrillation, endocarditis and congestive heart failure represent the most common CVD entities in many Middle East countries. Next in frequency is mitral valve prolapse (MVP), then congenital heart disease with expected adult survival.

An example of such rank of prevalence of CVD was obtained from the records of Al-Zahraa University Hospital, Al-Azhar University in Egypt. Among 4286 patients proved to have CVD by echo examination over 5-year period (from 1996 to 2001), 2568 cases (59.9%) were females. These females with CVD included 1006 (39.9%) with rheumatic heart disease, 568 (22.1%) with MVP and 242 (9.4%) with congenital heart disease. 208 women (8.1%) had ischemic heart disease (IHD) while 544 (21.2%) had other forms of CVD including hypertensive heart disease, hypertrophic cardiomyopathy, dilated cardiomyopathy . . . etc. (1).

In the postmenopausal age group, the CVD profile in women in the Middle East is nearly similar to that elsewhere as regards the disease entities, with IHD and hypertension being the commonest in occurrence. However, the lifestyle issues and environmental settings affect the morbidity and mortality of CVD among Middle East women.

In this article, results of some studies involving CVD in women will be briefly represented with special emphasis on prevalence and risk factor profile in some Middle East countries including Egypt.

A study based on the national death records over a 16-year period in 24 cities in Iran, showed a 38% and 24.8% decline in all-cause and CVD mortality in men compared to 35% and 34.9% in women (2).

Another study on 1567 cases in an urban setting in Lebanon over 10-year follow-up period, revealed total mortality (all-cause) of 33.7 and 25.2 per 1000 person years among men and women respectively. In 60% of deaths in both sexes, the leading cause of mortality was circulatory, and men were at higher mortality risk than women in particular for IHD (3).

Records of 4832 cardiac surgery patients in Nasser institute in Egypt (4), from January 1995 to May 2001 included 1257 (26%) women undergoing cardiac surgery. The female mortality was 6.4% compared to 4.8% male mortality (Figure 1). The

Cardiac Surgery in Nasser Institute
From Jan. 1998 to May 2001 *(Females vs. Males)*
Total No of pts: 4832, Females: 1257 (26%)

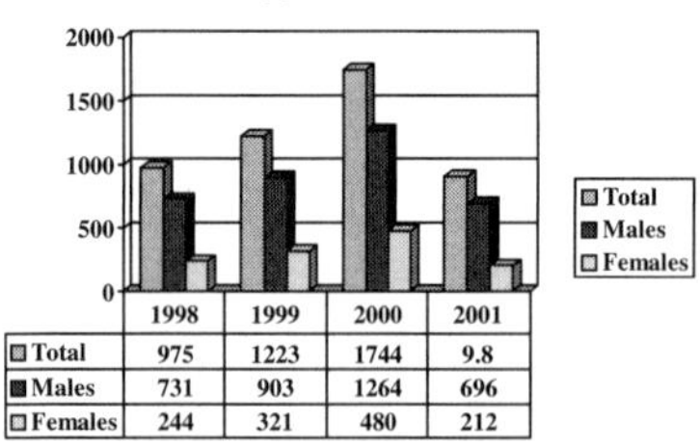

Cardiac Surgery Dept, Nasser Institute, June 2001

(a)

Cardiac Surgery Mortality in Nasser Institute
(From Jan. 1998 to May 2001) *(Females vs. Males)*
Total No of pts: 4832, Females: 1257 (26%)
Total Mortality:5.2% (F: 6.4% - M: 4.8%)

	1998	1999	2000	2001
Total	4.7%	5.5%	5.1%	5.5%
Males	4.4%	4.7%	5.0%	4.9%
Females	5.7%	7.8%	5.4%	7.6%

Percentage Mortality

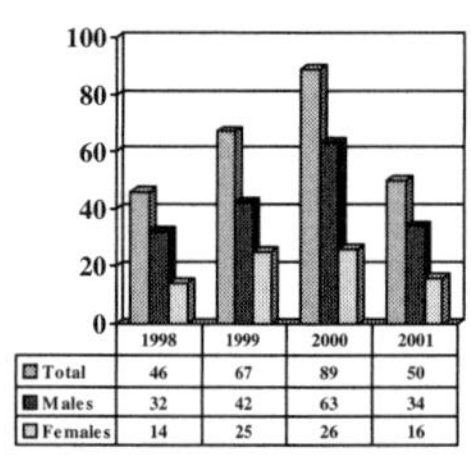

Cardiac Surgery Dept, Nasser Institute, June 2001

(b)

Figure 1. Percentage of cardiac surgery (a) and cardiac surgery mortality (b) in Nasser Institute, Egypt.

Cardiac Surgery in Nasser Institute

***From Jan. 1998 to May 2001** (Type of Surgery)*

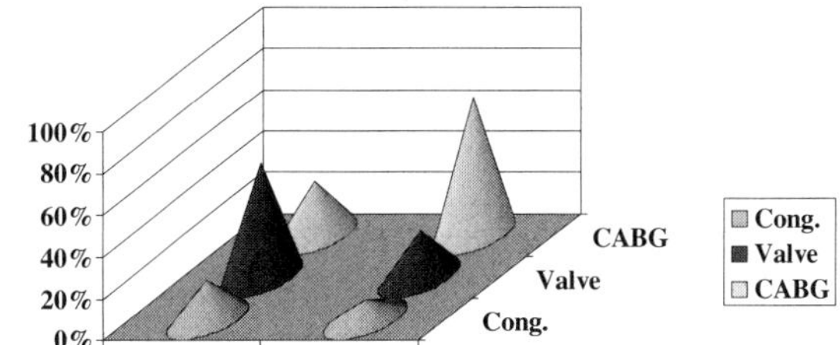

	Females	Males
Cong.	19%	10%
Valve	55%	23%
CABG	26%	67%

Cardiac Surgery Dept, Nasser Institute, June 2001

Figure 2. Types of cardiac surgery and their relation to sex in Nasser Institute, Egypt.

percentage of women undergoing valvular surgery was higher than that of men (55% vs 23%), while that of women undergoing coronary artery bypass grafts was lower than men (26% vs 67%), Figure 2.

CORONARY ARTERY DISEASE AND ITS RELATED RISK FACTORS IN WOMEN

It was reported that coronary artery disease (CAD) is responsible for more deaths in women each year than all other causes combined. Women have different cardiac presentation than men, and are more likely to be under-diagnosed and under-treated for CAD (5).

In the Lebanese myocardial Infarction study (6) which was conducted on 433 cases comprising 99 females, women were older, presented later, smoked less, but tended to have higher frequency of hypertension. Other CAD risk factors were similarly prevalent in males and females. In this study, the inotropic agents were used more commonly in women as they tended to develop more heart failure. Women also had significantly higher incidence of recurrent ischemia, myocardial infarction, high level of AV block and atrial arrhythmias in comparison to men. The overall mortality rates were higher in females (16.2% vs 8.1% in males, $p = 0.037$). This finding was attributed to the late arrival to hospital and occurrence of more complication compared to males.

Another study conducted in Turkey has described the CAD deaths and non-fatal coronary events over 5-year follow-up period in a cohort of random sample population including 2259 adults and comprising 1146 women (7). In this study there were 55 coronary deaths of which 26 were women. The annual rates of new coronary events in both males and females were 7.2 and 5.8 per 1000 respectively. High systolic blood pressure strongly predicted coronary deaths and high cholesterol levels predicted new coronary events in both men and women, whereas high diastolic blood pressure was of predictive value for combined outcome of coronary death and events in women but not in men.

The proportion of smoking is quite different in men and women in the majority of countries and it differs across cultures and may be related to environmental factors.

A study on 3859 Kuwaiti adults including 2061 women (8), showed 1.9% prevalence of smoking among women compared to 34.4% among men. In this study, 33% of smoker women began smoking when younger than 20 years (vs 70% of smoker men). The incidence of smoking was higher among lower levels of education, lower employment grades, being separated, divorced or widowed woman.

Another study on 608 couples in Kuwait revealed 0.5% current smoker wives vs 37% current smoker husbands (9).

In Bahrain, the prevalence of smoking in 516 subjects was 20.7% among women compared to 32.1% among men, and smoking was associated with less exercise and more television watching (10).

Obesity is an independent risk factor for all-cause mortality. It is highly associated with diabetes, hyperlipidaemia and hypertension. Obesity is a major risk factor for the development of type 2 diabetes, which is the most important risk factor for CAD in women. CAD generally presents at an older age in women than in men, but diabetes wipes out this gender protective effect. Furthermore, CAD is more likely to be fatal in women with diabetes (11).

At least one third of Arabs are obese as defined by body mass index (BMI) more than $30\,g/m^2$, and women have particularly high rates of obesity which is clearly associated with increased risk for mortality. Recent studies on the prevalence of obesity among population of the Arabian Peninsula revealed 17–43% prevalence ranges in women compared to 16–25% in men. In these studies, the most prevalent chronic diseases related to obesity were diabetes, hypertension and CAD (12).

A population-based cross-sectional survey in an urban Palestinian community showed that the prevalence of obesity defined as BMI $\geq 30\,g/m^2$, was found to be 49% in women compared to 30% in men. In contrast central obesity defined as waist-to-hip ratio (WHR) >0.90 in men or >0.85 in women, was found to be lower in women than men (25% vs 59% respectively). Both obesity and central obesity were found to be significantly associated with diabetes, low HDL-cholesterol and elevated triglycerides. Central obesity was also significantly associated with hypertension. These associations with diabetes, dyslipidaemia and hypertension pointed to a potential rise in CVD (13).

Another cross-sectional population-based study including 958 Turkish men and 1014 Turkish women aged 25–74 years was conducted to investigate the distribution of waist circumference (WC) and WHR and their relationship with established risk factors and their relevance to CVD morbidity in a random sample of Turkish general adult population. The overall mean values of both WC and WHR were lower in women than men (88.6 ± 13 vs 93 ± 12 respectively for WC) and (0.82 ± 0.07 vs 0.92 ± 0.08 respectively for WHR). Both WC and WHR were strongly associated with parameters reflecting insulin resistance such as diastolic blood pressure and plasma triglycerides. WHR was significantly associated with CAD in Turkish women (14).

The prevalence of obesity among 3435 Kuwaiti adults was found to be higher than reported elsewhere in the world being 70.2% grade 1 and 36.4% grade 2, and it was found to be significantly higher among women (15).

A cross-sectional study of 1385 Saudi females attending 15 health centers in urban and rural areas in Riyadh region was conducted to determine the prevalence of obesity and its associated factors among Saudi females. This study showed that only 26.1% of subjects were of ideal weight (BMI $<25\,g/m^2$), while a 26.8% were overweight (BMI $25–29.9\,g/m^2$), 41.9% were moderately obese (BMI $30–40\,g/m^2$), and 5.1% were morbidly obese (BMI $>40\,g/m^2$). High risk groups for obesity were mostly middle aged, multiparous, housewives and those living in rural areas (16).

In a study conducted on a small number of obese Egyptian population, both gender showed the same degree of LV diastolic dysfunction in the centrally obese patients whereas in peripherally obese patients, men had more LV diastolic dysfunction than women (17).

RHEUMATIC HEART DISEASE AND MITRAL VALVE PROLAPSE STUDIES IN SOME MIDDLE EAST COUNTRIES

A study comprising 9418 school-children in Saudi Arabia showed rheumatic heart disease prevalence of 24 per 10,000 with higher prevalence in females and in rural areas (18).

Another study conducted in Egypt on 1337 cases comprising 932 females with rheumatic mitral valve disease (MVD), showed that females had higher incidence of rheumatic MVD, with female to male ratio of 2.3 : 1, but they have less severe affection than males as evidenced by higher mitral valve area, lower echo score, lower mean diastolic pressure gradient across the mitral valve and lower left atrial size compared to males. In contrast neither mitral regurgitation severity nor LV function showed sex predilection (19).

Among 6609 patient (3570 women and 3039 men) referred for echo examination in Egypt, 317 cases had mitral valve prolapse (MVP). The prevalence of MVP among Egyptian female patients was 4.7% compared to 4.9% among male patients. This study revealed no sex difference in the incidence or etiology of MVP, in mitral regurgitation (MR) presence or absence, or in MR grade (20).

The incidence of MVP among 232 healthy Saudi women was found to be 12% of which 75% had mid to late systolic prolapse and 25% had holosystolic prolapse (21).

To sum-up, sex differences do exist in the incidence of CVD in Middle East. So, health care providers must co-ordinate their effort to effectively manage and prevent CVD in women taking into account the unique biological, physiological and epidemiological characteristics of CVD among women. Dealing with medical problems in the context of demographic trends is apparently the big challenge now and in the near future. New strategies must be developed targeting at an acceptable health status and appropriate lifestyle.

REFERENCES

1. Records of cardiology department, Al-Zahraa University Hospital, Al-Azhar University. Form 1996 to 2001, Cairo, Egypt.
2. Sarraf-Zadegan N, Boshtam M, Malekafzali H, Bashardoost N, Sayed-Tabatabaei FA, Rafiei M, Khalili A, Mostafavi S, Khami M, Hassanvand R. 1999. Secular trends in cardiovascular mortality in Iran, with special reference to Isfahan. Acta Cardiol 54:327–333.
3. Sibai AM, Fletcher A, Hills M, Campbell O. 2001. Non-communicable disease mortality rates using the verbal autopsy in a cohort of middle aged and older populations in Beirut during wartime, 1983–93. J Epidemiol Community Health 55:271–276.
4. Records of cardiac surgery department, Nasser Institute. From Jan 1998 to May 2001. Cairo, Egypt.
5. Jneid H, Thacker HL. 2001. Coronary artery disease in women: different, often untreated. Cleve Clin J Med 68:441–448.
6. Sawaya JI, Jazra C, Eid EV, Sabra RF. 1999. Gender differences in the diagnosis and treatment of acute myocardial infarction in Lebanon. J Med Liban 47:2–6.
7. Onat A, Dursunoglu D, Sansoy V. 1997. Relatively high coronary death and event rates in Turkish women. Relation to three major risk factors in five-year follow-up of cohort. Int J Cardiol 61:69–77.
8. Memon A, Moody PM, Sugathan TN, el-Gerges N, al-Bustan M, al-Shatti A, al-Jazzaf H. 2000. Epidemiology of smoking among Kuwaiti adults: prevalence, characteristics, and attitudes. Bull World Health Organ 78:1306–1315.
9. Radovanoric Z, Shah N, Behbehani J. 1999. Prevalence of smoking among currently married Kuwaiti males and females. Eur J Epidemiol 15:349–354.
10. Hamadeh RR, Musaiger AO. 2000. Lifestyle patterns in smokers and non-smokers in the state of Bahrain. Nicotine Tpb Res 2:65–69.
11. Braunwald E, Antman EM, Beasley JW, Califf RM, Cheitlin MD, Hochman JS, Jones RH, Kereiakes D, Kupersmith J, Levin TN, Pepine CJ, Schaeffer JW, Smith EE, Steward DE, Theroux P, Alpert JS, Eagle KA, Faxon DP, Fuster V, Gardner TJ, Gregoratos G, Russell RO, Smith SC. 2000. ACC/AHA Guidelines for the management of patients with unstable angina and non-ST-segment elevation myocardial infarction. J Am Coll Cardiol 36:970–1062.
12. al-Mahroos F, al-Roomi K. 1999. Overweight and obesity in the Arabian Peninsula: an overview. J R Soc Health 119:251–253.
13. Abdul-Rahim HF, Abu-Rmeileh NM, Husseini A, Holmboe-Ottesen G, Jervell J, Bjertness E. 2001. Obesity and selected co-morbidities in an urban Palestinian population. Int J Obes Relat Metab Disord 25:1736–1740.
14. Onat A, Sansoy V, Uysal O. 1999. Waist circumference and waist-to-hip ratio in Turkish adults: interrelation with other risk factors and association with cardiovascular disease. Int J Cardiol 70:43–50.
15. al-Isa AN. 1995. Prevalence of obesity among adult Kuwaitis: a cross-sectional study. Int J Obes Relat Metab Disord 19:431–433.
16. al-Shammari SA, Khoja TA, al-Maatouq MA, al-Nuaim LA. 1994. High prevalence of clinical obesity among Saudi females: a prospective, cross-sectional study in the Riyadh region. J Trop Med Hyg 97:183–188.
17. Eteiba WB, Mokhtar NM. 1997. The impact of obesity on left ventricular diastolic performance: new insight into the anthropometric classification of obesity. Egyp Ht J 49:45–52.
18. al-Sekait MA, al-Sweliem AA, Tahir M. 1990. Rheumatic heart disease in schoolchildren in western district, Saudi Arabia. J R Soc Health 110:15–16.
19. Hamdy A, Shaheen S. 1997. Age and Sex Relation to the Severity of Rheumatic Mitral Valve Disease First International Meeting of the Egyptian Echocardiography Working Group, Dec 17th–19th, Cairo, Egypt.
20. Hamdy A, Moshref I. 2001. Mitral Valve Prolapse: Echocardiographic Descriptive Analysis of 317 Patients. Sc J Az Med Fac (Girls) 22:599–608.
21. Noah MS, Alharthy SS, Joharjy IA, Alsedairy RM. 1987. Prevalence of mitral valve prolapse in healthy Saudi Women. Int J Cardiol 14:65–69.

Frontiers in Cardiovascular Health, edited by
N.S. Dhalla, A. Chockalingam,
H.I. Berkowitz & P.K. Singal
Kluwer Academic Publishers, Boston, 2003

Hypertension and Diabetes Situation in the Eastern Mediterranean Region: With Special Reference to Iran

Nizal Sarraf-Zadegan and Firoozeh Sajady

Isfahan Cardiovascular Research Center, Isfahan University of Medical Sciences

Summary. The incidence of hypertension (HTN) and diabetes mellitus (DM) appear to be increasing in the Eastern Mediterranean (EM) region. To initiate efforts to establish national or regional programs for the prevention and control of cardiovascular diseases (CVD) in EM countries, policy makers need more epidemiological data on HTN and DM. This study was undertaken to assess the current extent of HTN and DM prevalence and to identify the degree of awareness, treatment and control of HTN and DM.

These data were collected from most studies conducted since 1970 on the prevalence, awareness, treatment or control rates of HTN or DM in Iran and other EM countries. We searched for papers published in medical journals by using the MEDLINE database since 1970. The prevalence of HTN ranges between 7.7% and 31% in different cities in Iran and has been reported up to 33.6% in some urban areas in the EM region. The frequency of awareness of HTN ranges from 62% in Iran down to 23.5% in Saudi Arabia. On the contrary the treatment and control of HTN was better in Saudi Arabia of 76% and 20%, respectively compared to Egypt at 24% and 8%, respectively.

While it is estimated that 2 million Iranians have diabetes now, the prevalence of DM in different populations in the EM region varied between 0.1% in Sudan to as high as 25.5% in Bahrain.

While most of the surveys in the EM region showed that over 50% of diabetics are undiagnosed, high rates of DM awareness from Iran (70%) and Egypt (50%) were reported. The wide range obtained from these studies may be explained by the lack of standardization of the blood pressure or plasma glucose measurements, varied definitions, different age groups or sample size of the studied population and finally different dates of the studies. In summary,

Address for Correspondence: Isfahan Cardiovascular Research Center, P.O. Box: 81465-1148, Isfahan, Iran., Tel: +98-311-4460807, 4461826, Fax: +98-311-4459023, E-mail: isf.carvasrc@Hotmail.com.

our analysis indicates that although there are many reports from EM countries and Iran concerning the epidemiological views of HTN and DM, it is obvious that still there is more need to conduct a national or regional surveys using highly standardized methodology in the EM region.

***Key words*:** Hypertension, Diabetes mellitus, prevalence, treatment, awareness, diagnosed, control rate, population survey, developing world.

INTRODUCTION

Hypertension (HTN) is one of several risk factors for cardiovascular disease (1). The incidence of HTN appears to be increasing in the Eastern Mediterranean (EM) countries, affecting up to 30% of the adult population in some countries (2). The prevalence of HTN in many cities of Iran was different, having a range between 7.7% in Boshehr (a city located in the southern part of Iran) and 31% in Gonabad (one of the eastern cities in Iran) (3). According to the results of one big community-based study in Isfahan using the World Health Organization (WHO) standardized criteria, the age-adjusted prevalence rate was 18% (4) and the estimated figures for Iranian hypertensive men and women were 4,539,817 and 4,442,162, respectively. It has been shown that the reduction of highly or moderately elevated blood pressure (BP) level results in a decrease in cardiac, renal and cerebrovascular morbidity and mortality (5–7).

Diabetes Mellitus (DM) is another major cause of morbidity and mortality in the world, of which non-insulin dependent diabetes mellitus (NIDDM) is by far the most common form and thus accounts for the most disability (8–9). According to the WHO reports, it seems that nearly 40 million individuals are affected by diabetes in developing countries. It has become a major public health problem also in the EM region. Some studies have demonstrated that DM affects up to 10% of the population aged 20 years and older (10–12). In Iran, several epidemiological studies have been conducted. It is estimated that 2 million Iranians suffer from DM and the prevalence rate is reported to be 7% (13).

Many studies including community-based studies in western countries have shown that the awareness, treatment and control levels of HTN is far from optimal (14), and probably the rule of halves (that is half of hypertensive population is undetected, half of those detected are not treated and half of those treated are not controlled) may be still valid. It seems that undiagnosed, untreated and uncontrolled hypertensive cases outnumber the diagnosed cases in developing countries. This subject may be true also for DM, as NIDDM is often asymptomatic and many cases in the community remain undiagnosed, even in countries with good health care systems (15–16).

Unfortunately, rapid increase in the prevalence of some non-communicable diseases like HTN and DM have occurred in populations that are undergoing rapid changes in their life styles like westernization of their diet, decreased physical activity and increased smoking (17).

The available data from a recent WHO workshop held in Isfahan, Iran, Jan 5–8, 2002 indicates that two major common problems are facing the countries in the EM region, DM and HTN with a prevalence rate of 7 to 27% and 26% respectively.

This study has been conducted to help policy makers as they need more data on the prevalence, the number of diagnosed and non-diagnosed patients and levels of treatment and control for most diseases in order to assess the future needs for health care and preventive actions as circulatory diseases consist the main cause of mortality in Iran as well as other EM countries in the recent years (18).

METHODS AND DATA SOURCES

We compared studies on the prevalence, awareness, treatment and control rates of HTN or DM in Iran, and other EM countries attempting not only to review the differences, but also to gain some ideas regarding the differences in methodology, definitions, population under study etc, as well. The search was performed using the MEDLINE database of publications in medical journals since 1970 and by checking references in all detected publications (especially the national one). The keywords used were hypertension, diabetes mellitus, prevalence, awareness, treatment, control and population surveys.

RESULTS AND DISCUSSION

Epidemiology of hypertension in Iran and some Eastern Mediterranean Countries

Data on the prevalence or mean levels of systolic blood pressure (SBP) and diastolic blood pressure (DBP) would be very helpful in planning some primary preventive strategies.

Many community-based and sometimes national programs for detection or treatment of HTN were started in the EM countries in 1970s and 1980s. However the situation for comparison is further complicated by variability in classification criteria, methods of measurement, definition of HTN status (using different cut-points). Furthermore it is likely that in many EM countries such reports may be available in their local medical Journals but not through the MEDLINE search. Therefore the lack of standardization in these studies did not allow us to perform any valid statistical analysis. Table 1 provides HTN prevalence estimates from most of regional or national surveys in Iran (either urban or rural areas) in different years.

One of the reasons for the great differences observed in this table has been related mainly to the fact that some of these studies were done in urban and others in rural areas, as there is a widely accepted belief that blood pressure levels are lower in rural than urban environments (19–25). This difference was reported from other Mediterranean countries (like Egypt, Iraq, Pakistan) (26–28) and Iran as well (29). According to the data presented in Tables 1 and 2, the mean SBP and DBP as well as HTN prevalence seem to be higher among women. However the observed differences were not significant when the data were adjusted for body mass index (BMI) (4,30). On the other hand, available analysis showed that mean systolic & diastolic blood pressure and HTN prevalence in "Bandar Anzaly" one of the north

Table 1. The prevalence of hypertension by different regional and national surveys in Iran (1971–1996)

Cities	Date of the study	Sample size			Prevalence (%)			Definition Bp (mmHg)	Age (Year)	References No
		Female	Male	Total	Female	Male	Total			
Ramsar[n]	1970–1971			2,453	10.5	7.9	9.3	≥160/95	>15	3
Roodsar[n]	1971	381	192	573	10.6	11.5	11.2	≥160/95	35–65	3
Azarbayegan Sharghi[n]	1972	198	177	375	16.6	6.7	12	≥160/95	40–60	3
Bandar Anzali[n]	1973	202	384	586	29.3	17.2	23.3	≥160/95	>30	3
Isfahan[c]	1975–1976			1,830			16	≥160/90	>19	30
Boshehr[s]	1977	1,632	932	2,564	7.1	8.6	7.7	≥160/95	>15	30
Yazd[c]	1989			2,498	19	12	15	≥160/90	>15	3
Isfahan	1990	953	710	1,663			9.3	≥140/90	12–70	3
Iran*	1990	15,298	11,732	27,030	9.8	9.5	9.6	≥140/90	12–70	3
Tehran[c]	1992	4,742	4,950	9,692	17.9	17.6	17.7	≥160/90	>15	30
Isfahan	1994	4,860	3,242	8,102	19.4	16.8	18	≥160/95	>19	4
Hamedan[w]	1995	1,056	944	2,000	28.8	28	28.4	≥140/90	>20	3
Shiraz[c]	1995	2,440	1,754	4,194	28.7	26.5	27.7	≥140/90	>15	3
Gonabade	1996	501	749	1,250			31.3	≥90**	>18	3
Gilan[n]	1996	1,357	973	2,330	18.2	16.1	17	≥140/90	>25	3

*In 24 states.
**Diastolic blood pressure.
[n] *One of the northern cities in Iran.*
[c] *One of the central cities in Iran.*
[s] *One of the southern cities in Iran.*
[w] *One of the western cities in Iran.*
[e] *One of the eastern cities in Iran.*

Table 2. Sex-specified mean and standard deviation of systolic and diastolic blood pressure according to different studies in Iran (1971–1994)

Name of the cities	Date	Age (year)	SBP* Female	DBP** Female	SBP Male	DBP Male	Reference No
Roodsar[n]	1971	35–65	128.9 ± 19	73.1 ± 11	129.9 ± 21	73.1 ± 11.2	3
Azarbayegan Sharghi[n]	1972	40–60	130.5 ± 24	75.5 ± 15	121.9 ± 20	71.4 ± 13	3
Bandar Anzali[n]	1973	≥30	151.3 ± 9	81.7 ± 11	144.5 ± 24	82.3 ± 21	3
Isfahan[c]	1990	12–70	120 ± 20	75 ± 14	120 ± 18	75 ± 12	4
Iran	1990	12–70	119 ± 19	75 ± 14	121 ± 18	75 ± 12	4
Tehran[c]	1991	≥15	121 ± 18	75 ± 14	124.2 ± 20	75.8 ± 16	30
Isfahan	1994	≥19	125.8 ± 14	7.9 ± 8.9	127.4 ± 12.3	80.8 ± 7.6	4

*SBP: systolic blood pressure.
**DBP: Diastolic blood pressure.
[n] *One of the northern cities in Iran.*
[c] *One of the central cities in Iran.*

cities in Iran is high which is probably due to using salty smoked foods or special dietary patterns, genetic factors etc. It should be noted that although different methods were used, in the studies conducted in Tehran, Isfahan, Boshehr, all of them used the WHO standardized criteria for blood pressure measurement (31).

Epidemiological surveys on HTN in the EM region reported high prevalence rate in some countries. In Egypt, the Egyptian National HTN Project began its work to study the prevalence of HTN and its complications among the Egyptian population since 1991. Data from that project showed that HTN was common, affecting up to 30% of the studied adult population over 25 years of age. The cut-off level used for diagnosis was 140/90. HTN was more prevalent among urban areas, with Cairo having the highest prevalence rate (26). According to a study conducted in Iraq in 1979, the prevalence of HTN (defined as blood pressure of 160/90 or higher) was 13% among people aged 15 years and above (27). In Cyprus the Interhealth survey revealed the prevalence of HTN (BP ≥ 160/95) was 9.9% (17). The estimated prevalence rate of HTN (BP ≥ 160/95) among the population in Morocco was 10%. It would be higher if the WHO criteria for cut off level (140/90) was used (17). Considerable data were reported from studies conducted on patients, hospitalized for circulatory diseases in some of the EM countries showing higher prevalence rate of HTN (2).

Hypertension awareness, treatment and control rates in some developing countries, the EM region with special emphasis on Iran

This review assessed the current extent of HTN awareness, treatment and control in the community. It is based on many studies conducted on blood pressure in Iran and other countries in the EM region. Despite the recent increase in patients' awareness of HTN and participation in antihypertensive treatment, data from several countries indicate that fewer than 25% of all treated hypertensives currently meet the recommended goal blood pressure of less than 140/90 mmHg (32). Thus in industrialized countries the lack of awareness is not a major problem in attempts to control high blood pressure in the community. Conversely, the rate of awareness and treatment were much lower in the developing countries, resembling the one observed in developed countries nearly 20 years ago.

Unfortunately, there are few reports on the evaluation of prevalence, awareness and control rates of HTN in the general population. The frequency of HTN awareness, treatment and control in Thailand was 42%, 30% and 7% (33), in Egypt 37.5%, 24% and 8% (26) and in India 48%, 31% and 9% (34) respectively. The percentage of diagnosed (aware) hypertensives, those receiving drug treatment and those with their blood pressure controlled in five cities in Iran are presented in Table 3. The data in Table 3 shows results for the whole group (both men and women) while Table 4 showed the results in Isfahan among men and women separately. In Iran the awareness, treatment and control tended to be lower in areas with lower socioeconomic status (4), a finding similar to Egyptian experience (35). In Saudi Arabia one study reported 23.5% awareness level and, among known cases of HTN, 76% were receiving treatment, but only 20% were found to be controlled (36) (Table 5).

Table 3. Percentage of hypertension awareness, treatment and control rates in different cities of Iran (1991–1996)

City	Number of Samples	Date	Definition Bp (mmHg)	Number of hypertensives	Awareness* rate %	Treatment** rate %	Control*** rate %	References No
Tehran[c]	9692	1991	≥140/90	1938	38.7	19	6	30
Babol[n]	2000	1994	≥140/90		46	23	9	3
Isfahan[c]	8102	1995	≥160/95	1450	55	51	13	4
Hamedan[w]	2000	1995	≥140/90	576	30	25	15	4
Gonabad[e]	1250	1996	≥90	390	43	13	9.3	3

[c] *One of the central cities in Iran.*
[n] *One of the northern cities in Iran.*
[w] *One of the western cities in Iran.*
[e] *One of the eastern cities in Iran.*
* *Percent of hypertensives with previous history of hypertension.*
** *percent of hypertensives taking medication.*
*** *percent of treated hypertensives with blood pressure <140/90.*

Table 4. Prevalence, awareness, treatment and control rates of definite hypertension in Isfahan based on sex, 1995*

	19–29 (Yr) No (%)	30–39 (Yr) No (%)	40–49 (Yr) No (%)	50–59 (Yr) No (%)	60–69 (Yr) No (%)	≥70 (Yr) No (%)	Overall No (%)
Prevalence a							
Men	37 (9.0)	32 (7.4)	115 (21.8)	186 (27.9)	298 (40.3)	311 (47.5)	979 (28.5)
Women	19 (3.3)	68 (9.7)	254 (26.4)	586 (46.4)	669 (61.3)	426 (67.0)	2025 (38.7)
Aware[b]							
Men	4 (10.8)	4 (12.5)	34 (29.6)	72 (38.7)	145 (48.6)	170 (54.7)	429 (43.8)
Women	1 (5.3)	20 (29.4)	118 (46.4)	352 (60.1)	451 (67.4)	286 (67.1)	1228 (60.6)
Treated[c]							
Men	5 (13.5)	7 (21.9)	25 (21.7)	65 (34.9)	129 (43.3)	157 (50.5)	388 (39.6)
Women	4 (21.0)	23 (33.8)	110 (43.3)	292 (49.8)	425 (57.5)	288 (63.2)	1142 (53.4)
Controlled[d]							
Men	3 (8.1)	3 (9.4)	12 (10.4)	21 (11.3)	32 (10.7)	47 (15.1)	126 (12.9)
Women	4 (21.0)	12 (17.6)	38 (15.0)	42 (7.2)	94 (14.0)	62 (14.5)	255 (12.6)

*Reference: Prevalence of Hypertension and Associated Risk Factors in Isfahan, Islamic Republic of Iran. Eastern Mediterranean Health Journal, Vol 3, No. 5, 1999. Reference No. 4.
[a] The crude prevalence.
[b] Percent of hypertensives with previous history of hypertension.
[c] Percent of hypertensives taking medication.
[d] Percent of hypertensives with blood pressure <160/95 mmHg and reported currently taking antihypertensive medications.

Table 5. Hypertension prevalence, awareness, treatment and control rates in different populations in the Eastern Mediterranean regional countries (1990–1997)

Country	Sex	Age (Years)	Sample Size (No)	Definition Bp (mmHg)	Prevalence (%)	Awareness[α] (%)	Treatment[β] (%)	Control[γ] (%)	Year	References NO
Iran*	both	12–70	26,886	≥140/90	9.5	—	—	—	1990	94
Pakistan	Women	≥25	151	≥140/90	17	—	80	24	1994	45
Saudi Arabia	both	≥15	1,394	≥160/95	15.4	33.3	73	26	1994	95
Jordan	both	≥25	2,299	≥160/95	10.1	52.4	—	30	1995	96
Iran**,†	both	≥19	8,624	≥140/90	28.2	62.3	33.1	14	1996	4
Saudi Arabia	Men	≥10	1,936	≥140/90	10.6	—	—	—	1996	36
Saudi Arabia	Women	≥10	2,033	≥140/90	11.5	—	—	—	1996	36
Saudi Arabia	both	≥10	4,000	≥140/90	11.1	23.5	76	20	1996	36
Egypt	both	≥25	6,733	≥140/90	26	38	24	8	1997	35
Tunisia**	both	≥19	957	≥160/95	18.8	—	—	—	1997	97
Egypt	both	Adult	—	≥130/85	26.3	37.5	24	8	1998	98
Lebanon	Men	25–64	444	≥140/90	30.9	—	—	—	2001	99
Lebanon	Women	25–64	764	≥140/90	18.2	—	—	—	2001	99
Morocco**	Both	20–75	2,000	≥140/90	33.6	—	—	—	2001	100

* Rural.
** Urban.
† If the definition used is Bp ≥160/95 then the prevalence rate is 18%.
[α] Percent of hypertensives with previous history of hypertension.
[β] Percent of hypertensives taking medication.
[γ] Percent of treated hypertensives with blood pressure <140/90.

This review showed that, although the percentage of awared and treated patients in Iran is relatively high to moderate when compared to other developing or EM region, the control rate is low (one half of those actively treated for HTN are controlled) which is similar to other developing countries and far from developed countries (37–40). Most persons, whether hypertensives or not, aware or unaware of their disease, had good basic knowledge related to HTN determinents and consequences (41). The gap between the knowledge about HTN and it's control includes the concurrent cardiovascular risk factors affecting the overall heart health. The hypertensive patients knew well about these risk factors but reported making little actual change to control them (particularly regarding overweight and sedentary habits) (41).

One possible explanation for the gap between the potency of blood pressure control and the achievement of control is that HTN is an asymptomatic, chronic illness such that patients do not consider it as a problem to be treated or even diagnosed. Of the many reasons that treatment fails, drug side effects and costs, the periodic visits to the physicians office and the relationship between the patient and the physician are considered to be important ones. Another explanation, which may be true in Iran is the nonavailability of wide choice of antihypertensive drugs that allow the clinician to tailor the treatment to the patients' characteristics and the low efficacy of some antihypertensive drugs. Also, the complexity of the international guidelines for the management of HTN may discourage physicians to apply them. Some authors have shown that factors related to poor BP control are obesity (4,42–43) (which is relatively common among Iranian and other populations in the EM region (11,17,44–45) even among children from both sexes (45)), male sex (46), low education and occupation category (47–48) and alcohol intake (49). Finally BP measured at a single visit once or twice (which was used in most of the studies conducted in Iran and most of the EM region) may lead to overestimation of the prevalence of high BP and underestimation of the proportion of patients with adequately controlled BP (50).

Of particular interest was the fact that in Iran, hypertensive women tended to be more aware and achieved better treatment than men (Table 4). Nevertheless, when treatment for high BP is established, women (especially of older age groups) showed similar control rate to men (Table 4). The awareness and treatment findings are in agreement with results from previous studies in different western countries (14,51–55). The trends of the "North Karelia HTN control program" in Finland and the "Minnesota Heart survey" in the USA showed better improvements in HTN awareness, treatment and control among woman than men (56–57). The reduction in blood pressure among US women between 1960–62 and 1976–80 was greater than men (58). Similar findings were found among other communities in the EM region (17). The possible explanation for this sex difference may include a higher frequency of contact with general practitioners by women and their better compliance with treatment. Higher rates of awareness and control of HTN have been observed among people with higher level of education (47), but this cannot explain our findings since Iranian women had on average a lower educational level than did men. Another explanation for this finding could be the higher frequency of women visits to physicians due to the fact that the frequency of unemployed women is greater than unemployed men. Although few studies reported higher awareness level among hypertensive men (59), among established hypertensives, women achieved better treatment and control rates than men.

In general, many countries in the EM region reported high prevalence and low control levels either with moderate or low awareness levels of HTN.

Epidemiological considerations about Diabetes Mellitus in Iran and some of the Eastern Mediterranean countries

Epidemiological studies indicate that DM is a highly prevalent disease, which developing and nearly industrialized nations now facing the highest rates. There are currently 3.5 million people with DM type I worldwide, and this number is expected to increase to 5.3 million in the year 2011. For DM type II, the figures are 119.2 million and 212.9 million respectively (60).

To assess future needs for planning health services, policy makers need more information on the number of patients and changes in prevalence over time. In 1965, diagnostic criteria were first formulated by the WHO and revised and standardized in 1980 and 1985 (61–62).

Most epidemiological studies regarding the prevalence, awareness or treatment levels of DM dealt with the most common form of DM (type II), as this form is frequently undiagnosed for many years because the hyperglycemia is often not severe enough to provoke noticeable symptoms of diabetes (15,63). Nevertheless, such patients are at increased risk of developing macrovascular and microvascular complications.

It appears that, for many countries across the world, the incidence of IDDM is rising and in some cases in epidemic proportions. The areas with high incidence of the disease currently are Northern Europe and Sardinia (13). The prevalence of DM obtained by the same standardized method was 1.3% in France, 1.6% in Belgium, 1.7% in Sweden and 2.2% in Italy (64).

The majority of data regarding the incidence of IDDM comes from regions of high incidence i.e. Europe and North America. These studies reported low incidence in Asia, followed by Oceania (Australia and New Zealand), South and North America, and the highest rates were in Europe. The incidence varied from 0.6 per 100.000 in Korea and Mexico to 21.3 per 100.000 among US Navy personnel to 35.3 per 100.000 in Finland (65–66). Wide variation in IDDM prevalence rate was reported among European countries with Finland having the highest (35.3 per 100.000) and northern Greece with the lowest (4.6 per 100.000) (65). Epidemiological surveys from Moscow have shown that the incidence of type I DM markedly increases from birth to the age of 10–14, then persists up to age 40 (67).

Data on the IDDM in the EM region are scarce. There was very low incidence in the 1–14 and 1–19 year age groups (3.9 and 5.6 per 100.000 respectively) from Kuwait. Higher incidence rates come from Saudi Arabia (13), then from Sudan that reported increasing trend of IDDM in the recent years as the incidence rose up from 5.9 in 1987 to 10 per 100.000 in 1990 (13).

Few studies regarding the prevalence of IDDM have been conducted in Iran. Siddigh et al using the 50g-glucose test reported 0.06% abnormal screens out of 7017 school children (68). Another survey using the same method was done on 63,000 people of all ages and reported a prevalence rate of 0.5% among Iranian school children and 2.2% in adults aged 40 years and over in 1979 (69).

The prevalence studies on NIDDM are hard to interpret. Reported data even from one country may vary due to differences in population characteristics or differences in methodology. Surveys concerning NIDDM in some European countries revealed an age-adjusted prevalence of known diabetes between 30–64 years of age, which varies from 1.8% in Russia to 10.7% in Italy (8–9). In American surveys, the age adjusted prevalence rates among white population varies between 3 and 8% (8,70). The prevalence of NIDDM in developing countries is increasing because of changes in life styles, with migration of rural population to the cities (71). Previously reported data from Brazil showed prevalence rates of 7.1 and 9% for diabetes and intolerance glucose test (IGT), respectively (72). The prevalence varies from 4 to 8% in Singapore, and from 2 to 5% in Hong Kong recently (60). Data reported on the estimated and projected prevalence of DM for 1995 to 2025 for India was 3.8 to 6% and for China was 2 to 3.4%, respectively (73). During the last decade, community and hospital—based data on the epidemiology and clinical characteristics of DM have been reported from several countries of the EM region. Unfortunately, the varying methodologies and diagnostic criteria used have resulted in considerable discrepancies; therefore making comparison became more difficult. The prevalence rate in some countries in the EM region ranged from 4% to 25.5%. (10,13,74–75). Table 6 shows the prevalence rates of DM and IGT in different countries in the region. The overall prevalence rate of DM was higher among Bahraini than Kuwaiti or Omani people (76–77). It should be noted that many of the studies mentioned above did not use the recommended WHO criteria for diagnosis (62).

In Iran, it is estimated that currently 2 million people have DM (13,69). Table 7 showed different prevalence rates based on different age groups and several methodological studies [using either one fasting blood sugar (FBS) accompanied by clinical symptoms, two FBS measurements or 2-hour post load plasma glucose (2hpp)] conducted in several cities in Iran. Some of these studies have been done on urban and others on rural samples or special groups. These studies were done in different dates from 1977 to 1997 and among different age groups. None of these studies have used the self reported data alone, which may overestimate the prevalence rate. However when systematic screening with an oral glucose tolerance test (OGTT) was performed, the prevalence rate was 1.5 times higher (78).

Part of the differences in prevalence rate observed between the studies (even from one city) might be explained by the changes in case definition. The prevalence increase with age is clear. Table 7 also shows distinct geographical differences with the highest prevalence rates in urban areas and the lowest in rural areas. The effect of urbanization that have been increasing during the last two decades in most of the EM countries (including Iran) on the transition in dietary patterns and nutritional status that promote the development of non communicable diseases have been well documented before. In this analysis, we included studies conducted in the period 1977 to 1997; however, trends in this period of time were difficult to be interpreted. As noted before, case definitions, sample size, age groups and the geographical area in which the study have been done, may induce these variations. Furthermore true increase in the prevalence of DM in the recent years may be seen.

It was observed that the prevalence rate of DM among Iranian women was higher than men (Table 7), a finding that was reported in previous studies (72–73,76,79). However, some studies found no difference and the prevalence rate was equal among men and women (77) or even higher among men (80–81). A higher body mass index (BMI) among Iranian women compared to men (44) can be considered an additional explanation for the sex difference in DM prevalence as the incidence of DM increases with obesity which is becoming much more prevalent in urban areas. While the majority (>80%) of patients with NIDDM present in Europe and America are obese, in some developing countries like India, most people with NIDDM (>60%) are non-obese and many are actually lean with a BMI of <18.5 (82). It seems that the rarity of obesity may explain the low prevalence of DM in some populations (Like Hanoi, Vietnam) (8,79), however, the prevalence of obesity among individuals with NIDDM in the EM region varies between 46% among Sudanese to 75% in Iraqi Diabetics (13).

Available data on diagnosed or non-diagnosed diabetics demonstrate that overall, approximately 3% of the US population have diagnosed DM and an equal number have DM that is undiagnosed (70). This represents a significant health problem, since at the time of diagnosis several patients already have retinopathy, neuropathy or nephropathy (83). In addition, most of the surveys showed that over 50% of diabetics were undiagnosed (8,84–86).

In this analysis, the percentage of diabetics with known disease in Iran was relatively higher compared to other Mediterranean countries (87–88), and there was less variation between different regions (Table 7). Studies from Iraq, Kuwait and Sudan showed that the prevalence rates of known DM were about 50% (13,87) or even less than that (88). While other reports from Saudi Arabia (10) and Bahrain (77) demonstrated that 86% and 67.6% of diabetics were diagnosed prior to the surveys. The frequency of known DM depends on the way the prevalence rate is measured. Systematic screening with an OGTT yields higher prevalence rates of known DM, but our explanation for the high prevalence rate of known to unknown diabetes in Iran may be attributed to the easy accessibility of health care services for most people (especially in rural areas) and the high frequency of visits in health service centers. Recently the national plan for DM prevention and control have been started by the national committee for DM control related to the office of non-communicable diseases of the ministry of health, treatment and medical education which lead to better awareness among qualified general physicians in the primary health care centers and awareness of those people with positive family history of DM concerning the disease.

Table 6. Prevalence rate of diabetes mellitus (DM) and impaired glucose tolerance (IGT) in different countries in the Eastern Mediterranean Region (1982–1998)

	Prevalence %							IGT			Awareness %			
Countries	Men	Women	Total	Age (year)	Sample Size	Period	Definition	Men	Women	total	Men	Women	total	Ref No
Saudi Arabia (both)			0.3	25–34	1,358	1982	OGTT*							101
			2.6	35–44	1,358	1982	OGTT							
			9.6	45–54	1,358	1982	OGTT							
			11	55–64	1,358	1982	OGTT							
Sudan (both)			0.1	7–14	42,981	1985	OGTT						7	102
Saudi Arabia (a)	2.9	5.9	4.3		5,222	1987	CBG**							103
Saudi Arabia (both)		1.9		≥15	368	1988	2hpp***		8.4					104
Tunisia (a)	2.3	0.6			1,787	1988	FBS† & Δ							105
Tunisia (b)	4.6	3.5			3,826	1988	FBS & Δ							105
Oman (both)	9.7	9.8	10	≥20		1992	2hpp & CPG	8	13					10
Southern Saudi Arabia (a)	5.5	3.6	4.6	≥10	1,419	1992	2hpp	14	7.4	1.6			15	106
Egypt (both)			4.3	≥10		1992	OGTT							74
Egypt (a)			4.1	≥10		1992	OGTT							74
Egypt (b)			5.7	≥10		1992	OGTT							74
Pakistan (b)	16.2	11.7	25††	≥25	967	1994	2hPP	8.2	14.3		9	6.3		107

Egypt (a)			4.9	≥20		1995	2hPP&Δ						50	108
			13.5†††		6,052									
Egypt (b)			20#	≥20		1995	2hPP&Δ							108
			9.3##											
Kuwait (both)	14.7	14.8	14.8	≥20	3,003	1995	OGTT							76
Tunisia (a)	0.8	3.9		35–50	692	1996	FBS&Δ							109
Tunisia (b)	8.8	10.4		35–50		1966	FBS&Δ							109
Bahrain (both)	26.4	25	25.5	≥20	573	1996	2hpp	10.9	16.7	14.7	18.4	16.7	17.3	110
Kuwait (both)			7.6	≥20	8,336	1996	OGTT							87
Mauritania (Both)	1.30	2.29	1.88	≥20	744	1996	CBG						29	111
Iran (b)	6.3	6.7	6.6	20–60	800	1997	2hpp	7.8	7.7	8.4	66	86	70	78
Saudi Arabia (a)	7	7.7		≥15	13,177	1997	OGTT							112
Saudi Arabia (b)	12	14		≥15		1997	OGTT						44	112
Bahrain (both)			12.9	≥48		1998								113
Jordan (both)	14.9	12.5	13.4	≥25	2,836	1998	2hpp	9	10.8	9.8				114
Sudan (both)	9.9	7.5	8.3	≥25	724	1998	OGTT	4.1	9.7	7.9			3.2	115
Pakistan (a)	10.3	4.8	6.5	≥25		1999	OGTT	7.4	19	11.2				116
Pakistan (b)	11.1	10.6	10.8	≥25		1999	OGTT							116

Both, Rural & urban; a, Rural; b, Urban; *Oral glucose tolerance test; **Capillary blood glucose; ***2 hour post load plasma glucose ≥11.1 mmol/l; †Fasting blood sugar ≥7.8 mmol/l; Δ, Previously diagnosed diabetes; ††total glucose intolerance: Diabetes and IGT contained; †††Lower urban socioeconomic status; #Higher Urbans socioeconomic status; ##Diagnosed and nondiagnossed diabetes.

Table 7. Prevalence of non insulin dependent diabetes mellitus in some cities of Iran based on different diagnostic criteria (1977–1997)

City	Year of Study	Studied Population	No. of sample	Age	Prevalence (%)			Diagnostic Criteria	Reference No
					Men	Women	Total		
Tehran[c]	1977	Employee	3,677	>20	10.4			FBS*	68
Tehran	1977	Employee	3,677	>20	0.4	0.9		FBS	68
Iran	1980	Students	2,200	6–17			0.5	2hpp**	68
Iran	1980	Urban	14,500	>40			2.2	2hpp	3
Isfahan[c]	1992	Urban	1,800	10–40	1.09	3.7	2.04	FBS	3
Isfahan	1993	Urban	3,970	≥40	7.54	8	7.5	FBS	3
Tehran†	1994	Urban	2,128			4.5		2hpp	69
Tehran	1994	Rural	820			2.2		2hpp	69
Islamshahr[c]	1994	Urban	2,033	>30	7.1	7.2	7.1	2hpp	69
Kashan[c]	1994	Urban	19,259	>15			7.0	2hpp	3
Brojen[c]	1994	Urban	20,096	>15			3.0	2hpp	3
Bidgol in Kashan[c]	1994	Urban	1,220	>40			6.5	FBS	3
Tehran	1996	Urban	2,800	>20	7.9	8.3	7.2	2hpp	78
Tehran	1996	Rural	2,000	>30	4.9	10.4	4.3	2hpp	78
Tehran	1997	Students	7,017	2–14			0.06	2hpp	78
Isfahan	1997	Urban	800	20–69	6.8	7.7	6.9	FBS∇	78
Isfahan	1998	Urban	800	20–69	6.3	6.7	6.6	2hpp	78
Bosher[s]	1998	Urban	1,039	30–64	9.7	12.9	13.6	2hpp	3

* Fasting blood sugar ≥7.8 mmol/l.
** 2 hour post load plasma glucose ≥11.1 mmol/l.
† Gestational diabetes.
∇ Fasting blood sugar ≥7.8 mmol/l or using hypoglycemic therapy.
[c] *One of the central cities in Iran.*
[s] *One of the southern cities in Iran.*

Finally it appears that for many countries across the world, the incidence of DM is rising, and in some cases is in epidemic proportions. There are evidences to suggest that the prevalence is becoming higher in the EM countries like Iran, in which western nutritional life style (89), hyperlipidemia (90) and less physical activity (44) are considered as important environmental risk factors to influence the increasing prevalence of DM and HTN leading to the increasing prevalence of coronary heart disease among Iranian young people (91). On the other hand, as life expectancy has increased in most of the developing countries as well as Iran (92), most non-communicable diseases emerge as major health problem. Unfortunately these dramatic changes in life-style are affecting children living in these countries as well, as the prevalence of hyperlipidemia and obesity are increasing among Iranian children during the recent years (93).

CONCLUSION

High blood pressure and DM are two major risk factors for cardiovascular diseases and stroke. The pattern of HTN and DM prevalence in westernized population is decreasing now. The recent reports from many countries of the EM region as well as Iran demonstrated that most of the population are at increased risk of HTN and DM (or other non communicable disease) as they are considered among major causes of mortality, morbidity and premature death.

Experimental and observational studies indicate that HTN and DM and their consequences can be prevented. Continued public health efforts will be required to achieve better levels of awareness, treatment and control rates of both diseases which will ultimately lead to further decline in coronary heart disease or stroke. Therefore, the preventive strategies should be applied in the form of a comprehensive and well-coordinated activities together with healthy public policies.

ACKNOWLEDGEMENTS

This work was conducted and supported by Isfahan Cardiovascular Research Center. The authors are grateful to the following persons who cooperated in this study: M. Amiri, R. Hassanwand, S. Zarfeshani, M. Rafie, M. Mortazavi from Isfahan Cardiovascular Research Center and Dr. A. Alwan, Director, Management of Non-communicable Diseases, World Health Organization. Geneva, Switzerland, Dr. Arun Chockalingam, Health Canada, Health Promotion and Programs Branch, Ottawa, Ontario K1A 1B4.

REFERENCES

1. Martin MJ, Hulley SB, Browner WS, Kuller CH, Wentworth O. 1986. Serum cholesterol, blood pressure, and mortality: implications from a cohort of 361662 men. Lancet II:933–936.
2. Alwan A. 1993. Cardiovascular diseases in the Eastern Mediterranean Region. World Health Statistics quarterly 46(2):97–100.
3. Sajady F, Sarraf-Zadegan N, Mohamady-Fard M. 1997. Review of blood pressure changes in Iran from 1971–1996 In: The 1st Eastern Mediterranean Congress on Preventive Cardiology (2–5 May), Iran: Isfahan Cardiovascular Research Center.

4. Sarraf-Zadegan N, Boshtam M, Mostafavi S, Rafiei M. 1999. The prevalence of hypertension and associated risk factors in Isfahan, Iran. Eastern Mediterranean Health J 5(5):992–1001.
5. Medical Research Council Working Party. 1992. MRC trial of treatment of hypertension in older adults: principle results. Br Med J 304:405–412.
6. Neaton JD, et al. 1993. Treatment of Mild Hypertension Study. Final results. JAMA 270:713–724.
7. Dollery C. 1995. Hypertension trial results: consensus and conflicts. J Hum Hypertens 9:403–408.
8. King H, Rewers M. 1993. Global estimates for prevalence of diabetes mellitus and impaired glucose tolerance in adults. Diabetes Care 16:157–177.
9. Alberti KGM. 1993. Problems related to definitions and epidemiologies of type 2 (non-insulin-dependent) diabetes mellitus: studies throughout the world. Diabetologia 36:978–984.
10. Alwan A, King H. 1992. Diabetes in the Eastern Mediterranean Regions, World Health Statistics Quarterly 45:355–359.
11. Binhemd T, Larbi EB, Absood G. 1991. Obesity in a primary health care center: a retrospective study. Annals of Saudi Medicine 11:163–166.
12. Clinical disorders arising from dietary affluence in the EMR. 1989. Alexandria, WHO Regional office for the Eastern Mediterranean (Technical; publications No. 14).
13. Alwan A. 1993. Diabetes prevention and control: A call for Action. World Health Organization-EM/DIA/3/E/G.
14. Smith WG, Lee AJ, Crombie IK, Pedoe HT. 1990. Control of blood pressure in Scotland: the rule of halves. Br Med J 300:981–983.
15. Mooy JM, Grootenhuis PA, de Vries H, Valkenburg HA, Bouter LM, Kostense PJ. 1995. Prevalence and determinants of glucose intolerance in a Caucasian population: the Hoorn study. Diabetes Care 18:1270–1273.
16. Kalmijns S, Feskens EJ, Tuomilehto J, Stengard JH, Launer LJ, Stjnen T, Komhout D. 1995. Hypertension and overweight associated with hyperinsulinaemia and glucose tolerance: a longitudinal study of the Finnish and Dutch cohorts of the seven countries study. Diabetologia 38:839–847.
17. Alwan A. 1995. Prevention and control of Cardiovascular diseases. Alexandria. World Health Organization (EMRO technical publications, No. 22).
18. Sarraf-Zadegan N, Boshtam M, Malkafzali H. 1999. Secular trends in cardiovascular mortality in Iran: with special reference to Isfahan. Acta Cardiologica 54(6):327–333.
19. Mbanya JC, Minkoulou EM, Salah JN, Balkan B. 1998. The prevalence of hypertension in rural and urban Comeroon. Int J Epidemiol 27:181–185.
20. Bruce NG, Cook DG, Shaper AG, Thomson AG. 1990. Geographic variations in blood pressure in British men and women. J Clin Epidemiol 4:385–398.
21. Langford HG, Watson RL, Douglas BH. 1969. Factors affecting blood pressure in population groups. Trans Assoc Am Phys 81:135–146.
22. M'Buyamba-Kabangu JR, Fagard R, Staessen J, Lijnen P. 1987. Correlates of blood pressure in rural and urban Zaire. J Hypertens 5:371–375.
23. Poulter NR, Khaw KT, Hopwood BC, Mugambi M, Peart WS, Rose G. 1984. Blood pressure and associated factors in a rural Kenyan community. Hypertension 6:810–813.
24. Epstein FH, Eckoff RD. 1967. The epidemiology of high blood pressure: Geographic distributions and etiological factors. The epidemiology of hypertension. New York: Grune and Stratton 155–166.
25. Sever PS, Gordon D, Peart WS, Beighton P. 1980. Blood pressure and it's correlates in urban and tribal Africa. Lancet II:60–64.
26. Ibrahim M. 1993. The Egyptian National Hypertension Project: preliminary results from phase 1. Unpublished data.
27. Alwan A. 1982. Studies on the prevalence of hypertension in Iraqi rural and urban communities. Iraqi Medical J, 29:99–104.
28. Faruqi AM. 1983. Heart disease in South Asia: Experiences in Pakistan. In: Hurst JW, clinical essays on the heart, vol. 2. New York, MC Graw-Hill.
29. Sarraf-Zadegan N, Amini-Nik S. 1997. Blood pressure pattern in Urban and rural areas in Isfahan, Iran. Journal of Human Hypertension 11(7):425–428.
30. Marashi S. 1990. The preliminary report of the national study on hypertension in Iran. 300–515.
31. Working group on Risk and High Blood Pressure. 1985. An epidemiological approach to describing risk associated with blood pressure levels: Final report. Hypertension 7:457–468.
32. The fifth report of the joint committee on detection, evaluation and treatment of high blood pressure. 1993. Arch Intern Med 153:154–183.

33. Achananuparp S, Suriyawongpaisal P, Suebwonglee S, Sakdisawasdi O, Nanna P, Khumthong N, Limsuuan A. 1989. Prevalence, detection and control of hypertension in Thai population of a central rural community. J Med Assoc Thai 72:66–75.
34. Ghadha SL, et al. 1996. Prevalence, awareness and treatment status of hypertension in urban population of Delhi. Indian J Med Res 92:233–240.
35. Ibrahim M, Apple LJ, Ibrahim AS, Welton PK. 1995. Hypertension prevalence, awareness, treatment and control in Egypt. Hypertension 26:886–890.
36. Adolfotouh MA, Abu-zeid HA, Abdel Aziz M, Alakija W. 1996. Prevalence of hypertension in south western Saudi Arabia. East Mediterranean Health J 2:211–217.
37. Salomaa V, Tuomilehto J, Nissinen A, Korhonen HJ, Vartiainen E, Kartovaava L, Puska P. 1989. The development of hypertension care in Finland from 1982 to 1987. J Hypertens 7:837–844.
38. Joffres MR, et al. 1992. Prevalence, control and awareness of high blood pressure among Canadian adult. Can Med Assoc J 146:1997–2005.
39. Hense HW, Stieber J, Filipiak B, Keil U. 1993. Five-year changes in population blood pressure and hypertension prevalence. Results from the MONICA Augsburg surveys 1984/85 and 1989/90. Ann Epidemiol 3:410–416.
40. Burt VL, Cutler JA, Higgins M, Horan MJ, Labarthe D, Whelton P, Brown E, Roecella EJ. 1995. Trends in the prevalence, awareness, treatment and control of hypertension in the adult US population. Hypertension 26:60–69.
41. Sarraf-Zadegan N, Tavassoli A, Mortazavi M, Alikhasi H. 1995. The knowledge, attitude and practice of Isfahan population concerning the risk factors of cardiovascular diseases. J of Nabz 5:18–23. (Persian).
42. Vezu L, La Vecchia L, Vincenzi M. 1992. Hypertension, obesity and response to antihypertensive treatment: results of a community survey. J Hum Hypertens 6:215–220.
43. Liu L. 1993. Hypertension in China. Clin Exp Hypertens 15:1015–1094.
44. Sarraf-Zadegan N, Boshtam M, Rafiei M. 1999. Risk factors for coronary heart disease in Isfahan. Eur J Pub Health 9(1):20–26.
45. Akatsu H, Aslam M. 1996. prevalence of hypertension and obesity among women over age 25 in low income area in Karachi, Pakistan. JPMA 46:191–193.
46. Nieto FJ, Alonso J, Chambless LE, Zhong M, Ceraso M, Romm FJ, Cooper L, Folsom AR, Szklo M. 1995. Population awareness and control of hypertension and hypercholesterolemia. Arch Intern Med 155:677–684.
47. Lang T, Pariente P, Salem G, Tap D. 1988. Social, professional conditions and arterial hypertension: an epidemiological study in Dakar, Senegal. J Hypertense 6:271–276.
48. Fouriaud C, Jacquinet-Salord MC, Degoulet P, Aime F, Lang T, Lapurugne J, Main J. 1984. Influence of socioprofessional conditions on blood pressure levels and hypertension control. Am J Epidemial 120:72–86.
49. Lang T, Degoulet P, Aime F, Devies C, Jacquinet-Salord MC, Fouriaud C. 1987. Relations between alcohol consumption and hypertension prevalence and control in a French population. J Chron Dis 40:713–720.
50. Birkett NJ, Donner AP, Maynard MD. 1987. Assessing hypertension control in the community: the need for follow-up measurements to ensure clinical relevance. Can Med Assoc J 136:595–600.
51. Marques PV, Arveiler D, Amouyel PH, Bingham A, Ferrieres J. 1997. Sex differences in awareness and control of hypertension in France. J Hypertens 15(11):1205–1210.
52. Plans P, Pardell H, Salleras L. 1993. Epidemiology of cardiovascular disease risk factors in Catalonia (Spain). Eur J Epidemiol 9:381–389.
53. Wagner EH, James SA, Beresford SA, Strogatz DS, Grimson RC, Klienbaum DG, et al. 1984. The Edgecombe County high blood pressure control program. Correlates of uncontrolled hypertension at baseline. AM J Public Health 74:237–242.
54. Pica LA, Boucher MM, Grignon R. 1990. The prevalence, awareness and control of hypertension in Laval, Quebec, 1986. Can J public Health 81:427–430.
55. Burt VL, Whelton P, Roccella EJ, Brosn C, Cutler JA, Higgins M, et al. 1995. Prevalence of hypertension in the US adult population. Hypertension 25:305–313.
56. Nissinen A, Toumilehto J, Korhonen H, Pika T, Salonen J, Puska P. 1988. Ten year results of hypertension Care in the community. 127:488–498.
57. Spfka JM, Burke GL, Folsom AR, Luepker RV, Blackburn H. 1990. Continued decline in cardiovascular disease risk factors: Results of the Minnesota Heart Survey. American J of Epidemiol 132: 489–500.

58. Dannenberg AL, Drized T, Horan MJ, Haynes SG, Leavereton PE. 1987. Progress in the battle against hypertension: Changes in blood pressure levels in the United States from 1960 to 1980. Hypertension 10:226–223.
59. Marques PV, Tuomilehto J. 1997. Hypertension awareness, Treatment and control in the community: Is the rule of halves still Valid? J Hum Hypertens 11:213–220.
60. Bloomgarden ZT. 1998. International Diabetes Federation Meeting, 1997. Diabetes care 21:860–865.
61. World Health Organization. 1980. World Health Organization Expert Committee on Diabetes Mellitus. Second part. Geneva: WHO.
62. World Health Organization. 1985. Diabetes mellitus: report of a study group. Geneva: WHO, (Technical Report series No. 727).
63. Harris MI. 1993. Undiagnosed NIDDM; clinical and public health issues. Diabetes Care 16: 642–652.
64. Jirovec M, Teuscher A, Burgi U, Diem P. 1993. Prevalence of diabetes in Switzerland: Calculation based on drug sales. Schweiz-Med-Wochenschr 123:2247–2250. (WHO-EM/DIA/3/E/G).
65. Karvonen M, Toumilehto J, Libman I, Laporte R. 1993. A review of the recent epidemiological data on the worldwide incidence of type 1 (insulin-dependent) diabetes mellitus. World Heath Organization Project Group. Diabetologica 36:883–892.
66. Gorhan ED, Garland FC, Barrett-Conner E, Wingard DL, Pughn WM. 1993. Incidence of insulin-dependent diabetes mellitus in young adults: experience of 1,587,630 US Navy enlisted personnel. Am J Epidemiol 138:984–987.
67. Kuraeva TL, Sergeev AS, Lebedev MB, Babadzhanova GI, Kerimi NB. 1993. Diabetes mellitus incidence and it's prevalence in Moscow. Probl-Endokrinol-Mosk 39:4–7.
68. Seddigh G, Ghazanfarpoor M, Yasai M, Naghibi A. 1996. A report on the national survey of diabetes in Iran, National Institute of Nutrition.
69. Azizi F. 1996. Diabetes Mellitus in the Islamic Republic of Iran. IDF Bulletin 41:38–39.
70. Harris MI, Hadden WC, Knowler WC, Bennet PH. 1987. Prevalence of diabetes and impaired glucose tolerance and plasma glucose levels in US population aged 20–74 yr. Diabetes 36:523–534.
71. Zimmet PZ, Kelly west lecture 1991. 1992. Challenges in diabetes epidemiology from west to the rest. Diabetes Care 15:232–252.
72. Oliveira JP, Milech A. 1996. The prevalence of diabetes in Rio de Janeiro, Brazil Diabetes Care 19:663–666.
73. Gupta R. 1998. India leads in global diabetic count. South Asian preventive Cardiology 19:83–85.
74. Arab M. 1992. Diabetes mellitus in Egypt, World Health Statistics quarterly 45:334–337.
75. Dowse GK, Zimmet P. 1992. Amodel protocol for diabetes and other non communicable disease field survey. World Health Statistics quarterly 45:360–372.
76. Abdulla N, Al Arouj M, Al Nakhi A, Al Assoussi A, Moussa M. 1998. Non-Insulin-dependent diabetes in Kuwait: prevalence rates and associated risk factors. Diabetes Res Clin Pract 42:187–196.
77. Al Zurba F, Al Garf A. 1996. Prevalence of diabetes mellitus among Bahrainis attending primary health care centers. Eastern Mediterranean Health J 2:274–282.
78. Sajadi F, Sarraf-Zadegan N, Ali-Khassi H, Mohammadi-fard N, Abdar N. 1999. The prevalence of diabetes in Iran during 1976–1997. J of Uromia University of Medical Sciences 10(2):129–139. (Persian).
79. Quoc PS, Charles MA, Cuong NH, et al. 1994. Blood glucose distribution and prevalence of diabetes in Hanoi (Vietnam). Am J Epidemiol 139:713–722.
80. Ohmura T, Ueda K, Kiyohara Y, Kato I, et al. 1993. Prevalence of type 2 (non-insulin-dependent) diabetes mellitus and impaired glucose tolerance in the Japanese general population: the Hisayama study. Diabetologia 36:1198–1203.
81. Cockram CS, Woo J, Lau E, Chan AY, Lau J. 1993. The prevalence of diabetes mellitus and impaired glucose tolerance among Hong Kong Chinese adults of working age. Diabetes-Res-Clin-Pract 21:67–73.
82. Mohan V, Vijayaprabha R, Rema M, Premalatha G, Poongothai S, Deepa R. 1997. Clinical profile of lean NIDDM in South India. Diabetes-Res-Clin-Pract 38:101–108.
83. Engelgau MM, Aubert RE, Thompson TJ, Herman WH. 1995. Screening for NIDDM in non-pregnant adults: a review. Diabetes cares 18(12):1606–1618.
84. World Health Organization, 1992. Ad hoc diabetes reporting group. Diabetes and impaired glucose tolerance in women aged 20–39 years. World Health statistics quarterly 45:321–327.
85. American Diabetes Association. 1992. Screening for diabetes. Diabetes Care 15(52):7–9.

86. Sekikawa A, et al. 1993. Prevalence of diabetes and impaired glucose tolerance in Funagata area. Japan. Diabetes Care 16:570–574.
87. Abdulla NA, Khogali MM, Salman AD, Ghneimi SA, Bajaj JS. 1995. Pattern of non-Insulin dependent diabetes mellitus in Kuwait. Diabetes Res Clin Pract 29:129–136.
88. El Mahdi EM, Abdul Rahman IM, Mukhtar SD. 1989. Pattern of diabetes mellitus in the Sudan. Trop Geogr Med 41:353–357.
89. Mohammadifard N, Sarraf-Zadegan N, Jalali A, Alikhassi H, Rafiei M. 1998. Food and nutrient intake among adults of Isfahan, Iran. South Asian J preventive Cardiology 2:59–63.
90. Rfiei M, Boshtam M, Sarraf-Zadegan N. 1999. Lipid profiles in Isfahan population: Isfahan CVD Risk Factor Survey, 1994. East Mediterranean Health J 5(4):54–65.
91. Sarraf-Zadegan N, Tabatabaei F, Bashardosst N, Stodehmaram E, Tafazoli F, Karimi A, Maleki A, Totonchi M, Habibi HR. 1999. The prevalence of coronary artery disease in urban population in Isfahan, Iran. Acta Cardiologica 54(5):257–263.
92. Malek Afzali H. 1996. The life expectancy of Iranian men and women in 1996. Hakim Research J 1:107–110. (Persian).
93. Kelishadi R, Hashemipoor M, Sarraf-Zadegan N, Amiri M. 2001. Trend of Atherosclerosis risk factors in children of Isfahan (1993–1999). Journal of the Asian Cardiovascular & Thoracic Annals 9(1):36–40.
94. The ministry of Health and Treatment in Iran—The activity file of the Vice chancellor for Research in the ten year developing plan from 1988–1998.
95. Wahid Saeed AA, AL shammary FJ, Khoja TA, Hashim TJ, Anokute CC, Khan SB. 1996. The Prevalence of hypertension and sociodemographic characteristics of adult hypertensives in Riyadh city. Saudi Arabia. J Hum Hypertens 10(9):583–587.
96. Jaddou HY, Batieah AM, Ajlouni KM. 1996. Prevalence and associated factors of hypertension: results from a three community-based surveys, Jordan. J Hum Hypretense 10(12):815–821.
97. Ghannem H, Hadj-Fredj A. 1997. Prevalence of cardiovascular risk factors in the urban population in Tunisia. J Public Health Med 19(4):392–396.
98. Ibrahim M. 1998. Egyptian physicians' knowledge and Attitudes Towards Hypertension. Egyptian physicians hypertension survey. The Egyption hypertension society 4(2):1.
99. Khogali M. 2002. The cardiovascular disease prevention initiative. First attempt to a community based approach in the Arab World (1998–2001).
100. Cardiovascular and Neoplasic service non-communicable diseases division epidemiology direction. Moroccan survey on cardiovascular disease risk factor 2001.
101. Bacclus RA, Bell JL, Madkour M, Kilshaw B. 1982. The prevalence of diabetes mellitus in male Saudi Arabs. Diabetologia 23(4):330–332.
102. Elamin A, Cmer MI, Hofrander Y, Taemot T. 1989. Prevalence of IDDM in school children in khartoum sudan. Diabetes care 12(6):430–432.
103. Fatani HH, Mira SA, El Zubier AG. 1987. Prevalence of diabetes mellitus in rural Saudi Arabia. Diabetes Care 10(2):180–183.
104. Al-shawaf T, Akiel A, Moghraby SA. 1988. Gestational diabetes and impaired glucose tolerance of pregnancy in Riyadh. Br J Obstet Gynaecol 95(1):84–90.
105. Papoz L, Ben Khalifea F, Esch Wege E, Ben Ayed H. 1998. Diabetes mellitus in Tunisia: description in urban and rural population. Int J Epidemiol 17(2):419–422.
106. Abuzeid HA, Kassab AS. 1992. Prevalence and health-care features of hyperglycemia in semiurban-rural communities in southern Saudi Arabia. Diabetes care 15(4):484–489.
107. Shera AS, Rafique G, Khwaja IA, Ara J, Bagai S, King H. 1995. Pakistan National diabetes survey: prevalence of glucose intolerance and associated factors in shikarpur, sind province. Diab Med 12(12):1116–1121.
108. Herman WH, Ali MA, Auber RF, Engelgau MM, Kenny SF, Gunter EW, Malarcher AM. 1995. Diabetes mellitus in Egypt: risk factors and prevalence. Diabetes Med 12(12):1126–1131.
109. Gharbi M, Belhani A, Aouidet A, Ben Rayana C, Achour A, Nasraoui A, Tritar B. 1996. Level of cardiovascular risk factors in the urban and rural populations of Cap-Bon: Tunisia. Rev Epidemiol Sante publique 44(2):125–132.
110. Farouq I, Alzubra F, Algraf A. 1996. Prevalence of diabetes mellitus among Bahrainis attending ptimary health care centres. Eastern Mediterranean Health J 274–284.
111. Ducorops M, Baleynaud S, Mayaudon H, Castagne C, Bauduceau B. 1996. A prevalence survey of diabetes in Mauritania. Diabetes Care 19(7):761–763.
112. Al-Nuaim AR. 1997. Prevalence of glucose intolerance in urban and rural communities in Saudi Arabia. Diabet Med 14(7):595–602.

113. Musaiger AO. 1992. Diabetes mellitus in Bahrain: an overview. Diabet Med 9(6):574–578.
114. AJlouni K, Jaddou HY, Batieha AM. 1998. Diabetes and impaired glucose tolerance in Jordan: Prevalence and associated risk factors. J inter Med 244(4):317–323.
115. Elbagir MN, Eltom MA, Elmahadi EM, Kadam IU, Berne C. 1998. A high prevalence of diabetes mellitus and impaired glucose tolerance in the Danagla community in northern Sudan. Diabet Med 15(2):164–169.
116. Hamed K, Kadir M, Gibson T, Suitana S, Fatima Z, Syed A. 1995. The frequency of known diabetes, hypertension and ischemic heart disease in affluent and poor urban population of Karachi. Diabet Med 12:500–513.

Frontiers in Cardiovascular Health, edited by
N.S. Dhalla, A. Chockalingam,
H.I. Berkowitz & P.K. Singal
Kluwer Academic Publishers, Boston, 2003

Coronary Artery Disease in Developing and Newly Industrialized Countries: A Scientific Statement of the International College of Cardiology

Daniel Pella,[1] Ram B. Singh,[2]
Brian Tomlinson,[3] and Chee-Woon Kong[4]

International College of Cardiology, Safaric University, Kosice, Slovakia[1], Medical Hospital and Research Centre, Moradabad, India[2], The Chinese University of Hong Kong, Prince of Wales Hospital, Shatin, Hong Kong[3], Taiwan Society of Cardiology, Taipei, Taiwan[4]

Summary. Coronary risk factors such as hypertension, tobacco consumption, hypercholesterolemia and diabetes as well as coronary artery disease (CAD) have become a major health problem in developing and newly industrialized countries despite a moderate increase in fat intake and low rates of obesity. It is a paradox that in some of these countries the increased risk of people to diabetes and CAD, especially at a younger age, is difficult to explain by conventional risk factors. It is possible that the presence of new risk factors especially higher lipoprotein (a) (Lp(a)), hyperhomocysteinemia, insulin resistance, low high density lipoprotein cholesterol and poor nutrition during fetal life, infancy and childhood may explain at least in part, the cause of this paradox. The prevalence of obesity, central obesity, smoking, physical inactivity and stress are rapidly increasing in developing and newly industrialized countries due to economic development and affluence. Many countries in Eastern Europe (such as Slovakia, Poland, and Hungary) and Hong Kong, Singapore and Taiwan that are more affluent have greater prevalence of these adverse effects in comparison to less developed countries such as Philippines, China, Thailand, and Brazil. Hypertension, diabetes and CAD are very low in the rural population of India, China, and in the African sub-continent which has less economic development. However, in urban and immigrant populations of India and Chinese origin, the prevalence of hypertension (>169/95, 12–20%), diabetes (6–18%) and CAD (7–14%) are significantly higher than they are in some of the developed countries.

Correspondence to: Dr. R.B. Singh, MD, Professor of Medicine, Subharti Medical College, Civil Lines, Moradabad-10(UP) 244001, India. E-mail: icn@mickyonline.com.

Mean serum cholesterol (180–200 mg/dl), obesity (5–8%) and dietary fat intake (25–30% en/day) are paradoxically not very high and do not explain the cause of increased susceptibility to CAD and diabetes in some South Asian countries. The force of lipid-related risk factors appear to be greater in these populations due to the presence of the above factors and results into CVD at a younger age in these countries. Available studies support the consensus that people of poor economic origin on rapid nutritional transition may develop CVD at a younger age. They should therefore have lower desirable limits of serum cholesterol, body mass index, dietary fat intake and should also decrease the new risk factors for prevention of CAD. These findings may require modification of the existing guidelines of the International Task Force for Prevention of CAD.

Key words: hypertension, diabetes, ethnicity, prevalence, angiotensin converting enzyme.

INTRODUCTION

In majority of populations, chronic diseases of affluence develop due to interaction of gene and environmental factors (1,2). These problems, which are usually related to economic development, follow a sequence during the transition from poverty to affluence or on migration from rural to urban environments. Although diseases of poverty are not yet controlled, a mounting epidemic of cardiovascular disease (CVD) is now sweeping the urban areas of the developing world (1–5). Studies in developed countries have demonstrated that epidemiological evolution of CVD can be classified into six stages derived from population levels of acculturation, urbanization, affluence, saturated fat intake, salt intake, and tobacco consumption. The prevalence of CVD initially increases with a rise in these factors and then stabilizes due to the lack of health education and finally decreases on learning the message of prevention (1). Presently, in developing countries, these socioeconomic indices are at a stage of transition from poverty to affluence and hence explain the increasing risk of CVD. Whereas, in newly industrialized countries, these indices have reached the final stage of transition resulting in stabilization of coronary artery disease (CAD) and diabetes. The decrease in strokes appears to be due to the reduction in blood pressure and salt intake in the newly industrialized countries.

Chronic degenerative ailments, generally associated with affluent societies, constitute a major cause of death in impoverished countries of the developing world. In 1990, two thirds of the 14 million cardiovascular fatalities worldwide occurred in developing countries (1–6). These numbers are likely to increase as more than half the population is under 15. Furthermore in the developing world, CVD is emerging at an earlier age. In 1990, the proportion of CVD deaths occurred below the age of 70 years was 26.5% in rich countries as compared to 46.7% in poor countries (4–8). The causes for the increase in CVD are known. One important factor is the rising life expectancy. Other factors relate to rapid and chaotic urbanization with accompanying lifestyle changes as well as powerful economic and cultural influences of globalization (5–11). The shift in agricultural production from small farmer to large corporation, distribution from shopkeeper to supermarket, and consumption from fresh to processed foods, promote drastic changes in nutrition.

Dietary fiber and the complex carbohydrates rich whole grains, fruits and vegetables are substituted by junk foods. Consumption of fat and salt increase while consumption of phytochemicals diminishes. Energy intake multiplies while physical activity lessens due to market forces and rapid changes in lifestyle. The mismatch between energy intake and energy output manifests in a pandemic of overweight and central obesity with underlying hyperinsulinemia and higher angiotensin converting enzyme activity (1,6). Crowding, mass unemployment and violence engender social and psychological stresses causing additional risk factors for CVD and diabetes. Additionally, the rising consumption of tobacco and alcohol, in which the outcome is tragic, is causing an emergence of CVD, diabetes, gall stones and cancer.

In the 1990's, the retreat of cigarette companies has become a near route in some developed nations. To make up for lost revenue, the tobacco industry forged a long range global strategy to maintain sales roughly constant where they were under siege, while investing mammoth resources to increase market share in the Third World. In the past decade, United States tobacco consumption dropped 17 percent while exports have sky-rocketed by 259 percent (11). Tobacco consumption and promotion are pursued aggressively in developing countries, with advertising budgets frequently surpassing national funds appropriated for leading disease. Among the primary targets are women and children. These vulnerable groups are all ill equipped to cope with the slick marketing techniques and the dirty tricks perfected by the tobacco industry. Most developing countries have no advertising controls, lack adequate health warning requirements and have a dearth of pressure groups campaigning for stricter tobacco controls. They have set no age limits, nor imposed restrictions on smoking in public places. Their populations are poorly educated on the health hazards and no information is provided to the burgeoning numbers of teenagers who are most susceptible to the advertising hype (9–11). The higher tar and nicotine content purveyed to the developing world makes their cigarettes far more addictive and therefore more lethal. When the spreading tobacco habit is coupled with the rapid rising prevalence of sedentary behavior, obesity, hypercholesterolemia and high blood pressure, there is a definite firestorm spread of coronary heart disease, diabetes and cancer.

How should the developing world respond to this challenge? Current position indicates that it will follow stereotypically the pattern evident worldwide. The role models are the industrial nations, particularly in the USA and the UK. The emulation is in part driven by the fact that most developing countries have weak or nonexistent public health infrastructures (9), by their embrace of medical residency training programs aimed to impart proficiency in interventional technologies and the high incomes offered to those servicing wealthy clienteles in super-specialized sectors. Corporate sponsored medical emporia are now mushrooming in urban centers all over the developing world. Coronary artery bypass surgery and interventional cardiology is a lucrative business. To attract "customers", no costs are spared in acquiring cutting edge equipment serviced by highly trained professionals. Highlighted in these centers is specialized tertiary care treatment for those with ischemic heart disease while preventive strategies are largely ignored. In addition to the exorbitant social cost of such medical practice, it short-changes the individual patient by promoting unnecessary procedures which exact inevitable and unjustified burdens of morbidity as well as death.

It is possible that halfway technologies applied to advanced stages of disease are counter productive strategies for containing an ever-mounting epidemic (9). An important warning sign about "the road not to travel" is now being provided by the USA, chief advocate of a technological approach to health. The American people are now dealing with a health care crisis.

In most populations of the world, starvation and poor energy intake, as well as physically demanding occupations are associated with low plasma insulin, glucose, triglycerides, cholesterol and low angiotensin converting enzyme activity. Thus, contributing in lower blood pressure, as well as a lower risk of CAD and diabetes. However, socioeconomic development in these populations may predispose overweight, central obesity, higher angiotensin converting enzyme activity and hyperinsulinemia initially, followed by other problems including CAD and diabetes (1,12). CAD has become a major health problem in the developing world. The increased susceptibility to developing CAD at a younger age is not explained by conventional risk factors alone. Possibly, the interaction of genetic and environmental factors may explain the cause of the higher prevalence and CAD mortality which appears at a younger age in these countries.

The region of the Indian subcontinent (also known as South Asia) comprises India, Pakistan, Bangladesh, Sri Lanka, Nepal, Bhutan and Afghanistan. In these countries, we find nearly one quarter of the total world population in the process of nutritional transition, from poverty to affluence due to rapid economic development (1,2). Developed countries such as Japan, New Zealand, Australia, Southern Europe, Canada, and the United States have demonstrated a reduction in CAD mortality and incidence. However, Singapore, Hong Kong, Taiwan, and other newly industrialized countries such as Eastern Europe have an increased mortality and risk due to CAD. Reliable population-based data on coronary mortality are not available from Asia and other parts of the developing world. However, current epidemiological evidence (3–15) indicates that CAD has become a public health problem in these countries.

With its population over one billion, India already has a major and rapidly increasing CAD problem. In the Indian urban population, there has been a ten-fold increase in CAD prevalence in the last 3 decades (5). A similar situation appears to exist in Pakistan, Sri Lanka, Bangladesh, and Nepal as revealed by the World Health Organization estimates (1,2). In urban areas (14–26), the CAD is as common as in developed countries and the prevalence varies between 7–14%. Studies from rural areas (10–14) have shown a three-fold lower prevalence as compared to cities, however a rising trend has been observed in both rural and urban areas. The prevalence of CAD is significantly higher in the south as compared to North India (8,14–19) in both rural and urban areas. The risk of CAD in south Asians is higher among upper social classes (7–10). The Five City Study provides more useful evidence that CAD and coronary risk factors have become an important concern in

India. CAD incidence, case fatality and mortality have been reported (24–29) to be unusually high among people of South Asian origin living in industrialized countries. These reports come from Singapore, Uganda, South Africa, Fizi, Trinidad, Mauritius, United Kingdom, and United States where South Asians are more affluent. Therefore rich foods and the luxurious lifestyle of developing countries are within their reach even in the lower social classes (20–35). In England and Wales between 1979–1983, coronary mortality was 36% higher in men and 46% higher in women born in South Asia than in the general population (27). In South Africa, in 1985, the relative risk of coronary death in Indians compared with Europeans was 1.3 in men and 1.7 in women (28). The relative risk of CAD in men of Indian origin, under 40 years of age, was more than twice the national average. The high coronary mortality is common to Gujrati Hindus, Punjabi Sikhs, and Muslims from Pakistan and Bangladesh (29). The increased susceptibility of South Asians to CAD has been difficult to explain by conventional coronary risk factors, diet, and lifestyle factors (31–35). The prevalence of hypertension type II diabetes and hyperlipidemia follow a similar pattern among Indians. In rural Indians, energy intake from fat is <15% and mean serum cholesterol levels are <4.1 mmol/1(160 mg/dl), whereas in urban areas, fat intake accounts for 20–30% energy intakes and mean serum cholesterol are 4.9 mmol/1(190 mg/dl) with a two-fold higher prevalence of CAD. Similar situations to a lesser extent exist in many developing countries and may result into CAD in younger age groups (35).

PROPOSED MECHANISM

Most experts agree that South Asians are genetically susceptible to CAD (20–23,26–28) due to a presence of a "thrifty" genotype (which may have developed in a time of scarcity due to poverty and undernutrition). This may explain the cause of the higher risk of central obesity and diabetes (19), although insulin sensitivity cannot fully account for the increased coronary mortality in Indians (28,29). It is also possible that the "thrifty" genotype may also have selected the ability to store fatty acids, cholesterol and calcium in the coronary arterial cells for optimal physiological function during times of food scarcity and undernutrition. This phenotypic expression for health becomes a disadvantage during times of affluence resulting in phenotypic expression for disease. A modest increase in dietary fatty acids, cholesterol, iron and calcium although within prescribed limits for physiological function, may be misdirected along with lipoprotein a (Lpa), angiotensin II and lipid soluble pesticides, to arterial walls resulting in the development of atherosclerosis. Accumulation of cholesterol and calcium is damaging to endothelial cells and may in conjunction with higher Lp(a) and insulin, angiotensin II and other risk factors including antioxidant deficiency, enhance the process of atherosclerosis (26–36). In one study (33), the higher case fatality among South Asians was significantly associated with diabetes and thus indicated that diabetes and its associated risk factors, dyslipidemia, hyperinsulinemia and oxidative stress may be important in the pathogenesis of higher coronary mortality among South Asians.

Table 1. Prevalence % of coronary artery disease and coronary risk factors in south asians (means)

	North Indians		South Indians	Sri Lanka	UK South	British
	Rural	Urban	Urban	Urban	Asians	Native
Coronary Artery Disease	3.0	9.0	13.9	11.5	15.0	11.0
Smoking (%) (Men)	30	25.6	44.6	57.4	22	30
Diabetes (%)	2.3	6.0	8.0	5.8	19.0	5.0
Hypertension (<160/95 mmHg) (%)	4.0	15.0	18.0	17.2	18.0	20.0
Total Fat (kcal daily)	14.8	24.7	28.8	28.0	38.8	42.2
Saturated Fat (% kcal daily)	4.9	9.2	14.4	13.6	13.7	18.5
Cholesterol in diet (mg daily)	53	166	240	210	200	405
Body Mass Index (kg/m^2)	21.6	22.9	22.7	21.0	26	26
Waist-Hip Ratio (Male)	0.86	0.89	0.89	—	0.98	0.94
Fasting Plasma Insulin (Male) (mU/L)	4.8	5.1	16.6	—	9.8	7.2
2-Hour after Glucose (mU/L)	11.8	24.2	60.6	—	41.0	19.0
Serum Cholesterol (mg/dl)	168	190	210	196	230	236
HDL Cholesterol (mg/dl)	43.5	44.2	45.1	45.2	45.0	46.2
Angiotensin Converting Enzyme (IU)	37.5	63.4	72.0	—	80.0	—

Modified from Singh et al.[24] Lancet, 1995.
HDL = High Density Lipoprotein Cholesterol.

CORONARY ARTERY DISEASE PREVALENCE AND ITS RISK FACTORS

CAD is three times more common in the urban North Indians (9.0%), four times in urban South Indians (13.9%) and Bombay (11.6%), while significantly higher in Nagpur (10.0%) and Calcutta (8.2%) than in the rural (3.2%) population as revealed by the Five City Study (8–10,24). The paradox is that the total and saturated fat intake, fasting and 2-hour plasma insulin levels, serum cholesterol levels, hypertension, diabetes and smoking alone does not explain all the differences in risk of CAD in five Indian cities and in the other studies from South Asia (Tables 1–3). Increased susceptibility to CAD in South Asians may be due to decreased beta cell functions, insulin resistance, hyperinsulinemia, increased prevalence of type II diabetes, increased Lpa, increased plasminogen activator inhibitor-1 and apo B, decreased tissue plasminogen activator and low HDL-cholesterol (26), (Table 2). Recently, inflammatory markers, infections, heart rate and blood pressure variability as well as increased angiotensin converting enzyme activity (1,35,37) in urban compared to rural subjects (39.5 vs 65.5 IU) (30–34) have been demonstrated to be important risk factors of CAD. The prevalence of CAD in other countries varies from 3–4% in China to 4–5% in the Philippines, Thailand, Malaysia while approximately 5% in Singapore, Hong Kong, Taiwan and the newly industrialized countries. CAD

Table 2. Genetic and other specific risk factors common in south asians

Genetic or Environmental	Other Risk Factors
1. Insulin resistance and hyperinsulinemia	1. Increased plasminogen activator inhibitor-1
2. Poor beta cell function	2. Decreased tissue plasminogen activator
3. Increased prevalence of type II diabetes	3. Decreased antioxidant vitamins A, C, beta-carotene, E, Se, Zn, flavinoids, other polyphenolic substances
4. Increased lipoprotein(a)	4. Low high density lipoprotein cholesterol
5. Increased angiotensin converting enzyme	5. Elevated homocysteins
6. High Apo-B	6. Low Apo A1
	7. Increased heart rate variability
	8. Increased small dense LDL cholesterol

Table 3. Dietary guidelines and desirable level of risk factors for developing populations

Factors	Desirable Values
Energy (k calories/day)	1900–2300
Total Carbohydrate (k calories/day)	65.0
Complex Carbohydrate (k calories/day)	55.0
Total Fat (k calories/day)	21.0
Saturated Fatty Acids (k calories/day)	7.0
Polyunsaturated Fatty Acids (k calories/day)	7.0
Polyunsaturated/Saturated Fat Ratio	1.0
n 6/n-3 Fatty Acid Ratio	<5.0
Dietary Cholesterol (mg/day)	100
Whole Grains (wheat, rice, corn, legumes) (g/day)	400–500
Fruit, vegetables and nuts (g/day)	400–500
Salt (g/day)	<6.0
Brisk Walking (km/day)	9.0
Meditation (minutes/day)	30.0
Body Mass Index (kg/m^2)	
Range	19.0–23.0
Average	21.0
Waist-Hip Girth Ratio	
Male	<0.88
Female	<0.85
Serum Total Cholesterol (mg/dl) (4.42 mmol/L)	<170
Mild Hypercholesterolemia (mg/dl) (4.42–5.20 mmol/L)	170–200
Hypercholesterolemia (mg/dl) (>5.20 mmol/L)	>200
Low Density Lipoprotein Cholesterol (mg/dl) (2.32 mmol/L)	<90
Borderline High (mg/dl) (2.32–2.84 mmol/L)	90–110
High (mg/dl) (2.84 mmol/L)	>110
Triglycerides (mg/dl) (1.7 mmol/L)	<150
High Density Lipoprotein Cholesterol (mg/dl) (0.9 mmol/L)	>40
Blood Pressure (mmHg)	<140/90

Modified from Indian Consensus Group 27 J Nutr Environ Med, 1996.

prevalence is much greater in Eastern Europe and is rapidly rising above 5–6% in various countries of South America.

It is possible that variations in conventional risk factors in conjunction with the above risk factors along with the background of antioxidant vitamin deficiency, enhanced ACE activity and the thrifty genotype (37–46) may explain the cause of increased susceptibility and the variable prevalence of CAD in people of South Asian origin and possibly in other developing populations. The sources of atherogenic saturated fat in South Asian diets are hydrogenated fat, Indian ghee, cholesterol oxide, butter, milk and meat (Muslims) in North India (30), ground nut oil and trans fatty acids in West, East and Central India, and coconut oil in South India (8,31,38,39). Hepatic handling of insulin is modulated by habitual fat intake and a high fat diet especially due to saturated fatty acids and enhanced ACE activity. Insulin secretion can rise to suppress hepatic glucose production resulting in insulin resistance, higher angiotensin enzyme activity and decreased heart rate variability (39–57). This mechanism may have more adverse effects in South Asians because of widespread malnutrition during pregnancy causing fetal undernutrition (43) and may be associated with phenotypic expression for diabetes and CAD in adults. There is evidence that the relative increase in coronary risk with an increased intake of saturated fat, or an increase in serum cholesterol even in low cholesterol cultures was comparable in different cultures in the Seven Countries Study (2,36). However, the force of the risk factors varied from culture to culture since the absolute level of coronary risk differed substantially due to other risk factors among cultures (35). It is possible that the force of conventional risk factors is greater in South Asians compared to other populations due to the presence of genetic susceptibility including increased ACE activity and other new risk factors which would require different strategies for prevention (Table 3) (38).

ACE GENE AND CORONARY ARTERY DISEASE

Genetic factors are known to play an important role in the development of hypertension and atherosclerosis. Some of the most commonly studied polymorphisms in this field are those of the renin-angiotensin system (RAS) particularly the angiotensin-converting enzyme (ACE) insertion/deletion (I/D) polymorphism, the genes for angiotensinogen (AGT) M235T and the angiotensin type 1 receptor (AT1R). Our studies have found no relationship with baseline blood pressure levels and the ACE gene I/D polymorphism in Chinese populations (51–56) and most other studies in Chinese have found similar results. However, we found that polymorphisms in other genes such as the insulin receptor (55) and dopamine D2 receptor (42) were associated with blood pressure in Hong Kong Chinese subjects.

The DD genotype of the ACE gene has been reported to increase the risk of athersclerosis in some populations. There are large variations in the frequency of this genotype between populations and is low in Chinese populations (10–14%) as compared to Caucasians (25–43%) (43). An analysis of the frequencies of the DD genotype in various populations with lower rates of CAD suggested the DD genotype frequency may contribute to the interethnic differences in CAD mortality rates

(56). Homozygotes for the deletion (DD) have levels of circulating ACE approaching twice that of those homozygous for the insertion (II). This strong relationship between the I/D genotype and circulating ACE levels has been observed repeatedly in studies in white populations; similar findings have been noted in other ethnic groups. It was found that plasma ACE levels rather than ACE genotype correlated with lipids, plasma glucose and blood pressure in the Native American Pima Indians (56). Elevated plasma ACE levels may contribute to the link between insulin resistance and CAD disease which is becoming so prevalent in people of South Asian origin. This finding also poses the possibility that enhanced ACE activity can predispose insulin resistance.

PREVENTION OF CORONARY ARTERY DISEASE

If we compare the rural population of developing countries to other population groups, it is clear that the prevalence of CAD is still very low. This may be acceptable although it may be further decreased (Table 2). The risk of CAD is proportional to increases in affluence in urban and immigrant populations and from lower social classes to higher social classes (6–16). This is against the findings in developed countries where lower social classes have greater risk of CAD than higher social classes (1–3,47,48). Comparison of the lifestyle between rural and urban subjects, including lower and higher social classes, shows that the most striking difference is that rural and lower social classes have higher occupational physical activities (6–15,47,48) compared to other population groups. Rural and lower social classes also consume low fat, cereal based diets (10–20% daily), have lower serum cholesterol (150–180 mg/dl), triglycerides (100–130 mg/dl) and lower body mass index (19–21 kg/m^2) which indicates a graded increase in these risk factors in urban and immigrant populations (9–12,37,47,48). Low levels of risk factors and higher physical activity leads to a low risk of CAD despite greater levels of smoking and a lower intake of protective fruit and vegetables (50–100 g/day) (37,46). It is possible that cessation of tobacco intake and an increase in fruit and vegetable intake can further decrease the risk of CAD in the rural population and lower social classes (47). Cessation of smoking may also be important for the prevention of CAD in Southern Indians and Sri Lankans where 30–45% men smoke. However, these populations should be educated not to increase their fat intake and to continue physical activity which may be crucial for the prevention of CAD in people of South Asian origin (47–49).

PRIMORDIAL PREVENTION

It is important to avoid the development of risk factors for primordial prevention of CAD as defined by WHO (57). Primordial prevention is not unrealistic, however success requires further research and efforts at ensuring that the public knows the magnitude of health problems caused by risk factors. It calls for changing the socioenconomic status of the society and health education. The International College of Cardiology (ICC) has made some modifications to the guidelines of WHO:

ICC, TEN POINT PROGRAM

1. Greater emphasis on health education rather than economic status which is more difficult to improve due to more aggressive business policies of developed countries.
2. Encouragement of positive health behavior, prevention of adopting risk behavior, elimination of established risk behavior and promotion of the concept of health.
3. Encouragement to achieve spiritual well-being apart from physical and mental well-being of family, people and population.
4. General education, consisting of established principles and practice of health, should be included in a public health program.
5. Healthy lifestyles should be respected in society and further encouraged by improved community facilities.
6. Schools should play a decisive role in health education by stressing new social and behavioral values.
7. Close cooperation is necessary between all levels of the health and teaching professions.
8. Health education should emphasise the satisfaction and joy of healthy living.
9. The mass media should play a major role in health education programs by maintaining a close collaboration between health personnel and media representatives.
10. Special target groups should be considered; in particular, children and adolescents, the family unit, the under-privileged, the affluent and high risk groups.

Primordial prevention is concerned with the improvement in eating and exercise habits, as well as the decline of tobacco consumption in families, particularly in childhood when health risk behavior begins. Parents, teachers, doctors, and peer groups are important in imparting health education to children. In developing countries, there is a higher prevalence of obesity, high fat diets, tobacco consumption and hypertension among school-aged children. These risk factors can be prevented by the cessation of tobacco intake, changes in dietary habits and psychosomatic modulation by regular exercise and yogasans.

PRIMARY PREVENTION

The decline in CAD in the United States, Canada, Southern Europe, Australia and New Zealand is attributed to the reversal of risk factors that precipitated the epidemic of heart disease after World War II. The population strategy and high risk approach are two important methods for primary prevention of CAD (57–59). The population means of blood pressure, body weight and serum cholesterol reflect deviant individuals; the higher the mean, the greater the prevalence of that risk factor. Mean blood pressure of a population accurately predicts the number of hypertensive individuals and the mean body weight predicts the number of obese subjects. Population-wide approach corrects the underlying risk factors related to the cause of the epidemic and is both safer and more cost effective than the high risk approach. The criteria for the diagnosis of high risk subjects are given in Table 3. Physical inactivity and an increase in dietary fat intake (although still within desirable limits), in conjunction with psychosocial stress, brain-heart dysfunction, hypertriglyceridemia, hypercholesterolemia (especially small dense LDL), and homocysteine appear to be the most important determinant factors in the increased susceptibility to CAD in developing populations (60–67). Therefore, moderate physical activity such as brisk walking and jogging may be important for the prevention of CAD (1,66). Increased consumption of milk (calcium, lactose and saturated fat) and an inverse association of whole grain intake with CAD risk indicate that Asians should continue to eat low fat foods (21% daily) and more whole grains which may be protective (Table 3). Increased physical activity as well as a decrease in trans fatty acids and a higher consumption of n-3 fatty acids, such as mustard and soyabean oils, may decrease insulin resistance and dyslipidemia.

ICC, FIVE POINT PROGRAM

1. Follow the guidelines of the International College of Nutrition (Table 3) for a population strategy.
2. For a high risk approach, assess the risk factors such as the family history of premature CAD, diabetes, hypertension, hyperlipidemia, stroke and peripheral vascular disease (57–60).
3. A reduction in salt, meat, and caloric intake while increasing servings of fish (3–4 servings/week), whole grains such as rice, corn, legumes, millets, wheat (400–500 g/day), fruits, vegetables and nuts (400–500 g/day) in conjunction with 25–30 g/day of oils such as canola, rape seed, mustard, and olive oil, consistent with an Indo-Mediterranean diet (67).
4. An increase in exercise such as brisk walking and/or jogging (30–45 min/day) to prevent a sedentary lifestyle. Furthermore, a reduction in alcohol consumption to 50–100 ml on alternate days would provide multiple beneficial effects.
5. Hypercholesterolemia (statins, nicotinic acid, and fibrates), hypertension, diabetes, and CAD should be corrected by lifestyle changes, with or without drug therapy, during a treatment period of 24 weeks. Drug therapy should include drugs with proven efficacy through long-term randomized trials (beta blockers, ACE inhibitors, aspirin, clopidogrel, insulin, etc.). Statins (cerivastatin) should be used with caution preferably in conjunction with coenzyme Q10 to prevent deaths due to myopathy. Administration of statins above lower desirable level of cholesterol would be useful in the prevention of statin intoxication because only lower doses of statins would be used in such situations.

As South Asians have higher triglycerides, Lpa, low high density lipoprotein cholesterol (HDL-C) levels, high total cholesterol HDL-C ratios (13–26,37) and nicotinic acid (62), known to decrease Lpa and triglycerides and to increase HDL-C, may be useful for the prevention of CAD in these subjects. However, for secondary prevention, statins (59) should be administered with nicotinic acid in conjunction with diet and lifestyle changes to achieve serum cholesterol (<170 mg/dl), triglycerides (<130 mg/dl) and HDL-C (>40 mg/dl) levels similar to low risk rural populations. It is unlikely that statins are the answer for new risk factors common in developing populations (1–3,9,63). It seems that simply reducing the conventional risk factors to below those of the general population may not be the answer (68,69). There is a need to find out the role of trace elements, chromium, copper, zinc, magnesium, folic acid, pyridoxine, B12 n-3 fatty acids and ACE-inhibitors in the prevention of CAD and diabetes in Indians in view of the extraordinary results of the Hope Study (46,64,67).

CAD in the South Asian population is due to the interaction of genetic and environmental risk factors and the gap between desirable and undesirable levels of risk factors appears to be very low. Therefore, criteria for desirable levels of risk factors based on data for developed countries may be inappropriate (1,2,27,34) for South Asians due to the differences in body frame size, fat distribution and lower levels of risk factors observed in the low risk rural population (Tables 1, 2, 3). However, these guidelines are modifications of the existing guidelines for developed countries (61); missing data from longitudinal epidemiological studies and intervention trials (45) in South Asians would be of great value. The efficacy of weight loss, a decrease in central obesity, physical activity, reversed insulin resistance and a significant reduction in cardiac events in patients with CAD was observed in Indians (45,67).

Low maternal body weight and small size at birth is associated with risk of CAD. In developing countries, higher postpandial plasma insulin responses in low birth weight children indicate that improving the nutrition of pregnant mothers and infants appears to be important for the prevention of CAD (43). It may be necessary to control the lipid tetrad index (total cholesterol × triglycerides × lipoprotein(a)/HDL) in South Asians with due consideration to hyperinsulinemia, homocystenemia and ACE activity, especially for secondary prevention of CAD. Since the main victims are higher social classes of urban and rural populations, it may be prudent to simply avoid tobacco consumption in lower social classes and increase their intake of seasonal fruit and vegetables for the prevention of CAD. South Asians appear to be at greater risk than any other developing and newly industrialized country. Therefore, additional specific strategies are necessary for prevention (1,35,38).

REFERENCES

1. Singh RB, Tomlinson B, Thomas N, Sharma R. 2001. Coronary heart disease and coronary risk factors: The South Asian paradox. J Nutr Environ Med 11:43–51.
2. Janus ED, Postiglion A, Singh RB, Lewis B. 1996. Coronary heart disease in Asia. Circulation 94: 2671–2676.
3. Reddy KS, Yusuf S. 1998. Emerging epidemic of cardiovascular disease in developing countries. Circulation 97:596–601.
4. Murray CJ, Lopez AD. 1997. Mortality by cause for eight regions of the world: Global Burden of Disease Study. Lancet 349:1269–1276.
5. Murrey CJ, Lopez AD. 1997. Global mortality, disability and the contribution of risk factors: Global Burden of Disease Study. Lancet 349:1436–1442.
6. The World Heart Report. 1995. Bridging the Gaps. Report of the Director General, World Heart Organization, Geneva.

7. World Heart Organization Study Group. 1990. Nutrition and Prevention of Chronic Diseases. WHO, Geneva.
8. Chockalingam A, Balaguer-Vintro I. 1999. Impending global pandemic of Cardiovascular Disease World Heart Federation. Prous Science, SA. Barcelona, Spain.
9. Lown B. 2001. Cardiology at a crossroad: Challenge for India. Ind Heart J 53:38–41.
10. Drewnowski A, Popkin BM. 1997. The nutrition transition: New trends in the global diet. Nutrition Reviews 55:31–34.
11. Weissman R. 1997. Tobacco's global reach. The Nation, July 7, p. 5.
12. Gillum RF. 1996. Editorial, The epidemiology of cardiovascular disease in black Americans. N Engl J Med 335:1597–1599.
13. Hughes K, Aw TC, Kuperan P, Choo M. 1997. Central obesity, insulin resistance, syndrome X, lipoprotein(a) and cardiovascular risk in Indians, Malays and Chinese in Singapore. J Epidemiol Commu Health 51:394–399.
14. Enas EA, Senthikumar A, Jutura V, Gupta R. 2001. Coronary artery disease in women. Ind Heart J 53:282–292.
15. Gupta R, Kaul V, Prakash H, Sarna M, Singhal S, Gupta VP. 2001. Lipid abnormalities in coronary artery disease: A population based case control study. Ind Heart J 53:332–336.
16. Gupta R, Gupta VP. 1996. Metaanalysis of coronary heart disease prevalence in India. Ind Heart J 48:241–245.
17. Mendis S, Ekanayake EM. 1994. Prevalence of coronary heart disease and cardiovascular risk factors in middle aged males in a defined population in Sri Lanka. Int J Cardiol 46:135–142.
18. Chadda SL, Radhakrishan S, Ramchandran K, Kaul U, Gopinath N. 1990. Epidemiological study of coronary heart disease in urban populations of Delhi. Indian J Med Res 92:424–430.
19. Beegom R, Singh R. 1995. Prevalence of coronary heart disease and its risk factors in the urban population of South India. Acta Cardiol 50:227–240.
20. Singh RB, Niaz MA, Thakur AS, Janus ED, Moshiri M. 1998. Social class and coronary artery disease in an urban population of North India in the Indian Lifestyle and Heart Study. Int J Cardiol 64:195–203.
21. Chadda SL, Radhakrishnan S, Ramachandran K, Gopinath N. 1981. Epidemiological study of coronary heart disease in rural population of Gurgaon district (Haryana State). Ind J Comm Med 14:141–148.
22. Gupta SP, Malhotra KC. 1975. Urban, rural trends in the epidemiology of coronary heart disease. J Asso Phys India 23:585–587.
23. Wander GS, Khurana SB, Gulati R, Sachar RK, Gupta RK, Khurana S, Anand IS. 1994. Epidemiology of coronary heart disease in a rural Punjab population. Prevalence and correlation with various risk factors. Ind Heart J 46:319–323.
24. Gupta R, Gupta VP, Alhuwalia NS. 1994. Educational status, coronary heart disease and coronary risk factor prevalence in a rural population of India. Br Med J 309:1332–1336.
25. Singh RB, Ghosh S, Niaz MA, Gupta S, Bishnoi I, Sharma JP, Agarwal P, Rastogi SS, Beegom R, Chibo H, Shoumin Z. 1995. Epidemiologic study of diet and coronary risk factors in relation to central obesity and insulin levels in the urban population of North India. Int J Cardiol 47:245–255.
26. Raman Kutty V, Balakrishnan KG, Jayashree AK, Thomas J. 1993. Prevalence of coronary heart disease in the rural population of Thiruananthapuram district, Kerala India. Int J Cardiol 39:59–70.
27. Balarajan R. 1991. Ethic differences in mortality from ischaemic heart disease and cerebrovascular disease in England and Wales. Br Med J 302:560–564.
28. Steinberg WJ, Balfe DL, Kustner HG. 1988. Decline in the ischaemic heart disease mortality rates of South Africans, 1968–1985. S Afr Med J 74:547–550.
29. Balrajan R, Adelstein AM, Bulusu L, Shukla V. 1984. Patterns of mortality among migrants to England and Wales from the Indian subcontinent. Br Med J 289:1185–1187.
30. Singh RB, Rastogi SS, Rastogi V, Niaz MA, Madhu SV, Chen M, Shoumin Z. 1997. Blood pressure trends, plasma insulin levels, and risk factors in rural and urban elderly populations of North India. Coron Art Dis 8:463–468.
31. Enas EA, Yusuf S, Sharma S. 1998. Coronary artery disease in South Asians. Ind Heart J 50:105–113.
32. Mulhilal. 1996. Transition in diet and health implications of modern lifestyles in Indonesia. Asia Pac J Clin Nutr 5:132–134.
33. Wilkinson P, Sayer J, Laji K, Grundy C, Marchant B, Kopelman P, Timmas AD. 1996. Comparison of case fatality in South Asian and white patients after acute myocardial infarction, observational study. BMJ 312:1330–1333.

34. Mckeigue PM, Marmot MG, Adelstein AM. 1985. Diet and risk factors for coronary artery disease in Asians in North-West London. Lancet 11:1086–1090.
35. Singh RB, Niaz MA. 1995. Coronary risk factors in Indians. Lancet 346:778–779.
36. Monique Verschuren WM, Jacobs DR, Bloember BPM, Kromhout D, Menotti A, Aravanis C, Blackburn H, Buzina R, Dontas AS, Fidanza F, Kawomen MJ, Nodeljkovic S, Nissinen A, Toshima H. 1995. Serum total cholesterol and long term coronary heart disease mortality in different cultures. Twenty-five year follow-up of the Seven Countries Study. JAMA 274:131–136.
37. Enas EA, Dhawan J, Petkar S. 1997. Coronary artery disease in Asian Indians: Lessons learnt and the role of lipoprotein(a). Ind Heart J 49:25–34.
38. Indian Consensus Group. 1996. Indian consensus for prevention of hypertension and coronary artery disease. A joint scientific statement of Indian Society of Hypertension and International College of Nutrition. J Nutr Environ Med 6:309–318.
39. Bhatnagar D, Anand IS, Durrington PN, Patel DJ, Wander GS, Mackness MI, Creed F, Tomenson B, Chandrashekhar Y, Winterbotham, Brit RP, Keil JE, Sutton GC. 1995. Coronary risk factors in people from Indian subcontinent living in West London and their sublings in India. Lancet 345:405–409.
40. Singh RB, Ghosh S, Niaz Ma, Singh R, Beegum R, Chibo H, Shoumin Z, Postiglione A. 1995. Dietary intake, plasma levels of antioxidant vitamins and oxidative stress in relation to coronary artery disease in elderly population. Am J Cardiol 76:1233–1238.
41. Singh RB, Niaz MA, Ghosh S, Beggom R, Agarwal P, Nangia S, Moshiri M, Janus ED. 1998. Low fat intake and coronary artery disease in a population with higher prevalence coronary artery disease. The Indian paradox. J Am Coll Nutr 17:342–350.
42. Singh RB, Beegum R, Verma SP, Haque M, Singh R, Mehta AS, De AK, Kundu S, Ray S, Krishnan A, Simhadri H, Paranjpe NB, Agarwal N. 2000. Association of dietary factors and other coronary risk factors with social class in women in five Indian cities. Asia Pac J Clin Nutr 9:298–302.
43. Stein CE, Fall CHD, Kumaran K, Osmond C, Cox V, Barker DJP. 1996. Fetal growth and coronary heart disease in South India. Lancet 348:1269–1273.
44. Singh RB, Sharma JP, Rastogi V, Niaz MA, Ghosh S, Beegom R, Janus ED. 1997. Social class and coronary artery disease in a rural population of North India. The Indian Social Class and Heart Survey. Eur Heart J 18:1728–1735.
45. Singh RB, Rastogi V, Rastogi SS, Niaz MA, Beegom R. 1996. Effect of diet and moderate exercise on central obesity and associated disturbance, myocardial infarction and mortality in patients with and without coronary artery disease. J Am Coll Nutr 15:592–596.
46. The HOPE Study Investigators. 2000. Effects of an angio-tensin-converting enzyme inhibitor, ramipril on cardiovascular events in high risk patients. N Engl J Med 342:145–153.
47. Singh RB, Beegom R, Mehta AS, Niaz MA, De AK, Mitra RK, Haque M, Verma SP, Dube GK, Siddiqui HM, Wander GS, Janus ED, Postigione A, Hague MS. 1999. Social class, coronary risk factors and undernutrition, a double burden of diseases in women during transition in five Indian cities. Int J Cardiol 69:139–147.
48. Singh RB, Verma SP, Niaz MA. 1999. Social class and coronary artery disease in India. Lancet 353: 154–155.
49. Kamath SK, Hussain EA, Amin D, Mortillaro E, West B, Peterson CT, Argyy F, Murillo G, Aleketl DL. 1999. Cardiovascular disease risk factors in 2 district ethnic groups. Indian and Pakistani compared with American premenopausal women. Am J Clin Nutr 69:621–631.
50. Singh RB, Rastogi V, Niaz MA, Ghosh S, Sy RG, Janus ED. 1998. Serum cholesterol and coronary artery disease in populations with low cholesterol levels: the Indian paradox. Inter J Cardiol 65:81–90.
51. Thomas GN, Young RP, Tomlinson B, Woo KS, Sanderson JE, Critchley JA. 2000. Renin-angiotensin-aldosterone system gene polymorphisms and hypertension in Hong Kong Chinese. Clin Exp Hypertens 22:87–97.
52. Thomas GN, Tomlinson B, Chan JC, Lee ZSK, Cockran CS, Critchley JA. 2000. An insulin receptor gene polymorphism is associated with diastolic blood pressure in Chinese subjects with components of the metabolic syndrome. Am J Hypertens 13:745–752.
53. Thomas GN, Tomlinson B, Critchley JA. 2000. Modulation of blood pressure and obesity by the dopamine D2 receptor gene TaqI polymorphism. Hypertension 36:177–182.
54. Young RP, Sanderson JE, Tomlinson B, Woo KS, Critchley JA. 1995. Angiotensin converting enzyme insertion-deletion polymorphism in Chinese. J Hypertens 13:1479–1480.
55. Young RP, Thomas GN, Critchley JA, Tomlinson B, Woo KS, Sanderson JE. 1998. Interethnic differences in coronary heart disease mortality in 25 populations: association with the angiotensin-converting enzyme DD genotype frequency. J Cardiovasc Risk 5:303–307.

56. Nagi DK, Foy CA, Mohamed-Ali V, Yudkin JS, Grant PJ, Knowler WC. 1998. Angiotensin-1-converting enzyme (ACE) gene polymorphism, plasma ACE levels, and their association with the metabolic syndrome and electrocardiographic coronary artery disease in Pima Indians. Metabolism 47:622–626.
57. WHO Study group. 1985. Primary prevention of coronary heart disease. EURO Reports and Studies 98. Geneva, Who.
58. Assmann G, Carmena R, Cullen P, Fruchart JC, Jossa F, Lewis B, Mancini M, Paoletti R. 1999. Coronary Heart Disease: reducing the risk: a world wide view. International Task Force for the Prevention of Coronary Heart Disease. Circulation 100:1930–1938.
59. Greenland P, Abrams J, Aurigemma GP, et al. 2000. Prevention Conference V. Beyond secondary prevention: identifying the high risk patients for primary prevention: noninvasive tests of atherosclerotic burden. Circulation 101:16–21.
60. Rozanski A, Blumenthal JA, Kaplan J. 2000. Impact of psychosocial factors on the pathogenesis of cardiovascular disease and implications for therapy. Circulation 99:2192–2217.
61. Singh RB, Weydahl A, Otsuka K, Watanabe Y, Yano S, Mori H, Ichimaru Y, Mitsutake G, Sato Y, Fanghong L, Zhao ZY, Kartik C, Gvozdjakova A. 2001. Can nutrition influence circadian rhythm and heart rate variability? Biomed Pharmacother 55:7–18.
62. O'Keefe JH, Harris WS. 1997. Nicotinic acid, the underused ally in the fight against coronary disease. J Cardiovasc Risk 4:161–164.
63. Eisenberg DA. 1998. Cholesterol lowering in the management of coronary artery disease: The clinical implications of recent trials. Am J Med 104:2–5.
64. Hughes K, Ong C. 2000. Homocysteine, folate, vitamin B and cardiovascular risk in Indians, Malays and Chinese in Singapore. J Epidemiol Comm Health 54:31–34.
65. National Cholesterol Education Program. 2001. Executive summary of the third report of the National Cholesterol Education Program Expert Panel on detection, evaluation and treatment of high cholesterol in adults (Adult Treatment Panel III). JAMA 285:2486–2497.
66. National Institute of Health (NIH) Consensus Development Program. 1996. Physical activity and cardiovascular health: NIH consensus statement. Bethesda, USA. National Institute of Health.
67. Singh RB, Niaz MA, Gal D, Ghose S, Singh R, Pella D, Berry EM. 2002. The Indomediterranean Diet Heart Study. Lancet 360:1455–1461.
68. Pella D, Thomas N, Tomlinson B, Singh RB. 2003. Prevention of coronary artery disease. Lancet 361:79.
69. Singhal A, Fewtrel M, Cole TJ, Lucas A. 2003. Low nutrient intake and early growth for later insulin resistance in adolescents born preterm. Lancet 361:1089–1097.

Frontiers in Cardiovascular Health, edited by
N.S. Dhalla, A. Chockalingam,
H.I. Berkowitz & P.K. Singal
Kluwer Academic Publishers, Boston, 2003

Social Inequalities, Nutrition and Health

Elisabetta Della Valle, Saverio Stranges, Antonio Cajafa,
Giovanni Guglielmucci, Maria Triassi, and Eduardo Farinaro

Department of Preventive Medical Sciences, School of Medicine, University of Naples Federico II, Italy

Summary. The health status of individuals as well as of entire populations can be influenced by social inequalities. The disparity between the copious wealth of industrialized nations and the extreme poverty of the developing countries has yet to be leveled. A large percentage of the world population lies on the edge of poverty and lacks the financial and human resources to deal with the vast demographic and epidemiological transition which is taking place and which will add to the excessive toll of disability and death from infectious diseases a further burden from the impending epidemic of chronic-degenerative diseases. The unequal economic progress has caused an alteration of the health status in different communities, leading to a clear distinction between diseases in affluence and diseases in poverty. But not always a rise in the average income level has lead to a similar improvement in life expectancy. So we can figure an absolute poverty of the developing countries and a relative poverty of industrialized nations in which the prevailing diseases seem to affect overall the less educated and the social classes at a lower income. Nowadays people in the developing countries still die of starvation. The planning of strategies to ameliorate health conditions and to overcome absolute poverty in the less affluent regions and relative poverty caused by social inequalities in the wealthier ones, must take into account the level of education and a more equable distribution of resources. In the next future the goal of the challenge will be to obtain successful achievements in improving life expectancy and quality of life.

***Key words*:** social inequalities, nutrition, health, chronic degenerative diseases, cultural factors.

Economic progress and consequently changes in social organization, have always marked deeply the disease profile of human societies. As a matter of fact, social conditionings have constantly modulated the risk profile of a population, determining remarkable differences in the distribution of various diseases and of the main health

Correspondence: Eduardo Farinaro, M.D., Professor of Medicine, Department of Preventive Medical Sciences, School of Medicine, University of Naples Federico II, Via S. Pansini 5, 80131 Napoli, ITALY. Telephone: ++39-081 7462123, Fax: ++39-081-8901728, E-mail: farinaro@unina.it and social indicators. The ameliorated hygienic and sanitary conditions, the general reduction of infectious disorders, the increase in life expectancy, as well as the increase in chronic-degenerative diseases, typical of the industrialized nations, symbolize the aspects of humanity's evolution (1–4).

A socio-economic grouping of the World's countries identifies three major areas: the Established Market Economies (EME), enclosing Northern America, Western Europe and most of Australia; countries with Economies in Transition (EIT), the former socialist nations of Central and Eastern Europe; the last area is where the majority of the World population resides, the so called Developing Countries (DC), which comprises most of Africa, Asia, Latin America and the Middle Eastern Crescent, an heterogeneous mixture of economical, social and political conditions all associated with the attempt at an initial industrialization. Each of these three categories holds a different and quite definite social and health profile, as documented by the sensitive indicators used to evaluate the health-status of a community. It must also be underlined that, inside each grouping, considerable differences can be noted both between countries as inside any specific nation because of the considerable influence played by social factors which, alone, often represent the main determinants of the health status of a population (5).

In many countries there is still a huge gap between health in affluent groups and in the lower socio-economic classes, even if some indicators, like medium life-expectancy, indicate an overall improvement in health for the total population. Some nations are capable of maintaining a good health at a relatively low cost. For example, life-expectancy in China, Sri Lanka and in Kerala (a State in southern of India) is over 70 years, in spite of a Gross National Product, in 1994, of merely one thousand dollars per capita. These data seem to be in contrast with the same resulting from the residents of Harlem, whose medium family income in 1990 was over 24,000 dollars but whose life expectancy remained well less than 70 (6).

This proves how in the industrialized nations, life expectancy is not only associated with medium income levels, but depends also from social and cultural factors which are at the basis of social inequalities. Considerable differences in health status appear among the different neighborhoods of the bigger cities; as a matter of fact in the United States, life expectancy for whites living in the affluent areas of cities such as Philadelphia, Baltimore or New York is over 76 years, while for black residents of the poorer areas in the same cities reaches only 58. Hence there is a difference of 20 years in life expectancy between rich and poor inhabitants of the same city but who live in different areas (7–8).

Living in a difficult community is certainly not healthy: the lack of entertainments, the difficulty of accessing preventive, diagnostic and therapeutical services, job precariousness, segregation, continuous fear of crime, associated with unhealthy life-styles like an excessive alcohol and cigarette consumption, an unbalanced diet, a lack of physical activity often favored by the absence of facilities, strongly affect life expectancy (9–10).

A clear relationship between mortality rates and socio-economic status is easily demonstrated, and in spite of a significant decline in mortality in the last 30 years, the poorer individuals without education still die in higher percentages in comparison with the more educated and at a higher income. To the extent that in 1991 the U.S. National Cancer Institute (NCI) stated "poverty is a cancerous factor"; in the US, the total incidence of cancers attributable to a low socio-economic status (a family income lower than $15,000 per year) is 16.5%. This means that these factors have the same importance than smoking and nutrition on the determinism of these diseases, outlining the necessity of integrating the existing preventive strategies with appropriate social policies, in order to address and cover in particular those groups that live along with major privations (11).

In developing countries the burden of infectious disorders is still a sanitary priority: infective diseases remain the leading cause of mortality and morbidity (over 40% of global deaths), but in the last years we have witnessed a gradual and constant spreading of the main risk factors for the development of chronic-degenerative diseases, typically rooted in the unhealthy life-styles and behaviours of Western Societies. This has led to a significant increase of cardiovascular and neoplastic diseases in accordance with the "epidemiological transition" theory formulated by the World Health Organization (12–13).

Nutrition certainly represents one of the major factors that affect growth, physical and psychological development, performance and individual productivity and after all the evolution and fortunes of a population; notable are nowadays the differences of dietary profiles over the world, diverse the availability of resources, socio-economic, ethnic and religious conditionings, that make the relationship between food and pathologies complex, controversial and of difficult comprehension. Moreover, man's health depends strictly on the food gathered from the environment and since not long ago humanity was greatly bound to famine and seasonal availability in its choices for food. Therefore, it is believed that selection has favoured those biological mechanisms capable of preventing starvation rather than those limiting excessive weight gain, by activating the so called "frugal genes" (14). Today the major availability and quality of food has developed an extremely high incidence of obesity, diabetes, ateriosclerosis and cancer (15–17).

The FAO, in the 50th anniversary of its foundation, gave the news that food production had become insufficient for the World population. So, as a general principle, the wide-spread genetic predisposition to the maximum assimilation and utilization of food can be useful in this historical phase of humanity. But the major problem is the distribution of nutritional reserves; it is estimated that the populations of the industrialized countries, less than 25% of humanity, consume 80% of the World total production of food and drugs. According to more recent data provided by the same international organization, the average availability of food in the world is 2720 Kcal per person per day: 66% made up of carbohydrates, 23% of fats e 11% of proteins. The industrialized nations dispose, in average, of a greater availability of food: a daily medium of 3340 Kcal per person; in the less affluent countries this medium is only 2060 Kcal. Countries whose economy is in transition reach 2850 Kcal. A various and balanced diet must supply different nutrients, carbohydrates, fats, proteins, vitamins and minerals essential for growth and development, for preventing infections and, in general, for maintaining health. The diet of the poorer countries is definitely less various than that of the more industrialized nations. In the former, cereals count for 62% of the total energy, whilst in the latter they represent only 27%; proteins constitute 10% and over 12% respectively; finally fats make up 15% of a total diet in developing countries against 35% of industrialized nations. Furthermore, over 800 million people in the developing countries are chronically underfed and about 2 billion are suffering deficiencies of micronutrients like vitamin A, iron and iodine (18).

The UNICEF in the 50th anniversary of the ONU document on Human Rights has revealed tremendous data on poverty. A sixth of the world population, corresponding to over one billion people suffer hunger and two billion pathologic conditions are caused by an incomplete diet. The illiteracy and malnutrition are alone the main determinants of the diseases in poverty distinguished by a deficiency of the immune system: parasitic and infectious diseases caused by poverty-related malnutrition (AIDS, malaria, TBC, pneumonia and rheumatic fever) being the most common (19).

So it appears clear that differences in social classes can influence the health status of singles as well as of entire populations. In recent years many have tried to calculate how much social inequalities could impact on a population's health: one of the principle indicators for this sort of discrimination is DALY (Disability Adjusted Life Years); it considers not only mortality, but also disabilities caused by acute and chronic-degenerative diseases. Taking into account this indicator, it emerges that 90% of the World's DALY comes from the developing countries, while most of health care expenditure, in absolute and in relative terms, belongs to the industrialized nations (20–21). Its containment is, or at least should be, the aim of any significant effort towards development. Moreover many International Organizations are showing a renewing interest on poverty. Such care has been extended by the awareness that a true and full progress can only be accomplished after the elimination of poverty and alimentary uncertainty. Nevertheless, even if the eradication of poverty is felt as an ethical, social, moral and political imperative, recent estimates seem to indicate that this goal is still far to be reached, if not impossible at all, in the light of the present trends. The 2001 World Bank Report, indicates that twelve hundred million people in the world are living on less than one dollar a day, a higher number than the previous decade. Of these, over five hundred million reside in South-Eastern Asia and about three hundred million live in Sub-Saharan Africa, representing, respectively, 40% and over 46% of the local population (22). It is evident that one of the most immediate and severe consequences of this economic precariousness is characterized by inadequate nutrition and by the challenging supply of food, aspects these that have recently been aggravated by the numerous military conflicts of so problematical resolution. Another central question is the strong role played by social inequalities in many developing countries as well as in the economies in transition. On this point it is obvious that reducing poverty cannot be separated from significant changes in the distribution of wealth.

On evaluating the relationship between nutrition and health in the developing countries, in comparison with the significant world-wide economic progress we are still far from reaching the goal of an adequate nutrition for all both from a qualitative than from a quantitative point of view. As previously stated, nearly a billion people, concentrated above all in Africa, South-East Asia and in Latin America, still today, cannot face their daily needs with sufficient quantities of availability of food.

Many countries, including some of the poorest, have adopted and are engaging in measures directed to strengthen the supply and quality of food, of agriculture, of dietary education at a family and at a community level, all things that could bear quite a positive fall on famine and malnutrition. The actual challenge is to accelerate the progress already begun. Along this line, in the last few years, a global action for feeding the World has been planned, with the objective of creating appropriate guidelines for the Governments that, together with non governmental agencies (OMS, FAO, UNESCO, UNICEF), with private and local communities, must formulate policies, strategies and activities capable of improving the total nutritional status of their people and relieving social disparities that embitter the nutritional matter, thus assigning to it a remarkable socio-anthropological significance. Among the aims of this Plan there is the will to assure, first of all, the possibility of a continuous access to food reserves, as well as a various choice of safe foods at affordable prices and of drinkable water for everyone; to maintain an adequate nutritional status in the wealthier populations and the wide-spread diffusion of the correct information for preventing those diseases more strictly correlated to abundance and to an unbalanced diet; the reinforcement of policies for development sustainable from a social and environmental point of view, in order to preserve the potentials of the future generations; at last to eliminate famine and starvation in the world.

On a total, if we analyze the differences in the trends of the consumption of the main nutrients traced by the FAO over the last decade, the most significant aspect that appears is the striking difference existing between Africa and Asia (except for Asiatic countries at a higher average income like Japan) on one side and Europe and Northern America on the other, in terms of distribution of total energy intake: in fact, while in the first group more than 50% of the total intake comes from cereals or, less often, from fruit and tuberous vegetables, in the second less than 25% of total calories origin from cereals. The consumption of fats, alcohol, meat, dairy products and refined sugar is inversely related to the intake of fibers. As a matter of fact, less than 10% of the total energy intake in the developing countries derives from meat, while in Western countries, including Australia and New Zealand, more than 15% of the total calories come from meat products.

Examining the data from the period analysis carried out by the FAO on the "food balance sheets" of the last 40 years, it appears that in general, all the countries of the world are tending to diminish the consumption of food of cereal origin in spite of a gradual and continuous increase of fat usage, in nearly all areas, except for Oceania. The intake of fruit and vegetables has not shown significant changes (23).

This last information suggests the appearance of a new public health problem that is steadily assuming the nature of a pandemic: the increasing prevalence of overweight and obesity, both in the industrialized nations, as well as in the developing countries, as seen in recent times. With regard to the latter, if it is true that obesity coexists with malnutrition and it is still quite rare in Asia and in Africa, it is also true that it is a condition that is becoming always more and more common among the affluent urban sections. The diffusion of all the traditional risk factors of a typical western life-style can predispose these communities in the close future, even if in a inhomogeneous manner, to cardiovascular and neoplastic diseases (15).

REFERENCES

1. Murray Ch JL, Lopez AD. 1996. The Global Burden of Disease. A Comprehensive Assessment of Mortality and Disability from Diseases, Injuries and Risk Factors in 1990 and Projected to 2020. Harvard School of Public Health on behalf of the WHO and the World Bank.
2. The World Health Report. 1997. Conquering, Suffering, Enriching Humanity. Geneva: World Health Organization.
3. Achutti A, Balaguer-Vintrò I. 1999. Impending Global Pandemic of Cardiovascular Diseases. Challenges and opportunities for the prevention and control of cardiovascular diseases in developing countries and economies in transition. Ed. Chockalingam A, Balanguez-Vintrò I, 1–163. Barcelona: Prous Science.
4. International Advisory Board. 1992. Victoria Declaration on Heart Health. Health and Welfare Canada, Victoria, Canada.
5. World Bank. 1997. Human Development and Network Strategy. Health, Nutrition and Population Division, World Bank, Washington DC.
6. Marmot MG. 2001. Inequalities in Health. N Engl J Med, Vol. 345, No 2, July 12.
7. Pappas G, Queen S. 1993. The increasing disparity in mortality between socio-economic groups in the United States, 1960 and 1986. N Engl J Med 329:103–109.
8. Lynch JW, Kaplan GA. 1998. Income inequality and mortality in metropolitan areas of the United States. Am J Public Health 88:1074–1080.
9. Lynch JW, Davey Smith G. 2000. Income inequality and mortality: importance to health of individual income psychosocial environment, or material conditions, BMJ 320:1200–1204.
10. Marmot MG, Wilkinson RG. 2001. Psychosocial and material pathways in the relation between income and health a response to Lynch et al., BMJ 322:1233–1236.
11. Labarthe DR. 1998. Social conditions in Epidemiology and Prevention of Cardiovascular Disease. A Global Challenge. Ed Labarth DR, 423–447 Gaithersburg (Ma) USA: Aspen Publication.
12. Hinkle LE. 1961. Ecological observations of the relation of physical illness, mental illness, and the social environment. Psychosomatic Med 23:289–296.
13. Olshansky SJ, Ault AB. 1986. The fourth stage of the epidemiologic transition: the age of delayed degenerative disease. Milbank Q 64:355–391.
14. Nesse R, Williams GW. 1999. Perché ci ammaliamo. Torino (Italy): Einaudi.
15. Farinaro E coordinator. 1992. European Atherosclerosis Society and International Task Force for Prevention of Coronary Heart Disease. Prevention of coronary heart disease: scientific background and new clinical guidelines. Nutr Metab Cardiovas Dis 2:113–156.
16. Assmann G, Schulte H. 1997. New and classical risk factors the Münster heart study (PROCAM). Eur J Med Res 6:237–242.
17. Willet WC. 2000. Diet and Cancer. The Oncologist 5:393–404.
18. FAO. 1998. Large gap in food availability between rich and poor countries. Press Release.
19. WHO. 1997. Obesity Preventing and managing the global epidemic, Report of a WHO Consultation on Obesity, Geneva.
20. Trevisan M. 2000. Fattori sociali e benessere psicofisico, Ann Ig Suppl. 1:7–10.
21. Hyder AA, Rotlant G. 1998. Measuring the burden of disease: healthy life-years. Am J Public Health 88:196–202.
22. The World Bank Annual Report. 2001. Vol. 1, year in review.
23. FAO. 2000. Food Balance Sheet Roma.

Frontiers in Cardiovascular Health, edited by
N.S. Dhalla, A. Chockalingam,
H.I. Berkowitz & P.K. Singal
Kluwer Academic Publishers, Boston, 2003

The Potential Impact of CardioVision 2020 and Three Other Risk Factor Scenarios on Population Rates of Coronary Heart and Cardiovascular Disease: A Call to Action

Lambert A. Wu,[1] Lee N. Brekke,[2] Mark J. Brekke,[2]
Rebecca S. Hoffman,[1] and Thomas E. Kottke[1]

[1] *Division of Cardiovascular Diseases, Departments of Internal Medicine and Health Sciences Research, Mayo Clinic and Mayo Foundation, Rochester, Minnesota, United States of America*
[2] *Brekke Associates, Inc., Minneapolis, Minnesota, United States of America*

Summary

Background: We are implementing CardioVision 2020—a comprehensive, population-wide initiative—in Olmsted County, Minnesota to reduce the population burden of coronary heart disease (CHD) and cardiovascular (CVD) disease. In this analysis we compare disease incidence rates expected with CardioVision 2020 to three other scenarios.

Methods: We use Framingham study risk functions to calculate CHD and CVD incidence for four scenarios in the year 2020: population risk factor levels are unchanged; the population meets CardioVision 2020 goals; diabetes and smoking rates rise (negative trend 1); and, diabetes and smoking rates rise, and blood pressure and cholesterol control declines (negative trend 2).

Results: In the year 2020, the incidence of CHD (per 100,000) will be 586 at current risk factor levels, 329 if the population meets CardioVision 2020 goals, and 707 and 916 if the two negative trend scenarios come to pass. The CVD incidence will be 834 with current risk factor levels, 427 if the population meets CardioVision 2020 goals and 1099 and 1456 if the two negative trend scenarios come to pass.

Conclusion: Compared to CHD and CVD incidence rates at current risk factor levels, incidence rates will be 44% and 49% lower if the population meets CardioVision 2020 goals in the year 2020. If diabetes and smoking continue to rise and hypertension and cholesterol

Correspondence to: Lambert A. Wu, M.D., Department of Internal Medicine, Mayo Clinic and Mayo Foundation, 200 First Street SW, Rochester, MN 55905. Tel: (507) 284-2511, Fax: (507) 266-0229, Email: wu.lambert@mayo.edu.

return to historically high levels, CHD and CVD rates would be expected to rise by 56% and 75%, respectively.

Key words: Cardiovascular Disease Prevention, Epidemiologic Methods, Health Services Research, Healthcare Delivery Systems, Risk Factors.

INTRODUCTION

A favorable risk factor profile is associated with lower rates of coronary heart disease (CHD) and cardiovascular disease (CVD), and up to a decade of increased life expectancy (1). Primordial and primary prevention—preventing the emergence of risk factors on the one hand and, on the other, modifying the risk factor profile of patients who have not yet manifested cardiovascular disease—represent significant opportunities to reduce the burden of CVD in a population. However, Americans appear not to have taken advantage of this fact. Although death rates from CHD have declined since 1960, the majority of the recent improvement has been due to improved survival after myocardial infarction and not from primary prevention (2–4). Not only is this a missed opportunity to control cardiovascular disease through risk factor modification, there are disturbing signs that the incidence of CHD and CVD will increase in the near future because of rising risk factor levels. The incidence and prevalence of diabetes are increasing (5,6), hypertension control is decreasing (7), use of tobacco is increasing rapidly among some subpopulations of young adults (8–10), the population is becoming obese and sedentary (11), and consumption of fat and calories is increasing (12). Small changes in risk factors among all individuals in a population can have a very large impact on disease rates, both positive and negative (13,14). CardioVision 2020 was therefore developed as a comprehensive, population-wide disease-reduction initiative for Olmsted County, Minnesota (15,16).

We undertook this simulation study to quantify the expected reduction or increase in CHD and CVD in the Olmsted County population given four different risk factor scenarios. Stochastic simulation, a mathematical process that can be used to predict the impact of changes in risk factor levels or treatment strategies on disease rates in a population (17), has been widely applied in the field of cardiovascular disease (18–25). In this paper, we use a simple stochastic simulation to predict the incidence of CHD and CVD in the year 2020 under four different risk-factor scenarios.

MATERIALS AND METHODS

Current risk factor level scenario

We base the current risk factor level scenario on published risk factor distributions from Olmsted County (16). We obtained diabetes prevalence and tobacco use data for this publication from a random digit dial telephone interview conducted in 1999 with a stratified random sample of 1232 Olmsted County residents. We calculated rates for each gender within 6 age categories (20–29, 30–39, 40–49, 50–59, 60–69, and 70+). We obtained blood pressure data from a sample of 3040 Olmsted County

Table 1. Risk factor levels assumed for CardioVision 2020 and the three comparison scenarios (for ages 30–83 years)

	Current risk factor level scenario	CardioVision 2020	Negative trend scenario 1	Negative trend scenario 2
Smoking prevalence (%)	18.8	0	53.3	53.3
Systolic BP (mm Hg)	mean = 129.0	Mean = 115.6 (all < 130)	mean = 129.0	mean = 138.9
Diastolic BP (mm Hg)	mean = 79.9	Mean = 72.9 (all < 85)	mean = 79.9	NA*
Serum Cholesterol (mg/dl)	mean = 202.6	Mean = 171.8 (all < 200)	mean = 202.6	mean = 229.3
Diabetes prevalence (%)	3.7	2.0	4.8	4.8
High density lipoprotein (HDL) (mg/dl)	53.3	51.7	53.3	53.3
Left ventricular hypertrophy on ECG (%)	0.77	0.77	0.77	0.77

*Not used. Only systolic blood pressure was used in the model.

residents who made an office visit to a Mayo Clinic primary care service between October 1994 and April 1999 to estimate the population distribution of blood pressure levels by age and gender. We obtained total serum cholesterol and HDL data for 29,553 unique Olmsted County residents from the Mayo Clinic laboratory database from the years 1995, 1996 or 1997.

For the current risk factor level scenario the mean prevalence of smoking for ages 30–83 is 18.8%, the mean systolic blood pressure is 129.0 mm Hg and the mean diastolic blood pressure is 79.9 mm Hg (Table 1). The mean total serum cholesterol value is 202.6 mg/dl and the mean HDL is 53.3 mg/dl. The prevalence of diabetes is 3.7%.

The CardioVision 2020 scenario

The CardioVision 2020 scenario assumes that no one smokes, that all systolic blood pressure levels are less than 130 mm Hg, and that all serum cholesterol levels are less than 200 mg/dl. To create this scenario we use the same data as with the current risk factor level scenario, but we exclude all systolic blood pressure levels greater than 129 mm Hg and all serum cholesterol values of 200 mg/dl or greater. Since CardioVision 2020 does not have a goal for HDL cholesterol, we do not explicitly change this value. Because of the correlation of HDL with total serum cholesterol, its mean value for this scenario declines slightly to 51.7 mg/dl.

Although blood sugar and diabetes prevalence are not among for CardioVision 2020 goals, the Framingham risk function does include diabetes in the risk function. We reason that, if the population meets the CardioVision 2020 personal goals, individuals will be physically active and eat a diet low in saturated fat. For this scenario we assume that diabetes prevalence in the population will be the same as in Olmsted County in 1970—2.0% (5).

Negative trend scenario 1

With negative trend scenario 1, diabetes and smoking rates in the population increase. We linearly extrapolate diabetes rates to the year 2020 on the basis of Olmsted County prevalence trends from 1970 to 1990 (5). We extrapolate the overall rate for each gender and then apply it to the 1990 age-gender distribution stratified by five age groups (45–54, 55–64, 65–74, 75–84, and 85+). We then use these projected year 2020 age-gender rates in the simulation. We set the rates for ages 30–44 equal to the 45–54 age group rates. We assume that the overall prevalence of diabetes in 2020 is 4.8%.

On the basis of smoking rates in Minnesotans who were 18 to 25 years old in 1999 and other groups in which smoking is highly prevalent (8–10), we set smoking rates at 53.3% for the entire population. We do not change blood pressure, total serum cholesterol or HDL levels from the current risk factor level scenario.

Negative trend scenario 2

We create negative trend scenario 2 to represent a "worst-case" scenario. For negative trend scenario 2, we set diabetes (4.8%) and smoking rates (53.3%) as in negative trend scenario 1. We base total serum cholesterol and blood pressure values on historically high national rates measured over the last 40 years. To implement the simulation, we construct a database of total serum cholesterol values that models mean national levels in 1960–1962 (stratified by gender and six age categories: 20–34, 35–44, 45–54, 55–64, 65–74, and 75+) (26). We create the database by scaling the 29,553 values in the database of Olmsted County values (as described in the current risk factor level scenario, above) to achieve the desired national means within each age-gender category. The overall mean value for total serum cholesterol is 229.3 mg/dl. We leave the corresponding HDL values at their original levels.

Similarly, we construct a database of 3040 blood pressure values that models national blood pressure distributions in 1976–1980 (26). In this case, we scale the systolic blood pressure values in the current risk factor level scenario within each age-gender category to recreate the corresponding national hypertension rates. Mean systolic blood pressure is 138.9 mm Hg. The diastolic blood pressure values are not used in the analysis since the risk functions offer the choice of using either, but not both, systolic blood pressure or diastolic blood pressure.

Application of the stochastic simulation program

For each scenario, we generate a simulated population of 108,000 people with one thousand people assigned to each one-year age-gender group, ages 30–83. We stochastically assign the risk factors (total cholesterol, HDL, blood pressure, smoking, and diabetes) to this population. We assign all risk factors independently except for total serum cholesterol and HDL. We randomly assign smoking and diabetes with probabilities equal to the age-gender dependent rates described above. We assign blood pressure and cholesterol values by selecting records from the appropriate databases in random order (within age-gender groups). After all the records within a particular age-gender group are selected, we repeat the process until values are assigned to the desired number of records. In addition to the risk factors described above, the CVD risk functions requires that a person is defined as having or not having left ventricular hypertrophy on their electrocardiogram (ECG-LVH). We randomly assign this variable to our population based on the age-gender dependent rates reported in the Framingham Heart Study (27,28).

We use Framingham-based risk functions to calculate the probability of developing CHD or CVD for each of the people in the simulated populations (27,28). Coronary heart disease includes death from CHD, non-fatal myocardial infarction, coronary insufficiency, and angina pectoris as defined by the Framingham investigators. Cardiovascular disease includes any CHD event, stroke, transient ischemic attack, congestive heart failure, peripheral vascular disease, and death from CVD. The CHD risk function that we use depends on age, gender, blood pressure, total serum cholesterol, HDL, diabetes, and smoking. The CVD function depends on age, gender, systolic blood pressure, total serum cholesterol, HDL, diabetes, smoking, and ECG-LVH. We modify the published multi-year risk functions to produce approximate one-year risk functions by assuming that all risk factors except for age remain constant over the period of time covered by the original risk functions (e.g., 10 years for the CHD risk function). We further modify the CHD risk function by adding a correction for risk factors changing over time based on the age dependence of baseline Olmsted County data. Because this correction was small we did not apply it to the CVD risk function.

Finally, we weight the individual probabilities of an event by the estimated year-2000 Olmsted County population free from CHD or CVD (depending on the event being simulated) by age and gender (ages 30–83 years). The weighted mean probabilities give the predicted incident CHD and CVD rates. The year 2000 Olmsted County population is based on 1997 Census Bureau population estimates aged to the year 2000 using mortality rate data (29,30). We estimate CHD and CVD prevalence by age-gender categories from the 1999 random digit dial telephone survey of Olmsted County residents. We subtract the prevalent cases from the population that we use for calculating incidence rates. All incidence rates are for the population ages 30–83 years and are age-gender standardized to the Olmsted County year 2000 population. This is done to isolate the effect of the control or loss of control of risk factors on the incidence of CHD and CVD from the effect of aging of the population on CHD and CVD incidence.

The rates for smoking, diabetes and ECG-LVH are set as listed in Table 1 for each scenario. These rates are used for randomly assigning risk factors to the simulated population. The resulting population means might vary slightly from the underlying rates due to the statistical fluctuations associated with a finite population of 108,000.

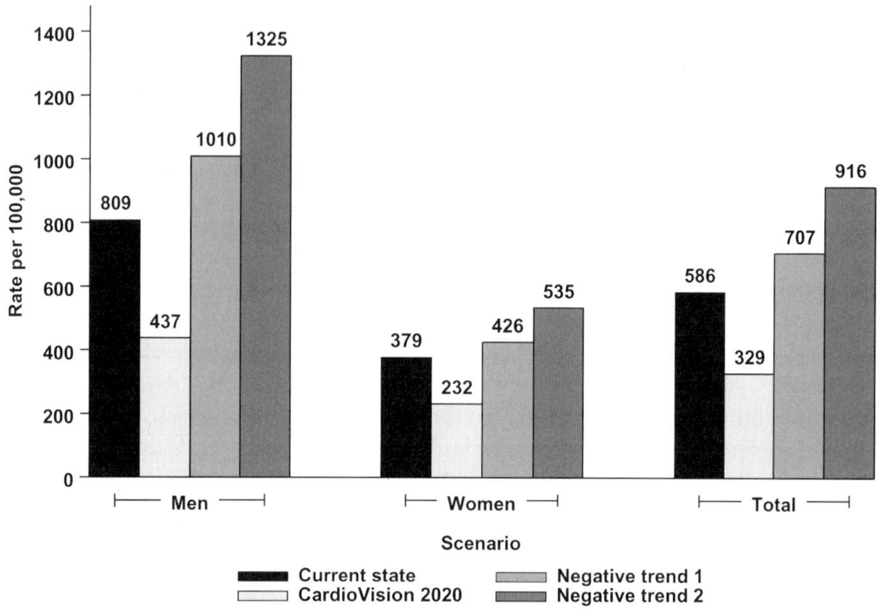

Figure 1. Predicted incidence rates of coronary heart disease by scenario for Olmsted County residents ages 30–83 years. Rates are age-gender standardized to the Olmsted County population in the year 2000. See text for the definitions of the four scenarios.

RESULTS

Coronary Heart Disease

Compared to the current rate of CHD for men (809/100,000), achieving the CardioVision 2020 goals would reduce rates by 45% (Figure 1). An increase in smoking and diabetes prevalence (negative trend 1) would be expected to increase CHD rates by 25% and an increase in smoking and diabetes prevalence plus loss of hypertension and hyperlipidemia control (negative trend 2) would be expected to increase CHD rates by 64%. The incidence rates with the worst case scenario (negative trend 2) would be three times as high as the incidence rates if the CardioVision 2020 scenario were met.

The absolute and relative impact of the four different scenarios would be less for women than for men. Compared to the current rate of CHD (379/100,000), the expected rate with CardioVision 2020 would be 39% lower. The rate with increased smoking and diabetes prevalence (negative trend 1) would be 12% higher and the rate with an increase in smoking and diabetes prevalence plus loss of hypertension and hyperlipidemia control (negative trend 2) would be 41% higher than current levels. The difference in rates between the CardioVision 2020 scenario and the worst case scenario (negative trend 2) would be 231%.

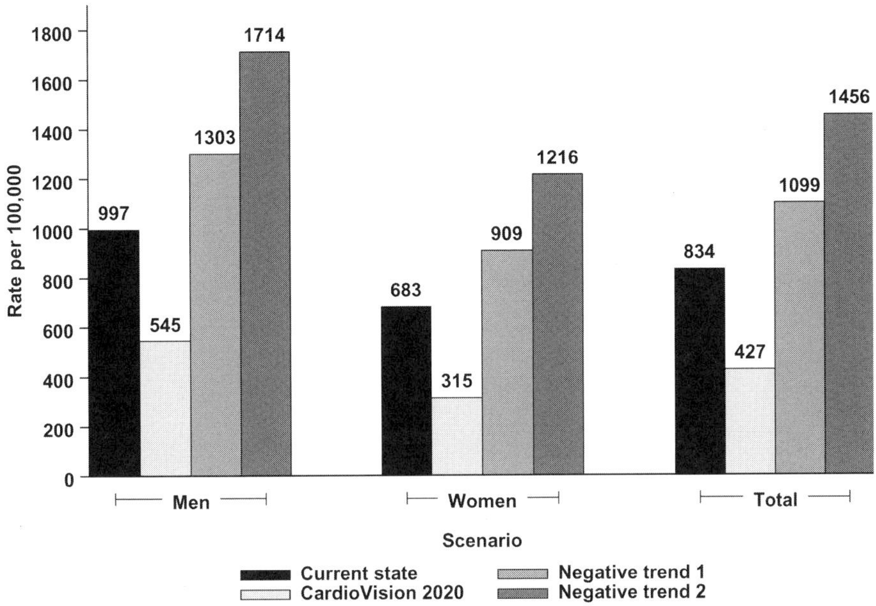

Figure 2. Predicted incidence rates of cardiovascular disease by scenario for Olmsted County residents ages 30–83 years. Rates are age-gender standardized to the Olmsted County population in the year 2000. See text for the definitions of the four scenarios.

The CHD rates for the genders combined would be 44% lower with the CardioVision 2020 scenario compared to the current rate scenario. Compared to the CardioVision 2020 scenario, the rates for the worst case scenario (negative trend 2) would be 278% higher.

Cardiovascular Disease

The impact of the risk factor changes on the CVD rates for men would be quite similar to the impact on CHD rates. Compared to the current rate of CVD for men (997/100,000), achieving the CardioVision 2020 goals would reduce CVD rates by 45% (Figure 2). An increase in smoking and diabetes prevalence (negative trend 1) would be expected to increase CHD rates by 31% and an increase in smoking and diabetes prevalence plus loss of hypertension and hyperlipidemia control (negative trend 2) would be expected to increase CHD rates by 72%. The incidence rates with the worst case scenario (negative trend 2) would be more than three times as high as the incidence rates if the CardioVision 2020 scenario were met.

The absolute and relative impact of the four different scenarios on CVD rates for women would be greater than the impact of risk factor differences on CHD rates for women. Compared to the current rate of CVD for women (683/100,000), the expected rate with CardioVision 2020 would be 54% lower. The rate with increased smoking and diabetes prevalence (negative trend 1) would be 33% higher and the rate with an increase in smoking and diabetes prevalence plus loss of hypertension and hyperlipidemia control (negative trend 2) would be 78% higher than current levels. The CVD incidence rates for women with the worst case scenario (negative trend 2) would be nearly four times as high as the incidence rates if the CardioVision 2020 scenario were met.

The CVD incidence rates for the genders combined would be 49% lower with the CardioVision 2020 scenario compared to the current rate scenario. Compared to the rates with the CardioVision 2020 scenario, the CVD incidence rates for the worst case scenario (negative trend 2) would be 341% higher.

DISCUSSION

This study estimates the potential impact of CardioVision 2020 on the incidence of CHD and CVD in the Olmsted County population. If the population could meet the CardioVision 2020 goals, incidence rates of CHD and CVD might be reduced by as much as 45% for men and 35% to 40% for women. If large unfavorable trends in cardiovascular risk factor levels develop (5–7,9,11,12) and are present in the year 2020, the model predicts that, compared to current levels, the incidence of CHD could be 50% higher for men and 35% higher for women. Given the same unfavorable trends, the incidence of CVD could be as much as 55% higher for men and nearly 60% higher for women. For men, there is nearly a 3-fold difference in CHD incidence rates depending on whether the CardioVision 2020 goals are met or risk factor control deteriorates. For women, the difference is more than 2-fold. Similar differences in CVD incidence rates are seen for men, but the differences for women are 4-fold.

Is this extreme range of risk factor differences within the realm of reason? The evidence indicates that our scenarios are realistic. The CardioVision 2020 goals are the Healthy People 2010 goals (31), and the changes predicted for the CardioVision 2020 scenario should be achievable: the North Karelia Project in Finland was associated with a 75% decline in death rates from cardiovascular disease over a 25 year period (32). Nearly all of the change is explainable by changes in risk factors (33). At the other extreme, total mortality rates and mortality from CHD and CVD rose rapidly in the former socialist economies of Eastern Europe (34). Between 1990 and 1994, the life expectancy of Russians declined five years in a four-year time span (35). About half of this decline was due to increasing CHD and CVD rates.

Even so, our predictions have limitations. The generalizability of our analysis is limited because we use the age- and gender-distribution of risk factors for the Olmsted County, year 2000 population. We obtain blood pressure values from random abstraction of patient charts and obtain cholesterol values from the Mayo Clinic laboratory database. These data might not be representative of all community members. We do not have cholesterol levels on a random sample of Olmsted County residents to compare with the values we obtained. However, for mean systolic blood pressure values, our baseline current community estimates are approximately 10 mm Hg less than those reported by Meissner et al. (7) for a random sample of community residents. Therefore, the model using current blood pressure levels (Scenario 1) actually underestimates CHD and CVD rates and lessens the expected difference between current and CardioVision 2020 scenarios. Because we model a population that is predominantly Caucasian and relatively well educated, we can expect the absolute risk to differ from that of other populations. However, a study group of the American Heart Association has concluded that the relative risk estimates that are generated from the risk functions of Caucasian populations are applicable across diverse populations (36). We also acknowledge that a different risk function may predict different rates of future events, and allowing for correlation among risk factors may change predicted outcomes somewhat. However, other investigators have shown that, while the absolute numbers may differ, the rank order of scenarios is stable when any one of several risk functions is used (37).

The fact that other simulation programs have been able to replicate historical trends in disease rates increases our confidence in our calculations (38). Assuming no correlation among risk factors appears to underestimate rather than overestimate the impact of risk factors on disease rates in the population (39). These calculations are a first step in the development of a much larger project to model the impact of risk factor changes and treatment interventions in a defined population (40). We plan to eventually place this tool in the public domain so that it can be used by health care planners and analysts.

Because these calculations demonstrate the critical importance of risk factor control in our population, we are implementing CardioVision 2020- a comprehensive, population-wide initiative aimed to produce outstanding risk factor control in our community. The personnel of CardioVision 2020 include a core group of health care professionals, specialists in marketing and communications, and lay community activists who work together on a range of community projects designed to motivate individuals to take responsibility for their personal health and to create environments that reinforce healthier choices for all. We recognize the importance of these complementary goals for optimum community health. The five CardioVision 2020 personal goals (zero exposure to tobacco and tobacco smoke; five servings of fruits and vegetables a day, only lean or extra lean meat, and only fat-free or 1% fat dairy products; 30 minutes of physical activity on most, if not all, days of the week; systolic blood pressure less than 130 mm Hg and diastolic blood pressure less than 85 mm Hg; and, total serum cholesterol less than 200 mg/dl or low density lipoprotein less than 100 mg/dl for individuals with coronary artery disease) are consistent with the goals set by Healthy People 2010 (31). CardioVision 2020 also seeks to create a community physical and social environment that enables and reinforces the personal goal behaviors. Examples of these efforts include teaming with restaurants and schools to provide healthier menu choices; working with the parks and recreation department to improve access to recreational/park facilities; and sponsoring periodic community activities to keep CardioVision 2020 and risk factor control in the public consciousness. CardioVision 2020 personnel also recently collaborated with the local medical society and other groups to precipitate the banning smoking in Olmsted County restaurants.

Based on our simulation, we conclude that risk factor control is important for any community. Optimal risk factor control could generate a significant decline in the incidence of coronary heart disease and cardiovascular disease. On the other hand, any community that loses control of its risk factor levels can expect to see a resurgence of the coronary heart disease and cardiovascular disease epidemics. We possess the technology and knowledge for coronary heart disease and cardiovascular disease prevention; whether we possess the personal and political will to prevent these diseases remains to be seen.

ACKNOWLEDGEMENT

This analysis was supported in part by an unrestricted research grant from McNeil Consumer Healthcare.

REFERENCES

1. Stamler J, Stamler R, Neaton JD, Wentworth D, Daviglus ML, Garside D, Dyer AR, Liu K, Greenland P. 1999. Low risk-factor profile and long-term cardiovascular and non-cardiovascular mortality and life expectancy. JAMA 282:2012–2018.
2. Salomaa V, Rosamond W, Mahonen M. 1999. Decreasing mortality from acute myocardial infarction: effect of incidence and prognosis. J Cardiovasc Risk 6:69–75.
3. Rosamond WD, Chambless LE, Folsom AR, Cooper LS, Conwill DE, Clegg L, Wang CH, Heiss G. 1998. Trends in the incidence of myocardial infarction and in mortality due to coronary heart disease, 1987 to 1994. N Engl J Med 339:861–867.
4. Goldberg RJ, Yarzebski J, Lessard D, Gore JM. 1999. A two decades (1975 to 1995) long experience in the incidence, in-hospital and long-term case-fatality rates of acute myocardial infarction: a community-wide perspective. J Am Coll Cardiol 33:1533–1539.
5. Leibson CL, O'Brien PC, Atkinson E, Palumbo PJ, Melton LJ 3rd. 1997. Relative contributions of incidence and survival to increasing prevalence of adult-onset diabetes mellitus: a population-based study. Am J Epidemiol 146:12–22.
6. National Diabetes Data Group. 1995. Diabetes in America. Bethesda: National Institutes of Health.
7. Meissner I, Whisnant JP, Sheps SG, Schwartz GL, O'Fallon WM, Covalt JL, Sicks JD, Bailey KR, Wiebers DO. 1999. Detection and control of high blood pressure in the community: Do we need a wake-up call? Hypertension 34:466–471.
8. Kopstein A. 2001. Tobacco Use in America: Findings from the 1999 National Household Survey on Drug Abuse, 122. (Analytic Series: A-15. DHHS Publication No. SMA 02-3622). Rockville, MD: Substance Abuse and Mental Health Services Administration, Office of Applied Studies.
9. http://www.cdc.gov/tobacco/youth.htm. CDC Tobacco Information and Prevention Source; Youth.
10. U.S. Department of Health and Human Services. 2001. Women and Smoking 2001. A Report of the Surgeon General. Executive Summary, 2. Atlanta: U.S. Department of Health and Human Services, Public Health Service, Centers for Disease Control and Prevention, National Center for Chronic Disease Preventon and Health Promotion, Office on Smoking and Health.
11. Flegal KM, Carroll MD, Kuczmarski RJ, Johnson CL. 1998. Overweight and obesity in the United States: prevalence and trends 1960–1994. Intl J Obesity 22:39–47.
12. Nutrition Insights, No. 5. 1998. Is total fat consumption really decreasing? Washington D.C.: USDA Center for Nutrition Policy and Promotion. http://www.usda.gov/fcs/cnpp.htm.
13. Rose G. 1985. Sick individuals and sick populations. Int J Epidemiol 14:32–38.
14. Kottke TE, Puska P, Salonen JT, Tuomilehto J, Nissinen A. 1985. Projected effects of high-risk versus population-based prevention strategies in coronary heart disease. Am J Epidemiol 121: 697–704.
15. Kottke TE, Roger VL, Nguyen TT, Dale LC, Burnett JC Jr, Tajik AJ. 1999. CardioVision 2020: A multidisciplinary cardiovascular disease prevention project. Euro Heart J 1(Suppl S):S14–S18.

16. Kottke TE, Brekke MJ, Brekke LN, Dale LC, Brandel CL, DeBoer SW, Hayes SN, Hoffman RS, Menzel PA, Nguyen TT, Thomas RJ. 2000. The CardioVision 2020 Baseline Community Report Card. Mayo Clin Proc 75:1153–1159.
17. Mooney C. 1997. Monte Carlo Simulation. Sage University Paper Series on Quantitative Applications in the Social Science. Thousand Oaks, CA: Sage.
18. Tsevat J, Weinstein MC, Williams LW, Tosteson AN, Goldman L. 1991. Expected gains in life expectancy from various coronary heart disease risk factor modifications. Circulation 83:1194–1201.
19. Weinstein MC. 1989. Methodologic issues in policy modeling for cardiovascular disease. J Am Coll Cardiol 14:38A–43A.
20. Weinstein MC, Coxson PG, Williams LW, Pass TM, Stason WB, Goldman L. 1987. Forecasting coronary heart disease incidence, mortality and cost: The coronary heart disease policy model. Am J Public Health 77:1417–1426.
21. Mackisack M, Dobson AJ, Heathcote CR. 1992. Predicting the prevalence of a disease in a cohort at risk. Stat Med 11:295–305.
22. Goldman L, Coxson P, Hunink MG, Goldman PA, Tosteson AN, Mittleman M, Williams L, Weinstein MC. 1999. The Relative Influence of Secondary Versus Primary Prevention Using the National Cholesterol Education Program Adult Treatment Panel II Guidelines. J Am Coll Cardiol 34:768–776.
23. Goldman L, Weinstein MC, Williams LW. 1989. Relative impact of targeted versus population wide cholesterol interventions on the incidence of coronary heart disease. Circulation 80:254–260.
24. Goldman L. 1990. Cost-effectiveness perspectives in coronary heart disease. Am Heart J 119: 733–740.
25. Grover SA, Abrahamowicz M, Joseph L, Brewer C, Coupal L, Suissa S. 1992. The benefits of treating hyperlipidemia to prevent coronary heart disease. JAMA 267:816–822.
26. Health, United States, 1999 With Health and Aging Chartbook. 2 ed. Hyattsville, Maryland: National Center for Health Statistics; 1999.
27. Anderson KM, Odell PM, Wilson PW, Kannel WB. 1991. Cardiovascular disease risk profiles. Am Heart J 121:293–298.
28. Wilson PW, D'Agostino RB, Levy D, Belanger AM, Silbershatz H, Kannel WB. 1998. Prediction of Coronary Heart Disease Using Risk Factor Categories. Circulation 97:1837–1847.
29. Compressed Mortality File: Office of Analysis and Epidemiology, Atlanta. National Center for Health Statistics, Centers for Disease Control and Prevention.
30. Estimates of the Population of Counties by Age and Gender: 1990–1997: U.S. Bureau of the Census; 1998.
31. U.S. Department of Health and Human S. Healthy People 2010. 2nd Ed. With Understanding and Improving Health and Objectives for Improving Health. 2 ed. Washington D.C.: U.S. Government Printing Office; 2000.
32. Puska P, Vartiainen E, Tuomilehto J, Salomaa V, Nissinen A. 1998. Changes in premature deaths in Finland: successful long-term prevention of cardiovascular diseases. WHO Bull 76:419–425.
33. Vartiainen E, Puska P, Pekkanen J, Tuomilehto J, Jousilahti P. 1994. Changes in risk factors explain changes in mortality from ischaemic heart disease in Finland. Brit Med J 309:23–27.
34. Thom T, Epstein F, Feldman J, Leaverton P, Wolz M. 1992. Total mortality and mortality from heart disease, cancer, and stroke from 1950 to 1987 in 27 Countries. Highlights of trends and Their Interrelationships Among Causes of Death. Bethesda. National Institutes of Health.
35. Notzon FC, Komarov YM, Ermakov SP, Sempos CT, Marks JS, Sempos EV. 1998. Causes of declining life expectancy in Russia. JAMA 279:793–800.
36. Grundy SM, Pasternak R, Greenland P, Smith S Jr, Fuster V. 1999. Assessment of Cardiovascular Risk by Use of Multiple-Risk-Factor Assessment Equations. Circulation 100:1481–1492.
37. Liao Y, McGee DL, Cooper RS, Sutkowski MB. 1999. How generalizable are coronary risk prediction models? Comparison of Framingham and two national cohorts. Am Heart J 137:837–845.
38. Hunink MG, Goldman L, Tosteson AN, Mittleman MA, Goldman PA, Williams LW, Tsevat J, Weinstein MC. 1997. The recent decline in mortality from coronary heart disease, 1980–1990. The effect of secular trends in risk factors and treatment. JAMA 277:535–542.
39. Kaplan RM. 1991. Imagine no coronary heart disease. Circulation 83:1452–1455.
40. Brekke MJ, Kottke TE, Brekke LN, Wu LA. 2003. The design and development of a coronary heart disease decision support tool. Int J Technol Assess Health Care 19(2):551–554.

Frontiers in Cardiovascular Health, edited by
N.S. Dhalla, A. Chockalingam,
H.I. Berkowitz & P.K. Singal
Kluwer Academic Publishers, Boston, 2003

Benefits of Exercise in Patients with Congestive Heart Failure

Koon K. Teo,[1] Mark Haykowsky,[2]
Catherine Demers,[1] and Robert S. McKelvie,[1]

[1] *The Division of Cardiology, Department of Medicine, and The Population Health Research Institute, McMaster University Hamilton, Ontario, Canada*
and
[2] *The Department of Physical Therapy, Faculty of Rehabilitation Medicine University of Alberta, Edmonton, Alberta, Canada*

Summary. A large majority of individuals with CHF suffer from fatigue and poor exercise capacity, the underlying cause of which is multi-factorial. These include central mechanisms such as cardiac dysfunction and poor cardiac output as well as peripheral maladaptations such as neurohormonal activation and abnormalities in skeletal muscle structure and metabolism. Studies in the last decades have shown that exercise training can reverse some of these adverse pathophysiological effects, which are both associated with poor exercise capacity and poor overall prognosis in CHF. Data from the EXERT study and other small clinical studies indicate that exercise training, based on individualized protocols and approaches geared toward each individual's capacity, is safe in selected patients. Although EXERT remains the largest randomized control trial of exercise training in CHF, these studies demonstrating the benefits of exercise are small. Conclusions on whether or not these observations can be translated into reductions in morbidity and mortality, despite the promise shown in the reversal of the pathophysiological mechanisms, remain unclear. Large adequately powered randomized controlled trials are needed to address this important question. Meanwhile, the traditional advice to CHF patients "to avoid physical exertion" should not longer be applied to all affected individuals.

***Key words*:** Congestive heart failure, pathophysiological mechanisms, physical limitations, poor exercise capacity, exercise training.

Corresponding Author: Dr. Koon K. Teo, Rm 3U4 McMaster University Medical Centre, 1200 Main Street West, Hamilton, Ontario, Canada L8S 3Z5. Tel: 905 521 2100 ext 76222, FAX: 905 521 5053, E-mail: teok@mcmaster.ca.

INTRODUCTION

Heart failure is a clinical syndrome in which the heart is unable to "pump blood at a rate commensurate with the requirements of the metabolizing tissues and/or to be able to do so only from an elevated filling pressure". This results in a complex clinical syndrome with multiple organ involvement, manifesting in a multitude of symptoms and physical signs (1). Acute myocardial infarction or myocarditis can present with acute heart failure, which often can evolve into chronic congestive heart failure (CHF). The left ventricle, scarred by the previous infarction or weakened by the myocarditis or ongoing myocardial ischemia undergoes remodelling, becomes unable to function effectively. Alternatively, CHF can gradually develop in the background of progressive pressure or volume overload as a result of hypertension, valvular stenosis or regurgitation. The final common pathway of all these various etiologies is the development of left ventricular cardiac enlargement, initial compensatory but chronic maladaptive activation of the neurohormonal system, which ultimately results in decreased efficiency of cardiac function.

CHF occurs more commonly in the elderly, with the incidence and prevalence of CHF increasing with age in western societies (1–4). In Canada and elsewhere, CHF is rapidly becoming a clinical and public health problem. Recent data indicate that 300,000 to 400,000 Canadians, 4.7 million U.S. residents, i.e., up to 2% of the adult North American population and more than 10% of those aged 75 years or older, suffer from CHF (2–4). Mortality and morbidity is significantly increased in individuals who have CHF compared to those who do not have the syndrome. CHF is the primary cause of 40,000 deaths (50% sudden) in the USA and contributes to another 25,000 deaths. Mortality remains unacceptably high at 50% over 5 years (2,3). Furthermore, CHF is associated with an increased frequency of hospitalization and a prolonged length of stay. In the U.S., it is the primary diagnosis in 900,000 hospitalizations, resulting in 6 million bed days and costing more than US$6 billion (3,4), which is more than the hospitalization costs for acute myocardial infarction or cancer. Patients with CHF are frequently fatigued and have limited exercise capacity. This physical limitation, in addition to the generally increased social isolation in the elderly, leads to depression, social withdrawal and a poor quality of life (5).

PHYSICAL LIMITATIONS IN CHF

Traditionally, patients with CHF are advised to rest and to avoid physical activities for fear that such activities may cause further harm. There are concerns that physical activities may worsen CHF and other cardiac symptoms, with increasing shortness of breath and fatigue, worsen the generally frail condition of the CHF patients and that dangerous complications may occur during exercise. Moreover, there is the perception that the exercise might cause worsening of the underlying disease, leading to deterioration of the ventricular shape and function, or result in further myocardial ischemia and subsequent cardiac damage (5). However, limiting regular physical activity may not only be unnecessary but detrimental as it may result in further deterioration of the fitness level of CHF patients. This would translate into further impairment of the CHF patients' ability to carry out activities of daily living and cause them to become more dependent unnecessarily.

Therefore, there is clearly a need to seek evidence whether exercise is beneficial in individuals with CHF, to examine the balance between benefit and harm in an exercise program, and to explore the boundaries within which exercise is safe and beneficial. A large number of studies have been carried out in the last two decades that have assessed the effects of exercise training on functional capacity in individuals with CHF (5–19). Some acute studies have examined the underlying pathophysiology of the poor exercise capacity in CHF patients. Other short-term studies, examining the effects of exercise and exercise training programs on patients with CHF, have demonstrated that exercise training may ameliorate partially the abnormal pathophysiological adaptations in CHF and suggested that such training may be beneficial.

The underlying cause of poor exercise capacity in CHF is multifactorial (6). Reduced cardiac output is an obvious and important component. This can be due to systolic and/or diastolic left ventricular dysfunction in a damaged heart. Recent studies also suggest that an abnormal pericardial-ventricular interaction associated with a dilated left ventricle can also lead to decreased cardiac output (7). Abnormal pulmonary hemodynamics, such as elevated pulmonary pressures, can also affect cardiac function. Generally, in advanced CHF, more than one of these mechanisms are operative and their additive effects worsen the clinical status. Of interest is the observation that poor systolic function of the left ventricle at rest, as indicated by a poor left resting ventricular ejection fraction, has no relation to an individual's exercise capacity (8). This suggests that the affected individual's ability to exercise may be related more to peripheral factors, which if corrected, may lead to improvement in the individual's exercise capacity, even if the underlying cardiac function remains impaired.

Numerous peripheral factors, which contribute to the symptoms and limitations in CHF, have been identified (5,6). These include abnormal blood flow to and in the exercising muscles, abnormalities in skeletal muscle structure and metabolism, abnormal neurohormonal system activation, and abnormalities of ventilation. While these abnormalities may be due, in part, to physical deconditioning/disuse or as a direct result of the CHF, the end result is that affected individuals are limited by and are fearful of their disability, and are not able or willing to undertake any exercise. Thus a vicious circle is maintained.

CLINICAL STUDIES—PATHOPHYSIOLOGY AND CLINICAL BENEFITS

The observation that peripheral mechanisms may be at least in part responsible for the reduction of exercise capacity supports the use of exercise training to improve the functional capacity of CHF patients. A number of clinical studies have demonstrated that exercise training in selected CHF patients may be beneficial and safe. Coats and colleagues studied 11 symptomatic CHF patients (NYHA classes II to III) with underlying coronary artery disease, average age 63 years and left ventricular ejection fraction 19%, in a random order cross over trial involving 8 weeks of home based bicycle exercise training and 8 weeks of rest (9). Following training, beneficial effects were found, with exercise duration increasing by 18% and peak oxygen consumption (VO_{2peak}), by 17%. There was an overall symptomatic improvement, with no adverse events reported. Based on these findings, it was concluded that exercise training was feasible, beneficial and apparently safe in individuals with severe left ventricular dysfunction and symptomatic CHF (9). Other investigators have reported similar benefits. In a series of studies, Sullivan et al reported their experience in 12 CHF patients, with average left ventricular ejection fraction of 24%, who underwent aerobic training for about 4 hours per week for 4 to 6 months (10,11). They reported a number of beneficial effects following the exercise training, including increased $V0_{2peak}$, and improved performance during maximal and submaximal exercise, with no deterioration of left ventricular function. These improvements in exercise capacity may be due to reversal of some of the peripheral maladaptations. Specifically, the investigators noted an improved peak blood flow to the exercising muscles, and decreased lactate accumulation at submaximal exercise. Ventilatory anaerobic threshold occurred at higher oxygen consumption levels. Exercise duration during the constant workload protocol increased significantly by nearly 50%. These peripheral adaptations were independent of central hemodynamics (10,11).

These peripheral maladaptations, have also been reported to be reversed in another study on 17 symptomatic (NYHA II to III) CHF patients, with underlying coronary artery disease and average left ventricular ejection fraction of about 20% (12). The patients underwent a random order cross over exercise training study, which consisted of 8 weeks of home-based bicycle exercise and 8 weeks of rest. Exercise tolerance increased by 19%, with reduced minute ventilation, by 11%. There was also a beneficial and significant shift of the sympathovagal balance from sympathetic towards enhanced vagal activity after exercise training. The increases in cardiac output associated with the training, 17% at submaximal and 13% at maximal exercise (12), were similar to the findings of another study. In this other study, 25 men post infarction or bypass surgery, average left ventricular ejection fraction 32%, were randomized to high intensity aerobic training or usual activities (13). Patients who underwent training had a 29% improvement in $V0_{2peak}$ and a 20% increase in maximal cardiac output, which were not found in the controls on usual activities. Of interest also is the observation that resting/exercise hemodynamics and resting left ventricular ejection fraction, did not change within or between groups, suggesting that the high intensity training did not cause further myocardial damage (13).

At a more basic level, the improvement in exercise capacity appears to be partly associated with an enhancement in endothelial function following exercise training (14–16). Using non-invasive methods, several studies have reported that (1) exercise training restored flow dependent dilatation measured in the radial artery, (2) regular exercise improved basal endothelial nitric oxide formation, (3) endothelial dependent vasodilatation of skeletal muscle vasculature was associated with increases in exercise capacity and, (4) exercise training improved endothelial dependent vasodilatation in the epicardial and resistance coronary arteries. This restoration of endothelial function can also improve the responsiveness of the vasculature in the regulation of blood flow (14–16).

That exercise training can reverse skeletal muscle metabolism and structure have been observed in several studies. In one such study, the effects of exercise training on skeletal muscle metabolism in one arm was compared with that in the non-exercising control arm in 10 CHF patients, using 31P-magnetic resonance spectroscopy (17). In the trained arm, but not in the control arm, there were increases in maximal voluntary contraction (by 6%), submaximal exercise duration (by 19%) and improved pH at submaximal exercise. The estimated effective rate of mitochondrial ATP synthesis was increased, indicating that the impaired oxidative capacity of the skeletal muscle was improved by local exercise training (17). Along similar lines, Hambrecht et al. studied skeletal muscle structural and metabolism by obtaining percutaneous biopsies of the vastus lateralis muscle at baseline and after 6 months of aerobic exercise in a randomized study of 18 CHF patients (9 training, 9 control), NYHA classes II to III, aged 51 years, and left ventricular ejection fraction 27% (18). Following training, there was a shift from type II to the more efficient type I skeletal muscle fibbers, with increases in the surface density of the cytochrome c oxidase-positive mitochondria (by 41%), mitochondrial cristae (by 43%) and mitochondrial inner border membrane (by 95%). It was concluded that the exercise induced improvement in oxygen uptake and lactate levels were related to changes in the mitochondrial structure leading to enhanced oxidative enzyme activity (18).

The effects of aerobic training on neurohormonal activity were studied in 19 CHF patients, NYHA classes II to III, aged 62 years, and left ventricular ejection fraction 30%, who were randomized to a walking program or control (19). After 16 weeks, while peak exercise neurohormone levels were unchanged, resting neurohormone levels were reduced in the training group with no changes in the control group. In the training group, resting angiotensin was reduced by 26%, aldosterone by 32%, vasopressin by 30% and atrial natriuretic peptide by 27%. These observations suggest that exercise training in CHF can partially reverse activation of the neurohormonal system (19).

Thus the evidence from the mechanistic and small randomized clinical studies indicate that exercise training can reverse a number of the peripheral maladaptations that contribute to the poor exercise capacity in individuals with CHF. These studies also suggest that exercise is feasible and safe in selected symptomatic individuals.

THE EXERCISE REHAB TRIAL (EXERT)

Whether or not beneficial effects can be obtained in a broader group of individuals undergoing an exercise rehabilitation program was addressed by the Exercise Rehab Trial (EXERT) (20). This was a randomized controlled trial of exercise training in CHF patients carried out in 2 Canadian centres. The objectives of this study were to evaluate the effects of short-term (3 months) supervised, and long-term (12 months) unsupervised, combined aerobic and resistance training on functional status, quality of life and safety. Unlike previous studies, EXERT incorporated an element of resistance training into the training program because it was believed that improvement in muscular strength would improve an individual's ability to more adequately carry out activities of daily living. Prior to starting this program, it had been shown that resistance training was safe in patients with coronary artery disease, and that it was feasible to adapt the resistance exercise training in CHF patients.

Individuals eligible for EXERT had documented diagnosis of CHF, left ventricular ejection fraction <40%, NYHA classes II-III symptoms and a 6 minute walk distance of <500 m. They were excluded if they were unstable despite the use of angiotensin converting enzyme inhibitors, digoxin, and diuretics therapy, their exercise tests were limited by claudication or angina, there was an abnormal exercise blood pressure response, they had residual impairment from a previous stroke, had significant respiratory limitation (FEV_1/VC <60% predicted), had non-cardiac conditions affecting survival or training, were geographically inconvenient or unable to attend for regular training.

Study endpoint evaluations consisted of VO_{2peak} testing, dynamic muscle strength measurements, 6-minute walk test, quality of life assessments and radionuclide ventriculography measures of left ventricular ejection fraction. All eligible patients underwent baseline endpoints evaluation prior to randomization, at the end of supervised training at 3 months, and, except for the radionuclide ventriculography, at the end of the unsupervised home-based training at 12 months. Endpoint evaluations were carried out at the two study centres by individuals who were blinded to the training assignment. Radionuclide ventriculography measurement of left ventricular ejection fractions was processed in one central laboratory.

Prior to randomization, all eligible participants underwent a run-in period consisting of 4 exercise sessions in order to ensure that they could undergo training if they were randomized to active training. They were then randomized to exercise training or to usual care, which consisted of usual advice by their regular physicians regarding physical activities. Those assigned to exercise training underwent supervised training 3 times a week for 3 months. Each participant underwent aerobic exercise consisting of treadmill walking and exercising on the arm and leg cycle ergometers. The Universal Gym was used for resistance training, with each upper and lower limb trained individually. For each patient, the target heart rate and strength training resistance were set individually, based on the initial baseline assessments. On completion of the 3 months of supervised training, a cycle ergometer and dumbbell weights were provided to participants in the training group who were given exercise guidelines that were to be followed during the home training program. Where necessary, an exercise physiologist visited the individuals' homes to ensure that the exercises were carried out properly. Each individual kept a log of the home exercise activities for 12 months. All study participants attended a special clinic once a month for general assessment and to ensure that the participants assigned to usual care were being followed-up. Exercise training was not discussed during these visits.

Table 1. Pertinent baseline characteristics in EXERT study

	Training Group (n = 90)	Control Group (n = 91)
Age (years)	64.8 ± 1.1	66.1 ± 1.0
Males/Females (%)	82/18	80/20
NYHA classes I/II/III (%)	2/67/31	1/66/33
Etiology (%)		
Ischemic	79	73
Idiopathic	6	13
Hypertensive	7	6
Valvular	5	4
Other	3	4
Medications (%)		
ACE inhibitors	91	92
Diuretics	81	86
Digoxin	62	66
Beta-blockers	20	23

Table 2. Follow-up and clinical outcomes in EXERT study

	Training Group (n = 91)	Control Group (n = 90)
At 3 months		
Completed follow up evaluations	80	83
Did not complete follow-up, reasons:		
Death	1	3
Worsening heart failure	2	1
Withdrawal	6	0
Other	1	4
At 12 months		
Completed follow up evaluations	64	75
Did not complete follow-up, reasons:		
Death	9	8
Worsening heart failure	3	2
Withdrawal	7	3
Other	7	3

Overall a 3-year period, 181 patients were recruited into the trial, 90 in the exercise group and 91 in the control group. Average age was 65 years, 81% were male, average left ventricular ejection fraction was 28%, and about two-thirds were in NHYA class II, with the rest in class III. Most patients were on ACE inhibitors (>90%), digoxin (>60%) and diuretics (>80%) (Table 1). Most patients (85%) completed the 3-month and 77% completed the 12-month endpoints evaluation. The common clinical reasons for not completing follow-up endpoint evaluations were worsening heart failure or death (Table 2) with no between group differences in incidence of clinical events.

Changes in study outcomes between measurements at baseline and those after supervised training at 3 months and after unsupervised training at 12 months were examined and compared between the two groups. At 3 months, VO_{2peak} increased by 0.104 L/min in the training group compared to the minimal increase of 0.025 L/min in the control group. The intergroup difference was statistically significant ($p < 0.05$). This trend was observed at 12 months, the training group showing a gain of 0.154 L/min in VO_{2peak} while the control group, with a gain of 0.024 L/min, hardly changed (p = n.s.). Changes in dynamic muscle strength showed similar trends. At 3 months, the average arm strength in the training group increased by 1.2 kg, compared to 0.5 kg in the control group, ($p < 0.05$). At 12 months, the training group showed a gain of only 0.6 kg compared to a gain of 1.1 kg in the control group (p = n.s.). When average leg strength (knee extension) was assessed at 3 months, the training group increased by 2.8 kg, compared to the 0.7 kg gained by the control group ($p = 0.0001$). At 12 months, the training group showed a gain of 1.1 kg while the control group had a 0.5 kg gain (p = n.s.). Gains in distances walked in 6 minutes did not differ between the two groups at 3 months or 12 months. At 3 months, the training group gained 22 m in average distance walked and the controls gained 15 m, (p = n.s.); at 12 months, the gains were 17 m and 20 m, respectively, (p = n.s.) (Table 3).

Quality of life, assessed by the Living with Heart Failure Questionnaire, showed a non-significant trend toward a better improvement in the training group, compared to the control group. This trend in intergroup difference was not obvious when assessed at 12 months (Table 3).

No obvious change in left ventricular ejection fraction was observed in either group at 3 months and there was no intergroup difference in the change in ejection fraction (Table 3).

From the findings in EXERT, it can be concluded that regular exercise training resulted in improvements in exercise capacity and muscle strength over the short-term period of 3 months. Regular physical activity could be performed without risk of deterioration of cardiac function. From this randomized long-term controlled trial, it appeared that exercise training is safe and feasible for a large heterogeneous group of CHF patients.

The gains, however, appeared uneven. Thus, while the study outcomes, which assessed the modalities employed in training, i.e., aerobic exercise and strength training showed significantly greater gains in the training group compared to the control group, this was not observed with the 6 minute walk test. The reason for this failure to show a greater gain is unclear. One speculation is that increases in VO_{2peak} may not translate into a faster walking pace during the 6 minutes of walking. Secondly, it is quite possible that the control group, having found that they could do some exercise during the baseline assessments and run-in phase and, encouraged by the objectives of the study, have decided to continue with walking exercises of their own. Such positive changes due to life style modification have been seen in other trials of life-style modification such as the Multiple Risk Factor Intervention Trial. This positive change may also explain the lack of a significant difference in changes in quality of life between the two groups.

The observation that at 12 months, there were no differences in VO_{2peak} and in

Table 3. Baseline and changes at 3 and 12 months for EXERT study endpoints

	Baseline		Change at 3 months			Change at 12 months		
	Training (n = 90)	Control (n = 91)	Training	Control	P-value*	Training	Control	P-value
VO2 peak (L/min)	1.10	1.14	+0.014	+0.025	<0.05	+0.154	+0.024	n.s.
6 min Walk Test (m)	434	421	+22	+15	n.s.	+17.3	+20	n.s.
Arm Curl (kg)	8.8	8.1	+1.2	+0.5	<0.05	+0.6	+1.1	n.s.
Knee Extension (kg)	17.1	16.6	+2.8	+0.7	0.0001	+1.1	+0.5	n.s.
Leg Press (kg)	66.8	64.0	+2.28	+1.07	n.s.	+1.6	+1.6	n.s.
MLHF Questionnaire Score	32.5	28.6	−3.9	−1.2	n.s.	−3.4	−3.3	n.s.
LV Ejection Fraction (%)	28.2	27.7	+0.2	+1.6	n.s.			

Adapted from ref. 20.
• comparing the change between training and control groups; n.s. = not significant.

upper and lower limb strength between the two groups, could be due to several reasons. While there is no reason to think that the training group did not perform their exercises properly since they had all being trained during the 3 months of supervised training, compliance at doing these exercises was a problem. Examination of the training logs showed that during the early months of unsupervised home-based training, participants exercised for at least 2 or more sessions per week, but towards the later months, the frequency of training decreased to an average of about 1.5 sessions per week. A small proportion of these individuals have actually stopped training completely. At the final assessment at 12 months, a number of participants failed to have their assessments and the study may not have adequate statistical power to detect differences at that stage. These factors likely contributed to the failure to show intergroup differences at 12 months. Thus, failure of long-term compliance with the exercise training has resulted in a loss of the initial improvement in exercise capacity.

CONCLUSIONS

Individuals with CHF experience physical limitations due to fatigue and poor exercise capacity, the underlying cause of which is multi-factorial. These include central mechanism such as cardiac dysfunction and cardiac output, as well as peripheral maladaptations such as neurohormonal activation and abnormalities in skeletal muscle structure, blood flow and metabolism. Studies in the last decades have shown that exercise training can reverse some of these adverse pathophysiological effects, which are both associated with poor exercise capacity and poor overall prognosis in CHF. The results of EXERT and other small clinical studies indicate that exercise training, based on individualized protocols and approaches geared toward each individual's capacity, is safe in selected patients. However, although promising, conclusions cannot be drawn from these studies that the results can be translated in beneficial reductions in morbidity and mortality in CHF patients. While EXERT remains the largest randomized control trial of exercise training in CHF, all these studies are too small for such conclusions to be drawn. Large adequately powered randomized controlled trials are needed to address this important question. Meanwhile, the traditional advice to CHF patients "to avoid physical exertion" should no longer be applied to all affected individuals.

REFERENCES

1. Johnstone DE, Abdulla A, Arnold JMO, et al. 1994. Diagnosis and management of heart failure. Can J Cardiol 10:613–631.
2. Ho KKL, Pinsky JL, Kannel WB, Levy D. The epidemiology of heart failure: The Framingham Study. J Am Coll Cardiol 22 (suppl A):6A–13A.
3. Brophy JM. 1992. Epidemiology of congestive heart failure. Canadian data from 1970 to 1989. Can J Cardiol 8:485–498.
4. Massie BM, Shah NB. 1997. Evolving trends in the epidemiology of heart failure. Am Heat J 133: 703–712.
5. McKelvie RS, Teo KK, McCartney N, Humen D, Montague T, Yusuf S. 1995. Effects of exercise training in patients with congestive heart failure: a critical review. J Am Coll Cardiol 25:789–796.

6. Myers J, Froelicher V. 1991. Hemodynamic determinants of exercise capacity in chronic heart failure. Annal Intern Med 115:377–386.
7. Janicki JB. 1990. Influence of the pericardium and ventricular interdependence on left ventricular diastolic and systolic function in patients with heart failure. Circulation 81(suppl): III 15–20.
8. Franciosa JA, Park M, Levine TB. 1981. Lack of correlation between exercise capacity and indexes of resting left ventricular performance in heart failure. Am J Cardiol 47:33–39.
9. Coats AJS, Adamopoulos S, Meyer TE, Conway J, Sleight P. 1990. Effects of physical training in chronic heart failure. Lancet 335:63–66.
10. Sullivan MJ, Higginbotham MB, Cobb FR. 1988. Exercise training in patients with severe left ventricular dysfunction: hemodynamic and metabolic effects. Circulation 78:506–515.
11. Sullivan MJ, Higginbotham MB, Cobb FR. 1989. Exercise training in patients with chronic heart failure delays ventilatory anaerobic threshold and improves submaximal exercise performance. Circulation 79:324–329.
12. Coats AJS, Adamopoulos S, Radaelli A, McCance A, Meyer TE, Bernardi L, Solda PL, Davey P, Ormerod O, Forfar C, Conway J, Sleight P. 1992. Controlled trial of physical training in chronic heart disease: exercise performance, hemodynamics, ventilation and autonomic function. Circulation 85:2119–2131.
13. Dubach P, Myers J, Dziekan G, Goebbels U, Reinhart W, Muller P, Buser P, Stulz P, Vogt P, Ratti R. 1997. Effect of high intensity exercise training on central hemodynamic responses to exercises in men with reduced left ventricular function. J Am Coll Cardiol 29:1591–1598.
14. Hambrecht R, Fiehn E, Weigl C, Gielen S, Hamann C, Kaiser R, Yu J, Adams V, Niebauer J, Schuler G. 1998. Regular physical exercise corrects endothelial dysfunction and improves exercise capacity in patients with chronic heart failure. Circulation 98:2709–2715.
15. Hornig B, Maier V, Drexler H. 1996. Physical training improves endothelial function in patients with chronic heart failure. Circulation 93:210–214.
16. Hambrecht R, Wolf A, Gielen S, Linke A, Hofer J, Erbs S, Schoene N, Schuler G. 2000. Effect of exercise on coronary endothelial function in patients with coronary artery disease. N Engl J Med 342:454–460.
17. Stratton JR, Dunn JF, Adamopoulos S, Kemp GJ, Coats AJS, Rajagopalan B. 1994. Training partially reverses skeletal muscle metabolic abnormalities during exercise in heart failure. J Appl Physiol 76:1575–1582.
18. Hambrecht R, Fiehn E, Yu J, Niebauer J, Weigl C, Hilbrich L, Adams V, Riede U, Schuler G. 1997. Effects of endurance training on mitochondrial ultrastructure and fiber type distribution in skeletal muscle of patients with stable chronic heart failure. J Am Coll Cardiol 29:1067–1073.
19. Braith RW, Welsch MA, Feigenbaum MS, Kluess HA, Pepine CJ. 1999. Neuroendocrine activation in heart failure is modified by endurance exercise training. J Am Coll Cardiol 34:1170–1175.
20. McKelvie RS, Teo KK, Roberts R, McCartney N, Humen D, Montague T, Hendrican K, Yusuf S. 2002. Effects of exercise training in patients with heart failure: the Exercise Rehabilitation Trial (EXERT). Am Heart J 144:23–30.

Frontiers in Cardiovascular Health, edited by
N.S. Dhalla, A. Chockalingam,
H.I. Berkowitz & P.K. Singal
Kluwer Academic Publishers, Boston, 2003

Cardiac Adaptations to Swim Exercise with Administration of a Cysteine Protease Inhibitor

Gavin D. Arthur[1] and Angelo N. Belcastro[1,2]

[1] *Schools of Rehabilitation Sciences and Human Kinetics, University of British Columbia, Vancouver, B.C. Canada, V6T 2B5 and* [2]*Faculty of Health Sciences, The University of Western Ontario, London, Ontario, Canada, N6A 5C1*

Summary. Using administration of a cysteine protease inhibitor (E64c), the hypothesis that calpain activation is a pre-requisite for swim-induced changes in cardiac performance and hypertrophy was assessed. The effects of acute swim exercise (54 ± 5 minutes) (n = 10) and training (6 weeks) (n = 16), both with (n = 10) or without E64c (n = 16) were observed for calpain activity, [cAMP], myofibril ATPase and left ventricular (LV) function. Acute swim resulted in: a) lowered calpain activity for E64c-untreated (41.5%) and treated rats (38.9%) ($p < 0.05$); b) increased [cAMP] from 606.1 ± 124.1 pmoles/g to 987.1 ± 165.1 ($p < 0.05$) (no E64c) and 649.81 ± 234 (with E64c) ($p > 0.05$); c) increased max LVP ($p < 0.05$); and d) lowered +dP/dt and −dP/dt. Training resulted in cardiac hypertrophy ($p < 0.05$) with no changes for resting [cAMP] and calpain activity ($p > 0.05$). Maximum LVP, +dP/dt and −dP/dt were reduced with training ($p < 0.05$), with E64c responses being comparable. Although the training-induced hypertrophy index was reduced with E64c, the selectivity of the E64c effects on biochemical parameters do not support a role for calpain activation in alterations of cardiac function induced by chronic swim exercise.

Key words: Swim-exercise, cardiac hypertrophy, calcium-activated protease, ventricular function.

Corresponding Author: Dr. Angelo N. Belcastro, Faculty of Health Sciences, Rm 125-Health Sciences Bldg, The University of Western Ontario, London, Ontario, Canada, N6A 5C1. Tel: (519)-661-4239, Fax: (519)-850-2347, E-mail: anbelcas@uwo.ca.

INTRODUCTION

Indicators of cardiac performance have been reported to improve following a period of exercise training (1,2). Despite some characterizations of swim exercise in the literature the precise mechanism(s) underlying these changes are still unknown. In the rat, swim exercise training induces primary changes in cardiac hypertrophy and function by altering the capacity of at least one (if not all) of the major biochemical systems responsible for the functional characteristics of cardiac muscle. For example, changes in actomyosin ATPase activity, sarcoplasmic reticulum Ca^{2+} transport and sarcolemmal function have all been reported (3–5) with either acute and/or chronic exercise. Acute and chronic swimming is also associated with morphological changes, such as mitochondrial damage, dilation of sarcoplasmic reticulum and myofibrillar disruption (4,6,7). Because the changes in calcium transport or calcium regulated process(es) are associated with these acute and chronic responses to swim exercise, it may be argued that calcium-dependent process(es) are central to these adaptive responses.

One calcium-regulated process reported to be active in hindlimb muscles with run exercise is the calcium activated neutral protease, calpain (8). Calpain targets membrane and myofibrillar proteins (9,10) that are known to be modified with exercise (8,11), and may be a causal agent underlying skeletal muscle morphological and biochemical changes (12). Moreover the development of cardiac hypertrophy, which involves Z-line smearing and selective degradation of constituent proteins of the cytoskeleton such as desmin and vimentin (6,7), has been linked to calpain activation (13). Although calpain is present in cardiac muscle and its actions in pathological conditions such as ischemia (10) and stunning (10,14) are documented; no information exists in the literature in regard to whether swim exercise is accompanied by activation of cardiac calpain. Because myocardial contractility is controlled by calcium and calcium regulated processes (i.e. troponin complex / sarcoplasmic reticulum) which are calpain substrates; it may be hypothesized that any exercise induced change in calpain activity would impact on the functional characteristics of the heart to exercise. To test this hypothesis calpain-like activity of individual rat hearts were assayed after one hour (acute) and 6 weeks (trained) of swim exercise and contrasted with indices of myocardial contractility (+dP/dt, −dP/dt).

Although demonstrating changes in calpain protease activity during acute and/or chronic swim exercise is informative, its role in eliciting these changes could not be determined. Of particular interest was whether or not exercise induced alterations in cardiac function are dependent on calpain activity. Because the exercise induced changes in calcium regulated processes are reminiscent of calpain involved actions and/or processes, our second hypothesis is that calpain activation is a prerequisite for swim exercise induced changes cardiac hypertrophy and/or performance. Partial support for calpain's role in cardiac hypertrophy is evident from experiments involving the development of beta-agonist induced hypertrophy (13). Therefore to assess calpain's role in the functional responses of the heart to both acute and chronic swim exercise, rats were treated with the cell permeable cysteine protease inhibitor

(2S-3S)-trans-epoxysuccinyl-1leucylamido-3-methylbutane (E64c) for 1 hr and 6 weeks of swim exercise.

MATERIALS AND METHODS

Male Wistar rats (n = 96), with initial body weight of 275–300 g were randomly assigned to one of seven groups: a) control (n = 12), b) acute swim exercise (n = 18), c) acute swim exercise with cysteine protease inhibitor, E64c (n = 12), d) 6 wk control (n = 20), e) 6 wk control with E64c (n = 6), f) 6 wk swim training (n = 18), and g) 6 wk swim training with E64c (n = 10). The rats were housed in a constant temperature animal care facility and given standard rat chow and water ad libitum. The University Animal Ethics Committee in accordance with guidelines established by the Canada Council on Animal Care approved all procedures.

Exercise

Animals swam in a fiberglass tank (36″ by 18″ and 24″ deep), which was divided in half to create two swimming areas for 5 animals at any one time. The water was recirculated and maintained at 33 ± 1°C. The same conditions were used for the acute swims except no weighting was used and the animals swam for 60 minutes or until they were unable to keep their heads above the surface of the water for 5 seconds.

The chronic swim protocol started with 30 minutes of swimming 4 days per week with 1% of body weight attached to the base of the tail. Swim duration and weighting were gradually increased up to 75 minutes with 2% body weight. The body weights for all animals were recorded on each of the swim days prior to swimming and were used to determine each animal's tail weighting. After every swim session the animals were toweled off and placed in cages under a warm heat lamp for thirty minutes and checked for signs of respiratory infections before being returned to the animal room.

At the termination of each experimental protocol, the rats were given an injection of sodium pentobarbital (0.75 mg/kg). For the cardiac performance measurements, the hearts were perfused immediately upon removal. All other hearts removed for biochemical measurements were quickly excised (< 2 minutes), rinsed in PBS, the left ventricle dissected away, and flash frozen in liquid nitrogen and stored at −70°C.

E64c

E64c was prepared in phosphate buffered saline (PBS) (pH 7.3) and injected subcutaneously at a dosage of 1 mg/Kg body weight. For the E64c treated acute swimmers the E64c injections were given 1 hour the prior to the swim exercise. Control rats received a subcutaneous injection of PBS at the same time as the E64c swimming animals received their injections. For the E64c treated acute swimmers the E64c injections were given 1 hour the prior to the swim exercise. For the 6-wk E64c swim group, injections were given 1 hour prior to the first and third swim sessions of the week. The 6-wk E64c control group received PBS injections at the same times as their swimming counterparts. All untreated controls received an injection of PBS alone to simulate the injection protocol.

Measurement of calpain like activity of cardiac muscle

Extraction and determination of calcium-dependent, calpastatin-inhibited proteolytic activity (calpain-like activity) was accomplished on all tissue samples (12). Tissue samples (approximately 100 mg) were suspended with an Ultra-Turrax homogenizer (IKA Laboratories, model TR-10) for 20 sec at a setting of 65 in 10–15 vols of a buffer containing 80 mM KCl, 20 mM Tris (pH 7.5), 5 mM EGTA and 2 mM DTT. The suspension was centrifuged (4°C) at 22,000 × g for 15 min (Hermle, model Z 233-M) and the supernatant (soluble fraction) decanted and stored in polypropylene tubes on ice (20 min) for subsequent assay of calpain-like activity. Following this centrifugation the particulate material was homogenized with a 2 ml Wheaton glass homogenizer (10 strokes) in 10–15 vols of a similar buffer (as above) with the addition of 0.35% Triton-X 100 and re-centrifuged. The supernatant from the second centrifugation step (particulate fraction) was stored on ice and assayed for calpain-like activity. This procedure was judged to be adequate in removing the 80 kDa band from the first pellet, because the second pellet (following glass homogenization with Triton-X 100) contained negligible (if any) amounts of this protein as assessed by PAGE and immunoblotting (12).

The calcium-dependent proteolytic activities of the supernatant (soluble) and pelleted (particulate) fractions were determined by a microplate assay using casein as the substrate (12). Briefly, 200 µl of soluble and/or particulate fractions were added to reaction mixtures final volume = 500 µl) containing: 2 mg/ml casein, 50 mM Tris (pH 7.5) and 20 mM DTT (in duplicate). Following a 5 min pre-incubation at 30°C, 5 mM total calcium (800 µM free calcium as determined by IONS software program) was added to one of the duplicates while the other contained 5 mM EGTA (chelating agent). After 30 min at 30°C, an aliquot (100 µl) of each sample was assayed for proteolysis in a total volume of 325 µl using a Bio-Rad protein dye reagent concentrate (Bio-Rad Laboratories). The protein dye reagent is composed of 0.05% (w/v) Coomassie brilliant blue G-250, 23.5% (w/v) ethanol and 42.5% (w/v) phosphoric acid. The enzyme activities (carried out in the absence and presence of calcium) are determined from a casein—coomassie blue standard curve and expressed as caseinolytic activity, where 0.1 absorbance change at an optical density of 595 nm being equivalent to 1 unit of enzyme activity. The calcium-dependent, caseinolytic activities of the soluble and particulate fractions are expressed as calpain-like activities because minimal activity (< 5%) was observed when calpastatin (a specific calpain inhibitor) was added to the assay. The values for total calpain-like activity of rat skeletal muscle determined in this study are comparable to those reported for partially purified calpain preparation (8).

Measurement of cardiac cAMP levels

Cardiac muscle tissue (10–20 mg) was homogenized with a glass rod homogenizer (Polytron) in 2.0 mls of ice cold 6% TCA buffer for 20–30 seconds with the homogenizing tube in a beaker of ice. The homogenates were placed on ice before centrifuging. After centrifuging, the supernatant fractions were transferred to extraction tubes and each sample was extracted 4 times with 5 ml aliquots of water-saturated ether. After extraction the sample tubes are placed in a water bath at 60°C for 10 minutes to remove the ether. The cAMP levels were measured using a cAMP[^{125}I] scintillation proximity assay (SPA) system (dual range) obtained from Amersham.

Left ventricular function measurements

Following removal, the hearts were immediately placed in ice-cold Chenoweth-Koelle solution containing 120 mM NaCl, 6 mM KCl, 2.18 mM $CaCl_2$, 2.1 mM $MgCl_2$, 19.2 mM $NaHCO_3$, and 10 mM glucose. The aortic stump was located and tied to a 15-gauge stainless steel aortic cannula. Perfusion was initially in the retrograde manner through the aorta at a perfusion pressure of 19 ml/min using a Masterflex peristaltic pump with a model 7016 pump head and Cole-Parmer Tygon tubing 6408-43. The perfusion fluid was Chenoweth-Koelle buffer maintained at 37°C and bubbled with 95% O_2/5% CO_2

A 16-gauge stainless steel cannula was then inserted into and tied to the pulmonary vein. Left ventricular developed pressure was measured by means of a Stratham pressure transducer attached to polyethylene PE90 tubing. The PE90 tubing was attached to a 20-gauge needle. The needle was then inserted through the apex of the heart into the left ventricle to allow continuos measurement of left ventricular pressure.

Cardiac work was initiated by switching the perfusion system from the mode to the working heart mode. In the working heart mode the perfusate entered the heart via the left atrium and was pumped out through the aortic stump by the left ventricle. The aortic outflow was subjected to an afterload of a 19 cm (7.5 in) column of H_2O inside PE160 tubing. Stratham pressure transducers attached to sidearms of the left atrial cannula and of the aortic outflow system are used to measure left atrial pressure and intraaortic pressure. Left ventricular pressure, left atrial pressure, intraaortic pressure, and the first derivative of left ventricular pressure were recorded on a Grass model 79D polygraph. Each heart was paced at 300 beats per minute by means of a stainless steel electrode placed on the left atrium at twice the threshold voltage with square wave pulses of 5-msec duration from a Grass model SD9D stimulator. The above preparation allowed us to measure indices of cardiac function across a range of left atrial filling pressures by changing the pump speed and therefore the perfusion pressure. Maximal rate of rise of left ventricular developed pressure (+dP/dt), rate of decline of left ventricular developed pressure (−dP/dt), and the maximum left ventricular pressure (max LVP) were recorded and analyzed on computer.

Ca^{2+} stimulated ATPase activity

Calcium stimulated cardiac myofibrillar ATPase was measured from cardiac myofibrils isolated and assayed according to the procedures as previously outlined (11).

Table 1. Morphological data of rats undergoing 6 weeks of chronic swim training, with and without administration of E64c (a cell permeable cysteine protease inhibitor (2S–3S)-trans-epoxysuccinyl-1leucylamido-3-methylbutane). The results are mean ± standard deviation

	n	Body Weight	LV Weight	LV Weight / Body Weight
Control	20	479 ± 35	1.154 ± 0.109	2.41 ± 0.201
Swim	16	478 ± 23	1.386 ± 0.123*	2.898 ± 0.24*
E64c Swim	9	469 ± 25	1.262 ± 0.101	2.69 ± 0.12
E64c Control	6	497 ± 24	1.163 ± 0.098	2.34 ± 0.155

* = Significantly different from control ($p < 0.05$).

Statistical analysis

All results presented are reported as mean values with the corresponding standard deviation. Ventricular weight to body weight ratios, calpain like activities and cAMP content of cardiac muscle were compared within the acute and chronic studies across the groups with a one way analysis of variance and a Tukeys post hoc test for individual group differences. The values for each of the three groups at each filling pressure in the functional measurements were compared using an one-way analysis of variance with a Tukeys post hoc test to determine the group(s) responsible for any significant differences. An α level of $p < 0.05$ was considered statistically significant.

RESULTS

Rats in the acute exercise groups completed 54 ± 5 minutes of swimming during the single session of exercise. Administration of E64c did not alter this swim time ($p > 0.05$). The training groups (with and without E64c) completed their program as described, with an average attrition of 6% across all training groups. No training or behavioural differences were observed as a result of chronic E64c administration.

Upon completion of the 6-wk program, left ventricular weight was significantly increased in the swim-trained animals and the E64c treated swimmers compared to the controls (Table 1). The E64c injected controls were not significantly different from normal controls ($p > 0.05$). Swimming did not produce any significant changes in body weight (Table 1). Therefore, the swimming groups showed increased left ventricular weight to body weight ratios from 2.41 ± 0.201 in controls to 2.898 ± 0.24 in the swim group ($p < 0.05$). The E64c treated animals had a left ventricular to body weight ratio of 2.69 ± 0.12, which is also greater than that of the control group ($p < 0.05$).

Biochemical Parameters

An acute single exhaustive swim decreased the total net cardiac calpain like activity from control levels of 27.26 ± 4.64 (U/g-wet wt) to 15.96 ± 2.37 after swimming ($p < 0.05$). The E64c preinjected animals showed a similar decrease to 16.66 ± 2.99 (Figure 1). The cardiac calpain levels were not significantly different across all of the chronic swim groups (Figure 1). Chronic control animals showed slightly

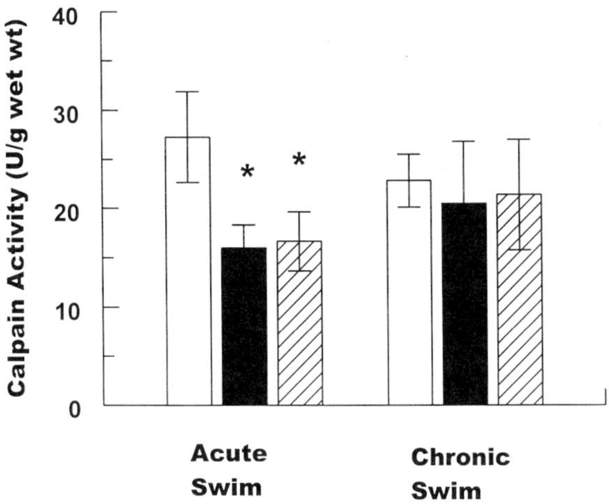

Figure 1. Calcium-stimulated, calpastatin-inhibited protease activity of extracts prepared from cardiac muscle following: a) acute swimming exercise (54 minutes-controls = open bars (n = 5); swimmers = solid bars (n = 5); E64c = hatched bars (n = 6)); and b) 6 weeks of chronic swim training rats (controls = open bars (n = 6); swimmers = solid bars (n = 7); E64c = hatched bars (n = 4)). Total calcium-dependent proteolytic activity was determined with a microplate assay where, 100 µl of extract was added to reaction mixtures containing: 2 mg/ml casein, 50 mM Tris (pH 7.5), 20 mM DTT and 0.75 mM free Ca^{2+} (containing EGTA). Values shown are means ± s.d. ⋆ = significantly different from control, $p < 0.05$.

lower calpain like activity than the acute controls with total net calpain like activity of 22.83 ± 2.7 while the chronic swimmers had levels of 20.49 ± 6.33 and the E64c chronic swimmers were also not significantly different at 21.39 ± 5.63 U/g-wet weight ($p > 0.05$).

An acute swim session resulted in a significant increase in the left ventricular cAMP content from 606.03 ± 124.1 (pmoles/g-wet wt) in controls to 987 ± 165.1 in swimmers ($p < 0.05$). The left ventricular cAMP content from rats injected with E64c prior to the swim was 649.81 ± 234, which is not significantly different from, controls (Figure 2). The chronic swim training groups showed minimal differences from each other in left ventricular cAMP levels (Figure 2).

The measurement of Ca^{2+} stimulated Mg^{2+} myofibrillar ATPase activity revealed no effect of either acute exercise (0.167 ± 0.020 umol Pi/g/min) or chronic training (0.167 ± 0.028 umol Pi/g/min), compared to controls (0.180 ± 0.040 umol Pi/g/min) ($p > 0.05$). E64c treatment did not affect the activity of any of the groups studied ($p > 0.05$).

Functional Parameters

The rate of rise of left ventricular pressure (+dP/dt) after acute exercise was decreased across an increasing range of left atrial filling pressures, at 8.1 mmHg of

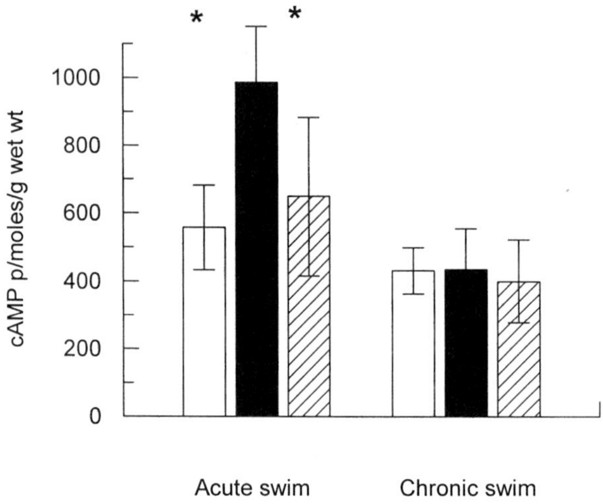

Figure 2. Left ventricular cAMP concentration (p/moles/g wet weight) of extracts prepared from cardiac muscle following: a) acute swimming exercise (54 minutes-controls = open bars (n = 5); swimmers = solid bars (n = 5); E64c = hatched bars (n = 6)); and b) 6 weeks of chronic swim training rats (controls = open bars (n = 6); swimmers = solid bars (n = 7); E64c = hatched bars (n = 4)). The cAMP levels were measured using a cAMP[^{125}I] scintillation proximity assay (SPA) system (dual range) obtained from Amersham. Values shown are means ± s.d. * = significantly different from control, $p < 0.05$.

left atrial filling pressure (LAFP) this was a 26.7% drop compared to control values ($p < 0.05$). Hearts from the E64c injected animals showed similar depression in +dP/dt values, with a 33.7% decrease at 8.1 mmHg LAFP (Figure 3). Hearts from chronically trained swimmers showed a similar depression from control levels of +dP/dt with a 26.7% decrease at 8.1 mmHg LAFP ($p < 0.05$), and those treated with E64c also showed depressed +dP/dt values to 33.7% ($p < 0.05$) (Figure 3).

Acute swim exercise also depressed the rate of relaxation for left ventricular pressure (−dP/dt) by 15.3% at 8.1 mmHg LAFP and generally over the entire range of filling pressures measured (Figure 4). The E64c treated rats showed a greater decrease in −dP/dt at 8.1 mmHg LAFP of 33.4% from controls; this decrease was also significant when compared to swimmers ($p < 0.05$). Swim training resulted in a lesser but still significant decrease in −dP/dt of 18.6% ($p < 0.05$), while training with E64c had an intermediate 11.4% decrease when compared to 6 wk controls ($p < 0.05$).

The only functional parameter to increase was found in the acute swimmers. The maximum left ventricular pressure (max LVP) as compared to control animals being increased by 12.6% at 8.1 mmHg LAFP (Figure 5) ($p < 0.05$). E64c injected swimmers showed max LVP 6.2% higher than controls at 8.1 mmH LAFP. Chronic swim trained rats on the other hand showed decreased max LVP by 15.1% at 8.1 mmHg

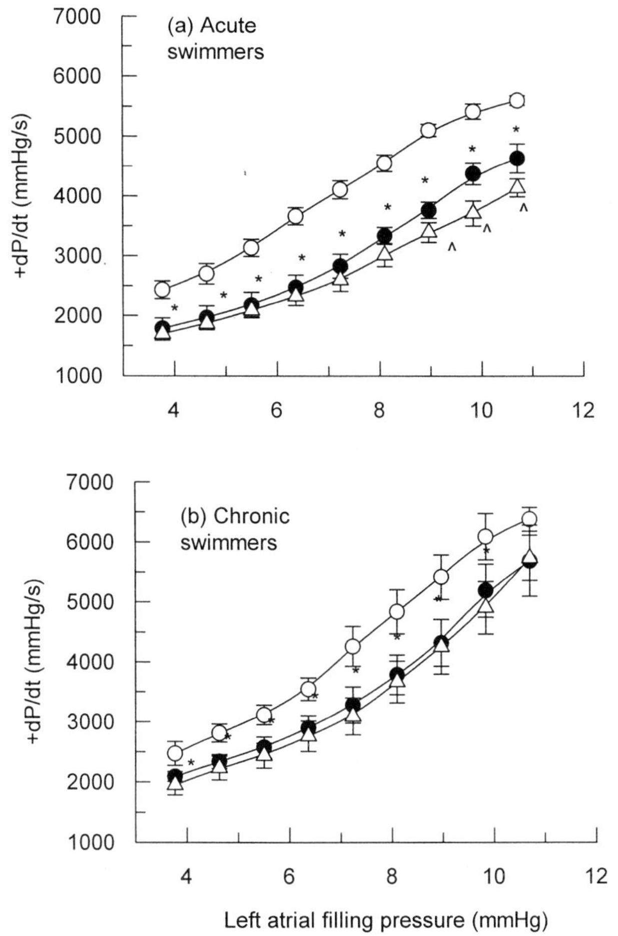

Figure 3. Rate of rise of left ventricular pressure; +dP/dt (mmHg/s) was determined using a working heart preparation. The open circles correspond to controls (acute n = 7, chronic n = 4), the solid circles are the swimmers (acute n = 5, chronic n = 5) and the filled triangles are the E64c treated swimmers (acute n = 4, chronic n = 4). Each heart was paced at 300 beats per minute by means of a stainless steel electrode placed on the left atrium at twice the threshold voltage with square wave pulses of 5-msec duration from a Grass model SD9D stimulator. Values expressed are means and standard deviations. ⋆ = significantly different from control, ∧ = significantly different from swimmers.

LAFP ($p < 0.05$). This decrease was also found in the chronic swimmers given E64c who showed a 14.3% decrease from controls ($p < 0.05$) (Figure 5).

DISCUSSION

Acute swimming lowered cardiac calpain like activity, with this effect also occurring in E64c treated rats. Similarly, the increased max LVP, lowered +dP/dt and

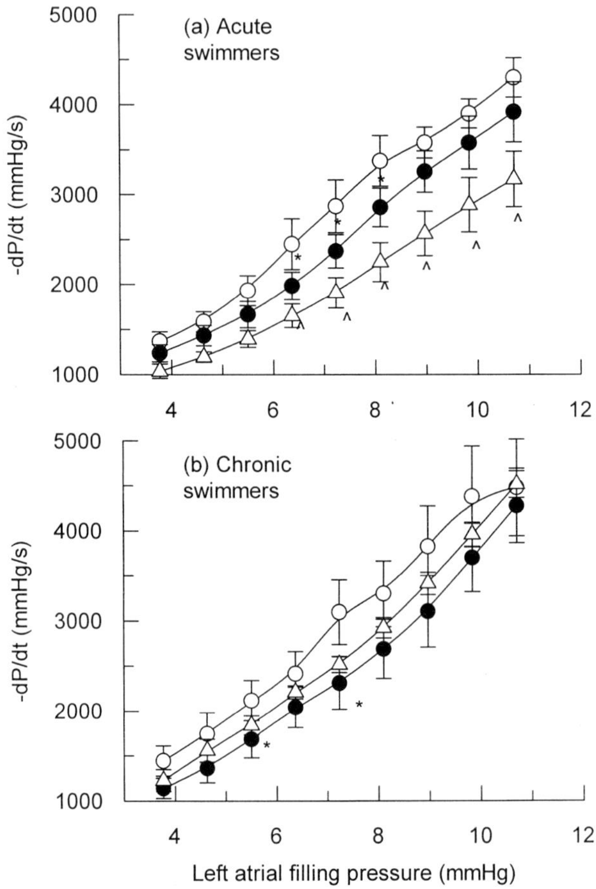

Figure 4. Rate of decline of left ventricular pressure; –dP/dt (mmHg/s) was determined using a working heart preparation. The open circles correspond to controls (acute n = 7, chronic n = 4), the solid circles are the swimmers (acute n = 5, chronic n = 5) and the filled triangles are the E64c treated swimmers (acute n = 4, chronic n = 4). Each heart was paced at 300 beats per minute by means of a stainless steel electrode placed on the left atrium at twice the threshold voltage with square wave pulses of 5-msec duration from a Grass model SD9D stimulator. Values expressed are means and standard deviations. ⋆ = significantly different from control, ∧ = significantly different from swimmers.

–dP/dt observed for acute swimmers were not altered by E64c administration. In contrast, E64c treatment did prevent the elevated cardiac levels of cAMP following acute swim exercise. The cardiac hypertrophy observed after swim training was attenuated with E64c administration, while resting [cAMP] and calpain like activities were not different among any chronic swim groups. In general the biochemical and functional responses of the heart to a single session of exercise were only

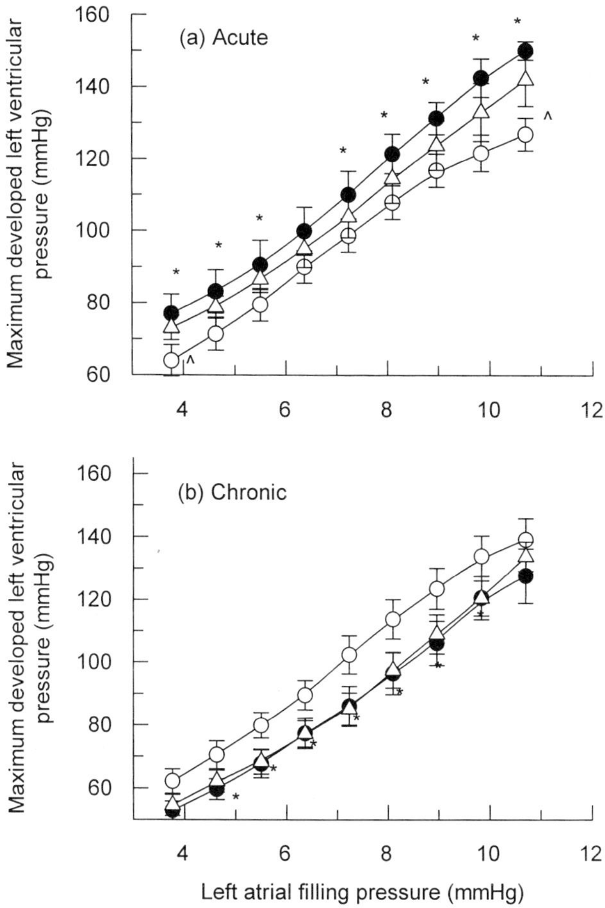

Figure 5. Maximum developed left ventricular pressure; Max LVP (mmHg/s) was determined using a working heart preparation. The open circles correspond to controls (acute n = 7, chronic n = 4), the solid circles are the swimmers (acute n = 5, chronic n = 5) and the filled triangles are the E64c treated swimmers (acute n = 4, chronic n = 4). Each heart was paced at 300 beats per minute by means of a stainless steel electrode placed on the left atrium at twice the threshold voltage with square wave pulses of 5-msec duration from a Grass model SD9D stimulator. Values expressed are means and standard deviations. ★ = significantly different from control, ∧ = significantly different from swimmers.

selectively modified with E64c. As with the acute swimmers, max LVP, +dP/dt and −dP/dt were reduced by chronic swimming, compared to controls, while E64c administration did not change these responses. Although E64c reduced somewhat the degree of hypertrophy, the absence of any specific, well defined E64c effects on cardiac related parameters does not therefore support an overall role for calpain in moderating long term swim exercise responses.

Cardiac hypertrophy in the rat is generally represented by increase in left ventricular to body weight ratio despite only small increases left ventricular mass, RNA content or fiber size (15,16). Reports of exercise-induced increases in left ventricular mass (2), are less common. Presumably this reflects the many different aspects of exercise protocols used. The protocol used in this study was sufficient to induce significant increases in left ventricular weight alone. The notable differences in hypertrophy response between swim exercise and treadmill exercise reported in the literature demonstrate how model specific exercise induced cardiac adaptations are (2,17,18). The importance of the exercise protocol is demonstrated when data from free running wheel exercise is considered. This "voluntary" form of exercise is equally as likely to produce some degree of hypertrophy or none at all (16). E64c administration (1 mg/Kg body weight) 1-hour prior to swimming attenuated the cardiac mass gains expected with chronic swimming. Whether increasing the dosage and or mode/time of delivery (19), would have completely blocked the increase in cardiac mass cannot be determined from the results of this study. The cardiac mass gains, induced by injection of isoproterenol and associated with increased total calpain like activities, are reduced with the administration of E64c (13). The ability of E64c to partly attenuate the swim induced cardiac mass increases suggests that further investigation is warranted, perhaps focusing on appropriate timing and dosage of E64c in the hypertrophy process.

With the acute swim exercise model it was hypothesized that total cardiac calpain like activity would be elevated, particularly since beta-adrenergic stimulation (elevated cAMP levels) hypoxia (14), myocardial stunning (10,14), and run exercise (20), all activate cardiac calpain. It was therefore surprising to observe acute swim exercise actually decreasing total net calpain like activity in contrast to the run exercise model (20). In this study, 6 weeks of chronic swim training did not alter the resting levels of calpain in the heart. These results may reflect the differences in myocardial response or demand placed on the heart during the swim exercise as opposed to running (21). In the rat, the blood flow distribution to the active muscle mass results in a decrease in total peripheral resistance with running but not in swimming. Swimming also induces much less tachycardia as compared to running (21). Such differences may be due to the vagal effects of partial or complete submission and the fact that air breathing mammals experience bradycardia as a response to diving (22). Whether these different acute physiological responses underlie the opposite responses of cardiac calpain to exercise is uncertain. To date however, the effects of chronic physical training on the activation characteristics of calpain are not available in the literature thus these results represent novel findings. An important consideration is also how this decreased net calpain activity with acute swimming is achieved, i.e. by lower calpain isoform activity or increased endogenous calpain inhibitor, calpastatin (9) or by some other regulatory factor(s). Although the conclusions that can be drawn from the net total calpain like activity with exercise alone and in combination with E64c are limited, it is clear that the calpain system responds quite differently to both acute running (8) and swimming exercise and to both isoproterenol (13) and chronic swimming models of cardiac hypertrophy. These differences may indeed reflect model specific situations that may prove useful in determining how calpain activity is regulated in vivo.

cAMP is known to be a candidate for regulating the hypertrophy response with beta adrenergic agonist stimulation (23,24), and swim exercise is known to increase cAMP in both skeletal and cardiac muscle (25). This increased cAMP content after swim exercise is thought to be mediated by an adrenal hormone as exercise does not promote increased cAMP in animals that have been adrenalectomized and because the exercise induced increases can be blocked by the non-specific beta blocker propranolol (25). Therefore E64c's ability to prevent the increase in cAMP in both this study and a previous study using isoproterenol (13), suggest a possible role of a calpain mediated effect upstream of adenylate cyclase, possibly at the level of the beta-adrenergic receptor / G-protein / adenylate cyclase complex. While such a selective proteolytic enzyme at the sarcolemmal membrane could act upon substrates such as receptors, sarcoplasmic reticulum, ion channels etc, this remains speculative and requires some well designed experiments to determine any role for calcium induced calpain mediated influence(s). Exercise training has been shown to either increase or not affect cAMP levels (26). Because of the differences between run and swim exercise, the precise mechanism(s) underlying the cAMP changes also require further investigation. It is of interest however that despite elevated cAMP in the myocardium of the acutely exercised animals there was a decrease in contractile function. Elevated cAMP is usually associated with improved contractile function due to PKA mediated regulation of Ca^{2+} regulatory and contractile (27,28) proteins. In this case the deleterious effects of the exercise, possibly such as depressed Ca^{2+} uptake (4) and lowered Ca^{2+} stores of the sarcoplasmic reticulum (29) may have depressed function despite PKA's inotropic actions. Also of consideration is evidence that the "functional pool" of cAMP involved in contractile regulation may not be well represented by total cellular [cAMP] because, as with β_2 adr or prostaglandin receptors, not all cellular pools of cAMP effected will alter Ca^{2+} dynamics or contractility of the heart (30).

In regard to the functional responses of the myocardium, the acute swimming protocol of this study resulted in depressed +dP/dt and −dP/dt, which is in agreement with data showing, depressed function (3) and even acute endocardial ischemia with swimming (31). Biochemical evidence from swim studies also show that sarcoplasmic reticulum calcium uptake is depressed significantly in rats that have swum to exhaustion (32). This would suggest a depression in the absolute capacity of the SR to take up Ca^{2+}. On subsequent excitation a depression in Ca^{2+} loading would tend to lower Ca^{2+} stores therefore the observed depression in SR Ca^{2+} transport may be associated with the impaired rate of tension development and relaxation in cardiac muscle preparations from acute exercise exhausted rats (31). The maximum rate of contractile force of hearts after 1 exercise bout is increased despite a slower rate of rise of pressure and relaxation of pressure. Therefore the fact that our chronic swimmers developed impaired contractile function goes against the data most often reported in the swim exercise model. The lack of any change in myofibrillar ATPase supports this conclusion. Chronic swimmers also showed little change in ATPase activity and suggests that the functional changes seen for +dP/dt and −dP/dt in the acute and chronic swimmers is likely due to factors other than myofibrillar ATPase.

Swim exercise training typically results in increased contractile function (1,2,18,33) although this is by no means a consistent finding. Data showing no improvement in functional parameters can be cited from run exercise studies (15), but generally swim studies result in some increases cardiac performance (2,33). The ATPase measures from the acute and chronic swimmers, both with and without E64c showed no significant alterations of the contractile metabolism. The lack of any increase in myofibrillar ATPase supports the functional data from the chronic swimmers, and suggests that the functional changes seen for +dP/dt and −dP/dt in the acute and chronic swimmers is likely due to factors other than myofibrillar ATPase. This reinforces the lack of conclusive E64c effects and suggests that the swim-induced adaptations shown in this study are not dependent on the calpain system.

ACKNOWLEDGEMENTS

The authors would like to express their gratitude to the Natural Sciences and Engineering Research Council of Canada for funds to complete this investigation. In addition GDA was a recipient of a Research Traineeship from the Heart and Stroke Foundation of British Columbia and Yukon. The support given by Dr. John McNeill and his laboratory in completing the working heart preparations and Mr. Tim Booker in completing the training programs are also generously acknowledged.

REFERENCES

1. Jacob R, Kissling G, Ebrecht G, Holubarsch C, Medugorac I, Rupp H. 1983. Adaptive and pathological alterations in experimental cardiac hypertrophy. In: *Advances in Myocardiology.* edited by E. Chazov, V. Saks, and G. Rona. p. 55–77, Plenum Publishing Corporation.
2. Moore LM, Korcick DH. 1995. Cellular adaptations of the myocardium to chronic exercise. Progress in Cardiovascular Diseases XXXVII:371–396.
3. Maher JT, Goodman AL, Francesconi R, Bowers WD, Hartley LT, Angelakos ET. 1972. Responses of rat myocardium to exhaustive exercise. American Journal of Physiology 222:207–212.
4. Pierce GN, Kutryk MJB, Dhalla KS, Beamish RE, Dhalla NS. 1984. Biochemical alterations in heart after exhaustive swimming in rats. *Journal of Applied Physiology: Respirat Environ.* Exercise Physiol 57:326–331.
5. Pierce GN, Sekhon PS, Meng H, Maddaford TG. 1989. Effects of chronic swimming training on cardiac sarcolemmal function and composition. Journal of Applied Physiology 66:1715–1721.
6. King DW, Gollnick PD. 1970. Ultrastructure of rat heart and liver after acute exhaustive exercise. American Journal of Physiology 218:1150–1155.
7. Watkins SC, Samuel JL, Marotte F, Bertier-Savalle B, Rappaport L. 1987. Microtubules and desmin filaments during onset of heart hypertrophy in rat: A double immunoelectron microscope study. Circulation Research 60:327–336.
8. Belcastro AN. 1993. Skeletal muscle calcium-activated neutral protease (calpain) with exercise. J Appl Physiol 74:1381–1386.
9. Goll DE, Thompson VF, Taylor RG, Zalewska T. 1992. Is calpain activity regulated by membranes and autolysis or by calcium and calpastatin? BioEssays 14:549–556.
10. Toya-Oka T, Morita T, Shin WS, Okai-Matsuo Y, Sugimoto T. 1997. Contribution of calcium activated neutral protease to the degradation process of ischemic heart. Japanese Circulation Journal 55:1124–1126.
11. Belcastro AN, Parkhouse W, Dobson G, Gilchrist JS. 1988. Influence of exercise on cardiac and skeletal muscle myofibrillar proteins. Mol Cell Biochem 83:27–36.

12. Raj DA, Booker T, Belcastro AN. 1998. Striated muscle calcium stimulated cysteine protease (calpain like) activity promotes myeloperoxidase activity with exercise. Pflugers Archive, European Journal of Physiology 435:804–809.
13. Arthur GD, Belcastro AN. 1997. A calcium stimulated cysteine protease involved in isoproterenol induced cardiac hypertrophy. Molecular and Cellular Biochemistry 176:241–248.
14. Iizuka K, Kawaguchi H, Yasuda H. 1991. Calpain is activated by beta-adrenergic receptor stimulation under hypoxic myocardial cell injury. Japanese Circulation Journal 55:1086–1093.
15. Nutter DO, Priest RF, Fuller EO. 1981. Endurance training in the rat I: Myocardial mechanics and biochemistry. Journal of Applied Physiology 51:934–940.
16. Perrault H, Turcottte RA. 1994. Exercise-induced cardiac hypertrophy: Fact or fallacy? Sports Medicine 17:288–308.
17. Hansen M, Rupp H. 1991. Cellular and molecular changes in the heart during stress or exercise. Methods and Achievements in Experimental Pathology 15:58–83.
18. Schiable TF, Scheuer J. 1985. Cardiac adaptations to chronic exercise. Progress in Cardiovascular Diseases XXVII:297–324.
19. Mehdi S. 1991. Cell-penetrating inhibitors of calpain. Trends in Biochemical Science 16:150–153.
20. Belcastro AN, Gilchrist JS, Scrubb J. 1993. Function of skeletal muscle sarcoplasmic reticulum vesicles with exercise. Journal of Applied Physiology 75:2412–2418.
21. Flaim SF, Minteer WJ, Clark DP, Zelis R. 1979. Cardiovascular response to acute aquatic and treadmill exercise in the untrained rat. Journal of Applied Physiology 46:302–308.
22. Prosser CL. 1973. *Comparative Animal Physiology*. p. 831–832. Philadelphia, PA, Saunders, USA.
23. Thomas DP, McCormick KM, Jenkins RR. 1988. Effects of B-adrenergic blockade on training induced structural adaptations in rat left ventricle. *European Journal of Applied Physiology* 57:671–676.
24. Yatani A, Brown AM. 1989. Rapid B-adrenergic modulation of cardiac calcium channel currents by a fast G protein pathway. Science 245:71–74.
25. Palmer WK. 1988. Effect of exercise on cardiac cyclic AMP. Medicine and Science in Sports and Exercise 20:525–530.
26. Noakes DT, Higginson LH, Oppie HA. 1983. Physical training increased the ventricular fibrillation threshold of isolated rat hearts during normoxia, hypoxia and regional ischemia. Circulation 67: 24–30.
27. Dunbar CC, Kalinski M. 1994. Cardiac intracellular regulation: exercise effects on the cAMP system and A-kinase. Medicine and Science in Sports and Exercise 26:1459–1465.
28. Sulakhe PV, Vo XT. 1995. Regulation of phospholamban and troponin-I phósphorylation in the intact rat cardiomyocytes by adrenergic and cholinergic stimuli: roles of cyclic nucleotides, calcium, protein kinases and phosphatases and depolarization. Molecular and Cellular Biochemistry 149/150: 103–126.
29. Dhalla NS, Das PJ, Sharma GP. 1978. Subcellular basis of cardiac contractile failure. Journal of Molecular and Cellular Cardiology 10:363–385.
30. Xiao RP, Lakatta EG. 1993. Beta-1-adrenoceptor stimulation and beta-2-adrenoceptor stimulation differ in their effects on contraction, cytosolic Ca^{2+}, and Ca^{2+} current in single rat ventricular cells. Circulation Research 73:286–300.
31. Barnard RJ, MacAlpin JR, Kattu AA, Buckberg GD. 1996. Ischemic response to sudden strenuous exercise in healthy men. Circulation Research. 48:936–942.
32. Sembrowich WL, Gollnick PD. 1977. Calcium uptake by heart and skeletal muscle sarcoplasmic reticulum from exercised rats. Medicine and Science in Sports and Exercise. 9:64.
33. Scheuer J, Tipton C. 1977. Cardiovascular adaptations to physical training. Annual Review of Physiology 39:221–251.

Frontiers in Cardiovascular Health, edited by
N.S. Dhalla, A. Chockalingam,
H.I. Berkowitz & P.K. Singal
Kluwer Academic Publishers, Boston, 2003

Reversal of Coronary Atherosclerosis by Yoga Lifestyle Intervention

S.C. Manchanda, R. Narang, K.S. Reddy, U. Sachdeva, D. Prabhakaran, S. Dharmanand*, M. Rajani, and R. Bijlani

All India Institute of Medical Sciences and Adhytma Sadhra Kendra, New Delhi, India

Summary. Yoga has potential for benefit for patients with coronary artery disease though objective, angiographic studies are lacking. We evaluated possible role of lifestyle modification incorporating yoga, on retardation of coronary atherosclerotic disease. In this prospective, randomized, controlled trial, 42 men with angiographically proven CAD were randomized to control (n = 21) and yoga intervention group (n = 21) and were followed for 1 year. The active group was treated with a user-friendly program consisting of yoga, control of risk factors, diet control and moderate aerobic exercise. The control group was managed by conventional methods i.e. risk factor control and American Heart Association step I diet.

At 1 year, the yoga groups showed significant reduction in number of anginal episodes per week, improved exercise capacity and decrease in body weight. Serum total cholesterol, LDL cholesterol and triglyceride levels also showed greater reductions as compared with control group. Revascularisation procedures (coronary angioplasty or bypass surgery) were less frequently required in the yoga group (1 versus 8 patients; relative risk = 5.45; $P = 0.01$). Coronary angiography repeated at 1 year showed that significantly more lesions regressed (20% versus 2%) and less lesions progressed (5% versus 37%) in the yoga group (chi-square = 24.9; $P < 0.0001$). The compliance of the total program was excellent and no side effects were observed.

Corresponding Author: Prof. S.C. Manchanda, Head, Department of Cardiology, Cardiothoracic Sciences Center, All India Institute of Medical Sciences, Ansari Nagar, New Delhi, India. E-mail: doctormanchanda@yahoo.com

Yoga lifestyle intervention retards progression and increases regression of coronary atherosclerosis in patients with severe coronary artery disease. It also improves symptomatic status, functional class and risk factor profile.

Key words: Atherosclerosis, Reversal, Yoga, Lifestyle.

INTRODUCTION

A number of studies have documented that a change in lifestyle (chiefly consisting of dietary modification, physical exercises and stress relaxation techniques) is beneficial to patients with coronary artery disease (CAD) (1–16). Yoga has potential for benefit for patients with CAD, as it includes dietary discretion, physical exercises, relaxation and stress management. However, objective, angiographic studies of yoga in patients with coronary artery disease are lacking. There is also a paucity of studies to determine whether lifestyle modification can result in regression of the coronary atherosclerotic plaques. Ornish et al (4,5) observed a regression of coronary atherosclerotic obstruction by strict lifestyle intervention. However, the coronary stenoses were mild (40% and 43% diameter stenosis in treatment and control groups, respectively) and the diet prescribed in their study was also very stringent with only 5 mg of cholesterol allowed per day. It is likely that such strict control of diet may not be practical for most patients.

The objective of this study was to determine whether a user-friendly yoga lifestyle intervention program (including yoga exercises, dietary management, moderate aerobic exercise and stress management) with control of risk factors can reverse atherosclerotic obstructions in patients known to have coronary artery disease. The effects on symptoms, exercise capacity, serum lipids and cardiovascular events were also analyzed.

MATERIAL AND METHODS

Forty-two male patients (mean age 51.0 ± 9.5, range 32–72 years) with angiographically proven CAD were included in this prospective, randomized, controlled trial. At baseline, detailed clinical assessment, serum lipid profile, treadmill exercise testing using modified Bruce protocol and coronary arteriography were performed. Patients in the control group (n = 21) were managed on conventional medical therapy (with control of risk factors, American Heart Association step I diet, moderate aerobic exertion), while those in the yoga group (n = 21) were advised strict lifestyle modification and yogic exercises as detailed below. The medications for angina were continued. No patient was receiving lipid-lowering drugs. The patients were followed for 1 year with regular assessments. At the end of 1 year, the patients again underwent detailed clinical assessment, serum lipid profile, treadmill exercise test and repeat coronary arteriography. Coronary arteriography was analyzed quantitatively using the caliper method. Two independent observers who were blinded to group allocation analyzed all arteriograms. The effect on individual lesions was compared in the 2 groups. Ethical clearance was obtained from the institutional ethics committee and all patients gave informed consent to take part in the study.

The baseline characteristics of the patient population are detailed in Table 1. Most patients were in NYHA functional class II (52% patients) or class III (41% patients). The patients in both groups had elevated mean total and low-density lipoprotein cholesterol. The study was conducted before the results of major trials of statins in coronary artery disease were published and none of the patients were on lipid lowering therapy. All patients had at least 1 mm ST segment depression during exercise testing. Coronary arteriography showed majority (81%) of patients to be having triple vessel disease.

Yoga lifestyle intervention program

After inclusion in the yoga group, patients, along with their spouses, spent 4 days at a yoga residential center, where they underwent training in various yogic lifestyle techniques. The yoga lifestyle intervention program consisted of:

- Yoga lifestyle methods (details about these methods are provided in the appendix):
  1. Health rejuvenating exercises: a set of exercises for improving general tone and flexibility of various parts of the body.
  2. Breathing exercises (*Pranayama*).
  3. Yogic postures for stretch relaxation (*Asanas*).
  4. Relaxation exercises (*Kayotsarg*): a method of complete relaxation to prepare the body and mind for meditation.
  5. Meditation (*Preksha*).
  6. Reflection and contemplation (*Anuvrat and Anupreksha*).
- Stress management (by relaxation, breathing exercises and *Preksha* meditation).
- Dietary control.
- Moderate aerobic exercises.

Patients visited the yoga center every fortnight for monitoring and evaluation. The compliance, as reported by patients themselves and by spouse, was recorded. In addition, the patients were followed every month in cardiac clinics of our hospital for clinical examination and investigations.

Dietary control

Patients were advised to take a low fat (mostly poly- or monounsaturated, providing 15% of calories), low cholesterol (<50 mg/d), high carbohydrate (mostly complex, providing 65% of calories) diet. Patients were also encouraged to have high soluble fiber diets (≥50 gm/d) consisting of vegetables and fruits, oat bran, soybeans, gram and other beans. They were also prescribed 15 gm psyllium husk (almost entirely fiber) daily. In addition, the diet advised was rich in antioxidants (carrots for beta-carotene, fruits for vitamin C, nuts like almonds and walnuts for vitamin E and flavenoids from colored fruits and vegetables). Illustrative recipes and menus with known nutritional values were provided to avoid monotony.

The compliance of patients was assessed using a questionnaire, which was analyzed to produce a quantitative score. The score could range from 0 to 100.

Table 1. Baseline characteristics of yoga and control groups

Parameter	Yoga group	Control group	P values (Yoga vs control)
Age (years)*	51 ± 9	52 ± 10	NS
Hypertensive	43%	38%	NS
Diabetic	29%	24%	NS
Smokers	19%	24%	NS
Previous MI	33%	29%	NS
Previous CABG	10%	5%	NS
NYHA functional class	2.62 ± 0.67	2.33 ± 0.58	NS
Anginal episodes/wk	6.71 ± 2.95	4.10 ± 2.14	0.002
Weight	72.1 ± 12.5	72.81 ± 9.84	NS
Total Cholesterol mg/dl	257 ± 43.6	236.86 ± 40	NS
LDL Cholesterol mg/dl	156 ± 32.7	145 ± 30.5	NS
HDL Cholesterol mg/dl	40.81 ± 6.25	38.81 ± 4.34	NS
Triglycerides mg/dl	193 ± 58.1	169 ± 47.13	NS
LDL / HDL ratio	3.84 ± 0.89	3.78 ± 0.87	NS
Exercise Duration	349 ± 147	430 ± 119.29	0.056
**Double Product achieved (10^3)	23.62 ± 2.66	24.13 ± 2.41	NS
ST segment depression during exercise test	2.62 ± 0.62	2.23 ± 0.53	0.044
Mean Lesion Severity	62.4 ± 14.5	59.7 ± 17.7	NS

NS = not significant.
*: All patients were men.
**: Product of heart rate and systolic blood pressure.

Statistical analysis

All data are presented as mean ± 1SD unless stated otherwise. The results at the end of 1 year were compared with those at the baseline. The changes in the yoga group were compared with those in the control group. The P values were calculated using student's t-test for paired data. Chi-square analysis using Yate's correction was performed wherever appropriate.

Results

Both groups were similar at baseline with respect to mean age, weight, serum lipid profile, and mean lesion severity (Table 1). However, patients in yoga group had significantly more anginal episodes per week (6.7 ± 3 vs 4.1 ± 2.1). On treadmill testing also, these patients could exercise for shorter duration (349 ± 147 vs 430 ± 119 seconds; P = 0.056) and had more ST segment depression (2.6 ± 0.6 vs 2.2 ± 0.5 mm, P = 0.04).

The compliance score varied from 50 to 95% (mean 79.5 ± 14.5%). Sixty seven percent patients had a compliance score of 80% or more. The results on various outcome variables are summarized in Table 2 and Figures 1–4.

Clinical profile

Patients in the yoga group showed an improvement in the NYHA functional class while patients in the control group showed an overall worsening ($p < 0.0001$). The

Table 2. Parameters at baseline and at 1 year in the yoga and control groups

	Yoga group					Control group					P values for Yoga vs control group
Parameter	Baseline	After 1 year	Change at 1 year	% Change	P (before vs after)	Baseline	After 1 year	Change at 1 year	% Change	P (before Vs after)	Change at 1 year
NYHA functional class	2.62 ± 0.67	1.43 ± 0.6	−1.19 ± 0.51	−46 ± 15%	<0.0001	2.33 ± 0.58	2.86 ± 0.57	0.52 ± 0.75	29 ± 37%	0.004	0.0001
Anginal episodes/wk	6.71 ± 2.95	2.14 ± 2.65	−4.57 ± 2.36	−73.2 ± 27%	<0.0001	4.10 ± 2.14	5.38 ± 2.29	1.29 ± 2.15	47 ± 67%	0.01	0.0001
Weight Kg	72.1 ± 12.5	66.5 ± 8.3	−5.62 ± 7.2	−6.8 ± 8.2%	0.0019	72.81 ± 9.84	72.4 ± 9.65	−0.38 ± 3.35	0 ± 5%	0.61	0.005
Total Cholesterol	257 ± 43.6	203 ± 33.9	−54.14 ± 36	−20.2 ± 12%	<0.0001	236.86 ± 40	236 ± 35.1	−1.29 ± 17.5	0 ± 8%	0.74	0.0001
LDL Cholesterol	156 ± 32.7	118 ± 29.8	−38.1 ± 33	−23.2 ± 17%	0.00004	145 ± 30.5	142 ± 27.17	−3.29 ± 16.83	−2 ± 12%	0.38	0.0002
HDL Cholesterol	40.81 ± 6.25	41.29 ± 4.47	0.48 ± 5.6	2.8 ± 14.9%	0.70	38.81 ± 4.34	39.8 ± 5.99	0.95 ± 4.41	3 ± 12%	0.33	0.76
Triglycerides	193 ± 58.1	148 ± 49.9	−45.7 ± 66	−20.1 ± 26%	0.005	169 ± 47.13	174 ± 51.06	4.76 ± 27.33	3 ± 17%	0.43	0.003
LDL / HDL ratio	3.84 ± 0.89	2.81 ± 0.66	−1.03 ± 0.99	−24.3 ± 22%	0.0001	3.78 ± 0.87	3.66 ± 1	−0.11 ± 0.53	−4 ± 13%	0.33	0.0008
Exercise Duration	349 ± 147	413 ± 132	63.8 ± 73.7	28.0 ± 44.7%	0.0008	430 ± 119.29	374 ± 150.88	−56.67 ± 117	−17 ± 23%	0.055	0.0007
Double Product achieved (10^3)	23.62 ± 2.66	23.79 ± 2.75	0.17 ± 2.08	1.0 ± 8.5	0.71	24.13 ± 2.41	23.6 ± 2.79	−0.57 ± 1.48	−3 ± 5%	0.12	0.14
ST segment depression during exercise test	2.62 ± 0.62	1.80 ± 0.82	−0.82 ± 0.59	−32.0 ± 25%	0.00001	2.23 ± 0.53	2.67 ± 0.56	0.44 ± 0.62	27 ± 49%	0.008	0.0001
Mean Lesion Severity	62.4 ± 14.5	60.9 ± 16	−1.5 ± 9.7	−1.5 ± 17%	0.23	59.7 ± 17.7	68.4 ± 16	8.7 ± 12.9	26.5 ± 80%	<0.0001	<0.0001

number of episodes of angina per week reduced by 73% in the yoga group, while they increased by 47% in the control group (Table 2).

The body weight showed a small but statistically significant decrease (7%; P = 0.002) in the yoga group while the control group which did not show any significant alteration. The lipid profile showed significant reduction in the level of total and LDL cholesterol as well as triglycerides in the yoga group (about 20% reduction in each of these; Table 2) while these parameters showed no significant change in the control group. Though there was no beneficial effect on the HDL levels, the atherogenic ratio (total/HDL cholesterol) reduced significantly in the yoga group.

Stress test

There was an improvement in the exercise duration and a reduction in the degree of ST segment depression occurring during the stress test in the yoga group. On the other hand patients in the control group showed a reduction in the exercise duration and an increase in the ST segment depression occurring during exercise (P = 0.0007 and 0.0001, respectively).

Coronary angiography

Coronary arteriography was repeated at 1 year in all patients. A total of 120 lesions were analyzed (61 in the yoga group and 59 in the control group). At baseline, there was no significant difference in the mean severity of lesions in the two groups (62.4% vs 59.7% diameter stenosis). At 1 year, there was progression of coronary stenosis in the control group (mean worsening of 9 ± 13% diameter stenosis) whereas the yoga group showed no significant change. This difference was highly significant (P < 0.0001) (Figure 3).

The change in the lesion severity was classified into regression (diameter stenosis reducing by ≥10 absolute percentage points), no significant change (diameter stenosis showing a change of <10 absolute percentage points) or progression (diameter stenosis increasing by ≥10 absolute percentage points). In the yoga group, 3 lesions showed progression, 46 lesions showed no change while 12 lesions showed regression. In the control group, 22 lesions showed progression, 36 showed no change while 1 showed regression (Figure 1). This difference was highly significant (chi-square 24.5; P < 0.0001).

Revascularisation procedures

Coronary artery bypass grafting (CABG) and percutaneous transluminal coronary angioplasty (PTCA) were markedly reduced in the yoga group as compared to controls. Only 1 in the yoga group needed revascularisation (PTCA) as against 8 in the control group (2 PTCA and 6 CABG) (relative risk 5.45; P = 0.01).

Determinants of clinical improvement

Since patients in the intervention group experienced a greater fall in the lipid levels and reduction in weight, we attempted to determine whether clinical benefit of

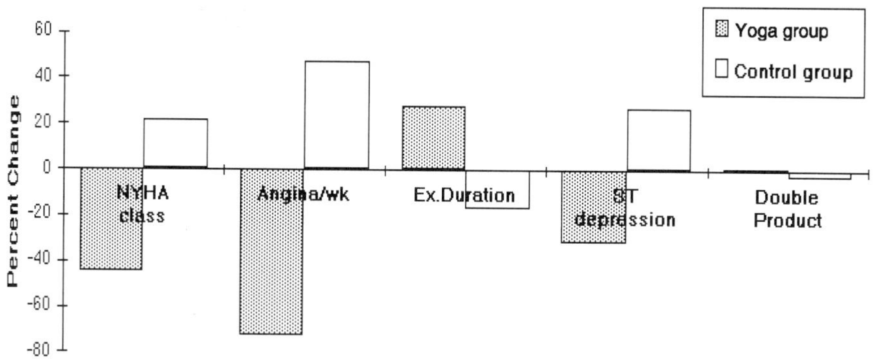

Figure 1. Change in symptoms, exercise capacity and other parameters of ischemia in yoga and control groups at 1 year of follow-up.

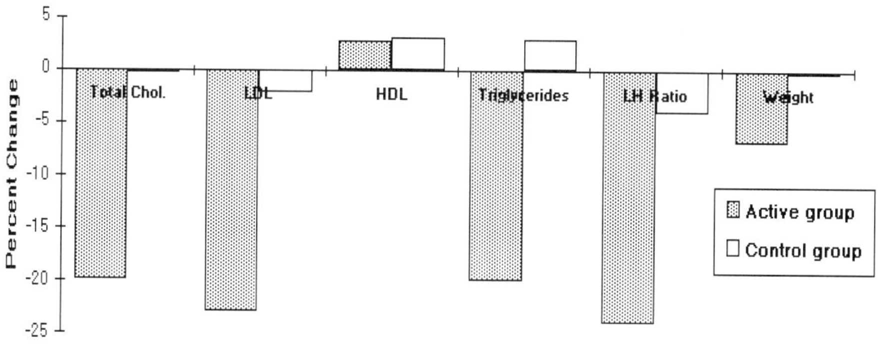

Figure 2. Effect on lipid profile and weight of patients in yoga and control groups at 1 year.

lifestyle intervention is mediated via reduction in weight &/or reduction in lipids. Univariate analysis showed significant correlation between reduction in number of weekly anginal episodes and reductions in weight, total cholesterol, LDL cholesterol and triglyceride levels (Table 3). Multivariate analysis was performed keeping the reduction in number of weekly anginal episodes as the dependent variable and reduction in weight, reduction in total cholesterol, reduction in LDL cholesterol, reduction in triglycerides and control/intervention group as predictor variables. The analysis showed that reductions in weight or lipid parameters were not independent predictors of reduction in anginal episodes, but the control/intervention group was ($P < 0.003$; Table 3). This indicates that the clinical benefit of yoga lifestyle intervention is not mediated through reduction in weight or lipids, but through other mechanism(s).

Table 3. Relation between reduction in anginal episodes per week and reductions in weight, total cholesterol, LDL cholesterol, and triglycerides levels

	Univariate analysis		Multivariate analysis	
Parameter	r	P	r	P
↓ **in wt.**	0.28	0.002	0.06	ns
↓ **in TC**	0.06	<0.0001	0.09	ns
↓ **in LDL**	0.06	0.0002	0.06	ns
↓ **in TG**	0.03	0.006	0.006	ns
Intervention group	5.9	<0.0001	4.52	0.003

DISCUSSION

There are a number of reports documenting favorable effect of lifestyle modification in patients with coronary artery disease (secondary prophylaxis of CAD) (1–7). However, effect of yoga on atherosclerotic coronary artery disease has not been studied in objective, angiographic studies. Ornish et al (1983) reported the short-term effects of stress management and dietary changes in patients with coronary artery disease (4). In this study of 46 patients (23 of whom received this intervention), there was 44% mean increase in exercise duration, 55% mean increase in total work performed and improved regional wall motion during peak exercise. These changes occurred at a mean of only 24 days of intervention. There was a remarkable 91% reduction in the frequency of anginal episodes. The mean reduction in plasma cholesterol levels was 21%.

Subsequently, in the Lifestyle Heart Trial, Ornish et al (1990) studied the effect of comprehensive lifestyle changes (low fat vegetarian diet, stress management training, moderate exercise and stopping smoking) on the severity of CAD determined by quantitative coronary arteriography (5). After 1 year of follow-up, analysis of 195 lesions in 48 patients (28 in the active group) showed that the average diameter stenosis regressed in the active group (from 40 ± 17% to 37.8 ± 16.5%) while it progressed in the control group (from 42.7 ± 15.5% to 46.1 ± 18.5%). Overall, 82% of active group patients had an average change towards regression. It was concluded that comprehensive lifestyle changes can produce regression of obstructive coronary artery disease after only 1 year, without the use of lipid-lowering agents. Gould et al (1992) from the same group subsequently showed that complex shape changes and stenoses moulding occur over a period of time (6). Such changes result in an overall regression of the severity of lesions with improved stenosis flow reserve with intensive lifestyle modification, while these changes result in overall progression of stenosis severity and worsening flow reserve in the control group.

In a recent study, Gould et al (1995) showed that such risk factor modification also results in a decrease in the size and severity of perfusion abnormalities on rest-dipyridamole positron emission tomography (PET), reflecting an improvement in the integrated flow capacity of the entire coronary arterial circulation (7). The size and severity of abnormalities increased in the control group over 5 year study period.

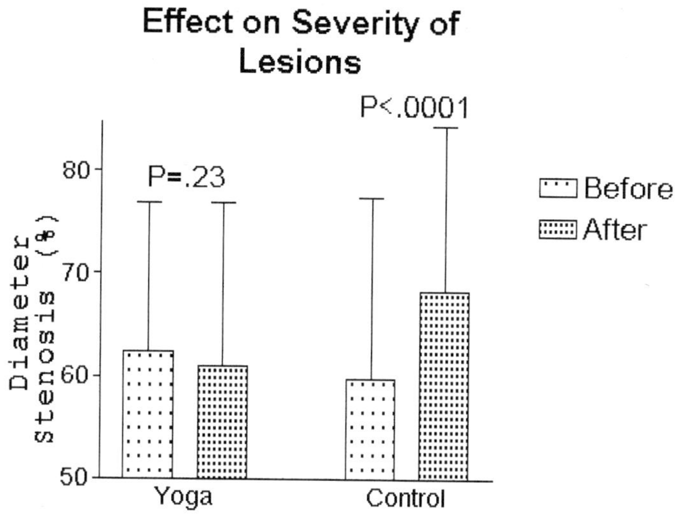

Figure 3. Effect of intervention on mean angiographic severity of coronary atherosclerotic lesions at 1 year of follow-up.

Studies from Heidelberg have also demonstrated the beneficial effects of comprehensive lifestyle changes (including diet and physical exercise) on the coronary anatomy in patients with CAD (8–14). Lipid lowering agents were not prescribed. After 1 year, the intervention group showed progression in 23% and regression in 32% patients, compared with 48% and 17%, respectively in the control group ($P < 0.05$) (8). The benefit persisted at 6 years of follow-up ($P < 0.0001$) (9). A multivariate analysis identified only physical work capacity as independently contributing to angiographic changes.

Effects of a comprehensive program of risk reduction involving both changes in lifestyle and medication were evaluated in the Stanford Coronary Risk Intervention Project (SCRIP) (15). Again, the risk reduction group showed a 47% reduced progression of coronary artery segments as compared with the "usual care" group ($P < 0.02$).

The results of our study are consistent with those of the above mentioned studies. Yoga lifestyle intervention was found to have several beneficial effects in patients with coronary artery disease, even when the disease was advanced. It markedly improved symptoms of angina and the exercise capacity of these individuals. It also reduced the body weight and favorably altered the lipid levels. It reduced total and low density lipid cholesterol as well as serum triglyceride levels, though the HDL cholesterol was not significantly affected. Coronary angiography showed retardation of progression of the disease as well as regression of significantly more lesions as compared to the control treatment. The revascularization procedures were significantly less in the yoga lifestyle group, though the numbers were small. This may be

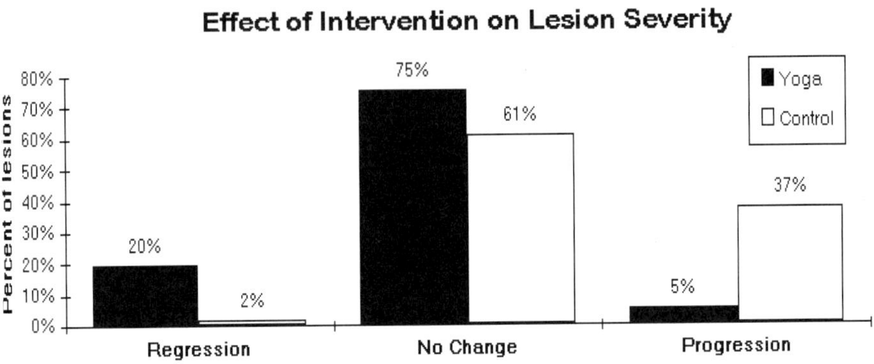

Figure 4. Proportion of coronary lesions showing regression (≥10% absolute reduction in percent diameter stenosis), no change (<10% absolute change in percent diameter stenosis) or progression (≥10% absolute increase in percent diameter stenosis) in yoga and control groups at 1 year of follow-up (overall chi-square = 24.5; $P < 0.0001$).

related to "stabilization" of the atheromatous plaques—similar to that thought to occur following statin therapy (17–24).

The main advantage of our program was that it was much more "user-friendly" than the interventions used in previous studies, such as those by Ornish and Gould. The dietary modification in our study was also more liberal as 15% of energy from fats and 50 mg of cholesterol per day were allowed, as compared with 10% energy from fats and only 5 mg of cholesterol per day in the study by Ornish et al (4,5). The patients included in our study also had significantly more severe disease (81% had triple vessel disease). Many of these patients had earlier declined to undergo revascularisation procedures. Moreover, ours is perhaps the only study which assessed the effects of yoga lifestyle intervention on the angiographic severity in patients with advanced CAD.

Limitations of the study

We recognize several limitation of this study. Relatively small number of patients has been studied. Though the results are encouraging, they need to be replicated in larger number of patients. By nature of the interventions involved, the study could not be blinded, and hence a placebo effect of yoga intervention cannot be excluded. However, independent observers blinded to group allocation interpreted the coronary angiograms. The compliance of diet and yoga exercises was monitored from the reports of patients themselves and was not directly observed by the investigators. However, the spouses of the patients in yoga group were also involved and they also monitored the compliance of patients. The differential effects of yogic exercises, dietary control and aerobic exercises, were not assessed. We considered yoga lifestyle modification program as a composite intervention incorporating all the above mentioned components.

However, despite above limitations, outcome variables in the two groups are significantly different and are likely to be clinically important.

CONCLUSIONS

The study shows that yoga lifestyle intervention program is feasible in the setting of advanced coronary artery disease with a high degree of compliance. It has favorable effects on angina, body weight, lipid levels and exercise capacity. It results in retardation of progression and increases regression of coronary obstructions as compared with control group. Yoga lifestyle may stabilize the atherosclerotic plaques resulting in reduced need for revascularisation procedures.

ACKNOWLEDGMENT

The study was supported in part by a grant from the Council of Yoga and Naturopathy, Ministry of Health, Government of India.

APPENDIX

Following is the outline of yoga component of lifestyle modification program:

A) Health rejuvenating exercises

These exercises are aimed mainly at improving the general tone and flexibility of various parts of body. These were also performed during warming up and to prepare for the next step, i.e. the *asanas*.

B) Asanas

These are the yogic postures and exercises mainly aimed at stretch relaxation. A number of *asanas* were taught including *Surya Namaskar, Tadasana, Padahasta asana, Vajrasana, Shasank asana, ardha-matsyendrasana, Paschimottantasana, Bhujangasana, Dhanush Ban asana, Shalabhasana, Uttanpadasana, Merudandasana, Pawan Muktasana, Sarwangasana, Matsyasana, Ardhamatsyasana* and *Pranayam*. The details of these asanas can be found in any book on yogic exercises.

C) Kayotsarg

A method of complete relaxation and preparation of body and mind for meditation. The literal meaning of *Kayotsarg* is to drop the body. In practice it is the conscious suspension of all gross movements of the body. As a result the muscles relax and the person becomes as restful as in sleep.

D) Preksha dhyana

Preksha means perception and *Dhyana* means concentration. *Preksha Dhyana* is performed in the sitting position and person first relaxes the body using *Kayotsarg*. He then concentrates on the breath and gradually and consciously reduces the rate of breathing from 15–17 / minute to 10–12 / minute. With practice, the rate may be reduced even to 4–6 / minute. By concentrating on the breath, the mental activity is controlled and the mind is prevented from being distracted.

E) Anuvrat and anupreksha

Anupreksha means contemplation or reflection or thoughtful consideration. *Anuvrat* is concerned with moral values which would include consideration for others, unity of mankind, communal harmony, non-violence, limitation of acquisition and consumption, integrity in behaviour and purity of means.

REFERENCES

1. Superko HR, Wood PD, Haskell WL. 1985. Coronary heart disease and risk factor modification: Is there a threshold? Am J Med 78:826–38.
2. Raichlen JS, Healy B, Achuff SC, Pearson TA. 1986. Importance of risk factors in the angiograhic progression of coronary artery disease. Am J Cardiol 57:66–70.
3. Glueck CJ. 1986. Role of risk factor management in progression and regression of coronary and femoral artery atherosclerosis. Am J Cardiol 57:35G.
4. Ornish D, Scherwitz LW, Doody RS, Kesten D, et al. 1983. Effects of stress management training and dietary changes in treating ischemic heart disease. JAMA 249:54–59.
5. Ornish D, Brown SE, Scherwitz LW, Billings JH, et al. 1990. Can lifestyle changes reverse coronary heart disease? The Lifestyle Heart Trial. Lancet 336:129–33.
6. Gould KL, Ornish D, Kirkeeide R, Brown S, Stuart Y, et al. 1992. Improved stenosis geometry by quantitative coronary arteriography after vigorous risk factor modification. Am J Cardiol 69:845–53.
7. Gould KL, Ornish D, Scherwitz L, Brown S, et al. 1995. Changes in myocardial perfusion abnormalities by positron emission tomography after long-term, intense risk factor modification. JAMA 274:894–901.
8. Schuler G, Hambrecht R, Schlierf G, Niebauer J, Hauer K, Neumann J, et al. 1992. Regular physical exercise and low-fat diet. Effects on progression of coronary artery disease. Circulation 86(1):1–11.
9. Niebauer J, Ilambrecht R, Velich T, Ilauer K, Marburger C, Kalberer B, et al. 1997. Attenuated progression of coronary artery disease after 6 years of multifactorial risk intervention: role of physical exercise. Circulation 96(8):2534–2541.
10. Niebauer J, Hambrecht R, Velich T, Marburger C, et al. 1996. Predictive value of lipid profile for salutary coronary angiographic changes in patients on a low-fat diet and physical exercise program. Am J Cardiol 78:163–167.
11. Niebauer J, Hambrecht R, Marburer C, et al. 1995. Impact of intensive physical exercise and low-fat diet on collateral vessel formation in stable angina pectoris and angiographically confirmed coronary artery disease. Am J Cardiol 76:771–775.
12. Niebauer J, Hambrecht R, Schlierf G, Marburger C, et al. 1995. Five years of physical exercise and low fat diet: effects on progression of coronary artery disease. J Cardiopul Rehabil 15:47–64.
13. Hambrecht R, Niebauer J, Marburger C, et al. 1993. Various intensities of leisure time physical activity in patients with coronary artery disease: effects on cardiorespiratory fitness and progression of coronary atherosclerotic lesions. J Am Coll Cardiol 22:468–477.
14. Schuler G, Hambrecht R, Schlierf G, et al. 1992. Myocardial perfusion and regression of coronary artery disease in patients on a regimen of intensive physical exercise and low fat diet. J Am Coll Cardiol 19:34–42.
15. Haskell WL, Alderman HL, Fair JM, Maron DJ, Mackey SF, Superko HR, Williams PT, et al. 1994. Effects of intensive multiple risk factor reduction on coronary atherosclerosis and clinical cardiac events in men and women with coronary artery disease. The Stanford Coronary Risk Intervention Project (SCRIP). Circulation 89(3):975–990.
16. De Feyter PJ, Vos J, Deckers JW. 1995. Progression and regression of the atherosclerotic plaque. Eur Heart J 16 (suppl I):26–30.
17. Shah PK. 1997. New insights into the pathogenesis and prevention of acute coronary syndromes. Am J Cardiol 79(12B):17–23.
18. Fuster V. 1997. Human lesion studies. Ann N Y Acad Sci 811:207–224.

19. Bjelajac A, Goo AK, Weart CW. 1996. Prevention and regression of atherosclerosis: effects of HMG-CoA reductase inhibitors. Ann Pharmacother 30(11):1304–1315.
20. Ganz P, Creager MA, Fang JC, McConnell MV, Lee RT, Libby P, Selwyn AP. 1996. Pathogenic mechanisms of atherosclerosis: effect of lipid lowering on the biology of atherosclerosis. Am J Med 101(4A):4A10S–4A16S
21. Stark RM. 1996. Review of the major intervention trials of lowering coronary artery disease risk through cholesterol reduction. Am J Cardiol 78(6A):13–19.
22. Shah PK. 1996. Pathophysiology of plaque rupture and the concept of plaque stabilization. Cardiol Clin 14(1):17–29.
23. Maher VM. 1995. Coronary atherosclerosis stabilization: an achievable goal. Atherosclerosis 118 Suppl: S91–S101.
24. Mancini GB. 1995. Mechanisms underlying reduction of clinical events in lipid lowering trials. Can J Cardiol 11 Suppl C:15C–17C.

Frontiers in Cardiovascular Health, edited by
N.S. Dhalla, A. Chockalingam,
H.I. Berkowitz & P.K. Singal
Kluwer Academic Publishers, Boston, 2003

Prevention of Heart Failure—A Clinical Reality?

Wilson Lee and J. Malcolm O. Arnold

Division of Cardiology
London Health Sciences Centre
Department of Medicine
University of Western Ontario

Summary. Heart failure is a major public health problem and has substantial economic impact. Over the past several decades, the mortality for most cardiovascular diseases has declined. In contrast, the incidence of and mortality for heart failure have increased. The key steps to approach an epidemic are prevention and early intervention. Effective prevention of heart failure can be achieved by modification of risk factors, aggressive management of coronary heart disease and hypertension, and early treatment of left ventricular dysfunction.

***Key words*:** heart failure, risk factors, hypertension, angiotensin converting enzyme inhibitors, β-adrenoceptor blockers.

INTRODUCTION

Cardiovascular disease is one of the leading causes of morbidity and mortality in the world. Heart failure is rapidly becoming one of the most prevalent cardiovascular disorders as the age of the population increases. A great deal of understanding into the pathophysiology of heart failure has been acquired over the last decade, leading to the development of new treatment strategies. Large scale clinical trials have provided significant insights with regards to evidence-based heart failure therapeutics and their effects on patients' outcome. Despite advances in pharmacologic and nonpharmacologic therapy, the prognosis of heart failure remains poor. To

Address for Correspondence: Dr. J. Malcolm O. Arnold, Division of Cardiology, London Health Sciences Centre, Lawson Health Research Institute, 375 South Street, London, Canada, N6A 4G5. Phone: (519) 667-6650, Fax: (519) 667-6526, E-mail: malcolm.arnold@lhsc.on.ca.

improve outcome, a more comprehensive management strategy which comprises prevention and early intervention should be implemented.

EPIDEMIOLOGY

Heart failure is an emerging epidemic and has evolved into a major public health problem. The magnitude of heart failure is well defined in the western society. In Canada, heart failure affects more than 350,000 individuals and its incidence is rapidly rising (1). In the United Kingdom, the prevalence of heart failure is estimated to be 15 per 1000 in the whole population and 80 per 1000 in those over 65 years old (2). In the United States, over 500,000 patients are newly diagnosed with heart failure each year. Data from the Framingham Heart Study indicate that the prevalence of heart failure increases with age (3). Approximately 80% of patients hospitalized with heart failure are older than 65 years (4).

Heart failure is the leading cause of hospitalization and the most common diagnosis in hospital patients over 65 years of age. In the last 10 years, the annual hospitalization rate has increased from approximately 570,000 to 870,000 for heart failure as the primary diagnosis (5). In addition, it accounts for 6.5 million hospital days each year in the United States (6).

In contrast to mortality declines for most cardiovascular diseases, the mortality rate for heart failure remains high. The one year mortality ranges between 25% to 40% after diagnosis (1). Fifty percent of the patients diagnosed with heart failure may die within 5 years (4). In patients with heart failure, the rate of sudden cardiac death occurs at 6 to 9 times the rate of the general population. Advances in the treatment of heart failure have resulted in substantial improvements in survival of patients in clinical trials but mortality remains high in the population at large.

Heart failure has a significant economic impact. The large number of hospitalizations with intense therapy make the management of heart failure very costly. Each hospitalization for heart failure averages 8 days of hospital stay in Canada, accounting for a total inpatient cost of over $1 billion per year (1). In the United States, heart failure accounts for a total inpatient and outpatient cost of approximately $38 billion annually (7). This financial burden will increase further as the age of the population and the incidence of heart failure continue to increase.

RISK FACTORS

Risk factors for the development of heart failure have been examined in the Framingham Heart Study (Figure 1) (3). The risk of heart failure increases with age. The combination of age-related changes in the cardiovascular system and a high prevalence of age-related cardiovascular disease increase the prevalence of heart failure in the elderly. Hypertension is a major risk factor and associated with a 2 to 4 fold increase in the incidence of heart failure. Left ventricular hypertrophy and diabetes are independent risk factors and associated with a significantly increased incidence of heart failure. Dyslipidemia characterized by a high total cholesterol to HDL ratio is strongly associated with the development of heart failure. Cigarette smoking increases the likelihood of heart failure in younger, but not in older individuals.

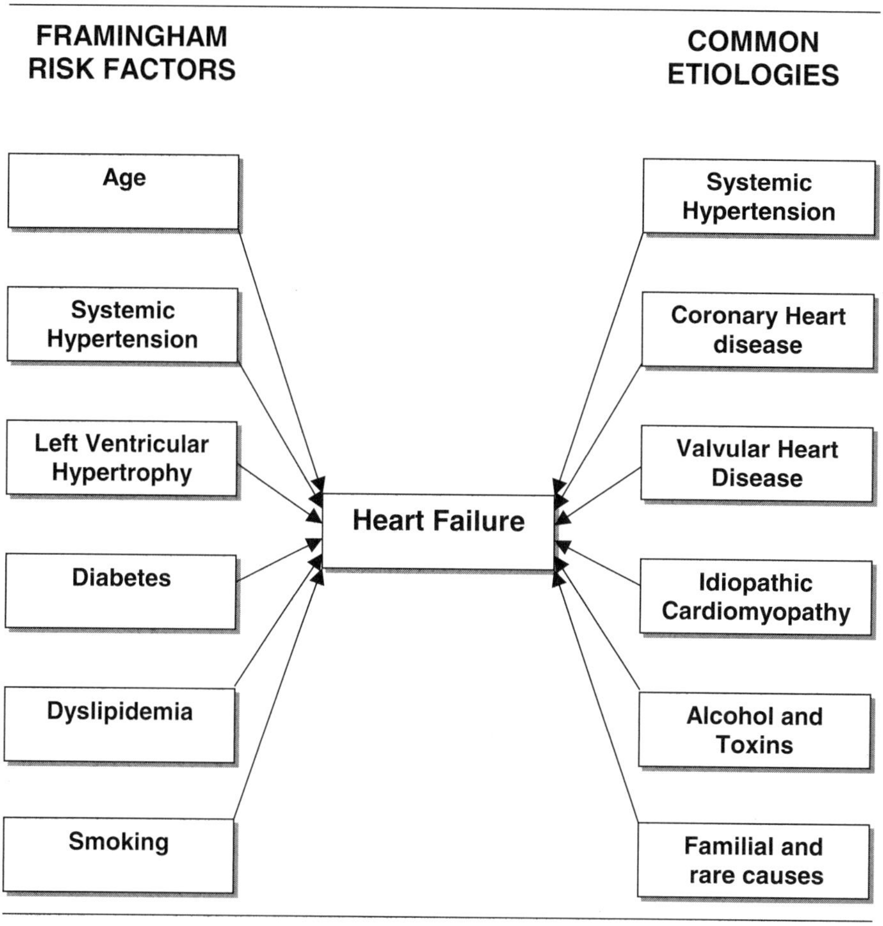

Figure 1. Risk factors and etiologies of heart failure.

ETIOLOGY AND PREVENTION

The most common etiologies of heart failure are systemic hypertension, coronary artery disease, valvular heart disease, and idiopathic cardiomyopathy (Figure 1). Other infrequent causes include myocarditis and nonischemic cardiomyopathy with an identifiable cause (e.g., alcohol, thyroid disease). Hypertension and coronary artery disease account for most cases of heart failure in the developed countries.

Hypertension

In the era prior to availability of antihypertensive agents, hypertension was the commonest cause of heart failure. Early data from the Framingham Heart Study revealed that hypertension was the only identifiable cause in 30% men and 20% women and a cofactor in another 33% of men and 25% of women (3). In subsequent analyses that evaluated both the original cohort and their offspring, substantial changes in the cause of heart failure were observed (6). Coronary artery disease has become the dominant etiology for heart failure as its prevalence increases over time. Although hypertension has declined in importance as the primary cause of heart failure, it remains a major predisposing condition to heart failure. Despite improvements in the pharmacologic treatment of hypertension, it has a high prevalence in the general population and carries the greatest attributable risk for heart failure. Risk of heart failure increases with the severity of hypertension and even moderate elevations of blood pressure will impose a substantial risk. In addition, hypertension predisposes the development of coronary artery disease and left ventricular hypertrophy, further increasing the risk of progressing on to heart failure.

Protective effects of antihypertensive therapy

Large scale, placebo controlled, trials of isolated systolic as well as systolic and diastolic hypertension have demonstrated the protective effects of antihypertensive treatment (Figure 2). In the Systolic Hypertension in the Elderly Program (SHEP) study, diuretic therapy (chlorthalidone) reduced the mean systolic blood pressure by 11.5 mmHg. There was a relative reduction of 48% in heart failure incidence from 4.6% patients in the control group to 2.4% patients in the treatment group (8). Other systolic hypertension trials show similar treatment benefits. In the Systolic Hypertension in China (Syst-China) study, calcium antagonist therapy (nitrendipine) reduced mean systolic pressure by 9.1 mmHg, resulting in a 58% reduction in heart failure incidence (9). In the Systolic Hypertension in Europe (Syst-Eur) study, calcium antagonist therapy (nitrendipine) decreased systolic blood pressure by 10.1 mmHg, resulting in a reduction of 29% in the incidence of heart failure (10). Despite a greater lowering in blood pressure, treatment of systolic and diastolic hypertension provided only a small additional protective effect compared to treatment of systolic hypertension alone. In the European Working Party on High Blood Pressure in the Elderly (EWPHE) and the Coope & Warrender trials, diuretic (hydrochlorothiazide/triamterene, bendrofluazide) and beta-blocker (atenolol) therapy reduced mean systolic pressure by 18 to 20 mmHg and mean diastolic pressure by 9 to 11 mmHg. There was a 33% to 63% reduction in the incidence of heart failure (11,12). In the Swedish Trial in Old Patients with Hypertension (STOP-Hypertension), diuretic (hydrochlorothiazide) or beta-blocker (atenolol, metoprolol, pindolol) therapy reduced mean systolic pressure by 19.5 mmHg and mean diastolic pressure by 8.1 mmHg, resulting in a 51% reduction in the heart failure incidence (13).

Not all antihypertensive agents improve heart failure outcome. In the Antihypertensive and Lipid-Lowering treatment to prevent Heart Attack Trial (ALLHAT), the doxazosin arm was terminated early because there was a twofold higher incidence of heart failure in patients receiving doxazosin compared to those receiving chlorthalidone (8.13% versus 4.45% at 4 years) (14). The underlying cause of the increased heart failure incidence remains controversial as to whether chlorthalidone decreases the rate or doxazosin increases the rate. In the recently published

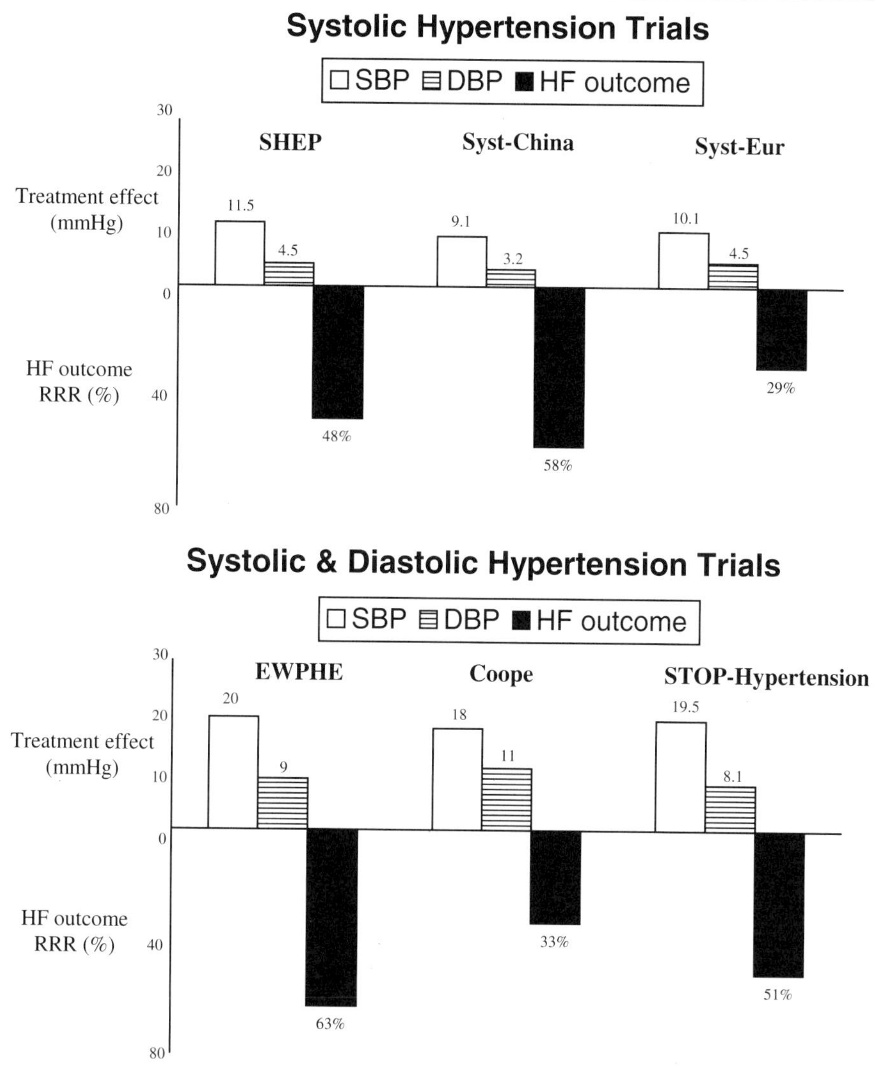

Figure 2. Treatment effect (placebo corrected reduction in blood pressure) and heart failure outcome of landmark hypertension trials: SHEP (8), Syst-China (9), Syst-Eur (10), EWPHE (11), Coope (12), STOP-Hypertension (13). HF = heart failure; RRR = relative risk reduction; SBP = systolic blood pressure; DBP = diastolic blood pressure.

Losartan Intervention For Endpoint reduction in hypertension (LIFE) study, there was no difference in blood pressure control or heart failure rate between losartan and atenolol in the treatment of hypertension and left ventricular hypertrophy (15).

Data from these hypertension trials with long follow up indicate that antihypertensive therapy is effective in the prevention of heart failure. The systolic blood pres-

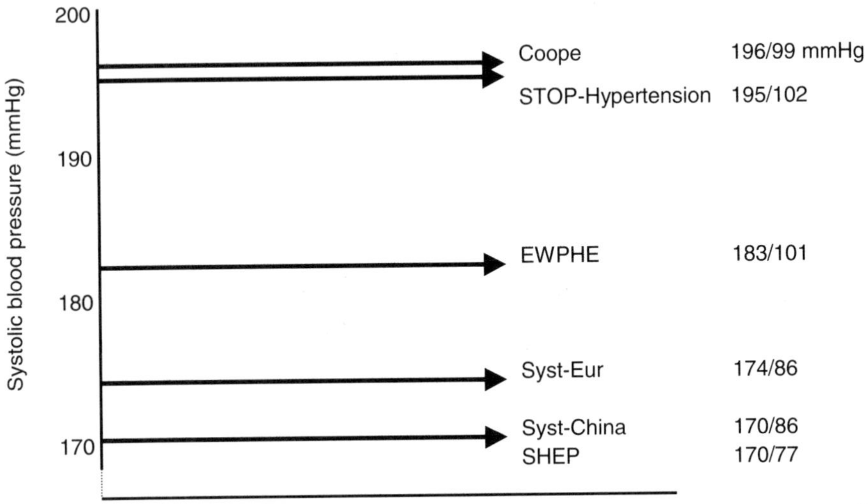

Figure 3. Landmark hypertension trials and blood pressure at entry: Coope (12), STOP-Hypertension (13), EWPHE (11), Syst-Eur (10), Syst-China (9), SHEP (8).

sure at entry to the studies was high and ranged from 170 to 196 mmHg (Figure 3). A relatively small reduction in blood pressure resulted in a substantial reduction in heart failure incidence. However, these studies were primarily designed to evaluate the effect of lowering blood pressure on the reduction of morbidity and mortality from myocardial infarction and stroke. Prevention of heart failure was defined differently amongst the studies and was analyzed as a secondary endpoint. This may be less precise in estimating the true benefit of treatment (16). The mean duration of follow up ranged from 2 to 5 years. However, the progression from hypertension to heart failure takes a chronic course and trials with a short follow up period would not allow adequate time for the full impact on heart failure to be observed. Echocardiograms were not performed in the studies; hence the results did not separate heart failure on the basis of systolic versus diastolic dysfunction. In addition, the studies demonstrated a strong relation between comorbidity (age and cardiovascular disease) and the incidence of heart failure. A higher rate of heart failure in the control group was observed in older patients and those with more comorbid cardiovascular disease.

Coronary artery disease

Significant changes in the etiology of heart failure have occurred over the last 2 decades. Coronary heart disease has become the most important cause of heart failure in western society and accounts for 68% of the heart failure cases (17). The prevalence of coronary artery disease before the diagnosis of heart failure has increased by 41% per calendar decade in men and 25% per calendar decade in women. Coronary artery disease was the primary attributable cause in 22% of patients in the 1950s and 67% in the 1980s (6). Given the magnitude of the problem, aggressive management of coronary artery disease plays an important role in the prevention of heart failure.

Protective effects of beta-blockers

Beta-blockers are first line antiischemic therapy in coronary artery disease and have been shown to reduce morbidity and mortality in patients after myocardial infarction (18). In management of established heart failure, beta-blockers have been demonstrated to improve patient survival, reduce sudden cardiac death, and decrease subsequent hospitalization for heart failure when added to standard therapy (19). Recently, the Metoprolol CR/XL Randomised Intervention Trial in Heart Failure (MERIT-HF) using metoprolol, the Cardiac Insufficiency Bisoprolol Study II (CIBIS-II) using bisoprolol, and the CarvedilOl ProspEctive RaNdomIzed CUmulative Survival (COPERNICUS) study using carvedilol have further supported the treatment benefits of beta-blockers (20–22). Although the benefits of beta-blockers in hypertension and heart failure therapy are well established, their role in the prevention of heart failure in patients with coronary artery disease is less clear.

Large scale trials in beta-blocker therapy after myocardial infarction have not demonstrated any significant protective effect in preventing heart failure. In the Norwegian trial, timolol was shown to reduce mortality and reinfarction. However, there was no difference in heart failure incidence between the treatment and control group (23). In the Beta-blocker Heart Attack Trial (BHAT) and the Metoprolol In Acute Myocardial Infarction (MIAMI) trial, the heart failure outcome was not significantly different between the treatment and control groups (24,25). These studies, however, were not specifically designed to study heart failure outcome and heart failure was not predefined as one of the major endpoints. Recently, the Carvedilol Post-Infarct Survival Control in Left Ventricular Dysfunction (CAPRICORN) trial demonstrated the benefits of carvedilol on outcome after myocardial infarction in patients with left ventricular dysfunction. Heart failure was evaluated as a secondary endpoint. However, the study failed to show any significant difference between the treatment and control group in hospital admission for heart failure (26). The mean duration of follow up of these studies ranged from 1 to 33 months. This short period of follow up may not allow adequate time to show the protective effect of beta-blockers in preventing heart failure. In a retrospective analysis of the Survival And Ventricular Enlargement (SAVE) study with a mean follow up of 42 months, beta-blocker therapy was associated with a 30% reduction in risk of developing severe heart failure. This beneficial effect of beta-blocker use was independent of the use of captopril (27).

Beta-blockers are effective cardiovascular therapy in management of established heart failure and left ventricular dysfunction. Nevertheless, there is inadequate prospective clinical trial evidence to quantify a beneficial effect of beta-blockers to prevent heart failure in patients with ischemic left ventricular dysfunction.

Protective effects of angiotensin converting enzyme inhibitors

Several large clinical trials have assessed the role of angiotensin converting enzyme (ACE) inhibitors for patients with acute myocardial infarction. The Survival And Ventricular Enlargement (SAVE), Acute Infarction Ramipril Efficacy (AIRE), and TRAndolapril Cardiac Evaluation (TRACE) trials were designed to evaluate the long term use of ACE inhibitors after myocardial infarction in high risk patients. The mean duration of follow up ranged from 15 to 42 months in these studies. In terms of heart failure outcome, ACE inhibitor therapy with captopril resulted in a 36% reduction in heart failure mortality and a 22% reduction in heart failure admission in the SAVE trial (28). In the AIRE study using ramipril and TRACE study using trandolapril, ACE inhibitor therapy was associated with a 29% and 27% reduction in occurrence of heart failure respectively (29,30). In a systematic overview of data from the three trials, there was a 23% reduction in heart failure admission. This corresponds to the avoidance of 36 cases of admission for heart failure per 1000 patients treated (Figure 4) (31).

Several other studies, including the COoperative New Scandinavian ENalapril SUrvival Study II (CONSENSUS-II), Gruppo Italiano per lo Studio della Sopravvivenza nell'Infarto miocardico (GISSI-3) study, Fourth International Study of Infarct Survival (ISIS-4), and Chinese Cardiac Study-1 (CCS-1), investigated the acute, short term use of ACE inhibitors in a broad patient population with acute myocardial infarction (32). The mean duration of follow up ranged from 1 to 6 months. In CONSENSUS-II with a mean follow up of six months, ACE inhibitor therapy with enalapril was shown to significantly reduce the incidence of worsening heart failure (33). In the other 3 studies, heart failure outcome was not significantly improved with ACE-inhibitor therapy (lisinopril in GISSI-3, captopril in ISIS-4 and captopril in CCS-1) (34–36). However, the duration of follow up in these studies was short and hence the opportunity in individual trials to detect a treatment effect would be compromised. A systemic overview was subsequently performed on these studies, demonstrating that ACE inhibitor therapy significantly reduced the incidence of nonfatal heart failure. This corresponded to the avoidance of 6.1 cases of heart failure per 1000 patients treated (Figure 4) (37).

The Studies Of Left Ventricular Dysfunction (SOLVD) prevention trial was designed to examine the long term effect of ACE inhibitor therapy in patients with left ventricular dysfunction (LVEF ≤ 35%). A substantial number of patients in the study had coronary artery disease and previous myocardial infarction. ACE inhibitor therapy with enalapril was shown to significantly reduce heart failure morbidity (hospitalizations for worsening heart failure) and mortality (38). This study indicates that ACE inhibitors can retard the progression to heart failure in asymptomatic patients with left ventricular dysfunction. Data from all of the above clinical trials confirm the crucial role of ACE inhibitor therapy in the prevention of heart failure events in patients after myocardial infarction with left ventricular dysfunction.

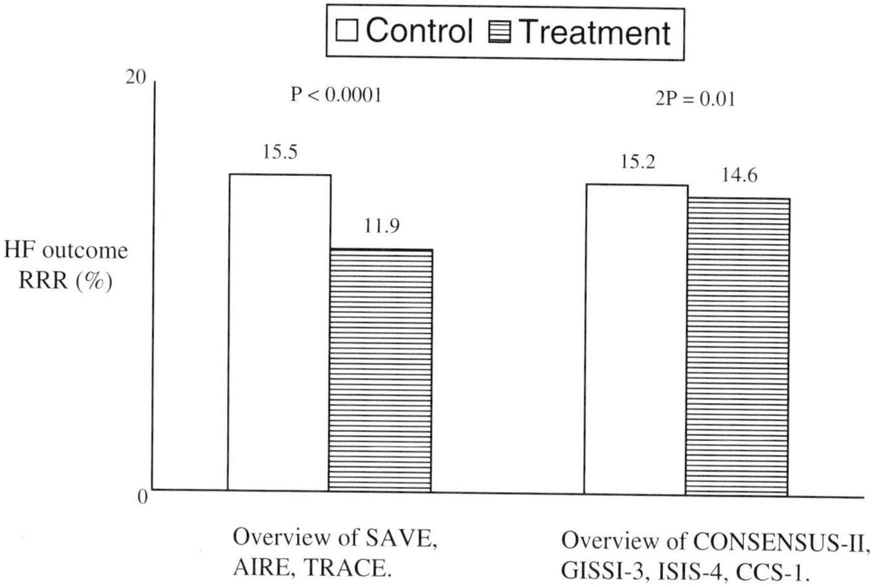

Figure 4. Systematic overviews (31,37) of post-MI ACE inhibitor therapy and heart failure outcomes. In SAVE (28), AIRE (29), TRACE (30), heart failure endpoint was defined as incidence of nonfatal heart failure. In CONSENSUS-II (33), GISSI-3 (34), ISIS-4 (35), CCS-1 (36), heart failure endpoint was defined as admission for heart failure. RRR = relative risk reduction.

Valvular heart disaese

Congenital heart disease and acquired valvular heart disease are strong contributors to the development of heart failure. However, they carry a relatively low attributable risk because they are much less prevalent than hypertension and coronary artery disease (39). During the past 2 decades, major advances have occurred in diagnostic techniques and surgical procedures for patients with valvular heart disease. The prevalence of valvular heart disease has dramatically declined due to improved detection, close monitoring, and earlier surgical intervention. Patients with valvular heart disease generally have a prolonged latent period in which morbidity and mortality are low. Eventually, symptoms of heart failure or left ventricular dysfunction may develop and the outcome becomes poor. Thus patients with valvular heart disease should be closely monitored for the development of symptoms and progression of disease. Follow-up clinical evaluation and serial echocardiogram for assessing left ventricular and valvular function should be performed on a frequency depending on the severity of the disease (40). Patients with valvular heart disease are at increased risk for bacterial endocarditis and should receive antibiotic prophylaxis prior to dental or surgical procedures.

For patients with chronic aortic regurgitation, afterload reduction therapy with ACE inhibitors has been shown to decrease the rate of left ventricular dilatation

Table 1. Vascular protection and heart failure prevention

Study	Eligibility	Treatment	HF Outcome RRR %
HOPE	Vascular disease, diabetes plus one risk factor	Ramipril	22%
RENAAL	Type 2 diabetes, nephropathy	Losartan	32%
4S	CHD, total chol >5.5 mmol/L	Simvastatin	19%

HOPE (45), RENAAL (46), 4S (48). CHD = coronary heart disease; chol = cholesterol; HF = heart failure; RRR = relative risk reduction.

(41,42). In a clinical trial of nifedipine, afterload reduction therapy reduced the need for valve replacement from 34% to 15% over 6 years (43). Since no heart failure outcomes were evaluated in the studies, the reduction of left ventricular dilatation, which should be beneficial in preventing heart failure, merely acted as a surrogate endpoint for heart failure outcomes. Among patients with chronic mitral regurgitation, the role of afterload reduction therapy is less certain as there are no large long-term studies to indicate that vasodilators are beneficial. Specific indications for surgical intervention are described in published national guidelines (40). However, the guidelines do not comment on whether surgical intervention will prevent heart failure.

Idiopathic cardiomyopathy

It is difficult to obtain reliable estimates of the prevalence and incidence of idiopathic cardiomyopathy because of the difficulty in diagnosis and its relative rarity in the general population (39). Several studies have suggested a potential link between viral myocarditis and idiopathic dilated cardiomyopathy. The incidence of viral myocarditis in dilated cardiomyopathy is estimated to be 10% to 20% (44). Unfortunately, there is no effective current treatment for viral myocarditis. Whether annual influenza vaccination in individuals at high risk reduces the risk of myocarditis is not known. Patients with idiopathic dilated cardiomyopathy should be monitored closely for progression of disease. ACE inhibitor therapy should be considered in all patients with dilated cardiomyopathy and impaired left ventricular systolic function to prevent the development of heart failure (38).

RISK FACTOR MODIFICATION

An effective preventive strategy for heart failure requires aggressive identification and correction of risk factors. The presence of multiple risk factors increases the risk of heart failure substantially. The Heart Outcomes Prevention Evaluation (HOPE) trial was conducted to evaluate the effect of ACE inhibitor therapy on preventing cardiovascular events in high risk patients (45). The study demonstrated that ramipril significantly reduced the incidence of heart failure by 22% (Table 1). Diabetes predisposes to heart failure at all ages and its prevalence has increased by more than 20% per decade (6). In patients with type 2 diabetes and nephropathy, the Reduction of Endpoints in NIDDM with the Angiotension II Antagonist Losartan (RENAAL) study showed that angiotensin II receptor antagonist therapy with losartan significantly reduced the rate of first hospitalization for heart failure by 32% (46,47). Larger clinical trials are needed to confirm this treatment benefit. The treatment of hypercholesterolemia with HMG-CoA inhibitor therapy has been shown to improve survival and heart failure outcome in patients with coronary artery disease. In the Scandinavian Simvastatin Survival Study (4S), simvastatin significantly reduced the incidence of heart failure by 19% (48).

CONCLUSION

Heart failure is a rapidly growing public health problem and has substantial economic impact. Aging of the general population will further increase the incidence of the disease syndrome in the near future. Heart failure continues to be a main cause of cardiovascular morbidity and mortality despite advances in diagnosis and treatment. The best management strategy for heart failure requires the combination of aggressive prevention and early intervention. Effective preventive management of heart failure can be achieved by treatment of coronary artery disease and hypertension and modification of risk factors. Diuretics, beta-blockers, and certain calcium antagonists are effective in the lowering of blood pressure and prevention of heart failure. In patients with myocardial infarction, ACE inhibitor therapy has been demonstrated to improve heart failure outcome when added to standard therapy. In addition, clinical trials have shown that ACE inhibitor therapy prevents heart failure and prolongs survival in asymptomatic patients with left ventricular dysfunction and in older patients at high risk of progressive atherosclerosis.

REFERENCES

1. Liu P, Arnold JMO, Belenkie I, et al. 2001. The 2001 Canadian Cardiovascular Society consensus guideline update for the management and prevention of heart failure. Can J Card 17(Suppl E): 5E–25E.
2. Mair FS, Crowley TS. 1996. Prevalence, aetiology and management of heart failure in general practice. Br J Gen Pract 46:77.
3. Ho KK, Pinsky JL, Kannel WB, Levy D. 1993. The epidemiology of heart failure: the Framingham study. J Am Coll Cardiol 325:293–302.
4. Hunt SA, Baker DW, Chin MH, et al. 2001. ACC/AHA guidelines for the evaluation and management of chronic heart failure in the adult: a report of the American College of Cardiology/American Heart Association Task Force on Practice Guidelines (Committee to Revise the 1995 Guidelines for the Evaluation and Management of Heart Failure). J Am Coll Cardiol 38(7):2101–2113.
5. Haldeman GA, Croft JB, Giles WH, Rashidee A. 1999. Hospitalization of patients with heart failure: National Hospital Discharge Survey, 1985 to 1995. Am H J 137:352–60.
6. Massie BM, Shah NB. 1997. Evolving trends in the epidemiology of heart failure: rationale for preventive strategies and comprehensive disease management. Am Heart J 133:703–712.
7. O'Connell JB, Bristow M. 1993. Economic impact of heart failure in the United States: Time for a different approach. J Heart Lung Transplant 13:S107–112.
8. SHEP Cooperative Research Group. 1991. Prevention of stroke by antihypertensive drug treatment in older patients with isolated systolic hypertension. JAMA 265:3255–3264.
9. Systolic Hypertension in China (Syst-China) Collaborative Group. 1998. Comparison of active treatment and placebo for older patients with isolated systolic hypertension. J Hypertens 16:1823–1829.
10. Staessen JA, Fagard R, Thijs L, et al. 1997. Randomised double-blind comparison of placebo and active treatment for older patients with isolated systolic hypertension. Lancet 350:757–764.
11. Amery A, Birkenhager W, Brixko P, et al. 1985. Mortality and morbidity results from the European Working Party on High Blood Pressure in the Elderly trial. Lancet 1:1349–54.

12. Coope J, Warrender TS. 1986. Randomized trial of treatment of hypertension in elderly patients in primary care. Br Med J 293:1145–1151.
13. Dahlof B, Lindholm LH, Hansson L, et al. 1991. Morbidity and mortality in the Swedish Trial in Old Patients with Hypertension (STOP-Hypertension). Lancet 338:1281–1285.
14. ALLHAT Collaborative Research Group. 2000. Major cardiovascular events in hypertensive patients randomized to doxazosin vs chlorthalidone: the antihypertensive and lipid-lowering treatment to prevent heart attack trial (ALLHAT). JAMA 283:1967–1975.
15. Wachtell K, Bella JN, Rokkedal J, et al. 2002. Change in diastolic left ventricular filling after one year of antihypertensive treatment: The Losartan Intervention For Endpoint Reduction in Hypertension (LIFE) Study. Circulation 105:1071–1076.
16. Moser M, Hebert PR. 1996. Prevention of disease progression, left ventricular hypertrophy and congestive heart failure in hypertension treatment trials. J Am Coll Cardiol 27(5):1214–1218.
17. Gheorghiade M, Bonow RO. 1998. Chronic heart failure in the United States: a manifestation of coronary artery disease. Circulation 97:282–289.
18. The ACC/AHA Task Force on Practice Guidelines. 1999. ACC/AHA guidelines for the management of patients with chronic stable angina: executive summary and recommendations. Circulation 99:2829–2848.
19. U.S. Carvedilol Heart Failure Study Group. 1996. The effect of Carvedilol on morbidity and mortality in patients with chronic heart failure. N Engl J Med 334:1349–1355.
20. MERIT-HF Study Group. 1999. Effects of metoprolol CR/XL in chronic heart failure: Metoprolol CR/CX Randomized Intervention Trial in Congestive Heart Failure (MERIT-HF). Lancet 353:2001–2007.
21. CIBIS-II Investigatiors and Committees. 1999. The Cardiac Insufficiency Study II: a randomized trial. Lancet 353:9–13.
22. Carvedilol Prospective Randomized Cumulative Survival Study Group. Effect of carvedilol on survival in severe chronic heart failure. 2001. N Engl J Med 344:1651–1658.
23. Norwegian Multicentre Study Group. 1981. Timolol-induced reduction in mortality and reinfarction in patients surviving acute myocardial infarction. N Engl Med 304:801–907.
24. Beta-Blocker Heart Attack Trial Research Group. 1982. A randomized trial of propranolol in patients with acute myocardial infarction. II. Morbidity results. JAMA 250:2814–2819.
25. MIAMI Trial Research Group. 1985. Metoprolol in acute myocardial infarction (MIAMI). A randomized placebo-controlled international trial. Eur Heart J 6:199–226.
26. The CAPRICORN Investigators. 2001. Effect of carvedilol on outcome after myocardial infarction in patients with left ventricular dysfunction: the CAPRICORN randomised trial. Lancet 357: 1385–1390.
27. Vantrimpont P, Rouleau JL, Wun CC, et al. 1997. Additive beneficial effects of beta-blockers to angiotensin-converting enzyme inhibitors in the survival and ventricular enlargement (SAVE) study. J Am Coll Cardiol 29(2):229–236.
28. Pfeffer MA, Braunwald E, Moye L, et al. 1992. Effect of captopril on mortality and morbidity in patients with left ventricular dysfunction after myocardial infarction: results of the survival and ventricular enlargement trial. N Engl J Med 327:669–77.
29. The Acute Infarction Ramipril Efficacy (AIRE) Study Investigators. 1993. Effect of ramipril on mortality and morbidity of survivors of acute myocardial infarction with clinical evidence of heart failure. Lancet 342:821–828.
30. The Trandolapril Cardiac Evaluation (TRACE) Study Group. 1995. A clinical trial of the angiotensin converting enzyme inhibitor trandolapril in patients with left ventricular dysfunction after myocardial infarction. N Engl J Med 333:1670–1676.
31. Flather M, Yusuf S, Kober L, et al. 2000. Long-term ACE-inhibitor therapy in patients with heart failure or left-ventricular dysfunction: a systematic overview of data from individual patients. Lancet 355:1575–1581.
32. Huckell VF, Bernstein V, Cairns JA, et al. 1997. Angiotensin-converting enzyme inhibition in myocardial infarction—Part 1: Clinical data. Can J Cardiol 13(2):161–169.
33. Sweberg K, Held P, Kjekshus J, et al. 1992. Effects of the early administration of enalapril on mortality in patients with acute myocardial infarction: results of the Cooperative New Scandinavian Enalapril Survival Study II (CONSENSUS II). N Engl J Med 327:678–684.
34. Gruppo Italiano per lo Studio della Sopravvivenza nell'Infarto Miocardico. 1994. GISSI-3: effects of lisinopril and transdermal glyceryl trinitrate singly and together on 6-week mortality and ventricular function after acute myocardial infarction. Lancet 343:1115–1122.

35. ISIS-4 Collaborative Group. 1995. ISIS-4: a randomised factorial trial assessing early oral captopril, oral mononitrate, and intravenous magnesium sulphate in 58,050 patients with suspected acute myocardial infarction. Lancet 345:669–685.
36. Chinese Cardiac Study Collaborative Group. 1995. Oral captopril versus placebo among 13,634 patients with suspected acute myocardial infarction: interim report from the Chinese Cardiac Study (CCS-1). Lancet 345:686–687.
37. ACE Inhibitor Myocardial Infarction Collaborative Group. 1998. Indications for ACE inhibitors in the early treatment of acute myocardial infarction: systematic overview of individual data from 100,000 patients in randomized trials. Circulation 97:2202–2212.
38. The SOLVD Investigators. 1992. Effect of enalapril on mortality and the development of heart failure in asymptomatic patients with reduced left ventricular ejection fraction. N Engl J Med 327:685–691.
39. Kannel WB, Ho K, Thom T. 1994. Changing epidemiological features of cardiac failure. Br Heart J 72(Suppl):S3–9.
40. Bonow RO, Carabello B, De Leon AC, et al. 1998. ACC/AHA Guidelines for the Management of Patients With Valvular Heart Disease: a report of the American College of Cardiology/American Heart Association Task Force on Practice Guidelines (Committee on Management of Patients With Valvular Heart Disease). J Am Coll Cardiol 32:1486–1588.
41. Lin M, Chiang HT, Lin SL, et al. 1994. Vasodilator therapy in chronic asymptomatic aortic regurgitation: enalapril versus hydralazine therapy. J Am Coll Cardiol 24:1046–1053.
42. Schon HR, Dorn R, Barthel P, Schomig A. 1994. Effects of 12 months quinapril therapy in asymptomatic patients with chronic aortic regurgitation. J Heart Valve Dis 3:500–509.
43. Scognamiglio R, Rahimtoola SH, Fasoli G, et al. 1994. Nifedipine in asymptomatic patients with severe aortic regurgitation and normal left ventricular function. N Engl J Med 331:689–694.
44. Sole MJ, Liu P. 1993. Viral myocarditis: A paradigm for understanding the pathogenesis and treatment of dilated cardiomyopathy. J Am Coll Cardiol 22(4) Suppl:99A–105A.
45. The Heart Outcomes Prevention Evaluation Study Investigators. 2000. Effects of an angiotensin-converting-enzyme inhibitor, ramipril, on cardiovascular events in high-risk patients. N Engl J Med 342:145–153.
46. The RENAAL Study Investigators. 2001. Effects of losartan on renal and cardiovascular outcomes in patients with type 2 diabetes and nephropathy. N Engl J Med 345(12):861–869.
47. The Heart Outcomes Prevention Evaluation Study Investigators. 2000. Effects of ramipril on cardiovascular and microvascular outcomes in people with diabetes mellitus: results of the HOPE study and MICRO-HOPE substudy. Lancet 355:253–259.
48. Scandinavian Simvastatin Survival Study Group. 1994. Randomized trial of cholesterol lowering in 4,444 patients with coronary heart disease: the Scandinavian Simvastatin Survival Study (4S). Lancet 344:1383–1389.

Frontiers in Cardiovascular Health, edited by
N.S. Dhalla, A. Chockalingam,
H.I. Berkowitz & P.K. Singal
Kluwer Academic Publishers, Boston, 2003

Diastolic Dysfuncion, Redox Stress, Extracellular Matrix Remodeling and Congestive Heart Failure in Diabetes Mellitus*

M.R. (PETE) Hayden[1] and Suresh C. Tyagi[2]

[1] *Department of cardiovascular atherosclerosis metabolism and aging Camdenton Community Health Center, Camdenton, Missouri USA 65020; and Department of Family and Community Medicine, University of Missouri-Columbia, MO, USA*
[2] *Department of Physiology and Biophysics, The University of Mississippi Medical Center, Jackson, MS 39216*

Summary. Congestive heart failure (CHF) is the one cardiovascular disease that has been increasing exponentially during the past decade. The current epidemic can only be expected to increase in the near future as our societies age. Hypertension (HTN), coronary artery disease (CAD), diabetes, and aging are currently the four big players and contribute to redox stress, myocellular and extramyocellular matrix (ECM) remodeling on the path to developing diastolic dysfunction (DD), systolic dysfunction (SD) and eventual CHF. The natural progression and history of CHF has a tendency to follow along two separate but interconnecting pathways as if tied together in a molecule. The roles of each of these factors will be discussed and the transition from DD to SD and overt CHF will be explored. Earlier diagnosis and compliance to current treatment paradigms by both the patient and physician are essential elements to slow or halt this progressive epidemic. Understanding the natural history of this morbid progressive disease will allow researchers and clinicians alike to develop novel treatment strategies and pave the way for newer developments in the diagnosis and treatment of CHF.

Key words: Congestive heart failure, diastolic dysfunction, systolic dysfunction, redox stress, and extracellular matrix remodeling.

Please correspondance to: Suresh C. Tyagi Ph. D., FAHA., Department of Physiology and Biophysics, The University of Mississippi Medical Center, Jackson, Mississippi, 39216-4505. Tel: 601-984-1899, Fax: 601-984-1817, E-mail: styagi@physiology.umsmed.edu.
*A part of this work was supported by NIU grants ML-71010 and ML-74185.

INTRODUCTION

Congestive heart failure (CHF) may be defined as any impairment that prevents the heart from adequately perfusing body tissues to meet metabolic demands. The natural history is one of complexity with a progressive nature. CHF may develop acutely following a myocardial infarction or insidiously over a continuum as with most chronic disease states. Hypertension (HTN) and coronary artery disease (CAD) are the two most common causes of CHF, with hypertension being the more common (1). As demonstrated in the Framingham Heart Study, HTN preceded 91% of heart failure cases with rising percentages associated with each decade from ages 50 to 80 years of age, which demonstrates that aging plays an additional important role in the overall picture of developing CHF (2). In the clinical setting these four: HTN, CAD, diabetes, and age all too frequently coexist. There are many in the field of cardiology, that feel CAD or ischemic heart disease is the most common cause of CHF in the Western world (3).

CHF is the most common cause for hospitalization in patients aged 65 and older in the U.S. There are 400,000 to 700,000 newly diagnosed cases per year (1.5% to 2% of the general American population, with 6%–10% of those 65 and older) and in excess of 4.8 million Americans suffer from this debilitating morbid disease. In excess of 20 billion dollars are spent annually in direct and indirect costs. Annual mortality is between 200,000–300,000 in the U.S. and the 5-year mortality rates are 62% in men and 42% in women (4,5). The statistical increases we have seen can only be expected to increase with the oncoming baby boom generation (approximately 80 million strong) transitioning to become the senior boom generation. Additionally, advances in the treatment of CAD with acute myocardial infarction (emergency interventional cardiology with thrombolytics, angioplasty, stenting, and interventional surgery with coronary artery bypass grafting) during the past two decades have created an increased number of survivors of myocardial infarction. These survivors now have entered the statistical arena to develop CHF (6). The role(s) of left ventricular hypertrophy (LVH), concentric (positive) remodeling, interstitial fibrosis (Figure 1) with associated impaired ventricular relaxation and filling will be discussed. Additionally, the more robust extracellular matrix remodeling of the transitioning phase, which results in the conversion of diastolic dysfunction to a thinned, flabby, eccentrically (negatively) remodeled heart typical of systolic dysfunction and CHF will be explored.

Diastolic dysfunction

The natural progression and history of CHF has a tendency to follow along two separate but interconnecting pathways as if tied together in a molecule (Figure 1). As mentioned in the introduction, HTN and CAD play important roles in the development of CHF. Let us first examine hypertension (both systolic and diastolic) from the standpoint of being a syndrome as it has a tendency to cluster with many other risk factors for the development of CHF (Figure 2) (7). These clustered abnor-

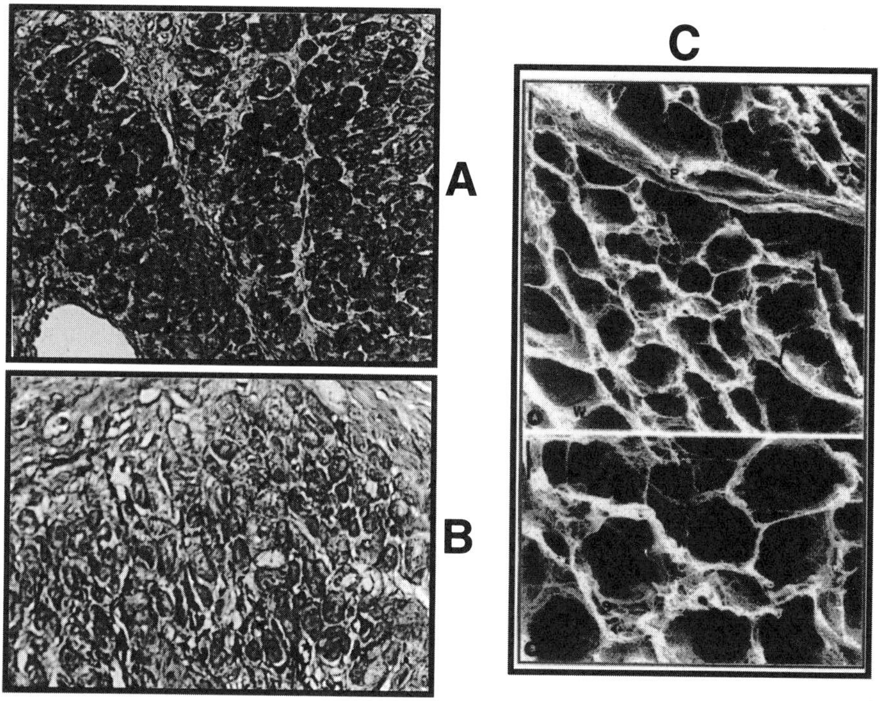

Figure 1. **A**. Representative trichrome stain of normal human heart: At 40 x magnification. Note: light collagen staining in between the myocytes. The myocytes are roundish and normal. **B**. Representative staining of human heart explant of a failing myocardium: At 40 x magnification. Note light staining of collagen between the myocytes. The myocytes are elongated, suggesting myocyte slippage and collagen disruption. **C.** Three dimensional image of ECM of the heart. In this image the endomysium (surrounding the absent myocyte), endomysial weave (W), and perimysium (P) are depicted. The collagen struts (s) connect individual myocytes and connect myocytes to interstitial microvessels (thin arrow) and to the perimysium(thick arrow). Courtesy of Marcos A. Rossi, M.D. (with permission).

malities (the insulin resistance state and the metabolic syndrome) contribute to a pattern of target organ damage, which involves the arterial vessel wall, heart, kidney, and brain.

LVH involves a concentric increase in left ventricular wall thickness as a result of myocyte hypertrophy and excessive formation of ECM. The change in architecture and structure of the left ventricle is a result of remodeling due to a pressure related increase in wall stress and mechanical strain. Additionally, the renin-angiotensin-aldosterone system (RAAS) is activated and directly involved in pathological myocyte hypertrophy and the subsequent deposition of ECM. Initially, this adaptive hypertrophy allows the heart to overcome increases in vascular resistance. Gradually there is a disruption of the normal myofibrillar architecture resulting in

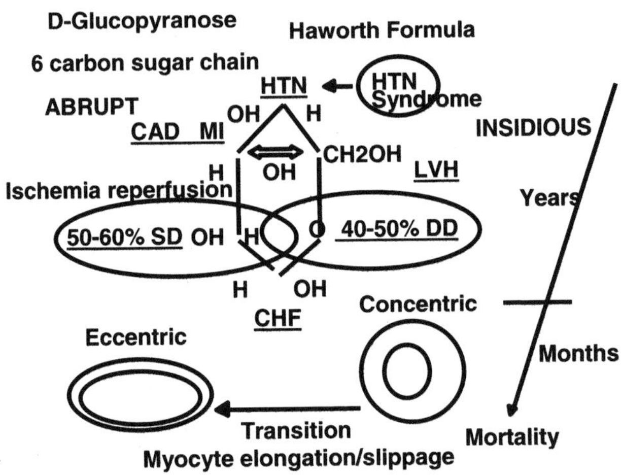

Figure 2. The conceptual D-glucopyronose six carbon sugar ring Haworth formula demonstrates how the various etiologies are interconnected and conform to a somewhat structured foundation for the transition to CHF.

Table 1. Etiologies of diastolic dysfunction

Common Etiologies	Less Common Etiologies
***AGING.**	**Hypertrophic cardiomyopathy.**
***DIABETES MELLITUS (types 1 and 2).**	**Infiltrative cardiomyopathy.**
(Diabetic Cardiomyopathy)	
***OBESITY.**	**Endocardial fibroelastosis.**
HYPERTENSION.	**Restrictive pericardial disease.**
CORONARY ARTERY DISEASE.	**Idiopathic hypertrophic subaortic stenosis.**
(atherosclerosis)	**(IHSS).**
AORTIC STENOSIS.	

impaired ventricular relaxation whereby the ventricle loses its ability to return to its normal resting state during diastole resulting in impaired filling.

Diastolic dysfunction (**DD**) is the heart's inability to properly fill as a result of impaired ventricular relaxation and is represented as an elevated end diastolic pressure in a normal or reduced sized chamber (concentrically, geometrically shaped) with a normal ejection fraction. In contrast systolic dysfunction (**SD**) is due to the heart's inability to properly empty and is represented by a reduced ejection fraction where the ratio of ventricular radius chamber to free wall ventricular width is increased (elliptical geometric shape) (8). DD has been found to be present in a large portion of patients with CHF approaching 50% (9–12). DD is an insidious disease and etiologies are numerous (Table 1). Aging, diabetes, and obesity have been marked with an asterisk to denote a marked increasing prevalence in our society

Table 2. Causes for progrssive systolic dysfunction simular to table 1 and decompensated CHF

Common Causes	Less Common Causes
NON COMPLIANCE OF MEDICATION AND DIET.	**ANEMIA.**
ARRHYTHMIAS.	**DECOMPENSATED COPD.**
INFECTION (SEPIS in particular).	**THYROID DISEASES.**
ISCHEMIA.	**RENAL FAILURE.**
UNCONTROLLED HTN.	**SURGICAL STRESS.**
IATROGENIC (hypokalemia, digoxin toxicity, coumadin toxicity)	**UNIDENTIFIED MEDS (OTC—NSAIDS)**
SOCIAL DEPRIVATION (social economic status).	**EMOTIONAL STRESS.**

and due to this recent trend we can only expect to see an acceleration in the development of DD. CAD is associated with an ischemia/ischemia-reperfusion injury to the myocardium which results in myocyte cellular loss through the process of ischemic necrosis and apoptosis. In a response to injury mechanism both local (passive fibrosis) and remote (active fibrosis) sites of the myocardium undergo interstitial fibrosis (13). With acute myocardial infarction these changes are abrupt in contrast to the insidious nature associated with HTN and LVH. However, the ischemia/ischemia-reperfusion injury may be insidious. Whether abrupt (MI) or insidious (ischemia/ischemia-reperfusion) CAD is associated more closely with SD (Table 2). While the conceptual model in Figure 1 attempts to simplify and compartmentalize a very complex, dynamic, interacting, progressive disease state, it is important to distinguish between SD and DD in order to provide appropriate therapy. Currently, noninvasive Doppler echocardiography allows clinicians to distinguish between SD and DD. It is important to understand the development of each of these two component diseases and how they progress to CHF as they may require different therapies at different points in time on this disease continuum.

DD is commonly found in both type 1 and 2 diabetes mellitus and is associated with a markedly increased interstitial, perivascular fibrosis of the ECM. Additionally, in the diabetic there is a considerable amount of Periodic Acid Schiff positive material (both in the interstitium and arterial vessel wall). It is felt that these histological abnormalities contribute to a distinct diabetic cardiomyopathy and the increased risk (up to 2.4 fold in males and 5.1 fold in females) of CHF seen in diabetes (14–17). This increased risk of heart failure persisted after adjustment for age, hypertension, obesity, hypercholesterolemia, and CAD. Zabalgoitia and collogues (18) found that DD in patients with type 2 diabetes mellitus free of cardiovascular disease was present in 41 of 86 (47%) of normotensive men and women by Doppler echocardiography. All subjects were asymptomatic for ischemic heart disease or heart failure. Global systolic function was normal (mean LV ejection fraction 58%, range 53% to 76%). This is why the D-glucopyranose Haworth ring structure of the 6-carbon glucose molecule was chosen as a foundation for the conceptual model in Figure 2.

Redox stress

Cellular respiration or the transference of electrons between oxygen species allows us to survive on this planet not only at the cellular level but also as an organism. *Redox Homeostasis* describes the normal physiologic process of reduction and oxidation in order to re-pair unstable, damaging, reduced, reactive oxygen species (ROS) or oxygen free radicals: [O2′ H2O2 and –OH′]. *Redox Stress* implies a loss of this homeostasis with an excess of ROS either through the process of reduction or oxidation whereas *Oxidative Stress* implies a loss of this homeostasis with an excess of ROS by the singular process of oxidation. It has been known for some time that ROS are detrimental and toxic to cells and tissues resulting in cellular injury to proteins, lipids, and nucleic acids. Our bodies are "hard wired" to utilize this mechanism of injury to fend off invading infectious organisms. Paradoxically, (when there is loss of homeostasis resulting in redox or oxidative stress) this protective mechanism turns on our own healthy tissues and causes damage to multiple organs, especially the heart in CHF.

ORIGINS OF REACTIVE OXYGEN SPECIES (ROS)

I. Excess O2 (Oxygen therapy).
II. Absorption of radiant energy (ultraviolet light) or ionizing radiation (radiotherapy).
III. Exposure to toxins: Carbon tetrachloride, (oxygen [I.]), many drugs.
IV. Reduction-oxidation (redox) reactions during normal physiologic processes.
V. Ischemia—Ischemia Reperfusion Injury.
VI. Inflammatory processes. Acute and Chronic.
VII. Once free radicals ROS form, they can react with membrane lipids, proteins, and nucleic acid to initiate auto catalytic reactions (ROS beget ROS).

In regards to the myocardium and CHF we are dealing with numbers: IV, V, VI, VII. Examples of number IV would be CHF associated with hyperthyroidism, sympathetic (neurohormonal) excess and the tachycardia paced animal models of CHF. Examples of number V and VI would be the ishcemia-ischemia reperfusion injury and the acute and chronic inflammatory process as a result of wound healing due to ischemic injury both being associated with CAD. Once there is an excess of ROS the viscous cycle of autocatalytic reactions develop (VII) and the stage is set for ROS begetting ROS. In addition, once the neurohormonal system is activated in HTN, LVH, and CHF we see the effects of angiotensin II activating the vascular intracellular NADH and the membranous NAD(P)H pathway (19). In this scenario we observe injury begetting injury and ROS begetting ROS, which contributes to the chronic viscous cycle of injury and repair associated with the wound healing response being chronically activated in the myocardium.

The ROS generated ([2O2 + 2H2O → 2 H2O2 + O2′ (super oxide)] dependent or independent of inflammatory and / or mitochondrial NADH/NAD oxidase and vascular NAD(P)H) overwhelms the activity of superoxide dismutase (SOD) and catalase (20–23). The ROS also negates the effect of eNOS and endothelial derived NO resulting in endothelial dysfunction within the myocardium. ROS activates latent resident myocardial matrix metalloproteinases (MMPs) and contributes to the ongoing chronic ventricular remodeling process within the myocardium (24,25). ROS are formed at an accelerated rate in post ischemic myocardium. Multiple cells (cardiac myocytes, endothelial cells, infiltrating neutrophils, and macrophages) contribute to ROS production. Exposure of these cellular components of the myocardium to endogenous or exogenous ROS can lead to cellular dysfunction and necrosis (26). The reaction of **[O2′ + NO → ONOO′ (peroxynitrite)]** supercedes and consumes NO. This in turn leaves an indelible footprint to test for the presence of oxidative stress. Recently in our laboratory, we have been able to demonstrate that percent endothelial cells were decreased (CD-31 labeling), ROS were increased (by spectrofluorometry), NO diminished (Greiss method), and nitrotyrosine levels increased (Western blot analysis) in human ischemic dilated cardiomyopathic hearts as compared to normal (unpublished data).

A quote by NS Dhalla and colleagues is appropriate: "The available evidence support the role of oxidative stress in ischemia-reperfusion injury and emphasize the importance of antioxidant mechanisms in cardio protection". Injury of myocardium due to ischemia-reperfusion includes cardiac contractile dysfunction, arrhythmias as well as irreversible myocyte damage. These changes are considered to be the consequence of imbalance between the formation of oxidants and the availability of endogenous antioxidants in the heart" (27). NO may be considered one of the hearts most potent natural occurring antioxidants as it readily consumes superoxide. NO, NO-generating compounds, and bradykinin all have the potential to suppress transforming growth factor-beta (TGF-beta 1) and inhibit the synthesis of collagen by the cardiac myofibroblast (28–30). ROS associated with ischemia / ischemia reperfusion injury play a central and key role in the development of ongoing myocardial damage and the development of cardiac hypertrophy and the transition from DD to overt SD and clinical CHF (31).

It is important to discuss homocysteine (Hcy) as it may be likened to a "Thief in the Night" as it consumes the endogenous antioxidant NO and the antioxidant enzymes: SOD-dismutation of O2′ → H2O2; Catalase-conversion of H2O2 → H2O + O2; and Glutathione peroxidase converts H2O2 and –OH′ (consuming GSH) to H2O + GSSG in turn GSSG is reduced by glutathione reductase to GSH at the expense of NAD(P)H. Hcy is not only a thief in the night but also acts as an accelerant to a fire where the fire is ROS and REDOX STRESS (Table 2). Independently, Hcy is a tough competitor and consumes endogenous myocardial antioxidants thus allowing for the other A-FLIGHT toxicities to take a greater toll. It becomes readily apparent that the multiple toxicities overwhelm the endogenous antioxidant mechanisms within the myocardium (32,33) (Table 2).

Extracellular matrix remodeling

The mammalian extracellular matrix (ECM) is classically made up of five major components: the collagens, the elastins, basement membranes, structural glycopro-

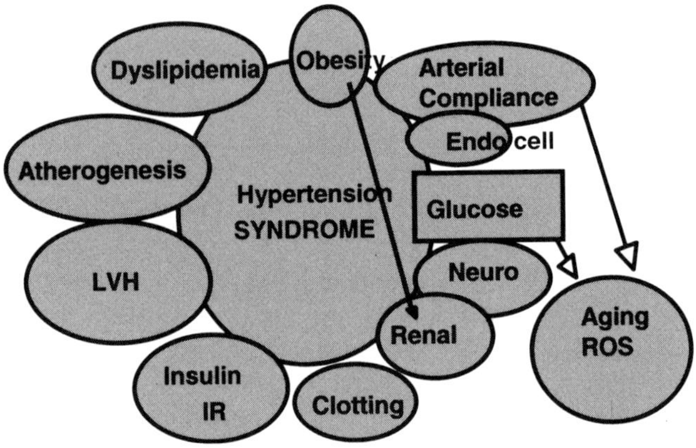

Figure 3. Hypertension Syndrome: Hypertension is only one risk factor of many. Global risk reduction is necessary to prevent the development of CHF (7).

teins, and proteoglycans. It exists in a wondrous and dynamic homeostasis, which involves degradation and repair (remodeling) in order to respond to its environment. It provides tissues with a scaffolding—structural support and is capable of exchanging information with surrounding cells and modulates numerous processes including development, cell migration, attachment, differentiation, repair, and recently cell survival (34). The myocardium is supported by an endoskeleton consisting of the ECM. The structural support of the myocardium is in dynamic homeostasis, which involves remodeling of this supporting structure; primarily types I and III collagen with interlacing elastin fibrils. When there is excessive remodeling and loss of this dynamic homeostasis we see the development of DD and SD and the progression to overt CHF.

In 1998, Rossi and colleagues (35) were able to demonstrate beautifully a three dimensional image of the ECM supporting the myocytes of the myocardium (Figure 3). From this image one can get a better concept of its contribution to ventricular function. The ECM provides the skeleton for the structure of the heart, its tensile strength or stiffness, the transmission of myocyte generated force allowing both shortening (contraction) and lengthening (relaxation). It is the ECM that allows for the shortening of sarcomeres of individual myocytes to be translated into myocardial pump function.

Remodeling may be defined as any change in an existing or native structure. In order to remodel any structure one must first tear down or degrade the structure in order to rebuild or change the existing structure. If there is robust degradation there will be robust synthesis. The matrix metalloproteinases (MMPs) are degrading enzymes responsible for the degradation of collagen (collagenolysis) and elastin (elastinolysis). MMPs are primarily synthesized by the cardiac myofibroblast (myoFb) and are stored in an inactive latent zymogen form (proMMPs) or a tissue-inhibitor complex or both within the ECM and are known to be activated to their active form by ROS and plasmin [tissue—urokinase plasminogen activating (t-PA, uPA) systems converting plasminogen to plasmin]. Once activated MMPs start degrading collagen within the ECM. Since collagen is stiffer and its turnover time is more rapid than elastin any remodeling will result in a stiffer matrix than before it was remodeled (thus decreasing ventricular compliance, ventricular relaxation and filling). Myocardial fibrillar collagen (types I, 80% and III, 11%) has the tensile strength of steel and is thus very stiff (13,24). The myoFb contains alpha smooth muscle actin and is the cell primarily responsible for the synthesis and deposition of types I and III collagen as the myocardium undergoes the process of rebuilding-repairing the myocardial architecture. It is important to describe two different types of fibrosis within the myocardium following an acute injury (MI—myocardial infarction).

Passive remodeling: occurs at the local site of MI and is related to myocyte necrosis and is also termed surrogate fibrosis. *Active remodeling*: occurs at sites remote from injury (MI) in non-infarcted areas, is not associated with myocyte necrosis, and is also termed interstitial fibrosis. The macophage, necrotic myocyte, and myoFb are sources for TGF beta-1, which is the most potent stimulus for the synthesis of myocardial collagen. TGF beta-1 activates interstitial fibroblasts and pericytes surrounding endothelial capillaries to undergo transformation to myoFbs. A fibrillar fibrin-fibronectin scaffolding forms soon after tissue injury and is a precursor to granulation tissue formation. The myoFb creates an attachment to this scaffolding via a fibronexus and starts laying down types I and III collagen due to the activation of TGF beta-1. Local or systemic AngII is a potent stimulus for the production of TGF beta-1 and the fibrotic process of repair (36,37).

The ECM is divided into three distinct structural subtypes. The endomysium (surrounds the individual myocytes and connects to capillaries), perimysium (surrounding myocyte bundles), and the epimysium (surrounding the individual components giving the heart its unique form including its valvular structures) [Figure 5]. A more robust activation of the MMPs allow for the initially positive adaptive remodeling to transition to maladaptive remodeling and allows for slippage of individual myocytes to result in a thinned myocardium (35–37). The myocytes are attached to the ECM through integrin (receptor)/matrix ligand binding (IMLB) sites. Collagen degradation is required for the creation of new integrin binding sites for cell (myocyte) survival. Excessive remodeling will allow for the myocyte to develop new IMLB sites, which helps to explain the myocyte elongation seen in the transition phase of adaptive remodeling to the thinned maladaptive remodeling of CHF. In addition, if there is an excessive degradation through continuous or robust MMP activation there will develop a complete disconnect between the matrix and the cell (myocyte), which will lead to apoptosis, slippage, dilatation and heart failure (Figures 1B & 4). In our laboratory we have been able to demonstrate an elevation of a disintegrin metalloproteinase (DMP) with an associated decrease in a cardiac inhibitor of metalloproteinase (CIMP) formally termed tissue inhibitor

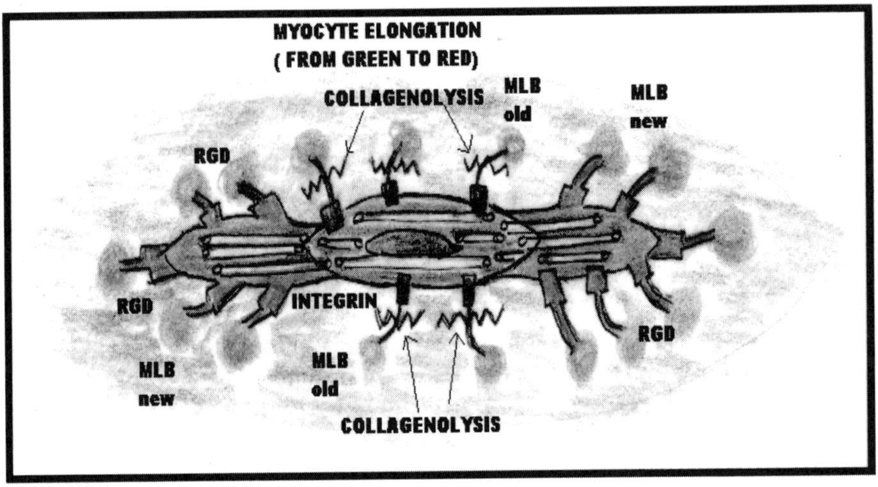

Figure 4. Myocyte elongation occurs as a result of excessive—robust MMP—DMP unabated activation which results in loss of Integrin binding to Matrix Ligand Binding (MLB) sites. If the loss of Integrin / MLB sites are excessive there will be a complete disconnect which results in apoptosis. As the myocyte is losing Integrin / MLB sites new ones will be formed and like a pseudopod a Caterpillar- like advancement of the myocyte will result in new MLB sites resulting in ELONGATION of the myocyte.

of metalloproteinase (TIMP-4) in human ischemic cardiomyopathic failing hearts. In these same hearts we noted an increase in synthesis and degradation of Beta 1- Integrin and connexin-43 as compared to normal human hearts (Figures 4, 5). These findings support the above discussion.

In summary, a pressure related increase in wall stress and mechanical strain, neurohormonal activation, redox stress, and injury—response to injury all play a significant role in the structural changes of cardiac ECM remodeling. Myocyte hypertrophy, excessive collagen deposition with fibrosis, apoptosis of myocytes, elongation of myocytes, and myocyte slippage all contribute to the architectural changes in the geometry of the left ventricle associated with the natural history of the failing myocardium (38). Whether these changes are abrupt or insidious they result in the morbid syndrome of CHF (Figures 1–5).

Congestive heart failure

The sympathetic-RAAS (neuroendocrine system)

The evidence for activation of the sympathetic-RAAS (neuroendocrine system) with excess norepinephrine, renin, angiotensin II, and aldosterone both systemically as well as local production discussed in the previous sections is overwhelming. Targeting treatment to interrupt this activated system has proved to be of great clinical value during the past two decades. The clinical improvement with decreased

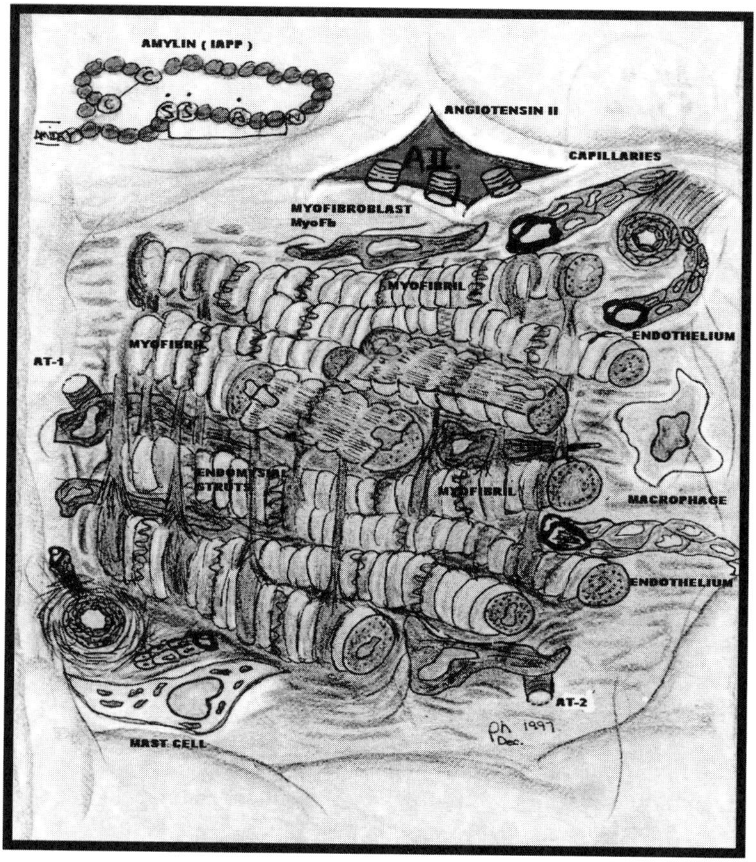

Figure 5. Individual myocardial muscle bundles (surrounded by the dark (trichrome) color of interstitial collagen and elastin. supported by endomysial cellular struts. Representing extracelluar matrix remodeling with interstitial fibrosis. When these struts are digested by robust MMP (DMP) expression and activation the myocardial muscle bundles may undergo slippage and contribute to the thinned, eccentrically remodeled myocardium of overt CHF. The importance of Ang II is noted to be central and superior in this image.

morbidity and mortality with the use of angiotensin converting enzyme inhibitors (ACEi) and adrenergic beta blockers (BB) have proved to be invaluable in the treatment of DD, SD, and overt CHF at each stage of development (Figure 1). Even with research and clinical evidence being so overwhelmingly positive there persists worldwide an "under treatment phenomenon" which is difficult to explain with the current available knowledge.

Decreased physician compliance to instigate treatment and patients' decreased compliance to maintain treatment certainly must play a role but do not totally explain the paradox of inadequately following the current treatment paradigms.

ACEi and BB certainly are not free of side effects (cough, metallic taste, rash, angioedema, hypotension, and malaise with ACEi and hypotension, malaise, and bradycardia with BB) and may add to the patient/physician under treatment phenomenon. If patients are unable to tolerate ACEi they may now substitute angiotensin receptor blockers (ARBs). Recently, spironolactone (an aldosterone receptor antagonist) has been shown to be quite effective in the treatment of SD and overt CHF (39). Review of the RALES (Randomized Aldactone Evaluation Study) data indicate that spironolactone decreases the collagen turnover within the myocardial ECM indicated by a decrease in N-terminal propeptide of type III procollagen as compared to placebo (40). Each of the above therapeutic regimens results in a positive effect on cardiac remodeling and serve to slow or halt the maladaptive architectural derangements associated with HTN, LVH, DD, CAD, SD, and CHF. Endothelin receptor blockers will soon be available to add to the clinical armamentarium as endothelin is activated by Ang II and therefore included in the neurohormonal system.

Before leaving this section it is interesting to note that compensated CHF is not associated with an activation of the systemic RAAS whereas decompensated CHF is associated with activation of the systemic RAAS and the sodium avid, fluid retention state. Also, activation of the neurohormonal system is an acute (short term) hemodynamically adaptive situation whereas activation of the local tissue RAAS is considered chronic (long term) and is felt to be more responsible for structural and functional influences on the myocardium, vasculature, and kidneys.

Diuretics

The clinical syndrome of CHF implies congestion of tissues as a result of a failing myocardium; centrally in regards to pulmonary congestion and peripherally in regards to dependent interstitial edema and as clinicians we would be hard pressed to treat a "wet patient" without the use of diuretics. They play an important central role in the acute and chronic treatment and stabilization of the decompensated patient with CHF. Both thiazides (chronic) and the loop diuretic furosemide (acute and chronic) play an extremely important role in the treatment of debilitating dyspnea, orthopnea, and peripheral edema.

Statins

The use of statins (HMG-CoA reductase inhibitors) play a tremendous role in the stabilization of vulnerable atherosclerotic plaques and prevention of acute events (MI) and the ischemia / ischemia reperfusion injury to the myocardium. In addition to the positive lipid effects (lowering the damaging substrate of LDL cholesterol, decreasing triglycerides, and raising HDL cholesterol) the importance of pleiotropic effects have emerged and we now have a better understanding of these positive roles thanks to multiple investigators in this exciting field (Table 2). Statins may be one of the best therapeutic modalities and be a great asset in helping to prevent the upcoming [baby boomer-senior boomer] boost to the exponential growth and current epidemic of CHF.

Rory Collins of Oxford University presented data from the heart protection study HPS (in late breaking clinical trials November 13th, 2001 Anaheim, California) at the 2001 American Heart Association meeting which were overwhelmingly positive and shed new light on the strategy of using statins. Benefits were unequivocal in patients who have normal or low cholesterol but are still considered to be at high global risk of CAD. Data included 20,000 patients ages 40–80. Statin dosage was 40 mg simvastatin. There were 4000 with diabetes, 5000 females, and 6000 aged 70 or older. The large numbers in these sub groupings helped to better understand the **global** benefits with statin treatment to prevent major coronary events (41).

Digoxin

Digoxin has been shown to improve symptoms, quality of life, functional capacity, exercise tolerance, and a decreased hospitalization rate of decompensated CHF. There have been no long-term studies to date to show a decrease in mortality. However, withdrawal of digoxin therapy has been shown to result in significant clinical deterioration.

Bed rest

The time-honored importance of complete bed rest cannot be overlooked when discussing the various treatments of CHF even though the current methods of reimbursement do not allow for such inpatient treatment as in the days of old. This method of treatment, which shuts down an activated systemic RAAS can still be entertained in the extended care facility and in the home with available home health agencies.

Potent inotropes

Stronger inotropes require hospitalization treatment with intravenous medications (dobutamine and nitroprusside) and are usually reserved for refractory CHF and to extend the time to transplantation.

Left ventricular assist devices: Automatic defibrillator implantation

Recently the use of left ventricular assist devices have been shown to be helpful and allow a (R and R) if you will to allow the myocardium to rest and rehabilitate. The possibility for some restoration of cardiac architectural remodeling is possible but there have been no definitive studies to date. Additionally the Multicenter Automatic Defibrillator Implantation Trial (MADIT) resulted in a 54% reduction in total mortality with the use of an implanted cardioverter-defibrillator in a defined subset of high-risk coronary patients (42).

Myocyte cell transplantation and myocardial cell cycling

Myocyte cell transplantation and myocardial cell cycling to allow the adult myocyte to undergo mitoses may be available in the very near future which would allow the myocyte to regenerate. Investigators (January 2002) have recently discovered that primitive cells from male recipients of female donor hearts can migrate to the newly transplanted heart and contribute to its remodeling and growth. These Y chromosome cells were more common in the atria than the ventricle and were negative for markers of bone marrow origin. Progenitor cells expressing MEF2, GATA-4, and nestin (which identify the cells as myocytes) and Flk1 (which identifies the cells as endothelial cells) were identified (43).

Naturally occurring MMP inhibitors

As mentioned earlier we have been able to show in our laboratory that a cardiospecific inhibitor of matrix metalloprotease we term CIMP is capable of inhibiting the excess collagenolysis of the robustly activated MMPs (especially DMP discussed previously) resulting in myocyte slippage and myocyte elongation. This naturally occurring MMP inhibitor (CIMP) could be sequenced and cloned and made available for gene transfection into the failing myocardium just as we have recently seen the positive results of angiogenesis induction as a result of the large body of work with cardiac gene transfer of phVEGF 165 by the late Jeff Isner and colleagues.

Synthetic MMP inhibitors

Many pharmaceuticals are now working at a rapid pace to develop various MMP inhibitors to slow, delay, or halt the robust MMP collagenolysis seen in CHF. The early studies are starting to look promising. The inhibition of one (MMP-9 by PD166793) (44) or multiple MMP inhibitors (BMS-275291) (45) are under development. These substances may also play a role in preventing the angiogenesis associated with tumor progression and metastasis.

Tetracycline family of MMP inhibitors

We have been interested in the tetracycline family of antibiotics in MMP inhibition. Tetracycline, doxycycline, and minocycline have all been shown to result in MMP inhibition. These MMP inhibitors remain to be tested in clinical trials as to their precise benefit in animal and human CHF models. If positive this treatment could be used in addition to the RAAS blockers and BBs. This area of research is very exciting and interest in this area could explode as pharmaceutical companies start to do clinical studies with their newly discovered MMP inhibitors. This area of research in the prevention of CHF could prove to be one of the more exciting areas of research in the 21st century.

In a left anterior descending coronary ligation rat model we have been able to show that doxycycline ameliorates cardiac fibrosis and collagen deposition in ischemic and non-ischemic groups post MI as well as improving endomyocardial endothelial dysfunction (unpublished data).

Vasopeptidase inhibitors: VPi

Soon to be clinically available is the class of drugs referred to as: Vasopeptidase inhibitors. The first to become available is called omapatrilat, Vanlev^{TM} and may be available for clinical use during 2003. This will be a potent ACEi with inhibition of the vasoactive—vasoconstrictor AngII and neutral endopeptidase inhibitor which will increase the endogenous cardiac vasoactive—vasodilator peptides atrial natriuretic peptide (ANP), B type natriuretic peptide (BNP), bradykinin (BK), and adrenomedullin (AM). Omapatrilat has been proven to be a potent antihypertensive and may play a major role in the prevention and stabilization of CHF.

Important role for atrial natriuretic peptides

The vasoactive vasodilatory cardiac atrial natriuretic peptides may be considered as markers for LVH and correlates very well with LVH and CHF (especially vessel dilator peptide (proAtrial Natriuretic Factor proANF 31–67) and B type Natriuretic Factor (BNP). It is possible that soon we may be checking these levels to screen for LVH, DD, SD and early asymptomatic or class I NYHA CHF to guide our therapy initially and use this test to monitor the success of our therapies and make adjustments based on their levels. Vasodilatory peptide is in phase II and III treatment clinical trials and appears to have a favorable impact on multiple parameters of cardiac function (46). In the future the measurement of DMP may be an effective means to screen and monitor these same patients.

Chronic anticoagulation

Chronic anticoagulation for the prevention of morbidity and mortality in those patients with CHF who have associated atrial fibrillation and those with normal sinus rhythm who have a very low ejection fraction should be strongly considered. However, patients would need to be carefully chosen due to the necessary frequent monitoring and compliance issues associated with the use of chronic anticoagulation.

Nontraditional risk factors: Hypertension syndrome: Metabolic syndrome

Approximately 50% of patients with ischemic heart disease are associated with an abnormality of lipid metabolism and therefore we need to look carefully at emerging risk factors of Hcy, Lp(a), hs-CRP, fibrinogen, von Willebrand factor antigen, Renin, and others.

Of historical note: During an interview of Dr. John Laragh by Dr. Michael Weber on February 5th 2001 posted on Heart Wire *www.theheart.org* Dr.Laragh stated: "My hope is . . . that renin testing will become a routine event all over the world . . . That's our final dream."

Hcy is now considered to be an independent risk factor for the development of atherosclerosis and its associated complications of CAD with subsequent MI, SD, and CHF (Figure 1). Hcy is proinflammatory (increasing ICAM and NFkappaB) and procoagulant (decreasing protein C and thrombomodulin). It is known to cause endothelial cell dysfunction with decreases in NO and endothelial toxicity with an associated increase in Redox Stress. Hcy is profibrotic and causes SMC proliferation and increased collagen synthesis and more recently induction of TGFbeta 1

Table 3. (52) a-flight toxicities: of the insulin resistant state—metabolic syndrome and type 2 diabetes mellitus

A	**Amylin** (Hyperamylinemia)/Amyloid toxicity*	ROS
	Ang II (Also induces PKC)	ROS plus PKC
	AGEs/AFEs (Advanced Glycosylation/	ROS
	Fructosylation Endproducts)	ROS
	*Atherosclerosis/Atherosclerosis/Atheroscleropathy → (prediabetes and overt T2DM)	ROS
F	**Free fatty acid toxicity.**	ROS
L	**Lipotoxicity**	ROS
I	**Insulin** (Hyperinsulinemia)/(Hyperproinsulinemia) toxicity (endogenous)*	ROS
G	Glucotoxicity **(compounds peripheral insulin resistance) Reductive stress.**	ROS plus PKC
	Sorbitrol/Polyol pathway	
	Pseudohypoxia (NADH/NAD increased)	
H	**Hypertension** toxicity (systolic/diastolic)	ROS
	t **Homocysteine (HCY)**	ROS
T	**Triglyceride** toxicity	ROS
	Reference (52)	

with intimal and perivascular fibrosis. All of these abnormalities contribute to and accelerate atherosclerosis. In regards to the effect on myocardial ECM remodeling the picture is not so clear-cut but soon we will better understand as many are working in this field. Accelerated epicardial atherosclerosis contributes to CHF (Figures 1, 3) and the perivascular fibrosis of intramyocardial arteries and arterioles would contribute to the ischemia/ischemia reperfusion injury which is known to result in redox stress and robustly increase MMP activity, which could result in increased collagenolysis and CHF.

Why devote this time to the emerging risk factor: Hcy? Hyperhomocyteinemia affects five to seven percent of the American population and this translates to approximately 10 million patients at risk for accelerated atherosclerosis and at a marked increased risk for the development of CHF. The first of many clinical trials regarding Hcy reduction with folic acid has recently been published and has shown that treatment with folic acid reduces the rate of restenosis 19.6% in the folate treated group verses 37.6% in the placebo group $p = 0.01$ in addition the need for revascularization of target lesions was 10.8% in the folate group verses 22.3 in the placebo group $p = 0.047$ (47). There are at least nine clinical trials which will be reported in the near future and if positive will reveal the importance given to this sulfur containing amino acid and how it fits in with SD, DD, Redox stress, and ECM remodeling and CHF (32,33,48). We need to continue reviewing the hypertensive syndrome and its association with the insulin resistant state and the metabolic syndrome and how it is playing a major role in the development of CVD and the development of CHF.

In the insulin resistance syndrome and early type 2 diabetes mellitus (T2DM) there are numerous toxicities resulting in elevated ROS (Table 3). Thus, the importance of redox stress cannot be overemphasized in the treatment and prevention of

Table 4. Summary: pleotropic effects of statins: (50,51) "the nifty nine" the positive role in the treatment and prevention of dd, sd, redox stress, ecm remodeling, and CHF

1. **Decreased TXA2.**
2. **Increased t-PA and Decreased PAI-1. D/RhoA.**
3. **Decreased Macrophage growth. D/RhoA.**
4. ***Decreased MMPs* and TF. D/RhoA.**
5. **Decreased hs-CRP.**
6. **Decreased Adhesion molecule.**
7. ***Decreased ROS*, SMC hypertrophy, and *Endothelial Dysfunction*. D/RAC 1.**
8. ***Increased NO. Decreased Endothelial Dysfunction*. And SMC proliferation. D/RhoA.**
9. ***Decreased ET-1 and AT-1 receptors with decreased vasoconstriction*. D/RhoA**

Table 5. The RAAS acronym for the prevention and treatment of DD, SD, redox stress, ecm remodeling and CHF

R—**Reductase inhibitors (HMG-CoA).** Decreasing modified LDL cholesterol, i.e. oxidized, acetylated LDL cholesterol. Improving endothelial cell (EC) dysfunction. Thus, decreasing the oxidative stress to the arterial vessel wall, myocyte, and myocardial interstitial space. ***Redox Stress Reduction.***

A—**ACEi–prils** and or **ARBS–sartans. Vasopeptidase inhibitors (Vpi)?** Inhibiting the effect of Angiotensin II locally as well as systemically. Affecting the hemodynamic stress through their antihypertensive effect as well as the deleterious effects of Angiotensin II on cells at the local level—injurious stimuli. Decreasing the A-FLIGHT toxicities. (table 2.) Plus the direct/indirect antioxidant effect within the myocardium. ***Redox Stress Reduction.***

Aldosterone Receptor Blockade Antagonist- Spironolactone. Local inhibition of ECM remodeling. **Aspirin and Adrenergic blockade.**

A—**Aggressive Control of Diabetes and Hcy.** Decreasing modified LDL cholesterol, i.e. glycated, oxidated LDL cholesterol and formation of AGEs. Improving endothelial cell dysfunction. Also decreasing glucose toxicity and the redox stress to the arterial vessel wall, myocyte, and myocardium. Aggressive control of Hcy with folic acid in addition to lowering Hcy folic acid restores the eNOS synthase reaction and aids in the restoration of endothelial NO production. ***Redox Stress Reduction.***

S—**Statins.** Improving plaque stability (pleiotropic) independent of cholesterol lowering. Improving endothelial cell dysfunction and preventing plaque angiogenesis associated with arterial vascular remodeling which destabilizes the unstable atherosclerotic plaque. Plus, the direct/indirect anti-oxidant effect within the islet promoting stabilization of the unstable, vulnerable islet. ***Redox Stress Reduction.***

Sympathetic adrenoreceptor blockade-BB. Reducing the effects sympathetic activation and its detrimental effects. ***Redox Stress Reduction.***

Screen for hyperhomocysteinia Hcy and treat aggressively with folic acid. ***Redox Stress Reduction.***

overt CHF. Even with the improved survival of MI mentioned in the opening remarks, it is important to note some staggering statistics: Within one year of an acute MI, mortality is as high as 10%; within 5 years 25% will have a second MI, and 20% will develop CHF (49).

These figures point out the importance of secondary prevention but cries out for an even more aggressive approach to primary prevention of MI and global risk reduction of cardiovascular disease to prevent the development of CHF. Every attempt should be employed to use the currently available treatment modalities and use them maximally. Earlier and accurate diagnosis with the use of Doppler echocardiography is mandated in all patients with CHF.

The closure of this chapter has briefly summarized the current treatment modalities and the newer methods of treatment rapidly becoming available for CHF. However, due to the scope of this chapter a detailed discussion of each treatment modality could not be accomplished. Use of the RAAS Acronym (Table 4) and the conceptual model (Figure 1) may help each of us to mentally compartmentalize the maximal treatment strategy for the prevention and treatment of HTN, LVH, DD, CHF and HTN, CAD, SD, CHF. The complex interaction of each of these entities and the interacting roles of redox stress and ECM remodeling will continue to fascinate researchers and clinicians alike in the coming years.

REFERENCES

1. Vasan RS, Levy D. 1996. The role of hypertension in the pathogenesis of heart failure: A clinical mechanistic overview. Arch Intern Med 156:1789–1796.
2. Levy D, Larson MG, Vasan RS, Kannel WB, Ho KK. 1996. The progression from hypertension to congestive heart failure. JAMA. May 275(20):1604–1606.
3. Remme WJ. 2000. Overview of the relationship between ischemia and congestive heart failure. Clin Cardiol. 23(7)(Suppl.IV):IV-4–IV-8.
4. American Heart Association. 1998. *1999 Heart and Stroke Statistical Update.* American Heart Association. Dallas, Texas.
5. Gomberg-Maitland M, Baran DA, Fuster V. 2001. Treatment of Congestive Heart Failure Guidelines for the primary care physician and the heart failure specialist. Arch Intern Med. Feb 161:342–352.
6. Bonneux L, Barendregt JJ, Meeter K, Bonsel GJ, van der Maas PJ. 1994. Estimating clinical morbidity due to ischemic heart disease and congestive heart failure: The future rise of heart failure. Am J Public Health. 84:20–28.
7. Glasser SP. 2001. Hypertension syndrome and cardiovascular events: High blood pressure is only one risk factor. Postgraduate Medicine November 110(5):29–36.
8. Vasan RS, Larson MG, Benjamin EF, Evans JC, Reiss C, Levy D. 1999. Congestive heart failure in subjects with normal versus reduced left ventricular ejection fraction: prevalence and mortality in population-based cohort. J Am Coll Cardiol. 33:1948–1955.
9. Mosterd A, Hoes AW, deBruyne MC, Deckers JW, Linker DT, Hofman A, Grobbee DE. 1999. Prevalence of heart failure and left ventricular dysfunction in the general population: the Rotterdam Study. Eur Heart J 20:447–455.
10. Kupari M, Lindroos M, Iivanainen AM, Heikkila J, Tilvis R. 1997. Congestive heart failure in old age: prevalence, mechanisms and 4-year prognosis in the Helsinki Ageing Study. J Intern Med 241: 387–394.
11. Senni M, Tribouilloy CM, Rodeheffer RJ, Jacobsen SJ. Evans JM, Bailey KR, Redfield MM. 1998. Congestive heart failure in the community: a study of all incident cases in Olmsted County, Minnesota, in 1991. Circulation. 98:2282–2289.
12. Vasan RS, Levy D. 2000. Defining diastolic heart failure: A call for standardized diagnostic criteria. Circulation. 101(17):2118–2126.
13. Weber KT. 1997. Extracellular matrix remodeling in heart failure: A role for de novo angiotensin II generation. Circulation. 96:4065–4082.
14. Chatham JC, Forder JR, McNeill JH. 1996. The Heart in Diabetes. Kluwer Academic Publishers, Boston.
15. Kannel WB, Hjortland, Castelli WP. 1974. Role of diabetes in congestive heart failure: The Framingham Study. Am J Cardiol 34:29.
16. Sowers JR, Epstein M. 1995. Diabetes mellitus and associated hypertension, vascular disease, and Nephropathy. Hypertension 26:869–879.
17. Sowers JR, Epstein M, Frohlich ED. 2001. Diabetes, hypertension, and cardiovascular disease: an update. Hypertension Apr 37(4):1053–1059.

18. Zabalgoitia M, Ismaeil MF, Anderson L, Maklady FA. 2001. Prevalence of diastolic dysfunction in normotensive, asymptomatic patients with well-controlled type 2 diabetes mellitus. Am J Cardiol Feb 1;87(3):320–323
19. Griendling KK, Sorescu D. Masuko U-F. 2000. NAD(P)H Oxidase Role in cardiovascular biology and disease. Circulation Research 86(5):494.
20. Babior BM. 1999. NADPH oxidase: an update. Blood 93(5):1464–1476.
21. McCord JM, Fridovich I. 1988. Superoxide dismutase: the first twenty years (1968–1988). Free Radic Biol Med 5(5–6):363–369.
22. Roos D, Weening RS, Wyss SR, Aebi HE. 1980. Protection of human neutrophils by endogenous catalase: Studies with cells from catalase-deficient individuals. J Clin Invest 65(6):1515–1522.
23. Lawrence RA, Burk RF. 1978. Species, tissue and subcellular distribution of selenium dependent, glutathione peroxidase activity. J Nutr 108(6):981-987.
24. Tyagi SC, Ratajska A, Weber KT. 1993. Myocardial matrix metalloproteinases: Localization and activation. Mol Cell Biochem. 126:49–59.
25. Rajagopalan S, Meng XP, Ramasamy S, Harrison DG, Galis ZS. 1996. Reactive oxygen species produced by macrophage-derived foam cells regulate the activity of vascular matrix metalloproteinases in vitro. J Clin Invest 98:2572–2579.
26. Lefer DJ, Granger DN. 2000. Oxidative stress and cardiac disease. Am J Med Sep 109(4):315–323.
27. Dhalla NS, Elmoselhi AB, Hata T, Makino N. 2000. Status of myocardial antioxidants in ischemia-reperfusion injury. Cardiovasc Res Aug 18;47(3):446–456.
28. Sigusch HH, Campbell SE, Weber KT. 1996. Angiotensin II-induced myocardial fibrosis in rats: Role of nitric oxide, prostaglandins and bradykinin. Cardiovasc Res 31:546–554.
29. Booz GW, Baker KM. 1995. Molecular signaling mechanisms controlling growth and function of cardiac fibroblasts. Cardiovasc Res 30:537–543.
30. Kolpakov V, Gordon D, Kulik TJ. 1995. Nitric oxide-generating compounds inhibit total protein and collagen synthesis in cultured vascular smooth muscle cell. Circ Res 76:305–309.
31. Hingtgen SD, Davisson RL. 2001. Gene therapeutic approaches to oxidative stress-induced cardiac disease: principles, progress, and prospects. Antiox Redox Signal Jun 3(3):433–449
32. Tyagi SC. 1999. Homocyst(e)ine and heart disease: Pathophysiology of extracellular matrix. Clin and Exper Hypertension 21(3):181–198.
33. Mujumdar VS, Hayden MR, Tyagi SC. 2000. Homocyst(e)ine induces calcium second messenger in vascular smooth muscle cells. Journal of Cellular Physiology 183:28–36.
34. Meredith JE Jr., Fazeli B, Schwartz MA. 1993. The extracellular matrix as a cell survival factor. Mol Biol Cell 4(9):953–961.
35. Rossi MA, Abreu MA, Santoro LB. 1998. Connective tissue skeleton of the human heart. A demonstration by cell-maceration scanning electron microscope method. Circulation 97:934–935.
36. Weber KT, Janicki JS, Pick R. Disruption of collagen tethers: Anatomic basis of muscle fiber slippage in the myocardium. Pages 18–35.
37. Jacob Seipel Zucker: Cardiac Dilatation. Gustav Fischer Verlag. Stuttgart. New York. 1990.
38. Weber KT. 1997. Extracellular matrix remodeling in heart failure: A role for De Novo angiotensin II generation. Circulation 96:4065–4082.
39. Francis GS. 1998. Changing the remodeling process in heart failure: basic mechanisms and laboratory results. Curr Opin Cardiol 13(3):156–161.
40. Weber KT. 2001. Aldosterone in congestive heart failure. Dec 345:1689–1697.
41. Heart Protection Study Collaborative Group. 2002. MRC/BHF Heart Protection Study of cholesterol lowering with simvastatin in 20,536 high-risk individuals: a randomised placebo-controlled trial. Lancet 360(9326):7–22.
42. Zannad F, Alla F, Dousset B, Perez A, Pitt B, RALES Investigators. 2000. Limitation of excessive extracellular matrix turnover may contribute to survival benefit of spironolactone therapy in patients with congestive heart failure: insights from the Randomized Aldactone Evaluation Study (RALES). Circulation 2000; 102: 2700–2706. [Erratum, Circulation 2001; 103:476.
43. Cohn JN, Bristow MR, Chien KR, Colucci WS, Frazier OH, Leinwand LA, Lorell BH, Moss AJ, Sonnenblick EH, Walsh RA, Mockrin SC, Reinlib L. 1997. Report of the National Heart, Lung, and Blood Institute Special Emphasis Panel on Heart failure Research. Circulation. 95:766–770.
44. Quaini F, Urbanek K, Beltrami AP, Finato N, Beltrami CA, Nadal-Ginard B, Kajstura J, Leri A, Anversa P. 2002. Chimerism of the transplanted Heart. NEJM January 3 346(1):5–15.

45. Li H, Simon H, Bocan TM, Peterson JT. 2000. MMP/TIMP expression in spontaneously hypertensive heart failure rats: The effect of ACE-and MMP-inhibition. Cardiovasc Res 46(2):298–306.
46. Naglich JG, Jure-Kunkel M, Gupta E, Fargnoli J, Henderson AJ, Lewin AC, Talbott R, Baxter A, Bird J, Savopoulos R, Wills R, Kramer RA, Trail PA. 2001. Inhibition of angiogenesis and Metastasis in two murine models by the matrix metalloproteinases inhibitor, BMS-275291. Cancer Res 61(23):8480–8485.
47. Vesely DL. 1999. Atrial natriuretic peptides in the diagnosis and treatment of congestive heart failure. Congestive Heart Failure 5:171–179.
48. Schnyder G, Roffi M, Pin R, Flammer Y, Lange H, Eberli FR, Meier B, Turi ZG, Hess OM. 2001. Decreased rate of coronary restenosis after lowering of plasma homocysteine levels. Nov 345(22): 1593–1600.
49. Homocysteine: The new risk factor: Introduction of patient management. March 1999; Professional Postgraduate Services ® (PPS), a division of Physicians World Communications Group, 400 Plaza Drive, Secaucus, NJ 07094.
50. Banas J. 1999. New insights into effects of statins on the atherosclerotic process. Cardiology Review Dec 16(12) (Suppl):1–4.
51. Takemoto M, Liao JK. 2001. Pleiotropic Effects of 3-hydroxy-3-methylglutaryl coenzyme A reductase inhibitors. Arteriosclerosis Thrombosis and Vascular Biology. Nov 21:1712–1719.
52. Hayden MR, Tyagi SC. 2001. "A" is for amylin and amyloid in type 2 diabetes mellitus. JOP. J Pancreas (Online) 2(4):124–139. *http://www.joplink.net*

Index

C